What's New in Cardiovascular Imaging?

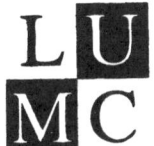

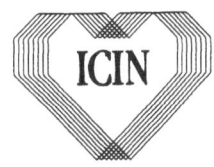

Developments in Cardiovascular Medicine

VOLUME 204

The titles published in this series are listed at the end of this volume.

What's New in Cardiovascular Imaging?

Edited by

JOHAN H.C. REIBER
Division of Image Processing,
Department of Radiology,
Department of Cardiology,
Leiden University Medical Center,
The Netherlands
and
Interuniversity Cardiology Institute of the Netherlands (ICIN),
Utrecht, The Netherlands

and

ERNST E. VAN DER WALL
Department of Cardiology,
Leiden University Medical Center,
The Netherlands
and
Interuniversity Cardiology Institute of the Netherlands (ICIN),
Utrecht, The Netherlands

This publication has been made possible with an educational grant from
Parke-Davis BV, Hoofddorp, The Netherlands
Pfizer BV, Capelle a/d IJssel, The Netherlands

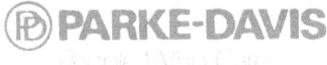 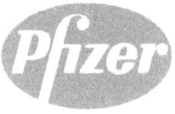

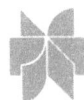

SPRINGER SCIENCE+BUSINESS MEDIA, B.V.

A C.I.P. Catalogue record for this book is available from the Library of Congress.

ISBN 978-94-010-6154-4   ISBN 978-94-011-5123-8 (eBook)
DOI 10.1007/978-94-011-5123-8

Printed on acid-free paper

Dedicated

to

Our Wives

Marjan and Barbara

and our Children

Beata   Hein

                         Sake and

                         Ernst Lucas

Table of contents

Part Five: **Nuclear cardiovascular imaging**

Part Six: **Echocardiography**

Part Seven: **Cine and spiral CT coronary imaging**

List of contributors

Wim R.M. Aengevaeren
Department of Cardiology, University Hospital Nijmegen, P.O. Box 9101, 6500 HB Nijmegen, The Netherlands
Coauthors: Gerard J.H. Uijen, Anton F.H. Stalenhoef[*], Tjeerd van der Werf
[*] Department of General Internal Medicine, University Hospital Nijmegen, Nijmegen, The Netherlands

Jeroen J. Bax
Department of Cardiology, Leiden University Medical Center, Albinusdreef 2, 2333 ZA Leiden, The Netherlands
Coauthors: Frans C. Visser[*], Jan Hein Cornel[**], Paolo M. Fioretti[***], Arthur van Lingen[*], Ernst E. van der Wall, Cees A. Visser[*]
[*] Free University Hospital, Amsterdam, The Netherlands
[**] Medical Center Alkmaar, Alkmaar, The Netherlands
[***] Instituto di Cardiologia, Udine, Italy

Nicolaas Bom[#*]
[#] Thoraxcenter, Erasmus University, Dr. Molewaterplein 40, 3015 GD Rotterdam, The Netherlands
Coauthors: Wenguang Li[#*], Stéphane Carlier[#], Ignacio Céspedes[# **], Antonius F.W. van der Steen[#*]
[*] Interuniversity Cardiology Institute of the Netherlands, Utrecht, The Netherlands
[**] Endosonics Corporation, Rancho Cordova, California, USA

Hans G. Bosch
Division of Image Processing, Department of Radiology, Leiden University Medical Center, Albinusdreef 2, 2333 ZA Leiden, The Netherlands
Coauthors: Gerard van Burken, Francisca Nijland, Johan H.C. Reiber

Michiel L. Bots[#*]
[#] Julius Center for Patient Oriented Research, Suite D.01.335, University Medical Center Utrecht, Universiteitsweg 100, 3584 CG Utrecht, The Netherlands
Coauthors: Antonio Iglesias[*], Diederik E. Grobbee[#]
[*] Department of Epidemiology and Biostatistics, Erasmus University Medical School, Rotterdam, The Netherlands

Albert V.G. Bruschke
Department of Cardiology, Leiden University Medical Center, Albinusdreef 2, 2333 ZA Leiden, The Netherlands
Coauthors: J. Wouter Jukema, Johan H.C. Reiber

Linda Cashin-Hemphill
Boston Heart Foundation, 139 Main Street, Cambridge, MA 02142, USA

Shuih-Yung James Chen
    Division of Cardiology, Department of Medicine, Campus Box B132, University of
    Colorado, Health Sciences Center, 4200 East Ninth Avenue, Denver, CO 80262, USA
Co-author: John D. Carroll

Jouke Dijkstra
    Division of Image Processing, Department of Radiology, Leiden University Medical
    Center, Albinusdreef 2, 2333 ZA Leiden, The Netherlands
Coauthors: Andreas Wahle[*], Gerhard Koning, Johan H.C. Reiber, Milan Sonka[*]
    [*] Department of Electrical and Computer Engineering, The University of Iowa, Iowa
    City, IA 52242, USA

Carlo Di Mario
    Cardiac Catheterization Laboratory, Centro Cuore Columbus, Via M. Buonarroti 48,
    20145 Milano, Italy
Coauthors: Joseph De Gregorio, Issam Moussa, Remo Albiero, Nobuyoshi Kobayashi, Marco
Vaghetti, Antonio Colombo

Berthe L.F. van Eck-Smit
    Department of Nuclear Medicine, Academic Medical Center, Meibergdreef 9, Amster-
    dam, The Netherlands

Pim J. de Feyter
    Coronary Imaging Unit, Dijkzigt-Thoraxcenter, University Hospital Rotterdam, Dr.
    Molewaterplein 40, 3015 GD Rotterdam, The Netherlands
Coauthors: Robert-Jan van Geuns, Peter van Ooijen, Fons Bongaerts[*], Benno Rensing, Hein
de Bruin[*], Pjotr Wielopolski[*], Matthijs Oudkerk[*]
    [*] Department of Radiology, Daniel den Hoed Kliniek, Rotterdam, The Netherlands

Stefan E. Fischer[#*]
    [#] Center for Cardiovascular MR, Cardiovascular Division, Barnes-Jewish Hospital at
    Washington University Medical Center, 216 South Kingshighway Blvd, St Louis, MO
    63110, USA
Co-author: Christine H. Lorenz[#]
    [*] Philips Medical Systems, Best, The Netherlands

Ernest V. Garcia
    Emory Center for PET, Emory University Hospital, 1364 Clifton Road, N.E., Atlanta,
    GA 30322, USA
Coauthors: Tracy L. Faber, C. David Cooke, Russell D. Folks

Junbo Ge
    Department of Cardiology, University Essen, Hufelandstrasse 55, 45122 Essen, Ger-
    many
Coauthors: Fengqi Liu, Rahul Bhate, Raimund Erbel

Peter Paul van Geel[#]

[#] Department of Clinical Pharmacology, Groningen University, Antonius Deusinglaan 1, 9713 AV Groningen, The Netherlands

Coauthors: Yigal M. Pinto[#], Aeilko H. Zwinderman[*], J. Wouter Jukema[**], Wiek H. van Gilst[#]

[#] Department of Cardiology, University Hospital Groningen, Groningen, The Netherlands

[*] Department of Medical Statistics, Leiden University Medical Center, Leiden, The Netherlands

[**] Department of Cardiology, Leiden University Medical Center, Leiden, The Netherlands

Rob J. van der Geest

Division of Image Processing, Department of Radiology, Leiden University Medical Center, Albinusdreef 2, 2333 ZA Leiden, The Netherlands

Co-author: Johan H.C. Reiber

Christopher J. Hardy

GE Corporate Research & Development, One Research Circle, Niskayuna, NY 12309, USA

Otto Kamp

Department of Cardiology, Free University Hospital, P.O. Box 7057, 1007 MB Amsterdam, The Netherlands

Coauthors: Gertjan Tj. Sieswerda, Cees A. Visser

Jacques Lespérance

Montreal Heart Institute, 5000 Belanger Street East, Montreal, Québec H1T 1C8, Canada

Coauthors: Luc Bilodeau, Johan H.C. Reiber[*], Gerhard Koning[*], Gilles Hudon, Martial G. Bourassa

[*] Division of Image Processing, Department of Radiology, Leiden University Medical Center, Leiden, The Netherlands

Jamshid Maddahi

Division of Nuclear Medicine and Biophysics, Department of Molecular and Medical Pharmacology, University of California at Los Angeles School of Medicine, 100 Medical Plaza #410, Los Angeles, CA 90095-7064, USA

Thomas H. Marwick

Department of Cardiology, F-15, Cleveland Clinic Foundation, 9500 Euclid Avenue, Cleveland, OH 44195, USA

Christoph A. Nienaber

Abteilung für Kardiologie, Innere Medizin II, Universitätskrankenhaus Eppendorf, Martinistrasse 52, D-Hamburg 20246, Germany

Coauthors: Klaus-Peter Schaps, Georg Stiel

Michael H. Picard
    Clinical Echocardiography, Massachusetts General Hospital, 55 Fruit Street VBK508,
    Boston, MA 02114, USA

Johan H.C. Reiber
    Division of Image Processing, Department of Radiology, Leiden University Medical
    Center, Albinusdreef 2, 2333 ZA Leiden, The Netherlands
    Coauthors: Jouke Dijkstra, Gerhard Koning, Pranobe V. Oemrawsingh[*], Martin J. Schalij[*],
    Bob Goedhart
    [*] Department of Cardiology, Leiden University Medical Center, Leiden, The Nether-
    lands

John A. Rumberger[#]
    [#] Department of Cardiovascular Diseases, Mayo Clinic and Foundation, 200 First Street
    SW, Rochester, MN 55905, USA
    Coauthors: Axel Schmermund[#*], Raimund Erbel[*]
    [*] Department of Cardiology, University Clinic Essen, Essen, Germany

Markus B. Scheidegger
    Institute of Biomedical Engineering, MR-Center USZ, 8091 Zürich, Switzerland
    Coauthors: Marcus Spiegel, Peter Boesiger

Milan Sonka
    Department of Electrical and Computer Engineering, The University of Iowa, Iowa
    City, IA 52242, USA
    Co-author: Xiangmin Zhang[*]
    [*] Boston Scientific Corporation, San Jose, California, USA

Jens C. Stollfuss
    Klinik für Nuklearmedizin, Technische Universität München, Klinikum rechts der Isar,
    Ismaningerstrasse 22, D-81675 München, Germany
    Coauthors: Frank M. Bengel, Markus Schwaiger

George R. Sutherland
    Department of Medicine and Care/Clinical Physiology, University Hospital, SE 581 85
    Linköping, Sweden

Jean-Claude Tardiff
    Intravascular Ultrasound Laboratory, Montreal Heart Institute, 5000 Belanger Street
    East, Montreal, Québec H1T 1C8, Canada
    Co-author: Hai Shiang Lee

Ernst E. van der Wall
    Department of Cardiology, Leiden University Medical Center, Albinusdreef 2, 2333 ZA
    Leiden, The Netherlands

Preface

What's New in Cardiovascular Imaging is a bibliographical "image" of a Symposium held June 22-24, 1998 in Leiden, the Netherlands. At this Symposium all the major advances in cardiovascular imaging in all the cardiovascular imaging modalities (X-ray, (intravascular) ultrasound, magnetic resonance, scintigraphy and CT) were addressed by the leading authorities in this field. Based on the presentations of the invited Faculty, this book consists of a compilation of manuscripts related to most of the topics discussed at this particular meeting. We express our gratitude to all authors and coauthors for having made great efforts in preparing their superb up-to-date chapters under a great time pressure, so that this book was available at the time of the Symposium. The authors are all excellent investigators in one or more fields of cardiovascular imaging and they have stimulated progress in cardiovascular imaging with the aim to improve patient care and clinical research.

This book consists of a total of 32 chapters subdivided into seven Parts. Each part describes a particular field in cardiovascular imaging. These Parts are: Coronary quantitation by QCA and intracoronary ultrasound (QCU), angiographic trials, progress in intravascular ultrasound, magnetic resonance (MR) coronary and vascular imaging, nuclear cardiovascular imaging, echocardiography, and cine and spiral CT coronary imaging. In general, each Part begins with a chapter that provides a broad overview of the advances in the field described in that particular Part, as well as a view towards the future. As such this introductory chapter provides the broader overview. In the following chapters in such a Part, individual topics are described in further detail by other experts. In this way, the book should be of great interest to the more "generalist" reader as well as to the more "specialist" reader.

It has been quite obvious for a long time that cardiovascular imaging is a field in which quantitative analysis of the corresponding images is a must for clinical research studies and which thereafter is often translated into routine practice. Particularly with the increasing use of three-dimensional (3D) data as well as 4D (3D plus time), it has been quite clear that the amount of information is so large that the conventional visual interpretation is not suitable anymore, and otherwise would result in unacceptably high inter- and intra-observer variabilities and underutilization of the data. Fortunately, (semi)-automated analysis techniques preferably with automated edge detection approaches provide a wealth of information with small systematic and random errors. These approaches can also be denoted "computer-aided" diagnosis or interpretation. With the rapidly increasing computer power of PC- and SUN-based workstations, the thresholds for the applications of these techniques in the clinical research and routine applications disappear. Also, the younger generations of scientists and medical specialists are brought up in this information technology era and are eager to use these approaches. It is also evident that the quality and robustness of these computer-aided approaches will only improve in the future, as more fuzzy logic, artificial intelligence, 3D and 4D model information, etc. approaches will be included into these processes.

In this book we have attempted to build a bridge between the image processing scientists and the physicists, and the medical specialists. It is of great importance that the technical scientists understand the needs of the medical doctors, and that the medical doctors try to understand the possibilities, the limitations and the complexity of these technological developments. Individual and isolated work by one party without involving the other party will lead in general to solutions that the other party cannot use, or only very minimally. The synergy of the ideas will lead to the innovative and well-validated solutions, that eventually will improve the quality of health care. Therefore, we hope that this book will assist the cardiologist, the radiologist, the nuclear medicine physician, the image processing specialist, the physicist, the basic scientist, and the fellow, who is in training for those specialties, in understanding the most recent achievements in cardiovascular imaging techniques and their impact on cardiovascular medicine.

Finally, we would like to acknowledge the significant contributions (in alphabetical order) from Mr. J.J. Beentjes, Mrs. A. van der Mey, Mr. J. Schoones, and Mrs. J.C. Tuinenburg, all from the Leiden University Medical Center, who all put a lot of effort in preparing, editing and realizing the entirely digitally formatted camera-ready version of this *What's New in Cardiovascular Imaging* within the very limited time available, and from Mrs. N. Dekker (Kluwer Academic Publishers, Dordrecht, the Netherlands) for the final publication process of the book. Lastly, this book would not have been possible without a generous educational grant from Parke-Davis BV (Hoofddorp, the Netherlands) and Pfizer BV (Capelle a/d IJssel, the Netherlands).

The Editors,

Johan H.C. Reiber and Ernst E. van der Wall

1. Current and future developments in QCA and image fusion with IVUS

Johan H.C. Reiber, Jouke Dijkstra, Gerhard Koning,
Pranobe V. Oemrawsingh, Martin J. Schalij & Bob Goedhart

Summary

Although quantitative coronary arteriography (QCA) has been around now for quite some time, research and development continue to take place along several directions. First of all, the imaging medium has changed from the traditional 35 mm analog cinefilm to the digital world with the CD-R as the preferred carrier. This required adaptations of the basic contour detection algorithms. Stimulated by these same changes, digital review stations or DICOM-Viewers have been developed. In addition, third-generation QCA algorithms have been designed and implemented, and applied to quantitate complex morphology and radiopaque stents.

Intravascular ultrasound has also found its place in interventional cardiology. Major developments include automated contour detection techniques in the individual cross-sections and in the 3D reconstructions obtained from (ECG-triggered) pullback approaches (quantitative coronary ultrasound or QCU). A great deal of attention is also given to improved 3D visualization of the vessel of interest. This will certainly be facilitated by the image fusion of biplane coronary arteriography and intravascular ultrasound, and the associated quantitative techniques QCA and QCU, respectively.

Introduction

Quantitative coronary arteriography (QCA) was developed in the 1970's to quantify vessel vasomotion and the effects of drugs on the regression and progression of coronary artery disease [1]. Initially, vessel contours were traced manually on optically magnified cineframes, later supported by semi-automated edge detection approaches [2,3]. Two major clinical developments from the early eighties which have grown exponentially since then have stimulated the use and interest in QCA: 1) the innovation and application in coronary recanalization techniques (PTCA, atherectomy, thrombolysis, stenting, laser, etc.); and 2) the increasing interest to study the effects of new drugs directed at the regression or no-growth of existing coronary artery disease, or the delay in the formation of new lesions [4]. Until recently these analytical approaches were used predominantly in clinical research trials with 35 mm cinefilm as the exclusive storage and exchange medium.

In the mid-1980's, digital systems were introduced into the catheterization laboratory to support the angiographer with the interventional procedures. Initially, only single digital

J.H.C. Reiber and E.E. van der Wall (eds.). What's New in Cardiovascular Imaging, 17–30.
©1998 Kluwer Academic Publishers.

frames could be displayed for road map purposes, later followed by cine loops, and facilities for on-line QCA [5]. As a result of the continuous evolution of digital angiographic technology, it has largely become accepted practice that interventional procedures should only be carried out in a laboratory with digital facilities. On-line QCA has been used predominantly for the selection of the optimal sizes of the interventional devices, and for the assessment of the efficacy of the procedure. However, the rapid dissemination of the digital technology and the resulting wide availability of the angiographic images in a digital format on CD-ROM's, plus the fact that these large number of images can be visualized on affordable PC technology, has created new and great opportunities for QCA, which will be discussed in this chapter.

The same is basically true for intravascular ultrasound (IVUS). IVUS has been very instrumental in the understanding of the morphology and the changes therein of the arterial wall, and particularly in the development of the optimal procedures for the stent placement [6]. It has been recognized that in particular immediately post-PTCA, IVUS may provide more reliable information about the vessel cross-section than QCA, because of the complex morphology and the fact that X-ray imaging is a shadow technology, while IVUS provides truly cross-sectional data. However, both techniques have their own strengths and weaknesses, and will provide complementary information. It is our belief that the combination of the two will provide the most complete information about the status of the disease in a particular vessel segment.

Off- and on-line QCA

In the new digital or DICOM (Digital Imaging and Communications in Medicine) era, there are clearly different ways that QCA is used, which we will refer to for simplification reasons by the notations "Off-line QCA" and "On-line QCA". These changes relative to the past have been due to the rapidly increasing availability of the so-called DICOM-Viewers or Digital Review Stations. The DICOM-Viewers will be discussed before these different QCA-usage's will be explained.

Digital review stations

We all have been so familiar with the 35 mm cinefilm and the fact that it is a worldwide standard, that viewing of such a patient record all over the world does not present any problem. However, as more and more cardiac catheterization laboratories were transformed in the past into digital laboratories in which all the angiographic runs were stored in a digital format, it became clear that a standardized exchange medium and image format had to be agreed upon to avoid a situation whereby angiographic runs could only be replayed at best in its own laboratory. This is where the ACC (American College of cardiology) and ACR/NEMA (American College of Radiology/National Electrical Manufacturers Association) later joined by the ESC (European Society of Cardiology) have carried out an enormously important task by bringing all parties together and agreeing upon the CD-R (Compact Disc - Recordable) as the exchange medium and the DICOM-3 format as the exchange format. With the introduction of these digital CD-R's, high quality digital review stations (also called "Digital Tagarno's" or "DICOM Viewers") had to become available to take the place of the traditional mechanical cineprojectors. It is obvious that such new digital viewers should minimally satisfy the same requirements as the conventional cinefilm projectors, and preferably even more. This sounds like a natural requirement nowadays, but to realize that taken into account the enormous amounts of digital data that needs to be read from the CD-R's and displayed onto the computer screen at high frame speeds, requires top quality hardware and software and lots of computer memory. A number of such requirements are: 1) review of image runs in real time, i.e. at least at the acquisition speed (12.5-30 frames/s) and preferably even faster up to 100 frames/s as on a cinefilm projector; 2) display of a still image at the original spatial resolution in a lossless format, while a small degree of lossy image compression may be allowed during the dynamic replay of a run. Due to the fact that these images are available in a digital format facilitates a number of features that are not available on the cineprojectors. Examples of these are: 1) adjustment of contrast and brightness; 2) zooming in on a region-of-interest; 3) providing an overview of all the runs on a particular disc using the so-called thumbnails; 4) allowing two or more runs to be displayed at the same time in separate windows, e.g. two views of the same artery or left ventricle, or a baseline and follow-up run of some artery; and 5) of course, the availability of analytical software for QCA and quantitative left ventriculography. The role of DICOM in the digital catheterization laboratory and an overview of digital review stations as of March 1998 is presented in ref. [7].

From this overview it is clear that there certainly are major differences in the qualities, usefulness, prices, etc. of all the workstations that are and will be made available commercially. To educate the cardiological community about DICOM, the Working Group 1 of the DICOM Standards Committee has published the so-called Primer [8].

Off-line QCA

With off-line QCA we mean one or more QCA-workstations which are not directly connected to the image generating X-ray system; on the other hand, it is possible that multiple QCA-workstations are connected to an internal network to exchange image data with a file-server for central storage purposes. Typical applications for such off-line workstations include Core Laboratory activities and smaller single center clinical research studies in a particular cardiology department. A schematic diagram of such a set-up is shown in the lower and right portion of Figure 1. Preferably, such a QCA-workstation should be able to accept the different image media now available, such as the traditional 35 mm cinefilm, as well as the CD-R's , and any other storage medium such as digital tape. This means that different acquisition modules must be available to accommodate the different storage media. A modern QCA-workstation will be based on at least the Pentium technology and preferably the Windows-NT operating system.

On-line QCA

With on-line QCA we mean the situation that the QCA-workstation is directly connected to the image generating X-ray system. The connection can be realized in different ways from a simple analog video connection to the output of the X-ray system, requiring a selected frame to be digitized by the QCA-workstation, to a preferred digital connection to the digital network of the imaging system. A schematic diagram of this on-line set-up is given in the upper portion of Figure 1. The typical applications of the on-line QCA include of course the

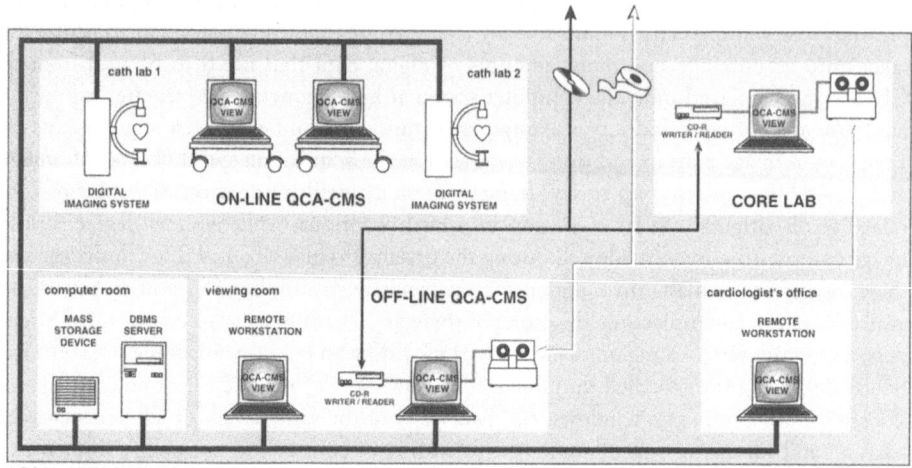

LOCAL AREA NETWORK

Figure 1. Schematic diagram of off-line and on-line applications of QCA workstations.

clinical decision making process about the therapeutic course to be taken during the catheterization procedure, such as the vessel sizing for the optimal selection of the interventional device (diameter and length of the balloon, stent, atherectomy device, etc.) in case of a coronary intervention, as well as the immediate assessment of the efficacy of the interventional procedure.

Basic principles of QCA

The general principles and characteristics of a modern QCA analytical software package can best be illustrated using the QCA-CMS (Cardiovascular Measurement System, MEDIS, Leiden, the Netherlands) algorithms developed in our laboratory [2,3]. Since these have been described extensively elsewhere, only a brief summary suffices; the latest version (4.0) facilitates DICOM support. If 35 mm cinefilm is the storage medium, a region of interest (ROI) in a selected frame is magnified optically on the cine-projector, converted into video format and digitized (analog to digital conversion) by a frame grabber and stored in memory of the QCA-workstation. A typical optical zoom factor is around 2.3 fold, such that the pixel size is in the range of 0.08-0.10 mm for a matrix size of 768×512 pixels. For a digital application, the ROI's are extracted from the digital matrix data (typically 512^2 pixels as prescribed by the DICOM format) and digitally zoomed again to a matrix size of 512^2 pixels using an interpolation approach.

To select the coronary segment to be analyzed in the selected ROI, the user only needs to define with the computer mouse the start and end point of that segment. In the next step, an arterial pathline through the segment of interest is computed automatically [3]. The contour detection technique is based on the so-called Minimum Cost Analysis (MCA), which uses the weighted sum of the first and second derivative values applied to the brightness levels measured along scanlines perpendicular to the pathline. To correct for the limited resolution of the entire X-ray system, the MCA algorithm is carried out in two iterations based on an analysis of the point spread function of the imaging chain, which is of particular importance for the accurate measurement of small diameters as in coronary obstructions.

Calibration of the image data is performed on a nontapering part of the contrast catheter following a similar MCA edge detection procedure as for the arterial segment; however, in this case, additional information is used in the edge detection process, knowing that this part of the catheter is characterized by parallel boundaries. It should also be recognized that the catheter calibration procedure is the weakest link in the analysis chain; for that purpose, restrictions have been formulated as to the size and the types of so-called QCA-approved catheters [9].

From the left- and right-hand contours of the arterial segment, a diameter function is determined. It should be noted that pincushion correction should not be applied as this may introduce more artefacts than resolve problems; for an extensive discussion of this point, see ref. [10]. From this calculated diameter function, many parameters are derived automatically, among others: the site of maximal percent stenosis, the obstruction diameter, the corresponding automatically determined reference diameter, and the extent of the obstruction. Additionally derived parameters include obstruction symmetry, inflow and outflow angles, the area of the atherosclerotic plaque, and functional information.

Complex vessel morphology

As explained above, the conventional or 2nd generation contour detection technique is based on the Minimum Cost Algorithm (MCA), which has been demonstrated to be fast and robust for images which may vary significantly in image quality. This approach has demonstrated to work very well in QCA as long as the vessel outlines are relatively smooth in shape. However, complex vessel morphology may occur post-coronary intervention, for example, when a dissection occurs. Also before intervention, obstructions with very sharp corners may be found.

The MCA technique in its design is hampered in tracing very irregular and complex boundaries. To be able to adequately analyze such very irregular stenoses, we have developed the Gradient Field Transform (GFT®), which does not have the limitations of the MCA algorithm [11] (Figure 2). As QCA is applied nowadays widely in interventional studies, the GFT is a *must* on a modern workstation; otherwise significant overestimations in the vessel dimensions may occur.

The GFT has been validated extensively on phantom images and on digital coronary arteriograms [11]. Our experiences with the GFT indicate that this approach is advocated for the analysis of ostial lesions and of radiopaque stents. With the appropriate optical zooming (in an off-line configuration), the GFT is able to follow the outer boundaries of the stent struts and the contrast lumen in between the stent struts.

Digital QCA

From the user's point of view, the analysis of digital images on the QCA-CMS is basically not different from the analysis of cinefilm frames described above. However, there are a number of important differences between the cinefilm and the digital media. These are: 1) cinefilm has a nonlinear density function, which differs between hospitals, and which may

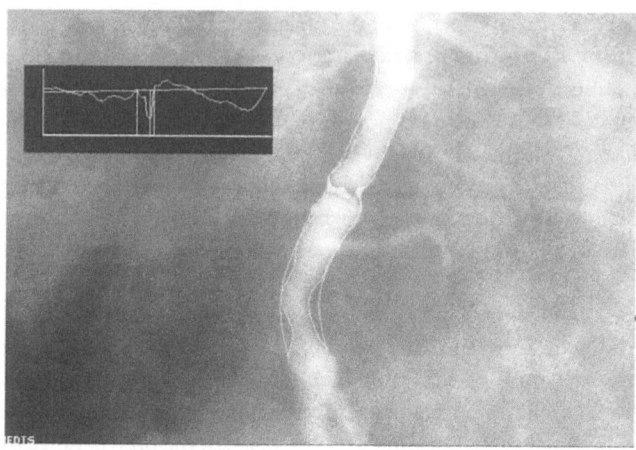

Figure 2. Example of the outcome of the Gradient Field Transform analysis on a vessel segment with a very severe complex stenosis. Conventional approaches with the MCA algorithm would not be able to follow automatically the abrupt changes in morphology.

also differ slightly from day to day or week to week, whereas the digital systems are characterized by a well-defined nonlinear function (the White Compression); 2) cinefilm is hampered by the presence of film grain noise, which is absent on the digital systems; 3) on cinefilm analyses we use an optical magnification, which is absent on the digital approach; 4) assuming a 2.3 fold optical magnification on the cinefilm, the effective matrix size on the cinefilm is 512^2 x 2.3 = 1180^2 pixels, whereas the matrix size for the digital images is 512^2 x 8 bits up to 1024^2 x 8, 10 or 12 bits depending on the equipment; 5) the pixel size in the optically magnified cinefilm images is 0.08 - 0.10 mm, and in the digital images before digital zooming 0.20 - 0.24 mm; 6) on the cinefilm the vessels are visible as bright structures on a dark background, and in the digital images as dark structures on a bright background; and finally 7) edge enhancement is not possible on cinefilm, while this is a frequently used option on the digital images. It will be clear that the MCA algorithm must be optimized for the image medium to take care of all these differences listed above; one just cannot apply 1st and 2nd derivative-functions (the kernels) derived for cinefilm applications to a digital image without modifications and expect the same systematic and random errors. Let us look at some more detail at the issue of optical and digital magnification.

The MCA edge detection algorithm has been optimized for the range of pixel sizes between 0.08 and 0.10 mm, which is achieved with an optical resolution of approximately 2.3 fold. To obtain pixel sizes in the same range for the digital images, we propose to use a similar value for the digital zoom on the digital images, i.e. approximately 2.3 fold. With a digital pixel size in the original image in the range of 0.20 - 0.24 mm, the magnified pixel size will therefore again be in the range of 0.08 - 0.10 mm.

Open issues with digital QCA

However, there are still a number of issues associated with digital QCA in general that need to be studied in great detail in the very near future. Questions have been raised whether the commonly used matrix size of 512^2 pixels and 8 bits of density resolution (256 gray levels) is really sufficient to appreciate the same fine details as visible on cinefilm. Should one use a matrix size of 1024^2 by 12 bits in stead? Are there any differences in QCA results between these different media (cinefilm and digital) and matrix sizes? Although various QCA studies carried out in the past have confirmed that there were only minor, nonsignificant differences between digital and cinefilm, these were based on phantom and clinical studies of relatively smooth vessels. We have also shown that QCA from cinefilm is associated with a smaller random error (by 10 - 15 %) than from digital [12]. With modern interventional cardiology, however, the requirements for proper viewing of these small devices and the subsequent quantitative analysis have increased, and with these goals in mind these resolution issues need to be revisited. It is to be expected that the requirements on the matrix sizes will depend on the kind of detail needed, i.e. one has to differentiate between smooth and complex lesions.

Edge enhancement and image compression

Other major issues of difference between the conventional cinefilm and the modern digital approach are edge enhancement and image compression. Edge enhancement is one of the major reasons why digital images look so much appealing to the user: the images have been sharpened and the degree of enhancement is even user-customizable! However, it has been demonstrated quite clearly that edge enhancement has a definite affect on the results of QCA [13]. Also, the edge enhancement cannot be undone using a deconvolution filter. As a result, it was concluded from that study that the raw digital data, as produced by the X-ray equipment, *must be used* for QCA and archival purposes! This is in accordance with the DICOM-3 exchange standard.

In an attempt to limit the enormous amount of digital data associated with a catheterization procedure, the use of image compression techniques has been considered. Lossless techniques allow only a compression factor of about two. To increase efficiency higher compression ratios are desired, which by definition become lossy, i.e. the original information cannot fully be recovered anymore. For these purposes the widely available JPEG techniques have been applied, although other modern compression schemes (e.g. Wavelets) may provide better results in the future. The highest acceptable lossy compression factor will be determined by the fact whether effects on the diagnostic interpretation of these images, and on the QCA results will still just not be noticeable. In a small pilot study on clinical images we have found that already at a JPEG compression factor of five, significantly increased random differences in QCA results were apparent although at unchanged systematic differences [14]. To come up with a widely acceptable standard, the Working Group 1 of the DICOM Standards Committee in which the ACC, ACR, NEMA and the ESC participate has set up an International Compression Viability Study (ICVS) which will answer these remaining questions in the course of 1998.

Future QCA directions

It must be clear that the DICOM-3 standard has been developed to exchange image data between machines from different vendors. It has never been meant to be an archive standard. The simplest archive of a digital laboratory is of course the same old shelve, now with the CD-R's on it in stead of the cinefilm boxes in the past. This may work for a small laboratory (e.g. less than 1000 cases/yr), but that is not exactly what we expect from a digital laboratory.

For the medium- and large-volume laboratories automated archives are preferred with different levels of access, for example an "on-line" short-term storage, a "near-line" long-term storage and an "off-line" storage. For an excellent overview of these archival issues, the reader is referred to [15].

Furthermore, we do expect extensive networking of digital review stations with and without QCA packages in the catheterization laboratory. Of course this network will be connected to the imaging network of the catheterization laboratories, thereby allowing images to be transferred to the cardiologist's office and also to referring hospitals. The selected images and the corresponding results can be saved on a central file server for later review and possibly reanalysis.

In terms of extension of analytical software packages, we anticipate further developments in the automated segmentation of parts of or the entire coronary tree from two preferably orthogonal views [16]. This will allow the selection of optimal views for selected coronary segments, and the assessment of the area at risk of the myocardial muscle [17]. For the near future, the integration with intravascular ultrasound can be expected; this will be discussed under the section Image Fusion.

With so many different approaches and devices for coronary recanalization now available (balloons: compliant and noncompliant; long, medium and short; perfusion balloon; hybrid balloon; ultralow profile balloon; local drug delivery balloon; stents: slotted tube, coiled, self-expanding with or without biocompatible coatings, etc.), it is likely that on-line QCA and/or IVUS will be used increasingly to help guide the logical choice of technology, based on lesion morphology and location in the coronary tree.

Quantitative coronary ultrasound (QCU)

Intravascular ultrasound (IVUS) is able to provide real-time high resolution images of sections of the arterial wall, in contrast to X-ray arteriography that provides a shadow image (luminogram) of the entire lumen. The accuracy and reliability of IVUS image data have been investigated extensively by correlation with both angiography [18] and histology [19]. IVUS has potentially a great strength in diagnostic and interventional procedures [20]. In the first application, IVUS is able to demonstrate the presence or absence of compensatory coronary artery enlargement, to assess the severity of intermediate lesions, to reveal occult left main disease, and angiographically 'silent' atherosclerosis. In interventional cardiology, IVUS may support the selection of the devices, i.e. rotablators in calcified lesions, and atherectomy devices in large plaque burden. The results of such procedures can be studied on-line, under the restrictions described later. In the current practice of IVUS-guided interventional cardiology, the lumen and the wall of a particular coronary segment are inspected visually by moving the intracoronary ultrasound catheter through the vessel. The global positioning of the catheter is guided by X-ray angiography. In this way the section with the narrowest lumen can be selected and analyzed quantitatively by using a manual caliper in its simplest approach, or by outlining the lumen and vessel wall contours in a more accurate approach. This will lead to the calculation of the percent cross-sectional area narrowing at that particular cross section, and minimal and maximal diameters. However, the associated inter- and intra-observer variabilities are definite limitations of this approach. Considering the irregularity of the lumen shape and the presence of artefacts in the individual cross-sections in the coronary artery, it will be clear that simple contour detection approaches, like simple edge detectors, will not work. More sophisticated automated contour detection algorithms which preserve the continuity of the contour using dynamic programming techniques like the minimum cost algorithm, or the active shape model or snakes have to be used for luminal boundary detection [21]. For the detection of dissection or ruptures, the techniques which are looking for more or less convex sections will not work; in such cases a technique with characteristics as the earlier mentioned Gradient Field Transform is needed.

3D reconstruction

Since IVUS is in principle a tomographic technique, the catheter can be pulled back, while at the same time the images are being digitized and stored in computer memory. To assure that the pullback speed is constant, several motorized pullback techniques have been developed. To avoid the artifacts caused by cardiac motion, the image acquisition for a pullback should be ECG-triggered. The individual cross-sections can be stacked in the computer memory and visualized. For visualization, at least two approaches have been developed, one being the display of the longitudinal cross-sections of the vessel segment (sagittal view) in combination with the corresponding cross-sections, and the other one the 'clam-shell' view which requires image segmentation. The three-dimensional reconstruction of a pullback series results in a straight tube representation, because the catheter does not provide information about the three-dimensional trajectory of its pullback path. In the majority of the cases this will, of course, not be correct. This may lead to misinterpretations of the location of the plaque, and to highly incorrect measurements of the lumen and plaque volumes due to expansion and compression of the reconstructed 3D data. With pullback techniques, the catheter movement is sensed at its proximal site, but it is the distal tip that produces the images. An excellent overview of the advantages and limitations of 3D IVUS imaging can be found in [22].

The sagittal views are regarded by many users as extremely helpful, as these provide the observer with important longitudinal perspectives, while maintaining the morphologic information [23]. Unless the true vessel curvature is taken into account, three-dimensional reconstruction may not offer more information to the interventional cardiologist than a series of longitudinal views. None of the currently available 3D-reconstruction techniques accounts for the vessel curvature; they all provide a simple 3D rendering of stacked IVUS slices.

3D quantitative analysis

Since the image quality of the individual cross sections is limited due to the fact that the image resolution and image contrast are relatively low, that the images are very noisy and drop-out regions are present, it is very difficult to develop a contour detection technique that is automated and robust in the individual cross sections. Therefore, one should try to make use of the continuity of the morphology in the individual cross sections. Li et al. have developed a very elegant and practical approach in this direction [24]. Their semi-automatic approach consists of three steps. First, two perpendicular cut planes which are parallel to the longitudinal axis are selected interactively. The second step is an interactive tracing procedure which defines the contours of the lumen and plaque in the longitudinal images. For each longitudinal image, two lumen and two media-adventitia contours are traced. The third step is the contour detection in each cross-sectional image thereby using the informa-

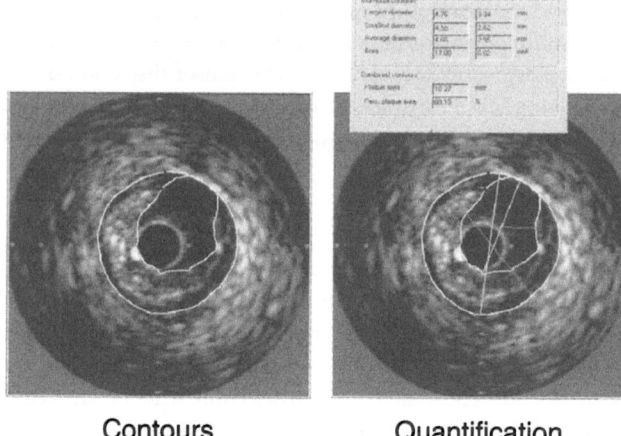

Contours   Quantification

Figure 3. First results of our automated contour detection approaches for the luminal and vessel boundaries in IVUS images on the QCU-CMS system.

tion from the longitudinal contours. By transforming the contours from the two longitudinal planes to the transverse plane, four pre-defined points per contour become available for each cross-section. These points indicate the locations through which the contours should go in that particular cross section. The automated contour detection in the cross section again is based on the minimum cost (MCA) contour detection technique. Once the contours are available, the clinically relevant data such as the volumes of the lumen and the plaque can easily be calculated.

The approach that we have taken is somewhat similar. Our QCU-CMS system is running under the Windows-NT operating system on a Pentium-II 233 MHz processor computer. For image manipulation purposes we have developed the MPIRE® software package, that allows standardized handling of images and contours and integration with other software modules developed in our laboratory. A part of the contour detection approach is similar to that developed by Li; the QCU-CMS system allows the user to select any longitudinal cross-section (more than two are allowed and they do not need to be perpendicular). The contour detection in the longitudinal images is based on the MCA approach. Recently, our MCA has been redesigned using the C++ computer language in an object-oriented approach. The advantage of the redesign is that it has become very flexible and therefore can be adapted very quickly to new applications. This redesigned MCA allows the incorporation of mathematical models of the structures to be detected and other physical or anatomical knowledge, which makes the contour detection procedure more robust. The approach by Li is based on a matching technique, whereby the information of the contours drawn in a first frame, will be matched as best as possible to the subsequent frames. We base the results from our contour detection on the local image properties and on additional information from models and knowledge about IVUS images. The information from adjacent slices is only used to guide the positions and directions of the scanlines for the resampling of the images. Figure 3 shows the first results of our automatically determined luminal and vessel contours and derived quantitative data. In addition, a Gradient Field Transform-like approach will be developed and implemented, allowing to detect irregularly shaped cross sections, especially for the lumen contour. In the three-dimensional reconstruction, corrections will be carried out for possible rotation of the catheter during pullback and catheter movement. An interesting approach in this direction has been described by Prause et al. [25].

Future IVUS directions

It will be clear that IVUS is complementary rather than in competition with arteriography. Arteriography provides an overall, critically important roadmap, while IVUS goes to the appropriate address and tells the investigator what is happening in the vessel wall at that particular place. QCA and IVUS pre-intervention can help to decide which interventional device to use and its size. It can also teach all sorts of things about the local environment inside the artery, that will help make the case go better and quicker. Preliminary results indicate that IVUS may allow the automated assessment of plaque composition in terms of soft and hard/shadowed plaques based on texture descriptors and automated classification techniques [26]. It is also clear that not in all cases the combination of QCA and IVUS will be necessary. In some vessels it will suffice to use only QCA, in others only IVUS and in the remaining cases the combination. Clinical trials need to be designed to sort out these choices, taking into account that IVUS adds to the cost and the length of a procedure. Anyway, the angiogram will always be needed to guide the 3D reconstruction procedure. Large prospective trials are underway to address the effects of IVUS on device selection or the predictibility of long-term results; these will provide answers to the cost-benefit ratio of peri-interventional intravascular ultrasound [20].

Image fusion

Safar we have addressed the current and future approaches for the individual image modalities. With all the data available in digital format, it will be clear, that attempts will be made towards image fusion. One of the most apparent applications, is the image fusion of coronary arteriography and intracoronary ultrasound in combination with their quantitative

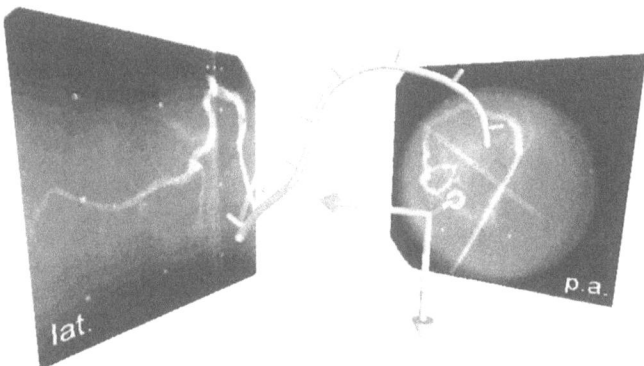

Figure 4. Biplane contrast angiogram of right coronary artery in a cadaveric pig heart with 3-D reconstructed centerline. Short vectors indicate the orientation of IVUS images along the pullback as derived by sequential triangulation; note the clockwise twist from front to back. One unit of the axes equals 10 mm in the real world (with permission from ref 25).

approaches of QCA and QCU, respectively. As was described earlier, at present 3-D reconstructions of coronary vessels are generated from IVUS by stacking up preferably ECG-gated and segmented IVUS frames of a pullback sequence. This simplified approach always results in straight vessel reconstructions, and therefore, provides an incorrect representation of bended and tortuous coronary arteries. From two biplane X-ray views, the pathlines of the relevant coronary segment can be traced by well-known pathline tracer techniques. Subsequently, the 3-D course of the vessel can be reconstructed three-dimensionally assuming that the correct geometric data of the X-ray gantries is available. The IVUS cross-sectional images can then be displayed around this 3D pathline, thereby providing a realistic view of the reconstructed coronary segment and allowing more accurate calculations of luminal and plaque volumes [27]. Figure 4 illustrates the basic concepts of this data fusion approach (with permission from ref. 25).

References

1.   Brown BG, Bolson E, Frimer M, Dodge HT. Quantitative coronary arteriography: estimation of dimensions, hemodynamic resistance, and atheroma mass of coronary artery lesions using the arteriogram and digital computation. Circulation 1977;55:329-37.

2.   Reiber JHC, Serruys PW, Kooijman CJ et al. Assessment of short-, medium-, and long-term variations in arterial dimensions from computer-assisted quantitation of coronary cineangiograms. Circulation 1985;71:280-8.

3.   Reiber JHC. An overview of coronary quantitation techniques as of 1989. In: Reiber JHC, Serruys PW, editors. Quantitative coronary arteriography. Dordrecht: Kluwer Academic Publishers; 1991. p. 55-132.

4.   Bruschke AVG, Reiber JHC, Lie KI, Wellens HJJ, editors. Lipid-lowering therapy and progression of coronary atherosclerosis. Dordrecht: Kluwer Academic Publishers; 1996.

5.   Reiber JHC, Van der Zwet PMJ, Koning G et al. Accuracy and precision of quantitative digital coronary arteriography: observer-, short-, and medium-term variabilities. Cathet Cardiovasc Diagn 1993;28:187-98.

6.   Di Mario C, Fitzgerald PJ, Colombo A. New developments in intracoronary ultrasound. In: Reiber JHC, Van der Wall EE, editors. Cardiovascular Imaging. Dordrecht: Kluwer Academic Publishers; 1996. p. 257-75.

7.   Goedhart B, Reiber JHC. The Dicom viewing stations: are they truly different. Int J Card Imaging. In press 1998.

8.   Kennedy TE, Nissen SE, Simon R, Thomas JD, Tilkemeier PL, editors. Digital cardiac imaging in the 21st century: a primer. Bethesda, Maryland: The Cardiac and Vascular Information Working Group, American College of Cardiology; 1997.

9.   Koning G, Van der Zwet PMJ, Von Land CD, Reiber JHC. Angiographic assessment of dimensions of 6F and 7F Mallinckrodt Softouch[R] coronary contrast catheters from digital and cine arteriograms. Int J Card Imaging 1992;8:153-61.

10. Van der Zwet PMJ, Meijer DJH, Reiber JHC. Automated and accurate assessment of the distribution, magnitude, and direction of pincushion distortion in angiographic images. Invest Radiol 1995;30:204-13.

11. Van der Zwet PMJ, Reiber JHC. A new approach for the quantification of complex lesion morphology: the gradient field transform: basic principles and validation results. J Am Coll Cardiol 1994;24:216-24.

12. Reiber JHC, Von Land CD, Koning G et al. Comparison of accuracy and precision of quantitative coronary arterial analysis between cinefilm and digital systems. In: Reiber JHC, Serruys PW, editors. Progress in quantitative coronary arteriography. Dordrecht: Kluwer Academic Publishers; 1994. p. 67-85.

13. Van der Zwet PMJ, Reiber JHC. The influence of image enhancement and reconstruction on quantitative coronary arteriography. Int J Card Imaging 1995;11:211-21.

14. Koning G, Baretta P, Zwart P, Reiber JHC. Effect of lossy image compression on QCA results [abstract]. Circulation 1995;92(8 suppl):I-22.

15. Cusma JT, Bashore TM. The digital catheterization laboratory - is it practical today? In: Reiber JHC, Van der Wall EE, editors. Cardiovascular Imaging. Dordrecht: Kluwer Academic Publishers; 1996. p. 157-70.

16. Dumay ACM. Image reconstruction from biplane angiographic projections[dissertation]. Delft: Delft University of Technology; 1992.

17. Seiler C, Kirkeeide RL, Gould KL. Basic structure-function relations of the epicardial coronary vascular tree. Basis of quantitative coronary arteriography for diffuse coronary artery disease. Circulation 1992;85:1987-2003.

18. De Scheerder I, De Man F, Herregods MC *et al.* Intravascular ultrasound versus angiography for measurement of luminal diameters in normal and diseased coronary arteries. Am Heart J 1994;127:243-51.

19. Nishimura RA, Edwards WD, Warnes CA *et al.* Intravascular ultrasound imaging: in vitro validation and pathologic correlation. J Am Coll Cardiol 1990;16:145-54.

20. Görge G, Ge J, Haude M *et al.* Intravascular ultrasound for evaluation of coronary arteries. Herz 1996;21:78-89.

21. Maurincomme E, Finet G, Reiber JHC, Savalle L, Magnin I. Quantitative intravascular ultrasound imaging: evaluation of an automatic approach [abstract]. J Am Coll Cardiol 1995;25special issue:354A.

22. Maurincomme E, Finet G. What are the advantages and limitations of three- dimensional intracoronary ultrasound imaging? In: Reiber JHC, Van der Wall EE, eidtors. Cardiovascular Imaging. Dordrecht: Kluwer Academic Publishers; 1996. p. 243-55.

23. Roelandt JRTC, Di Mario C, Pandian NG *et al.* Three-dimensional reconstruction of intracoronary ultrasound images. Rationale, approaches, problems, and directions. Circulation 1994;90:1044-55.

24. Li W, Bom N, Von Birgelen C *et al.* State of the art in ICUS quantitation. In: Reiber JHC, Van der Wall EE, editors. Cardiovascular Imaging. Dordrecht: Kluwer Academic Publishers; 1996. p. 79-92.

25. Prause GPM, DeJong SC, McKay CR, Sonka M. Towards a geometrically correct 3-D reconstruction of turtuous coronary arteries based on biplane angiography and intravascular ultrasound. Int J Card Imaging 1997;13:451-62.

26. Sonka M, Zhang X. Assessment of plaque composition using intravascular ultrasound. This book;

27. Evans JL, Ng KH, Wiet SG *et al.* Accurate three-dimensional reconstruction of intravascular data. Spatially correct three-dimensional reconstructions. Circulation 1996;93:567-76.

2.

Issues in the performance of quantitative coronary angiography in clinical research trials

Jacques Lespérance, Luc Bilodeau, Johan H.C. Reiber, Gerhard Koning, Gilles Hudon & Martial G. Bourassa

Summary

Quantitative coronary analysis remains the classical and most commonly used tool to assess the results of coronary pharmacological or mechanical intervention. The authors review the methodology of this type of analysis, highlighting the pros and cons of previous recommendations. Special interest has been devoted to catheter calibration and the choice of angiographic views for optimal measurement and reliability. Significant additional information in terms of acute gain, late loss or restenosis rate is not gained by the use of averaged orthogonal measurements as compared to the more simple single view approach. Also calibration procedures can be simplified by using tables of mean measured values for various types of catheters instead of measuring each catheter with a precision micrometer and by doing calibration measurements on contrast filled instead of flushed catheters. Moreover, specific *in vitro* and *in vivo* criteria have been proposed and tested for acceptance of catheter type and size in QCA analyses. Based on these criteria only catheters of sufficient size (6F or greater) and approved for QCA are recommended.

Thus, simplification in the calibration procedure and in measurements using the single view approach may lessen some of the burden of an angiographic laboratory without sacrifying precision and information.

Introduction

Randomized trials using angiographic endpoints instead of clinical events have the obvious advantages of requiring less patients, of being less time-consuming, and thus less expensive [1]. During the last 10 years, many studies have used angiographic measurements to evaluate the effect of pharmacological or interventional treatments on prevention of restenosis after coronary angioplasty or to study the efficacy of drugs on progression or regression of coronary atherosclerosis. The objective of angiographic measurements is to detect and quantify even small changes in the severity and extent of coronary stenoses. Assessment of the degree of change is closely dependent upon the overall variability of the method and of the instruments used to measure them. Quantitative coronary angiography (QCA) has been used extensively for this purpose.

J.H.C. Reiber and E.E. van der Wall (eds.), What's New in Cardiovascular Imaging, 31–46.
©1998 Kluwer Academic Publishers.

In this chapter we will briefly review some general QCA guidelines which are well accepted [2-7] such as availability of a robust QCA system, technical quality of angiograms, control of image acquisition and standardization in the choice of frame to analyze. In addition, we will discuss in more details other previously advocated methodological requirements such as the use of multiple or orthogonal views versus a single most severe view approach, measurements with a precision micrometer of each catheter utilized during the procedure and filming of saline flushed instead of contrast filled catheters for calibration purposes.

We will compare these specific recommendations with the most recent experience from our laboratories (Leiden and Montreal) and indicate how these methodologies can be simplified in order to lessen the burden to the activities of an angiographic laboratory without sacrifying precision and information.

Availability of a robust QCA system

Before undertaking such angiographic studies, one must have access to a system of quantitative measurements which is robust and in which the algorithms of automatic detection has been validated both *in vitro* and *in vivo*, according to currently accepted standards [8-15]. The precision of a state-of-the-art QCA system should be in the order of 0.10-0.13 mm for comparison with plexiglass models of known dimensions. Determination of the precision of repeated measures for an *in vivo* study may vary from 0.10-0.15 mm for measurements on a single frame (inter-or intra-observer) to 0.20-0.30 mm for repeated measurements on different frames or different examinations (short, mid-or long-term variabilities) [11].

Angiograms of good quality

Secondly, accurate measurements are directly influenced by the quality of the basic material available. We need angiograms of high technical quality. High contrast and high resolution must be obtained from high quality image intensifiers, with minimal distortion, using small focal spot of the X-Ray tube, optimal collimation of the field of interest, and control of quantum mottle with proper kV and mAs [16,17].

Control of image acquisition

The baseline and follow-up angiograms must be obtained under relatively comparable and well controlled study conditions and according to prerequisite guidelines [2,3,5-7,18,19]. These guidelines usually include the following steps:

Vasodilation

Maximal coronary artery dilation is an universally accepted prerequisite for adequate standardization. It is best obtained by an intracoronary bolus injection of 0.1 to 0.3 mg of nitroglycerin. Peak effect is rapid (1 minute), predictive and with minimal systemic effect. Nitrates increase artery diameters by up to 30%, depending upon their basal status [20,21].

Sublingual and intravenous nitroglycerin can also be used, but their vasodilator responses are less predictive.

Use of contrast media

Ionic contrast agents induce a coronary vasodilation that may reach 20%. In comparison, nonionic substances cause little coronary vasodilation, not exceeding 6% [20] and therefore their use has been advocated to minimize this supplementary variation [2]. However, one must realize that vasodilation is usually adequate after routine intracoronary nitroglycerin [7,21]. Nevertheless, the same contrast medium should be used for baseline and follow-up studies in order to avoid this potential cause of variability.

Vessel opacification

Hand-delivered opacification of the coronary arteries must be optimal in all angiographic views, leading to adequate mixing of contrast material with blood. Inadequate cannulation of the coronary ostium or insufficient force of injection can result in streaming and low concentration of contrast material in the segments opacified, leading to underestimation and lower precision of diameter measurements [5,16,22].

Angiographic views

The coronary arteries must be visualized in multiple transverse and sagittal views, in order to clearly separate stenoses from branches, to minimize foreshortening and to obtain views as perpendicular as possible to the long axis of the segments to be analysed [2,3,23,24].

Catheter calibration

The distal 2-3 cm of the straight non tapered portion of the catheter should be clearly visible on each cinerun to provide a reliable scaling device.

Information collection

The detailed technical parameters should be collected on specific worksheets in order to replicate at follow-up the same protocol as was used at baseline. These include: nitroglycerin dosage, angulations and rotation of the gantry, contrast medium, type and size of each catheter used [2,4,6]. In the early days of QCA, the levels of table height and image intensifier position were also requested. However, their recording for each cinerun significantly adds to the complexity of the procedure and hardly improves reproducibility. Differences in table height and image intensifier are corrected for by the calibration procedure: if the degree of magnification changes, then the projected size of the catheter changes, and as a consequence so does the calibration factor expressed in mm/pixel.

Choice of frame

Preferably, as previously mentioned, a frame from a view perpendicular to the long axis of the vessel must be selected in order to avoid foreshortening and overlap of branches. Whenever possible, an end-diastolic frame is chosen, where kinetic flow due to cardiac motion is minimized and vessel filling by contrast material is optimal [3,5,23]. However, since minor differences are detected in variation coefficients between end-diastolic frames and those from other phases of the cardiac cycle (4.5% vs 6%) [3,25,26] it is probably preferable to select a frame with optimal opacification allowing accurate identification of vessel boundaries in a segment free of branch overlap, regardless of the cardiac cycle. Moreover, since only a small variability (5% to 6%) has been observed between measures made on different frames of a same diastole and even between different cardiac cycles of a same injection [19,27], it does not appear useful to average measurements from 3 to 5 adjacent frames as suggested [28]. This prolongs the procedure with only slight reduction of measurements variability [19]. Other factors such as changes in degree of foreshortening, vessels pulsatility, subtle out-of-plane magnification and changes in vessel location resulting in variations of pincushion distortion may contribute, albeit minorly, to the variability of angiographic measurements. Variability in lesion assessment is caused primarily by incomplete control of vasomotor tone, by different mixing of contrast material with blood and most importantly by the quantum mottle of the X-ray images. The sharpness of the structures to be analysed, namely the coronary vessel and the catheter, is directly influenced by the level of the quantum mottle.

Measurement in single plane versus orthogonal views

Some QCA laboratories strongly advocate measurements in multiple or orthogonal projections [29-34]; whereas others prefer using the most severe view approach [35-43]. In our laboratory (Montreal), measurements are made in the single plane projection showing the best opacified and preferably most severe stenosis. This view is usually obtained in the same projection at baseline and at follow-up. Although multiple projections are available almost routinely, a second view is not always suitable for quantitative analysis because of vessel foreshortening, branch overlap, stenosis at a bifurcation or on a proximal segment. Moreover, optimal measurements obtained in the best visualized view should not be compromised by measurements in a second view of suboptimal quality, thus less reliable [3,44].

Furthermore, measurements in two truly orthogonal views are possible in only 50% to 60% of cases according to some investigators [45,46] or even less often (30% to 40%) as reported by others [28,47]. Data from our MVP (Multi Vitamins and Probucol) Restenosis Trial show that only 144 of 373 segments (39%) were suitable for orthogonal view analyses. For the remaining 229 segments, the decision was made not to perform measurements in orthogonal projections because, in the second available view, the stenosis was either not as clearly profiled or the film was of suboptimal quality and could compromise the best view measurements [43].

A major argument for measuring stenoses in two orthogonal views is that approximately 50% to 60% of them are somewhat eccentric [48]. More recently, Mintz et al. [49] have demonstrated that the concordance rate of detecting eccentricity is only 54%, when comparing angiography with intravascular ultrasound. Therefore angiography may not be an adequate tool for assessing plaque distribution and eccentricity.

Moreover, markedly eccentric lesions may not be adequately detected, even by biplane orthogonal projections [18,50] which in fact usually represent an hybrid view located more or less between maximal and minimal stenosis severity [51]. It is only by chance and in fact infrequently that, amongst the three to four projections usually performed for a given artery, two projections fall in a plane showing the more and the less severe diameter stenosis. We have previously shown only a small difference of 0.11 ± 0.09 mm in the minimal luminal diameter before PTCA, comparing the worst versus the average of two views in 147 lesions [44]. After PTCA, the difference was only slightly greater (0.15 mm ± 0.12 mm). The two methods were within ± 0.2 mm for absolute minimum luminal diameter in 96% of the lesions and within ± 10% in stenosis severity for all but 2.7% of cases. These results were confirmed by two more recent analyses done in Montreal, the first involving a comparison of 183 segments and showing again small differences between the worst view and the average of orthogonal views, i.e. 0.08 ± 0.07 mm for pre-dilatation and 0.13 ± 0.11 mm for post-dilatation MLD. The second was our recent MVP Restenosis Trial [43], in which 144 segments were analyzable in two views. Mean differences between the worst versus two views were even smaller than in the two previous studies with standard deviations of the same small magnitude, i.e. 0.09 mm for pre and 0.14 mm for post-PTCA measurements (Table 1).

Table 1: Comparison of mean minimal lumen diameters using 1 versus an average of 2 angiographic views (N = 144 segments) based on the MVP restenosis trial [43]

	Worst view	*Average of 2 views*	*Difference*
Mean minimal lumen diameter (mm)			
Pre-PTCA	0.89 ± 0.28	0.92 ± 0.27	0.03 ± 0.09
Post-PTCA	1.84 ± 0.39	1.88 ± 0.40	0.04 ± 0.14
At follow-up	1.53 ± 0.62	1.55 ± 0.63	0.02 ± 0.10

Table 2: Comparison of continuous and categorical changes using 1 versus an average of 2 angiographic views (N = 144 segments) based on the MVP restenosis trial [43]

	1 view	*Average of 2 views*	*Difference*	*P value*
Acute gain (mm)	0.96 ± 0.40	0.96 ± 0.41	0.002 ± 0.14	0.85
Late loss (mm)	0.32 ± 0.53	0.33 ± 0.54	0.011 ± 0.15	0.37
RS[a] >50%	54/144 37.50%	53/144 36.81%		
RS >50% with a minimal Change of 15%	40/144 27.78%	40/144 27.78%		

a. RS = restenosis

The magnitude of acute gain and late loss are almost identical using either method of analysis. This is also true for categorical definitions of restenosis rates (RS) either with or without a minimal change of 15% (Table 2).

A different opinion was recently expressed [34] in a paper reviewing data from the Intact Study on progression and regression of coronary disease, and evaluating the influence of angiographic projections on the results obtained. The authors concluded that changes should be preferably averaged over all angiographic projections available, in order to avoid the overestimation of progression and/or regression that may occur when selecting only the projection with maximal changes (i.e. most severe). However, changes in vessel diameter that have become apparent in only one view may be obscured by the averaging effect of measurements in multiple views [52].

The relative irrelevance of performing measurements in multiple views is again illustrated by comparing data from two recent clinical trials evaluating the effect of lipid-lowering drugs (Statins) on progression and regression of coronary artery disease [33,39]. Using the same QCA system (CMS) [10], measurements were performed on all analyzable segments at baseline and at 2-year follow-up. In the REGRESS Study [33], the average values of all adequately visualized orthogonal projections were calculated for each segment; the average number of angiographic views available for QCA was only about 1.4. Conversely the CCAIT study [39] selected the frame with identical angulation at baseline and follow-up that best showed the most severe stenosis. The primary angiographic endpoint i.e. the coronary change score, defined as the per patient absolute mean of minimum lumen diameter changes at 2 years, is almost identical in the two trials; 0.09 and 0.10 mm, respectively in the placebo groups, and 0.05 and 0.06 mm in the active treatment groups. A similar range of changes was observed in the SCRIP Study [38] which also chose only the most severe best view.

In our laboratory, using the single most severe lesion approach, the methodology for selecting projections is as follows: as a first step, the baseline, post-intervention (if present) and follow-up angiograms are first visualized by simultaneous, side by side projections. The single plane projection showing the best opacified and usually most severe lesion with minimal foreshortening and branch overlap at baseline is selected. Next, we verify if this single best (and usually more severe) projection can be matched with identical post-procedure (if present) and follow-up projections. In rare instances, the selected projection can differ if, at follow-up, the stenosis is better shown, better opacified or obviously more severe in a view definitively different from the one chosen at baseline. In this situation, one may reverse the process of selection by first choosing the follow-up frame showing the most severe lesion and trying to match this view with similar projections post-intervention and, if possible, at baseline [35]. In doing so, the quality of this second set of projections should remain as good as for the first choice in order to avoid compromising the accuracy of measurements. If this second baseline (or post-procedure) view is of less than optimal quality or does not show the lesion at its best, we then choose a post-intervention and/or follow-up projection that is different from baseline. In practice, this occurs very rarely.

This methodology of using the single most severe lesion at each step may slightly overestimate the measured changes at angioplasty and at follow-up [34,52,53]. However data from the MVP restenosis trial (Table 2) suggest that this bias is minimal, (small differences in acute gain or late loss). In the worst view approach, comparison is not made between the most severe versus less severe view but rather between one view versus an average of two views which includes the worst one by definition. This tends to minimize differences.

In summary, no significant additional information is gained by the use of orthogonal measurements in clinical trials assessing efficacy of either mechanical or drug interventions on angiographic endpoints. Not performing averaged measurements represents a lesser burden on the activities of a angiographic laboratory, without loss in reliability.

Catheter calibration

To obtain absolute vessel dimensions, calibration of the selected cineframes is performed using the guiding or diagnostic catheters. This calibration procedure is thus of utmost importance and the type of catheter, its size and whether it is filled with contrast or saline, may significantly influence the accuracy of each measurement. In the past, it has been recommended [2,4,6,54] to avoid calibration with 5F and even 6F catheters, to measure the actual size of all catheters employed in clinical trials with a precision micrometer and to use flushed instead of contrast filled catheters as the scaling device to obtain a more precise measurement of their outer walls.

The current status of these recommendations is discussed below.

Type and size of catheters acceptable in QCA analyses

For an automated edge detection of the catheter shaft or tip to be reliable and reproducible, it is necessary for the image contrast of the catheter, as well as the sharpness of the edges of the displayed catheter, to be sufficiently high; this last characteristic is denoted the edge strength. The visibility and the edge strength are determined by the material composition of the catheter and the presence of radiographic contrast dye in the catheter lumen. It should be emphasized that it is not the carrier material (like, for example, nylon or polyurethane), but the type and concentration of the radiopaque filler compound in the wall of the catheter shaft/tip that determines the radio-detectability of a catheter. These filler compounds are mostly combinations of different barium- bismuth-, or tungsten-compounds, kept a secret by the catheter companies.

To visualize the differences between the qualities of catheters with respect to the suitability for automated edge detection purposes, Figure 1 illustrates the gray level cross-sectional profiles along a line perpendicular to the centerline of a poor quality catheter (only nylon, no filler compound, Fig 1A) as well as of a high quality catheter (polyurethane carrier and radiopaque filler compound, Fig 1B), both saline and contrast-filled, and assessed under the same circumstances. Figure 1B clearly demonstrates that the slopes of the profiles of the saline- and contrast-filled catheter are very similar for this high quality catheter; in other words, the contrast material has a minimal effect on the slopes and only produces a higher "mountain top" on this inverse mountain-like profile. The edges to be detected will be at the same positions, resulting in the same calibration factor for the two situations. On the other hand, the image contrast of the empty nylon catheter in Figure 1A is very low (only 10 gray levels on a scale of 256 levels), which makes this catheter very difficult to detect in *in vivo* images. Also, the slopes of the contrast-filled nylon catheter are different from the empty catheter, which will lead to different edge points and therefore in different calibration factors.

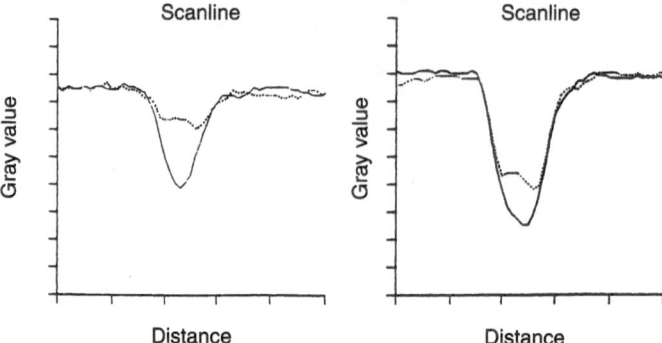

Figure 1. Cross-sectional density profiles taken perpendicular to the centerline of a poor quality catheter (Figure 1A) and of a high quality catheter (Figure 1B). In each figure the dotted profile represents the one for a saline-filled catheter, the continuous profile for a contrast-filled catheter.

Table 3: Current list of QCA-approved catheters

Catheters	cinefilm medium		digital medium	
	saline	100% contrast	saline	100% contrast
Cordis				
6F Infiniti™	√	√	√	√
6F Super Torque™	√	√	√	√
7F High Flow™	√	√	√	√
5F Infiniti™	√	√	√	√
5.2F Super Torque™	√	√	√	√
Goodtec				
6F Judkins	√	√	-	√
6F Amplatz	√	√	-	√
6F Multipurpose	√	√	-	√
5F Judkins	-	√	-	-
5F Amplatz	-	√	-	√
5F Multipurpose	-	√	-	-
5F Brachial	√	-	-	-
Mallinckrodt				
6F Softouch®	√	√	√	√
7F Softouch®	√	√	√	√

Over the last several years, we have tested several types of catheters for QCA purposes [55]. In these *in vitro* and *in vivo* acceptability studies, several requirements were set for a catheter to be acceptable. Among others, in the *in vitro* studies the absolute average difference in the angiographically measured mean diameters of the catheter with respect to the true value should be smaller than 5% under each of the individual circumstances and smaller than 3.5% as averaged over said conditions (which are: saline filling and 100% contrast medium filling, 5 and 7 inch image intensifier sizes, and 60, 75 and 90 kV-levels). Under these circumstances, the pooled standard deviation of the angiographically measured size of the catheter should be on the order of 0.1 mm or smaller. Based on these criteria, so far the following catheters were tested in our laboratory and accepted for QCA (Table 3); it should be noted that this is only a provisional list. Although some very small (5F) catheters were approved for QCA, in general, the smaller the catheter, the less pixels available for edge detection, which makes it less likely that the catheter will be approved. Based on these criteria and the data from Table 3, one can recommend to use catheters of sufficient size (6F or greater) and only those approved for QCA.

As the calibration procedure is the bottleneck in QCA, other approaches have been thought of. One such is the use of catheters or guidewires with radiopaque markers at regular distances. Instead of measuring the small diameters, one could then measure over larger length distances. In addition, the calibration object is in the vessel to be measured, so that also the out-of-plane error is absent. However, the foreshortening then becomes a limiting factor. We have recently tested the Cordis Stabilizer™ Marker Wire and concluded that relative errors are less than 7% for foreshortening angles < 20° [56]. If one can judge from the images under practical circumstances that the foreshortening is minimal, then this is an attractive alternative.

Measurement of catheter sizes by micrometer

Catheter size as specified by the manufacturer may vary from its true size. In some recent trials [4,29-31,33], a segment of the catheter was cut and sent with the cinefilm for more precise measurement of the outer diameter with a precision micrometer. This represents a significant effort in the activities of an angiographic core laboratory as well as for the participating clinical centers. In addition, these procedures can lead to errors in identifying the right catheters. To circumvent these problems, Reiber et al. [57] have measured with a micrometer more than 2000 catheters of various types and sizes from different manufacturers. Mean measured values were slightly smaller than their corresponding nominal French sizes. The variability of measurements was small (0.02-0.03 mm), representing an error of only 1% in average catheter size, showing that these catheters are manufactured very consistently. It was recommended that these mean measured values for various catheter types be used for calibration instead of using nominal French sizes, thus avoiding the need for repeated micrometer measurements.

It should be realized that this relatively cheap mechanical micrometer has one important drawback being that the catheter material is slightly compressed when measured, even when it is done very carefully. Also, catheters with thin walls are prone to a higher compressibility, and thus to an erroneous measurement. This effect can be assessed by comparison of the measured diameter of a catheter using a mechanical micrometer and a more expensive laser scan micrometer. The advantage of this last device is that there is no mechanical contact with the catheter. If the differences in measured diameters are large, then the catheter is too soft to

Table 4: Catheter sizes as measured with a precision mechanical micrometer and a laser scan micrometer

	True size (mm)	Measured size using a mechanical micrometer mean ± pooled s.d. (%diff)	Measured size using a laser scan micrometer mean ± pooled s.d. (%diff)
Cordis			
Super Torque JL4 5.2F	1.733	1.722 ± 0.003 (-0.6%)	1.734 ± 0.002 (0.1%)[a]
Super Torque JL4 6F	2.000	1.996 ± 0.002 (-0.2%)	2.007 ± 0.002 (0.3%)[a]
High Flow JL4 7F	2.333	2.226 ± 0.004 (-4.6%)	2.243 ± 0.001 (-3.9%)[a]
Infiniti JR4 4F	1.333	1.305 ± 0.003 (-2.1%)	1.321 ± 0.001 (-0.9%)[a]
Infiniti JL4 5F	1.667	1.620 ± 0.002 (-2.8%)	1.635 ± 0.002 (-1.9%)[a]
Infiniti JL4 6F	2.000	1.949 ± 0.003 (-2.5%)	1.964 ± 0.001 (-1.8%)[a]
Guiding catheter 8F	2.667	2.638 ± 0.007 (-1.1%)	2.650 ± 0.002 (-0.6%)[a]
Medtronic			
Cascade JL4 6F	2.000	1.956 ± 0.002 (-2.2%)	1.961 ± 0.006 (-1.9%)
Cascade JR4 6F	2.000	1.965 ± 0.002 (-1.8%)	1.965 ± 0.004 (-1.7%)
Cascade High Flow JL4 6F	2.000	1.970 ± 0.002 (-1.5%)	1.986 ± 0.004 (-0.7%)
Schneider			
Visiguide L4 8F	2.666	2.529 ± 0.018 (-5.2%)	2.785 ± 0.013 (4.4%)[a]

a. Measurements performed with a mechanical micrometer and laser scan micrometer were statistically significantly different (p << 0.05)

be measured by the mechanical micrometer. The results of a limited number of catheter measurements are presented in Table 4. From this table it can be observed that the laser measured diameters are in all cases larger than mechanically measured diameters, as expected. For the Cordis catheters these differences were only 0.015 mm (about 0.5%), although statistically significant. For the Medtronic Cascade catheters the differences are even smaller, showing that both these catheter product lines are hardly compressable by the mechanical device. However, the difference between the mechanical and laser measurements for the Schneider Visiguide catheters is about 0.25 mm, which makes this catheter unsuitable for mechanical measurements.

One can conclude from these results, that we should be aware of possible measurement errors with the mechanical device, which are absent with the more expensive laser scan micrometer.

Flushed versus contrast filled catheters for calibration

A few years ago, the use of empty (flushed) instead of contrast filled catheters was advocated as the scaling device in an attempt to measure more exactly the outer diameter of catheters and not only the column of contrast material inside the catheters [4,58]. This was supported by theoretical considerations in the sense that the edge detection algorithm should find the outermost edges of the gray level profiles as illustrated in Figure 1.

Depending on the quality and robustness of the edge detection technique used, as well as of the angiographic quality of the catheter, the detected edges may significantly be influenced and attracted by the contrast material in the catheter, leading to too narrow contours. The measurements of contrast filled catheters would then yield smaller pixel values and the derived calibration factors in mm/pixel would thus be larger than expected. According to data from the Rotterdam group [58,59], measurements were overestimated by an average of 8.5% to 9.1%. Thus, they strongly recommended the use of flushed catheters for calibration.

Fortin et al. [60] have also shown that radiographic diameters of catheters vary widely according to different composition and attenuation factor of their walls and may differ up to 27% if compared to micrometer measurements. More recently, Finet et al. [17] observed the same phenomenon and noted larger errors when the true diameters of the Medis phantoms were calibrated with the catheter filled with contrast agent. The average filled calibration factor was 0.247 mm/pixel and the average empty calibration factor was 0.211 mm/pixel, representing a significant difference of 17%. This higher calibration factor will cause overestimation of all subsequent measurements.

Discordant data were, however, presented by Herman et al. [61]. A total of 32 guiding catheters of different types and sizes were either filled with water or contrast media and were measured using a one centimeter grid as a calibration device. These measurements were compared to true values obtained by a precision micrometer. In contrast to a previous study from the same group [6] using the same methodology of analysis, they found that contrast filled catheters underestimate true size only very slightly by -0.8% as compared to an overestimation of +4.4% for flushed catheters. In this preliminary paper, they suggest that contrast filled catheters should be favored as a scaling device. They also recognize that new materials for guiding catheters do have sufficient radiopacity.

An easier approach to this problem is to optimize the edge detection algorithm such as to ensure a more appropriate detection of the outer diameter of a contrast filled catheter [10,62,63]. Using the CMS analysis package, Reiber et al. [55] have shown minimal differences between contrast filled and contrast empty catheters for Cordis 6F Super Torque and Cordis 7F High Flow catheters as compared with true size measurements (accuracy of -1.6% for 100% contrast vs +0.1% for saline 6F tip). The same group also analysed the tips of 6F and 7F Mallinckrodt catheters, and found that the average deviation of measured vs true size was low, varying from -0.4% to 2.1% on cinefilm images. Koning et al. [62] concluded that the content of catheters (either 100% contrast material or saline) did not have a significant effect on their measurement accuracy.

Table 5: Comparison of calibration factor and diameter stenosis measurements for contrast-filled versus contrast-empty 7F diagnostic (N = 16) and 8F guiding (N = 15) Cordis catheters

	Contrast-filled catheter	Contrast-empty catheter	Difference filled-empty	Deviation in % vs empty
Calibration factor (mm/pixel)	0.093 ± 0.004	0.088 ± 0.005	0.005 ± 0.003	+5.7%
Obstruction diameter (mm)	1.44 ± 0.54	1.36 ± 0.54	0.08 ± 0.34	+0.057
Reference diameter (mm)	3.09 ± 0.67	2.93 ± 0.62	0.15 ± 0.40	+5.2%
% stenosis	51.86 ± 19.06	52.37 ± 18.98	0.51 ± 12.03	-0.97%

Their results are also consistent with data obtained in Montreal. In a total of 128 *in vivo* measurements on contrast empty or filled 8F guiding catheters (120 Schneider, 8 Medtronic) the mean difference for calibration factor was 0.0008 ± 0.004 mm/pixel [55]. This represents a difference of only 0.87%, that can be explained by the good radiopacity of the walls of Schneider catheters.

We recently measured 31 Cordis catheters (15 guiding 8F and 16 diagnostic 7F) from current cineangiograms and showed that the calibration factor of contrast filled catheters was indeed slightly overestimated by +5.7% as compared to saline filled catheters, the difference being only 0.005 ± 0.003 mm/pixel. The measurements done on the same stenosis (same frame) obtained from these two calibrations factors showed a difference of 0.078 mm for the MLD measures, which is less than the variability of intra-observer repeated analysis (Table 5).

Filming flushed catheters offers the advantage of recording the calibration catheter routinely in the center field of the amplifier. This technique reduces measurement variability resulting from pincushion distortion [13,17], although this is less of an issue with modern image intensifiers [7]. However, this extra filming increases somewhat the length of fluoroscopy and cineruns. It adds an extra burden (but not necessarily negative) to an already complex procedure and offers benefits which are not readily evident when applied to *in vivo* studies. Moreover, this approach is applicable only to prospectively designed studies, such as restenosis trials. In most progression-regression studies, routinely acquired (catheter filled) angiograms must be relied upon for baseline measurements. As a consequence, only contrast filled catheter images should also be used in follow-up studies. There is also much more pressure from clinical centers to use 6F catheters for follow-up studies. The 6F flushed catheters are, however, sometimes more difficult to properly measure as compared to a contrast filled 6F, particularly if the cineangiograms are of suboptimal quality. Another issue with the measurement of flushed catheters, is that the straight line approach between the beginning and end points in the catheter must be used for the definition of the catheter segment. The automated pathline trace will not work in the absence of maximal gray values in the center of the catheter as seen in flushed catheters.

In conclusion, because of some controversial data in the variability of measurements between flushed or contrast filled catheters and because of the possibility of large differences in radiopacity of catheters, it appears to us that the most practical and simplest way to circumvent the possible problems in variation of calibration factors, is to use the same type of catheter material made by the same manufacturer at baseline and at follow-up, using as preference contrast filled catheters for easiest contour detection. As previously stated for the methodology of one versus two views, we must remember that the primary objective of QCA measurements in clinical trials is to allow more precise and reliable analyses of the real changes after interventions namely acute lumen gain and late lumen loss, expressed in millimeters. This is best achieved if exactly the same setting is applied during the procedure and at the follow-up studies: i.e. replication of same views, same doses of intracoronary nitroglycerin, same contrast media, same catheter type or material, and, if feasible, same catheterization room.

References

1. Waters D, Lespérance J, Craven TE, Hudon G, Gillam LD. Advantages and limitations of serial coronary arteriography for the assessment of progression and regression of coronary atherosclerosis. Implications for clinical trials. Circulation 1993;87(3 suppl):II38-47.
2. Reiber JHC, den Boer A, Serruys PW. Quality control in performing quantitative coronary arteriography. Am J Card Imaging 1989;3:172-9.
3. Herrington DM, Walford GD. Optimal frame selection for QCA. In: Reiber JHC, Serruys PW, editors. Advances in quantitative coronary arteriography. Dordrecht: Kluwer Academic Publishers; 1993. p. 125-35.
4. Hermans WRM, Rensing BJ, Pameyer J, Serruys PW. Experience of a quantitative coronary angiographic core laboratory in restenosis prevention trials. In: Reiber JHC, Serruys PW, editors. Advances in quantitative coronary arteriography. Dordrecht: Kluwer Academic Publishers: 1993. p. 177-92.
5. Lespérance J, Bourassa MG, Schwartz L *et al.* Definition and measurement of restenosis after successful coronary angioplasty: implications for clinical trials. Am Heart J 1993;125:1394-408.
6. Umans VAWM, Hermans WRM, Herrman JPR, Pameyer J, Serruys PW. Experiences of a quantitative coronary angiographic core laboratory in restenosis prevention trials. In: Serruys PW, Foley DP, de Feyter PJ, editors. Quantitative coronary angiography in clinical practice. Dordrecht: Kluwer Academic Publishers; 1994. p. 121-35.
7. Reiber JHC, Jukema JW, Koning G, Bruschke AVG. Quality control in quantitative coronary arteriography. In: Bruschke AVG, Reiber JHC, Lie KI, Wellens HJ, editors. Lipid-lowering therapy and progression of coronary atherosclerosis. Dordrecht: Kluwer Academic Publishers; 1996. p. 45-63.
8. Lespérance J, Waters D. Measuring progression and regression of coronary atherosclerosis in clinical trials: problems and progress. Int J Card Imaging 1992;8:165-73.
9. Haase J, Di Mario C, Slager CJ *et al.* In-vivo validation of on-line and off-line geometric coronary measurements using insertion of stenosis phantoms in porcine coronary arteries. Cathet Cardiovasc Diagn 1992;27:16-27.
10. Reiber JHC, van der Zwet PMJ, Von Land CD *et al.* Quantitative coronary arteriography: equipment and technical requirements. In: Reiber JHC, Serruys PW, editors. Advances in quantitative coronary arteriography. Dordrecht: Kluwer Academic Publishers;, 1993. p. 75-111.
11. Reiber JHC, Koning G, Von Land CD, van der Zwet PMJ. Why and how should QCA systems be validated? In: Reiber JHC, Serruys PW, editors. Progress in quantitative coronary arteriography. Dordrecht: Kluwer Academic Publishers; 1994. p. 33-48.
12. Beauman GJ, Reiber JHC, Koning G, Van Houdt RCM, Vogel RA. Angiographic core laboratory analyses of arterial phantom images: comparative evaluations of accuracy and precision. In: Reiber JHC, Serruys PW, editors. Progress in quantitative coronary arteriography. Dordrecht: Kluwer Academic Publishers; 1994. p. 87-104.
13. Ribichini F, Steffenino G, Dellavalle A *et al.* On-line quantitative coronary analysis in clinical practice: one step closer to reality? Cathet Cardiovasc Diagn 1994;31:102-9.

14.   Keane D, Haase J, Slager CJ *et al.* Comparative validation of quantitative coronary angiography systems. Results and implications from a multicenter study using a standardized approach. Circulation 1995;91:2174-83.

15.   Bell MR, Britson PJ, Chu A, Holmes DR Jr, Bresnahan JF, Schwartz RS. Validation of a new UNIX-based quantitative coronary angiographic system for the measurement of coronary artery lesions. Cathet Cardiovasc Diagn 1997;40:66-74.

16.   Herrington DM, Siebes M, Walford GD. Sources of error in quantitative coronary angiography. Cathet Cardiovasc Diagn 1993;29:314-21.

17.   Finet G, Liénard J. Parameters that influence accuracy and precision of quantitative coronary arteriography. Int J Card Imaging 1996;12:271-87.

18.   Hermiller JB, Cusma JT, Spero LA, Fortin DF, Harding MB, Bashore TM. Quantitative and qualitative coronary angiographic analysis: review of methods, utility, and limitations. Cathet Cardiovasc Diagn 1992;25:110-31.

19.   Herrington DM, Siebes M, Sokol DK, Siu CO, Walford GD. Variability in measures of coronary lumen dimensions using quantitative coronary angiography. J Am Coll Cardiol 1993;22:1068-74.

20.   Jost S, Rafflenbeul W, Reil GH *et al.* Elimination of variable vasomotor tone in studies with repeated quantitative coronary angiography. Int J Card Imaging 1990;5:125-34.

21.   Jost S, Sturm M, Hausmann D, Lippolt P, Lichtlen PR. Standardization of coronary vasomotor tone with intracoronary nitroglycerin. Am J Cardiol 1996;78:120-3.

22.   Reiber JHC, van Eldik-Helleman P, Visser-Akkerman N, Kooijman CJ, Serruys PW. Variabilities in measurement of coronary arterial dimensions resulting from variations in cineframe selection. Cathet Cardiovasc Diagn 1988;14:221-8.

23.   Finet G, Masquet C, Eifferman A *et al.* Can we optimize our angiographic views every time? Qualitative and quantitative evaluation of a new functionality. Invest Radiol 1996;31:523-31.

24.   Dodge T, Sparano AM, Ryan K *et al.* Best angiographic views to minimize coronary artery foreshortening [abstract]. Circulation 1997;96(supp 1):I78.

25.   Selzer RH, Hagerty C, Azen SP *et al.* Precision and reproducibility of quantitative coronary angiography with applications to controlled clinical trials. A sampling study. J Clin Invest 1989;83:520-6.

26.   Beauman GJ, Reiber JHC, Koning G, Vogel RA. Comparisons of angiographic core laboratory analyses of phantom and clinical images: interlaboratory variability. Cathet Cardiovasc Diagn 1996;37:24-31.

27.   Reiber JHC, van Eldik-Helleman P, Kooijman CJ, Tijssen JGP, Serruys PW. How critical is frame selection in quantitative coronary angiographic studies? Eur Heart J 1989;10(suppl F):54-9.

28.   Gibson CM, Sandor T, Stone PH, Pasternak RC, Rosner B, Sacks FM. Quantitative angiographic and statistical methods to assess serial changes in coronary luminal diameter and implications for atherosclerosis regression trials. Am J Cardiol 1992;69:1286-90.

29.   Serruys PW, Rutsch W, Heyndrickx GR *et al.* Prevention of restenosis after percutaneous transluminal coronary angioplasty with thromboxane A_2-receptor blockade. A randomized, double-blind, placebo-controlled trial. Coronary Artery Restenosis Prevention on Repeated Thromboxane-Antagonism Study (CARPORT). Circulation 1991;84:1568-80.

30.   Does the new angiotensin converting enzyme inhibitor cilazapril prevent restenosis after percutaneous transluminal coronary angioplasty? Results of the MERCATOR study: a multicenter, randomized, double-blind placebo-controlled trial. The Multicenter European Research Trial with Cilazapril after Angioplasty to Prevent Transluminal Coronary Obstruction and Restenosis (MERCATOR) Study Group. Circulation 1992;86:100-10.

31.   Serruys PW, de Jaegere P, Kiemeneij F *et al.* A comparison of balloon- expandable-stent implantation with balloon angioplasty in patients with coronary artery disease. Benestent Study Group. N Engl J Med 1994;331:489-95.

32.   Fischman DL, Leon MB, Baim DS *et al.* A randomized comparison of coronary- stent placement and balloon angioplasty in the treatment of coronary artery disease. Stent Restenosis Study Investigators. N Engl J Med 1994;331:496-501.

33.   Jukema JW, Bruschke AVG, Van Boven AJ *et al.* Effects of lipid lowering by pravastatin on progression and regression of coronary artery disease in symptomatic men with normal to moderately elevated serum cholesterol levels. The Regression Growth Evaluation Statin Study (REGRESS). Circulation 1995;91:2528-40.

34.   Jost S, Deckers J, Nikutta P *et al.* Influence of the selection of angiographic projections on the results of coronary angiographic follow-up trials. International Nifedipine Trial on Antiatherosclerotic Therapy Investigators. Am Heart J 1995;130:433-9.

35. Gordon PC, Gibson CM, Cohen DJ, Carrozza JP, Kuntz RE, Baim DS. Mechanisms of restenosis and redilation within coronary stents—quantitative angiographic assessment. J Am Coll Cardiol 1993;21:1166-74.
36. Kastrati A, Schömig A, Dietz R, Neumann FJ, Richardt G. Time course of restenosis during the first year after emergency coronary stenting. Circulation 1993;87:1498-505.
37. De Jaegere P, Serruys PW, Van Es GA *et al.* Recoil following Wiktor stent implantation for restenotic lesions of coronary arteries. Cathet Cardiovasc Diagn 1994;32:147-56.
38. Haskell WL, Alderman EL, Fair JM *et al.* Effects of intensive multiple risk factor reduction on coronary atherosclerosis and clinical cardiac events in men and women with coronary artery disease. The Stanford Coronary Risk Intervention Project (SCRIP). Circulation 1994;89:975-90.
39. Waters D, Higginson L, Gladstone P *et al.* Effects of monotherapy with an HMG- CoA reductase inhibitor on the progression of coronary atherosclerosis as assessed by serial quantitative arteriography. The Canadian Coronary Atherosclerosis Intervention Trial. Circulation 1994;89:959-68.
40. Sirnes PA, Golf S, Myreng Y *et al.* Stenting in Chronic Coronary Occlusion (SICCO): a randomized, controlled trial of adding stent implantation after successful angioplasty. J Am Coll Cardiol 1996;28:1444-51.
41. Mudra H, Regar E, Klauss V *et al.* Serial follow-up after optimized ultrasound- guided deployment of Palmaz-Schatz stents. In-stent neointimal proliferation without significant reference segment response. Circulation 1997;95:363-70.
42. Sharaf BL, Williams DO, Miele NJ *et al.* A detailed angiographic analysis of patients with ambulatory electrocardiographic ischemia: results from the Asymptomatic Cardiac Ischemia Pilot (ACIP) study angiographic core laboratory. J Am Coll Cardiol 1997;29:78-84.
43. Tardif JC, Côté G, Lespérance J *et al.* Probucol and multivitamins in the prevention of restenosis after coronary angioplasty. Multivitamins and Probucol Study Group. N Engl J Med 1997;337:365-72.
44. Lespérance J, Hudon G, White CW, Laurier J, Waters D. Comparison by quantitative angiographic assessment of coronary stenoses of one view showing the severest narrowing to two orthogonal views. Am J Cardiol 1989;64:462-5.
45. Dehmer GJ, Popma JJ, Van der Berg EK *et al.* Reduction in the rate of early restenosis after coronary angioplasty by a diet supplemented with n-3 fatty acids. N Engl J Med 1988;319:733-40.
46. Loaldi A, Polese A, Montorsi P *et al.* Comparison of nifedipine, propranolol and isosorbide dinitrate on angiographic progression and regression of coronary arterial narrowings in angina pectoris. Am J Cardiol 1989;64:433-9.
47. Brown BG, Bolson E, Dodge HT. Quantitative computer techniques for analyzing coronary arteriograms. Prog Cardiovasc Dis 1986;28:403-18.
48. Marcus ML, Harrison DG, White CW, McPherson DD, Wilson RF, Kerber RE. Assessing the physiologic significance of coronary obstructions in patients: importance of diffuse undetected atherosclerosis. Prog Cardiovasc Dis 1988;31:39-56.
49. Mintz GS, Popma JJ, Pichard AD *et al.* Limitations of angiography in the assessment of plaque distribution in coronary artery disease: a systematic study of target lesion eccentricity in 1446 lesions. Circulation 1996;93:924-31.
50. Spears JR, Sandor T, Als AV *et al.* Computerized image analysis for quantitative measurement of vessel diameter from cineangiograms. Circulation 1983;68:453-61.
51. Rosenberg MC, Klein LW, Agarwal JB, Stets G, Hermann GA, Helfant RH. Quantification of absolute luminal diameter by computer-analyzed digital subtraction angiography: an assessment in human coronary arteries. Circulation 1988;77:484-90.
52. Beatt KJ, Huchns TY, Zhang XF. Flawed methodology in assessment of restenosis? The relevance of multiple views and late loss index [abstract]. In: 5th International Symposium on Coronary Arteriography. Rotterdam, June 1993; p. 132.
53. Lincoff AM, Keeler GP, Berdan LG, Debowey D, Topol EJ. "Worst view" angiographic analysis in CAVEAT provided a "Worst Case" scenario of restenosis rates and vessel luminal diameters [abstract]. Circulation 1994;90(4 Part 2):I60.
54. Reiber JHC, Kooijman CJ, Den Boer A, Serruys PW. Assessment of dimensions and image quality of coronary contrast catheters from cineangiograms. Cathet Cardiovasc Diagn 1985;11:521-31.
55. Reiber JHC, Von Land CD, Koning G *et al.* Comparison of accuracy and precision of quantitative coronary arterial analysis between cinefilm and digital systems. In: Reiber JHC, Serruys PW, editors. Progress in quantitative coronary arteriography. Dordrecht: Kluwer Academic Publishers; 1994. p. 67-85.
56. Koning G, Kemppainen JS, Rothman MT, Reiber JHC. Suitability of the stabilizer™ marker wire for QCA calibration; in vitro study. Eur Heart J 1997;18(Abstr Suppl):391.

57.   Reiber JHC, Jukema W, Van Boven A, Van Houdt RM, Lie KI, Bruschke AVG. Catheter sizes for quantita-
       tive coronary arteriography. Cathet Cardiovasc Diagn 1994;33:153-55.

58.   Di Mario C, Hermans WRM, Rensing BJ, Serruys PW. Calibration using angiographic catheters as scaling
       devices - importance of filming the catheters not filled with contrast medium. Am J Cardiol 1992;69:1377-
       8.

59.   Herrman JR, Keane D, Ozaki Y, Den Boer A, Serruys PW. Radiological quality of coronary guiding cathe-
       ters: a quantitative analysis. Cathet Cardiovasc Diagn 1994;33:55-60.

60.   Fortin DF, Spero LA, Cusma JT, Santoro L, Burgess R, Bashore TM. Pitfalls in the determination of abso-
       lute dimensions using angiographic catheters as calibration devices in quantitative angiography. Am J Car-
       diol 1991;68:1176-82.

61.   Herrman JPR, Haase J, Den Boer A, Ligthart JMR, Amo D, Serruys PM. Assessment of radiographic qual-
       ity of coronary guiding catheters [abstract]. In: 5th International Symposium on Coronary Arteriography.
       Rotterdam, June 1993; p. 192.

62.   Koning G, van der Zwet PMJ, Von Land CD, Reiber JHC. Angiographic assessment of dimensions of 6F
       and 7F Mallinckrodt Softouch[R] coronary contrast catheters from digital and cine arteriograms. Int J Card
       Imaging 1992;8:153-61.

63.   Legrand V, Raskinet B, Martinez C, Kulbertus H. Variability in estimation of coronary dimensions from 6F
       and 8F catheters. Cathet Cardiovasc Diagn 1996;37:39-45.

3. The cost-effectiveness
of QCA in interventional cardiology

Christoph A. Nienaber, Klaus-Peter Schaps & Georg Stiel

Summary

In conjunction with interventional cardiovascular procedures, eye balling, especially when executed by the coronary angiographer, tends to infer self referral bias due to overestimation of stenosis severity in lesions of 40-60% diameter reduction in the attempt to justify angioplasty.

This inherent conflict which results in a bimodal distribution of stenosis diameter by eye balling instead of a gaussian distribution by quantitative coronary angiography has always been a strong argument to use QCA for selecting patients for interventional procedures. QCA is able to objectively differentiate stenosis of ≤ 50% diameter reduction from higher grade stenosis and is independent of individual bias, thus avoiding unnecessary procedures unlikely to have a meaningful impact on patient symptoms and outcome. This current study showed that QCA is able to more objectively select patients for angioplasty procedures and also to limit the use of expensive supplies such as balloons and even stents to a minimum which may be a reduction of up to 50% costs for medical supply, not even considering the amount of money saved by the process of better patient selection. In an idealized model calculation we could prove that savings of more than 50% and a substantial net reimbursement benefit for the health care provider may be achieved in a capitation model as long as on-line intraprocedural QCA is used to select the most appropriate angioplasty material (and balloon size) and thus limit the number of balloons per stenosis to one.

On the basis of price tags from 1996 to 1997, a critical volume of about 138 QCA-supported PTCA procedures are required to reach the break-even point of invested hardware for QCA and maximum savings derived from QCA-supported angioplasty. Thus, in busy catheterization labs with a considerable volume of PTCAs above 500, it is clear that substantial savings up to a multiple factor of the invested costs may be realized with optimized use of on-line QCA to select patients as well as balloon and stent equipment to achieve an optimal angioplasty result. It appears undoubtful that QCA may not only improve the quality of an interventional procedure but also the benefit for both the individual patient and the socio-economic system, especially the health care provider.

Introduction

Since the first publications on quantitative coronary arteriography (QCA), interest in this technique has grown substantially [1,2]. Two major clinical developments have stimulated

J.H.C. Reiber and E.E. van der Wall (eds.), What's New in Cardiovascular Imaging, 47–60.
©1998 Kluwer Academic Publishers.

this interest over the last 15 years. First, the clinical applications of interventional coronary revascularization techniques such as PTCA, atherectomy, thrombolysis, stent placement, and laser application, and second, the growing impact of chronic treatment strategies with new drugs directed at regression or no-growth of existing coronary artery disease, or the delay in the formation of new lesions [3-7]. Moreover, QCA has been shown to allow an objective evaluation of coronary lesions forming the base for a better treatment of coronary heart disease with interventional recanalization techniques [6,11]. Few data, however, are available with respect to both the impact of QCA on cost development, the appropriate use of expensive catheters for coronary interventions. Conceptually, QCA enables the operator to size the optimal balloon or stent diameter and length for a particular interventional proce-dure and to assess the success of the procedure in an operator independent manner rather than by eye balling [8-10]. It has also been demonstrated that residual stenoses < 20% mea-sured objectively after the procedure, lead to a lower event rate after 6 months [12]. Quanti-tative evaluation of angiograms is facilitated by the ongoing improvements in computer hardware (roughly a 100% increase in performance every 2 years) and software, by the opti-mization and invention of better suited algorithms for the analysis of coronary lesions, and the development of the better/faster user interfaces, so that results become available almost on-line, thereby minimizing any delay during an angiographic procedure. On the other hand, on-line applications significantly increase the demands on the QCA analytical soft-ware packages in terms of robustness, accuracy and precision, and the capability to follow even an irregular vessel morphology. Only if such demands are met in the near future, such packages are likely to be used as an inherent adjunct to a professional interventional proce-dure. Considering the high costs of the interventional devices, on-line QCA applications may stimulate widespread use as health insurance companies begin to focus their interest on cost-benefit aspects of interventional procedures.

Subjects to this scrutiny will be individual patients undergoing diagnostic catheterization to evaluate the possibility of significant stenosis or restenosis [3-6] and subsequent referral for angioplasty [3, 13-15].

Clinical scenario and emerging problem

There is no doubt, that newly developed digital imaging systems offer both on-line review of acquired angiograms and on-site assessment of stenosis morphology and thus invite to rou-tinely perform angioplasty as an extension of diagnostic angiography for many good reasons such as physical and psychological inconvenience to the patient, minimizing exposure to radiation and contrast media, and reduction of total direct and indirect costs [6].However, at stake is the objective decision-making for or against coronary angioplasty free of "self-refer-ral" bias [16,17] and based on precise assessment of angiographic findings. Conversely, visual interpretation"eye balling" = EB) of coronary angiograms and estimates of percent stenosis and vessel diameter, parameters on which most therapeutic decisions are often based, are known to be imprecise and poorly reproducible [10,12,18]. The American Col-lege of Cardiology/American Heart Association Task Force defined a (hemodynamically) sig-nificant stenosis as "one that results in a 50% reduction in coronary diameter as determined by caliper method" [15]. Accordingly, a borderline stenotic lesion (usually < 60% diameter stenosis) should not be dilated because of a demonstrated risk of accelerated restenosis with even greater severity [8].

Eye balling versus QCA

There is a growing body of evidence that demonstrates both, the risk of a consistent overestimation of stenosis severity with "eye balling", and therefore a bias for "self-referral" (even by experienced angiographers) to justify coronary angioplasty even of objectively moderate lesions. In addition, there is also evidence that QCA-supported decisions to guide interventional decisions have cost saving potential whose extent, however, is unknown. For this purpose an idealized projection of potential cost savings by better selection of patients and improved choice of PTCA-balloons is demonstrated.

Methods

We studied 62 consecutive patients (49 men and 13 women at age 62 ± 10 years), undergoing diagnostic coronary angiography. All patients met the criteria for coronary angiography according to the guidelines of the American College of Cardiology/American Heart Association Task Force [15], and were eligible for a variety of angioplasty procedures. Four attending experienced cardiologists were chosen to perform both, elective coronary angiography and coronary angioplasty, if considered necessary based on visual analysis of coronary angiograms. Immediately after coronary angiography each angiographer was requested to estimate on-site and from the acquired digital coronary angiogram, whether a hemodynamically significant or nonsignificant atherosclerotic lesion was present, and to assess visually (by "eye balling") the percent diameter stenosis (nearest 5%) and the diameter of the normal reference segment for the choice of the PTCA balloon (in 0.5 mm steps). Visual estimates were based on visual "catheter tip calibration". When performing visual "measurements" the operators were unaware of any objective computerized quantitative measurements.

Simultaneously, digital quantitative coronary angiography (DQCA) was carried out on-line, but off-site in a central core laboratory using an automated edge detection technique and a digital angiographic workstation (AWOS™ VA41A, Siemens Erlangen, Germany). Analyses were performed independently by an experienced operator not involved with patient care and unaware of any clinical characteristics of patients. The method was previously validated in a study on 104 vessel models (0.1 - 5.0 mm). Digital quantitative measurements from digital coronary images on AWOS have previously shown both, to reliably assess vessel diameters of dimensions as small as 0.4 mm, and to reproducibly quantify coronary artery stenosis from 5% to 90% diameter reduction ($y = 0.99x - 0.24$; $r = 0.99$; $p < 0.0001$) [19-21].

AWOS® system

The angiographic workstation (AWOS®) is an extended analysis system to realize on-site both the on-line and post-processing digital quantitative coronary angiography (DQCA) in a patient defined digital angiography environment [19, 21]. AWOS® can be connected via high speed link to HICOR® IS and via ETHERNET to POLYTRON® 1000 digital cardiac imaging system. It offers the possibility to display and to process digital angiograms direct from HICOR® IS or POLYTRON® 1000 or 35 mm cine images digitized by a framegrabber from an ARRIPRO®-35 cineprojector with television camera. AWOS® is operated by a (menu-in) windows technique. Analytic results are displayed on the SIMOMED® HD monitor; a standardized VHS/S-VHS (CCIR- or US-RS 170-Standards) and hardcopy printouts are also available. At present an individual digital archive for each patient is based on 525 MB streamer tape.

Hardware overview

AWOS® is based on the SMI®-5 image processor architecture. "Backbone" of this concept is a fast MULTIMUX bus capable of dealing with the transfer rates which occur with image and scene handling. On this bus reside task specific modules (boards). For AWOS® these boards are the SIAM, the IMAGER, the LISA and the D2. SIAM has double functionality. On one hand it carries the so-called host computer as the front-end to the programmer. On the other hand it also contains the coupling to the SMI®-S image processor and 8MB of dedicated image RAM, the P4 memory. This is the 8 or 16 bits deep working storage for image processing programs. Via SIAM all the other modules are addressed. IMAGER realizes both a sort of display buffer for gray scale image and for overlaying graphics with 8 independent graphics planes and the A/D-conversion and the monitor control. Image to be display actually is effected by a transfer from other image RAM into the IMAGER. Gray-scale-windowing is done by means of the input lookup table of the IMAGER. D2 is a scene memory as an image RAM of 128 Mbytes on one board. LISA is a board for image zooming by pixel interpolation in real-time. In the SIAM module a 32 Bit computer SUN SPARC ENGINE II has been integrated with 16 Mbytes of RAM.

Software overview

The software platform is SUN OS 4.1.2. is a version of Berkeley's UNIX (BSD 4.2). The corresponding C® compiler is recommended as implementation language, although, for compatibility with past developments, the SUN FORTRAN 77-compiler is supplied as well. The window surface is XView, contained in the Open Windows 2.0 release. It includes the screen editor, file manager, multiple command tools and many other utilities. Apart from TCP/IP, DECNET is also available as an ETHERNET "dialect" in the DNI-package.

The AWOS® workspace is shared by two areas. The large square area is the image area. It displays both the images and additional operating elements of the functions selected and messages. Images are displayed in squares. The white frame is the active square. When square one is active the next image or scene is loaded into square 2. The control is subdivided into several blocks: an actual block for display of actual patient data, a dynamic block to start and operation of the evaluation packages, a result block to display of already available evaluation results, a display block with monitor split mode, a postprocessing block with functions for image selection and image display and a message field. The following display modes are available: 1024-matrix or zoom 512-matrix and zoom 512-matrix to 1024-matrix. Zoom of the displayed image allows by pixel interpolation.

Image evaluation packages

There is a choice of the following analysis packages for single plane or biplane evaluation: geometric and densitometric ventricle evaluation, stenosis and crossline stenosis evaluation, time-density curves or myocardial flow ratio, geometric evaluation like distances, angles and calculation of average values and statistical evaluation of single frames like average, minimal and maximal gray value and number of pixels in a region of interest [21-24]. Catheter and distance calibration as manual input of calibration factor have been implemented as well.

Calculation of costs and savings

The traditional economic view of costs is that it represents the consumption of financial resources (used for medical, labor supplies and equipment expenses) that could have been used for another purpose. Society consumes resources to satisfy its wishes and needs (in this regard related to health care, especially cardiovascular health care). Resources are usually sub-divided into a large generic category such as labor, supplies, equipment and facilities. These resources can be combined to the use of technology to produce desired goods and services, especially relevant in the expensive section of cardiovascular medicine. However, it is difficult to summarize all the individual inputs to a particular health care service (such as for instance coronary angioplasty), in order to compare those alternative expenditures, each with their own unique list of resource inputs. However, based on relatively simple and major factors that contribute to the total expenditure calculated or individual angioplasty procedure, we used the major components of total procedural costs such as balloon costs, labor costs, cumulated supplies costs and the reimbursement as paid by the health care providers (capitation) and the cumulative reimbursement normalized to the number of procedures to eventually calculated hospital net benefits and estimate savings as derived from idealized projected calculations with optimal use of QCA considered to improve the selection of patients for angioplasty and limit the costs of supplies due to optimal choice of balloon catheters.

To identify the potential of QCA to reduce both the costs to perform coronary angioplasty and therefore improve the financial reimbursement for the hospital based on a capitation model, the calculations in a real group of 62 consecutive patients in which decisions have been based on eye balling estimation of stenosis severity are contrasted to calculation based on optimized selection of patients and equipment as dictated by QCA. For the calculation the standard figures as used in Germany in 1996 and 1997 were applied. Standard statistical methods were used to compare both approaches.

Procedural and angiographic results

With "eyeballing" 94 balloons were used for 62 lesions (1.54 balloons per stenosis; range 1 to 5) at the discretion of the angiographer, and up to 5 balloons in upsizing order (from 2.50 ± 0.53 to 3.81 ± 0.46 mm) were necessary to reach an optimal balloon size/reference diameter ratio of 1:1 and a satisfactory result (Figure 1). The mean reference lumen diameter as assessed by QCA was 2.80 ± 0.61 mm and was virtually identical to the maximum mean balloon size. With eye balling the initial balloon size chosen was in general too small (mean BS/RLD ratio = 0.93 ± 0.27) and was followed by bigger balloons (mean BS/RLD ratio = 1.04 ± 0.25) to reach an acceptable therapeutic result. Calibration of the image data is usually performed on a non-tapering part of the contrast catheter following a similar edge detection procedure as for the arterial segment; the additional information, that the projection of a circle-cylindrical structure is characterized by parallel boundaries was used in the definition of the catheter contours. During film analysis, regions of interest (ROI's) are magnified optically (± 2.3 fold) resulting in calibration factors in the range of 0.08-0.10 mm/pixel, which is optimal for the edge detection algorithm used for the cinefilm application. During digital

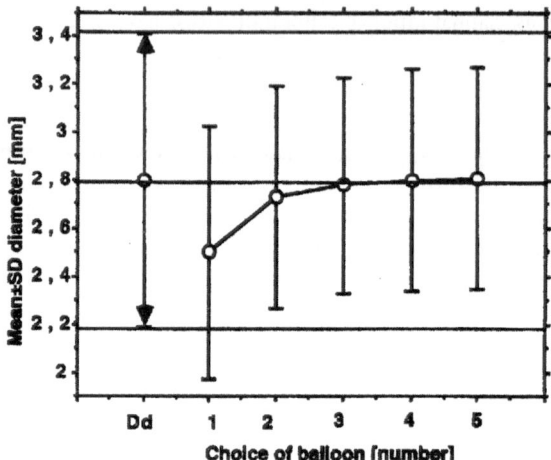

Figure 1. The graph demonstrates the relation between the diameter (mean and SD) of the normal vessel diameter adjacent to the target stenosis as measured by QCA (left, 2.8 mm ranging from 2.2 to 3.4 mm to be used for optimal selection of balloon size), and the angiographic result (QCA-derived) as obtained with the use of 1, 2, 3, 4 or 5 balloons selected on the basis of eye balling rather than pre-interventional QCA. With eye-balling up to 5 balloons in upsizing order were used to obtain an angiographically satisfying result; on average 1.54 balloons were required.

analysis, the ROI's are obtained by a bicubic two-fold interpolation approach resulting in calibration factors typically in the same range as for cinefilm for images acquired with a 7" image intensifier.

From the left- and right-hand contours of the arterial segment a diameter function is determined, on the basis of which the following parameters are automatically calculated: the site of maximal percent diameter stenosis, the obstruction diameter, the corresponding automatically determined reference diameter and the extent of the obstruction. Additionally derived parameters include obstruction symmetry, inflow and outflow angles, area of the atherosclerotic plaque and functional information in terms of the radiographic stenosis flow reserve (SFR-) value and transstenotic pressure gradients [25].

Visual assessment versus quantitative coronary angiography

By comparing the angiographic characterization of a given stenosis in a series of 62 consecutive patients, eye balling was identified to overestimate severity of the diameter reduction in the target lesion with 83.4 ± 9.9 as compared to the identical stenosis when evaluated by QCA (65.1 ± 13.4), p < 0.001. Moreover, the reference diameter in the normal adjacent segment was estimated 2.5 ± 0.5 mm by eye balling prior to PTCA as compared to 2.8 ± 0.6 in the identical segment as assessed by QCA. Only the estimated stenosis length was similar by both assessment techniques. In addition, as depicted in Table 1, QCA provides functional by the calculated stenosis severity flow reserve potentially useful as an alternative parameter for stenosis severity. Interestingly, 29 of 62 lesions, revealed normal stenosis flow reserve > 3 prior to PTCA; only 33 of 62 lesions had a significantly reduced stenosis flow reserve of less than 3. Both the high percentage of normal stenosis flow and significant minor target lesion diameter stenosis by QCA underline the obvious overestimation of less severity by eye balling (Table 1).

Table 1: Overestimation of less severity by eye balling

	pre-PTCA	post-PTCA	3 month F/U
ReferenceDiameter(range)	2.5±0.5	(1.5-3.5) *	
% Diameter Stenosis (range)	83.2±9.9 (40-100) *	30.3±12.5 (10-70)	46.9±19.8 (20-100)
EB			
Stenosis Length (range)	11.0±4.1	(< 20)	
ReferenceDiameter (range)	2.8±0.6 (1.04.1)	2.8±0.6 (1.2-4.1)	2.8±0.6 (1.5-4.5)
MLD[a] (range)	0.9±0.4 (0-1.8)	1.9±0.5 (1.0-3.1)	1.6±0.6 (0-3.2)
%Diameter-Stenosis(range)	65.1±13.4 (40-1003	31.7±13.5(1-60)	44.2±17.7(8-100)
QCA			
Stenosis Length (range)	9.9+3.4 (3-18)	10.3⊥4.0 (3-22)	9.8±4.3 (0-24)
SFR (range)	2.3±1.2 (0-4)	4.4±0.6 (2.6-5)	4.0±0.9 (0-5)
SFR ≥ 3	33	2	4
SFR > 3	29	60	58

a.   MLD = Minimal lumen diameter; SFR = stenosis flow reserve

Table 2: Distribution of target lesion stenosis severity

Target lesion stenosis		EB		QCA	
		n	%	n	%
% diameter stenosis	≥70%	60	(96)	22	(35)
	≥60%	60	(96)	38	(61)
	≥50%	62	(100)	56	(90)

Table 2 summarizes the distribution of target lesion stenosis severity; the Table shows that 60 patients (96%) had a diameter reduction of more than 70% and all patients (100%) had a diameter reduction of more than 50% in their target lesion. In contrast to these values derived from eye balling, QCA revealed 22 patients (35%) to have a diameter reduction of more than 70%, 38 patients (61%) with a diameter reduction of more than 60% and 56 patients (90%) with a diameter reduction of more than 50%; 10% of all patients had a diameter reduction of the target lesion of less than 50%. Thus with respect to stenosis severity of 60 and 70% diameter reduction the classification of patients into these groups was significantly different when eye balling was compared with QCA; this may be critical for the appropriate selection of patients before a coronary interventional procedure. With regards to the consumption of expensive supply in the 62 patients in whom angioplasty was performed according to the discretion of the operator based on eye balling, the total number of balloons was 95 or 1.54 balloons per patient.

As shown in Table 3 and in Figure 1 up to 5 balloons of incremental size were used to appropriately dilate the target lesion in a single patient. In another patient 4 balloons were necessary, in 2 patients three balloons and in 22 patients, 2 balloons were utilized to achieve the appropriate angiographic result.

Table 3: Target lesion delay in a single patient

		n	%
total # of lesions		62	100
total # of balloons		95	100
balloons/lesion		1.54	—
balloon/patient	1	36	58.1
	2	22	35.5
	3	2	3.2
	4	1	1.6
	5	1	1.6

When calculating the supplies cost in the test group of 62 consecutive patients in which decisions were based on eye balling only total balloon cost amounted 95.000 DM or 1.540 DM average cost for balloons per patient, based on a balloon price of 1000 DM (Table 4). With a reimbursement per patient for one PTCA procedure of 6.300 DM (capitation in 1996) the cumulative reimbursement by the health care providers (insurance companies) to the hospital amounts to 390.600 DM. Subtraction of the cumulative total cost for supplies of 187.150 DM may result in an average net hospital benefit of 203.450 DM for the total group of 62 patients. With the idealized projection of improved patient selection and balloon sizing based on QCA information, the balloon costs ideally would be only 1.000 DM or one balloon per patient, or 88.660 DM cumulative total costs for 62 procedures. With the same health care provider, reimbursement per patient of 6.300 DM the cumulative reimbursement by the health care providers would again be 390.600 DM; however, considering the idealized cumulative total costs of 88.660 DM for 62 patients, the total hospital net benefit would reach 301.940 DM reflecting a 48.2% increase in net hospital benefits for a group of 62 patients subjected to angioplasty under ideal conditions. These figures are also expressed in Euro, assuming 1 Euro to equal 1.92 DM.

Table 4: Supplies cost in the test group of 62 consecutive patients

	Eye balling		QCA		
	DM	Euro	DM	Euro	
Total balloon costs[a]	95.000	49.479	62.000	32.292	-53.2%
Balloon costs/ patient	1.540	820	1.000	521	-57.3%
Cumulative costs/ patient	1.970	1.026	1.430	745	-37.7%
Cumulative total- costs	187.150	97.474	88.660	46.177	—
Reimbursement/ patient (capitation)	6.300	3.281	6.300	3.281	—
Cumulative reim- bursement	390.600	203.437	390.600	203.437	—
Hospital net benefit	203.450	105.963	301.940	157.260	+48.2%

a. Assumption 1 Euro = 1.92 DM

Table 5: Relationship between invested costs and optimized savings with QCA

nPTCA/ annum	QCA investment/ annum[a]		net cost reduction with QCA		net savings	
	DM	Euro	DM	Euro	DM	Euro
100	75.000[a]	39.062	54.000	28.125	-21.000	-10.937
138	75.000	39.062	74.520	38.812	break even point	
500	75.000	39.062	270.000	140.625	195.000	101.562
1.000	75.000	39.062	540.000	281.250	465.000	242.187
1.500	125.000[b]	65.104	810.000	421.875	685.000	356.771

a. Invested annual costs for QCA (20.000 DM annual depreciation for hardware. 5.000 annual service fees, 50.000 DM costs for QCA technician)

b. 2 QCA technicians

Taking this simplified calculation one step further by relating it to the volume of a given cath lab, Table 5 summarizes the relationship between invested cost and optimized savings potential with QCA in various cath lab scenarios. Assuming a baseline investment for QCA equipment of 100.000 DM (or 20.000 DM per annum in a 20% annual depreciation model for hardware), 5.000 DM annual service fees and 50.000 DM annual expenses for 1

QCA technician, the annual investment would amount to 75.000 DM up to a volume of 1.000 PTCA's per year. In a scenario of 1.500 PTCA's per year, two QCA technicians would be required to handle this volume. As shown in Table 5, the net cost reduction with QCA are contrasted to the QCA investment per year and subsequent net savings per year are projected. QCA as a financial investment is not useful for a catheterization laboratory of less than 138 procedures in which QCA may be required for decision making. Above this break-even point of 138 procedures per year, the idealized net savings with QCA may be 195.000 DM, 456.000 DM or 685.000 DM in a scenario of 500, 1000 or 1.500 QCA-guided PTCA procedures per year. Thus, from the economics standpoint of a busy catheterization laboratory, the investment of QCA equipment and personnel may well be justified by reducing costs and increasing savings per year in a Germany based 1996 capitation model for coronary angioplasty.

Discussion

Previous comparative studies between QCA and eye balling assessment of coronary stenosis severity have show that QCA enables an operator-independent and less subjective assessment of stenosis severity as compared to eye balling; eye balling especially when executed by the coronary angiographer tends to infer self-referral bias due to overestimation of stenosis severity in lesions in the range of 50-60% diameter reduction in order to justify coronary angiography [5,8,26,27]. This inherent conflict resulting in a bimodal distribution of stenosis diameter reduction with eye balling instead of normal gaussian distribution of stenosis severity is well-known and has been always a strong argument to favor QCA for selecting patients for interventional procedures that are usually justified with a diameter reduction of at least 60% [6,8,28]. QCA is able to objectively differentiate stenosis of less than 50% diameter reduction from higher grade stenosis. Thus by avoiding eye balling to select patients for angioplasty procedures, mild and moderate stenosis with only marginal benefit from angiography can be better identified and separated from high grade lesions more likely to benefit from interventional procedures. QCA has shown to be an efficacious tool for better patient selection and thus for avoiding unnecessary procedures likely to result in cosmetic treatment of mild to moderate lesions and without any meaningful impact on symptoms and outcome. By better selection of patients expensive supplies such as balloons and even stents may be saved and resources be channeled to patients that really would benefit from coronary angioplasty.

The above mentioned model calculation shows that savings of more than 50% and a substantial net reimbursement benefit for the health care provider model can be achieved in a capitation, when both selection of patients for angioplasty procedures are optimized and balloons are selected based on quantitative measurements from on-line intraprocedural and independent QCA measurement in order to avoid incremental balloon sizes to achieve an optimal angioplasty result. Since costs for balloons are critical in an era of cost containment, a cost-saving potential of optimized selection of balloon material appears to be substantial as shown in both Tables 4 and 5. In addition, with QCA to be used to discriminate patients with high grade from those with moderate or mild target lesions, the element of quality control comes into play [16,28,29]. QCA is likely to enhance quality by improved selection of patients and avoidance of inappropriate procedures, and unlikely to benefit the individual health insured patient. As a general rule, rigid quality control and adherence to guidelines

[7,16,29] are highly likely to reduce costs, a concept which has been reconfirmed in various scenarios in the medical world. As calculated in our model scenario and based on public price tags on medical supplies in 1996 in Germany, a critical volume of 138 QCA-supported PTCA procedure is critical (under ideal conditions) to reach the break even point between cost saving and necessary annual investment in both hardware and manpower. The substantial savings that can potentially be obtained with strict adherence to angiographic selection criteria for targeting a stenosis with angioplasty, however, are derived under conditions of an ideal situation. Moreover, even with QCA on average more than just one catheter may be necessary to obtain an optimal angiographic result with PTCA. Thus, the substantial savings and critical reduction in costs may be less pronounced in the real world than calculated and shown in Tables 4 and 5. However, QCA is probably a useful tool, if used appropriately, to avoid unnecessary, or cosmetic interventions in subcritical lesions, that will not benefit from PTCA or even from stenting, as long as a critical diameter reduction has not been documented [30]. Eye balling alone, however, is likely to infer and facilitate self referral, and thus increase the number of patients subjected to angioplasty without clinical benefit. Although the setting of this model calculation is an ideal world, there is no doubt that even in the "real world" QCA may lead to substantial cost cutting and increase in net savings although not as pronounced as shown in our calculation. No other technique including intravascular ultrasound imaging has provided cost-cutting potential [31]. In addition, the investment necessary to perform QCA on a routine basis may be higher than projected in our model, whereas the investment for hardware and software may on the long line even be lower than in our model calculation , the expenses to train and to teach personnel and eventually to pay for a trained technician or QCA operator may be higher than assumed in our model. Furthermore, quantitatively less important factors may have been neglected in our calculation; but there may be both cost reducing and cost driving factors neglected in our calculation such as impact on hospital stay, quantity of contrast material, and service contracts. Irrespective, however, of additional (smaller) cost factors the allover message, that objective selection of patients for a costly procedure, and optimized selection of balloon material to execute this procedure professionally are critical factors to reduce costs. Independent on-line QCA and strict adherence to accepted inclusion criteria have the potential to contribute significantly both to reduce costs and eventually to produce net hospital savings, by simultaneously enhancing the quality of medical care in the clinical scenario of coronary angioplasty.

Thus it appears undoubtful that QCA is beneficial for both the individual patient and the socio-economic system, especially for the health care provider. The optimal selection of patients for the procedure certainly avoids unnecessary risks and expenses to patients that would not necessarily benefit from a cosmetic PTCA, better patient selection will also shorten the waiting list for urgent indicated procedures and thus reduce the associated mortality, morbidity and additional financial burden. In addition, optimized balloon selection in those patients who deserve PTCA may not only decrease procedural risks of multiple balloon changes, but also decrease procedural time and thus complications related to the duration of the procedure. For instance, vessel dissection and increased need for adjunct stenting is likely to prolong hospital stay and intensify post-interventional treatment besides the costs for the stents. These assumptions, however, have to be proven in randomized head-to-head comparative trials.

In summary, with independent objective assessment of coronary dimensions, there is substantial potential for cost reduction in a busy catheter laboratory, and with QCA even experienced operators are less likely to be affected by self referral bias and thus may deliver better medical care in a socio-economic scenario of cost containment.

References

1. Ryan TJ, Bauman WB, Kennedy JW *et al.* Guidelines for percutaneous transluminal coronary angioplasty. A report of the American Heart Association/American College of Cardiology Task Force on Assessment of Diagnostic and Therapeutic Cardiovascular Procedures (Committee on Percutaneous Transluminal Coronary Angioplasty) Circulation 1993;88:2987-3007.

2. Topol EJ, Ellis SG, Cosgrove DM *et al.* Analysis of coronary angioplasty practice in the United States with an insurance-claims data base. Circulation 1993;87:1489-97.

3. Feldman RL, Macdonald RG, Hill JA *et al.* Coronary angioplasty at the time of initial cardiac catheterization. Cathet Cardiovasc Diagn 1986;12:219-22.

4. Beatt KJ, Serruys PW, Luijten HE *et al.* Restenosis after coronary angioplasty: the paradox of increased lumen diameter and restenosis. J Am Coll Cardiol 1992;19:258-66.

5. Serruys PW, Foley DP, de Feyter PJ. Restenosis after coronary angioplasty: a proposal of new comparative approaches based on quantitative angiography. Br Heart J 1992;68:417-24

6. Lund GK, Nienaber CA, Hamm CW, Terres W, Kuck KH. Einzeitige Herzkatheterdiagnostik un Ballondilatation ("prima-vista"-PTCA): Ergebnisse und Risiken. Dtsch Med Wochenschr 1994;119:I69-74.

7. Umans VA, Hermans WR, Herrman JP, Pameyer J, Serruys PW. Experiences of a quantitative coronary angiography core laboratory in restenosis prevention trials. In: Serruys PW, Foley DP, De Feyter PJ, editors. Quantitative coronary angiography in clinical practice. Dordrecht: Kluwer Academic Publishers; 1994. p. 121-35.

8. Ischinger T, Gruentzig AR, Hollman J *et al.* Should coronary arteries with less than 60% diameter stenosis be treated by angioplasty? Circulation 1983;68:148-54.

9. Guidelines for coronary angiography. A report of the American College of Cardiology/American Heart Association Task Force on Assessment of Diagnostic and Therapeutic Cardiovascular Procedures (Subcommittee on Coronary Angiography). Circulation 1987;76:963A-977A.

10. Beauman GJ, Vogel RA. Accuracy of individual and panel visual interpretations of coronary arteriograms: implications for clinical decisions. JAm Coll Cardiol 1990;16:108-13.

11. Keane D, Haase J, Slager CJ *et al.* Comparative validation of quantitative coronary angiography systems. Results and implications from a multicenter study using a standardized approach. Circulation 1995;91:2174-83.

12. Faxon DP, Vogel R, Yeh W, Holmes DR Jr, Detre K. Value of visual versus central quantitative measurements of angiographic success after percutaneous transluminal coronary angioplasty. NHLBI PTCA Registry Investigators. Am J Cardiol 1996;77:1067-72.

13. O'Keefe JH Jr, Rutherford BD, McConahay DR *et al.* Myocardial salvage with direct coronary angioplasty for acute infarction. Am Heart J 1992;123:1-6

14. Stiel GM, Schaps KP, Lattermann A, Nienaber CA. On-line independent digital stenosis morphometry avoids self referral bias for interventional coronary therapy. Comput Cardiol 1995:141-44.

15. Ryan TJ, Klocke FJ, Reynolds WA. Clinical competence in percutaneous transluminal coronary angioplasty. A statement for physicians from the ACP/ACC/AHA Task Force on Clinical Privileges in Cardiology. J Am Coll Cardiol 1990;15:1469-74.

16. Relman AS: "Self-referral" - what's at stake? N Engl J Med 1992;327:1522-4.

17 Faxon DP: Is there a solution to the problem of self-referral for PTCA? Presented at the American Collegue of Cardiology, 42nd Annual Scientific Session. March 16, 1993.

18. Marcus ML, Skorton DJ, Johnson MR, Collins SM, Harrison DG, Kerber RE. Visual estimates of percent diameter coronary stenosis: "a battered gold standard". J Am Coll Cardiol 1988;11:882-5.

19. Stiel GM, Barth K, Eicker B, Vogel C, Towara U, Nienaber CA. AWOS: angiographic workstation for digital quantitative coronary angiography. Comput Cardiol 1994:599-602.

20. Stiel GM, Nienaber CA, Lattermann A, Barth K, Meinertz T. Comparison of coronary vessels edge detection and cross line methods to quantify the degree of stenosis as accessed by digital systems. Comput Cardiol 1995:473-5.

21. Hausleiter J, Jost S, Nolte CW *et al.* Comparative in-vitro validation of eight first- and second-generation quantitative coronary angiography systems. Coron Artery Dis 1997;8:83-90.
22. Gould KL. Quantification of coronary artery stenosis in vivo. Circ Res 1985;57:341-53.
23. Pijls NH, Lamfers E, van Leeuwen K, Uijen GJ, Van der Werf T. l. Klinische Anwendung und Bewertung der maximalen Myokardperfusion aus EKG-getriggerten digitalen Angiogrammen. Electromedica 1991;59:34-48.
24. Rigolin VH, Robiolio PA, Spero LA *et al.* Compression of digital coronary angiograms does not affect visual or quantitative assessment of coronary artery stenosis severity. Am J Cardiol 1996;78:131-5.
25. Kirkeeide RL, Gould KL, Parsel L. Assessment of coronary stenoses by myocordial perfusion imaging during pharmacologic coronary vasodilation. VII. Validation of coronary flow reserve as a single integrated functional measure of stenosis severity reflecting all its geometric dimensions. J Am Coll Cardiol 1986;7:103-13.
26. King SB 3rd, Weintraub WS, Tao X, Hearn J, Douglas JS Jr. Bimodal distribution of diameter stenosis 4 to 12 month after angioplasty: implications for definitions and interpretation of restenosis [abstract]. J Am Coll Cardiol 1991;17(Suppl A):345A.
27 Stiel GM, Stiel LSG, Barth K, Nienaber CA. Patient Defined Digital Angiocardiography (PDDA): a valid way for individual staging of coronary artery disease. In: Brody WR, Johnston GS, editors. Computer applications to assist radiology. Carlsbad, MD: Symposia Foundation; 1992. p. 712-3.
28. Rensing BJ, Hermans WRM, Deckers JW, De Feyter PJ, Tijssen JGP, Serruys PW. Lumen narrowing after percutaneous transluminal coronary balloon angioplasty follows a near gaussian distribution: a quantitative angiographic study in 1,445 successfully dilated lesions. J Am Coll Cardiol 1992;19:939-45.
29. Topol EJ. Quality of care in interventional cardiology. In: Topol EJ, editors. Textbook of interventional cardiology. Philadelphia: Saunders; 1994. p. 1354-67.
30. De Jaegere P, Hermans WR, Rensing BJ, Strauss BH, De Feyter P, Serruys PW. Matching based on quantitative coronary angiography as a surrogate for randomized studies: comparison between stent implantations and balloon angioplasty of native coronary artery lesions. Am Heart J 1993;125:310-9.
31. Prati F, Gil R, Di Mario C *et al.* Is quantitative angiography sufficient to guide stent implantation? A comparison with three-dimensional reconstruction of intracoronary ultrasound images. G Ital Cardiol 1997;27:328-36.

4.

3-D coronary angiography: improving visualization strategy for coronary interventions

Shiuh-Yung James Chen & John D. Carroll

Summary

Given the 3-D character of the coronary artery tree, it is expected that any projection will foreshorten a variety of segments. The visual perception provided by such a projection shows a variety of arterial segments with a degree of foreshortening that may or may not be appreciated. Due to the problem of vessel overlap and foreshortening, multiple projections are necessary to adequately evaluate the coronary arterial tree with arteriography in the form of coronary fluoroscopy or angiograms. The elimination or at least minimization of foreshortening and overlap is a prerequisite for an accurate quantitative coronary analysis such as determination of intra-coronary lengths in a 2-D display. Hence, the patient might receive additional radiation and contrast material during diagnostic and interventional procedures. This traditional trial-and-error method provides views in which overlapping and foreshortening are minimized, but only in terms of the subjective experience-based judgment of the angiographer. A method has been developed for on-line 3-D reconstruction of the coronary arterial trees based on two views acquired from routine angiograms at arbitrary orientation using a single-plane or biplane imaging system. Based on any coronary stenosis, a plane of gantry angulations minimizing the foreshortening of arterial segment is calculated yielding multiple computer-generated projection images among which a set of views with minimal vessel overlap are chosen. With the proposed technique, the spatial relationships and 3-D morphological structures of arteries can be clearly identified which are not easily achieved by other modalities such as interventional ultrasound or magnetic resonance imaging. A computer simulation confirmed the accuracy of 3-D reconstruction to within 2.1% error by use of a pair of actual angiograms of intra-coronary guide wire. The length of the wire is 105 mm with 8 markers of 15 mm inter-distance. More than 120 cases of coronary arterial trees have been completed for 3-D reconstruction including left coronary artery trees, right coronary artery trees, and bypass grafts among which more than 40 cases were performed in-room of our cardiac catheterization laboratory. With this 3-D coronary processing tool, assessment of lesion length and diameter narrowing can be optimized in both interventional cases and studies of progression and regression.

J.H.C. Reiber and E.E. van der Wall (eds.). What's New in Cardiovascular Imaging, 61–78.
©1998 Kluwer Academic Publishers.

Introduction

The linkage between the duration and outcome of the intervention and optimally visualizing the coronary segment being treated is a fundamental principle of interventional cardiology. Planning and performing a coronary intervention involves more than selecting equipment, but analyzing the diagnostic images to match the equipment to the anatomy and selecting the views that are optimal for performing the procedure. Thus an optimal visualization strategy has multiple components including:

- What view is optimal for choosing and placing a guiding catheter ?
- What view(s) is optimal for steering the guide-wire ?
- What views are optimal for assessing take-off angles and tortuosity in order to gauge the difficulties of performing the procedure ?
- What views are optimal for visualizing the diseased segment in order to characterize the nature of the lesion, its length and reference diameter ?
- What views are optimal for visualizing to facilitate the placement of intra-coronary stents in terms of locations close to ostia and side branches ?

In the past twenty years of coronary interventions, most developments have focused on new therapeutic devices and techniques rather than the visualization process used in performing the procedure. There has been a dramatic improvement of the X-ray imaging equipment that has provided better quality images which can be reviewed immediately and efficiently. Furthermore, the transition to digital storage and quantitative coronary analysis softwares to be used on the two-dimensional (2-D) images have provided additional functionality and efficiencies. Yet, the fundamental process of presenting 2-D images on monitors and the user-image interaction have remained unchanged over these decades. It is useful to step back and consider the visual environment that exists in the cardiac catheterization laboratory. Despite numerous attempts with all kinds of imaging modalities to define the presence, extent, and functional significance of coronary artery disease, coronary angiography remains the primary method of understanding the patient-specific anatomy of the coronary arterial tree, and the standard approach for determining the presence, extent, localization, and severity of coronary artery disease. Interventional coronary procedures are universally performed with fluoroscopy that is an extension of the coronary arteriographic diagnostic study. In the 1640 cardiac catheterization laboratories in the United States, there were 2.7 million procedures in 1996 alone. Of these 37% involved an intervention.

Unlike cardiac surgeons who directly see and touch the patient's heart, the coronary interventionalist manipulates distant miniaturized equipment and visualizes what she or he is doing on a monitor with flat 2-D projection images based on X-ray equipment. Multiple clues of the 3-D character of the artery are lost by the projection X-ray modality. Moving the X-ray source-image acquisition system is the solution that has circumvented some but not all of these problems. Cardiologists choose several views to perform the coronary intervention and document the results. Fluoroscopy is typically performed in projections suggested by arteriography as being good "working" views, defined as a projection that displays anatomic regions of interest in a fashion that helps the operator perform the procedure. Such a trial-and-error approach of traditional coronary arteriography and fluoroscopy has been used to determine optimal visualization (or standard views) for diagnostic and therapeutic coronary procedures for multiple decades. However, the diversity of human coronary anatomy and its exact location and orientation in the thorax precludes the uses of standard projections as anything but rough guides.

The clinical value and the scientific challenge of performing 3-D coronary reconstruction are not new to the cardiology and imaging science communities. Up until recently these approaches failed to be practical for the clinical world of interventional cardiology. Many endeavors of computer-assisted techniques for estimation of the 3-D coronary arteries from biplane projection data have been reported [1-11]. These methods were based on the known or standard X-ray geometry of projections, placement of landmarks, or the pre-determined vessel shape and on iterative identification of matching structures in two or more views. In [12], a method based on motion and multiple views acquired in a single-plane imaging system was proposed. The motion transformations of the heart model consist only of rotation and scaling. By incorporation of the center-referenced method and initial depth coordinates and center coordinates, a 3-D skeleton of coronary arteries was obtained. However, actual heart motion during contraction involves five specific movements: translation, rotation, wringing, accordion-like motion, and movement toward the center of the ventricular chamber [13]. Therefore, the model employed may not be general enough to portray the true motion of the heart, especially near end-systole.

Other knowledge-based or rule-based systems have been proposed for 3-D reconstruction of coronary arteries by use of a vascular network model [14-20]. Because the rules or knowledge base were organized for certain specific conditions, it is not likely to generalize the 3-D reconstruction process to arbitrary projection data. In [21], the 3-D coronary arteries were reconstructed from a set of X-ray perspective projections by use of an algorithm from computed tomography. Due to the motion of the heart, only a limited number of projections can be acquired. Therefore, accurate reconstruction and quantitative measurement are not easily achieved. Closed-form solution of the 3-D reconstruction problem using a linear approach was a significant development in [22-28]. Unfortunately, actual data are always corrupted by noise or errors and the linear approach based techniques may not be sufficiently accurate from noisy data. Hence, optimal estimation has been explicitly investigated. In [29-35], a two-step approach was proposed for an optimal estimation of 3-D object structures based on maximum-likelihood and minimum-variance estimation. Preliminary estimates computed by the linear algorithm were used as initial estimates for the process of optimal estimation.

In our proposed research, an on-line 3-D reconstruction technique has been developed to accurately reconstruct the coronary arterial trees based on two views acquired from routine angiograms at arbitrary orientation using a single-plane imaging system. In the proposed method, a new optimization algorithm is developed by minimizing the *image point* and *directional vector* errors associated with bifurcations in both views subject to the constraints derived from the intrinsic parameters of the employed single-plane imaging system. Given 6 or more corresponding object points in both views, a constrained nonlinear optimization algorithm is applied to obtain an optimal estimate of the transformation in the form of R and $\vec{t}$ which characterizes the position and orientation of one view relative to the other. The initial solution to the optimization process is calculated on the basis of the employed intrinsic single-plane imaging parameters. In the next section, an overview of the proposed on-line 3-D reconstruction algorithm will be presented. Afterwards, the process for determination of optimal views is explained. In experimental results, a pair of actual angiograms of intracoronary guide wire were employed for validation. The length of the wire is 105 mm with 8 markers of 15 mm inter-distance. The results confirmed that the accuracy of 3-D length measurement was within 2.1% error. More than 120 cases of coronary arterial trees have been completed for 3-D reconstruction including left coronary artery (LCA) trees, right coronary artery (RCA) trees, and bypass grafts among which more than 40 cases were performed in-room of our cardiac catheterization laboratory. Two typical examples of LCA and RCA reconstructions are chosen for demonstration in this chapter.

On-line 3-D reconstruction of coronary arterial tree

The proposed method of on-line 3-D reconstruction consists of four major steps: (1) acquisition of two standard angiogram sequences by use of a single-plane imaging system, (2) identification of 2-D coronary arterial trees and feature extractions including bifurcation points, vessel diameters, vessel directional vectors, and vessel centerlines in the two images, (3) determination of transformation in terms of a rotation matrix R and a translation vector $\vec{t}$ based on the extracted vessel bifurcation points and directional vectors, (4) calculation of 3-D coronary arterial trees based on the calculated transformations and identified vessel diameters and centerlines. These are detailed in the following subsections.

Image acquisition

After routine cardiac catheterization is initiated, a standard coronary arteriogram is completed in two standard views; two injections in a single-plane imaging system. The examination table may be moved horizontally and/or vertically between the acquisitions. "Panning the table" commonly happens in the routine angiography study in order that the magnified projections of the entire cardiac vasculature can be captured by the image intensifier. These images are acquired on the basis of 15 or 30 frames per second in each view with or without electrocardiogram (ECG) triggering acquisition mode. With the acquired two angiogram sequences, a pair of images are chosen corresponding to the same or close acquisition time instance (*e.g.*, end-diastole or end-systole) in the respective cardiac cycles. These are transferred to the computer workstation through the fiber optic link for analysis and reconstruction. The transfer rate is 2 seconds per image with the matrix size of 512×480 pixels and one byte storage for each pixel.

Segmentation and feature extraction of 2-D coronary arterial structures

A semi-automatic system [33] based on the technique of deformation model and segmentation technique is employed for identification of the 2-D coronary arterial tree in the given angiograms. The required user interaction involves only the indication of several points inside the lumen, near the projection of vessel centerline in the angiogram. Afterwards, a spline-curve is formed based on the selected points, which serves as the initial centerline of the vessel. A window with the size of m by m pixels (*i.e.*, a ridge operator) was applied to be convolved with the given image by which the pixel on image is selected as vessel centerline point if it is a local minimum on intensity within the window. By use of the deformation model, the identified pixels are served as the external forces to act on the initial model curve such that it will be gradually deformed and finally resides on the real centerline of vessel.

The identified centerlines and the branching relationships are used for construction of the vessel hierarchy in each angiogram by their labeling according to the appropriate anatomy and connectivity among the primary and secondary coronary arteries. The labeling process on the coronary tree is performed automatically by application of the algorithm of

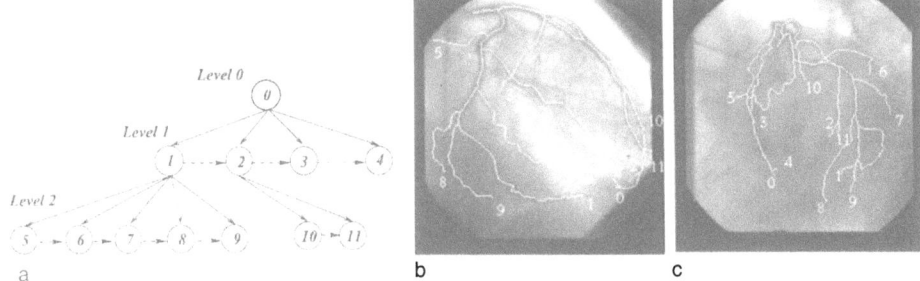

Figure 1. (a) The constructed vessel hierarchical digraph associated with the 2-D coronary arterial trees identified from the two standard angiograms (b) and (c), where the solid and dashed arrows denote the descendent and sibling arcs, respectively.

breadth-first search to traverse identified vessel centerlines and associated bifurcations. From each vessel of the coronary tree that is currently visited, this approach tries to search as broadly as possible by next visiting all of the vessel centerlines that are adjacent to it, and finally results in a vessel hierarchically <u>di</u>rected <u>graph</u> (digraph) containing a set of nodes with corresponding *depth levels* and two types of arcs (descendant and sibling arcs) defining the coronary anatomy. In the hierarchical digraph, each node represents a vessel in the coronary arterial tree, and the *descendent arc* connects the nodes between the vessel and its branch. If a vessel has multiple branches, the nodes associated with these branches are connected as a linked list by *sibling arcs* according to the branching locations relative to the ascendant vessel.

With the constructed hierarchical digraph, bifurcation points, directional vectors, and diameters are then calculated for all of the bifurcations and coronary arteries. The calculated results are saved into the nodes corresponding to the branching vessels in the hierarchical digraph. In Figure 1(a), a hierarchical digraph constructed corresponding to the coronary arterial trees identified from angiograms in Figures 1(b) and (c). Figures 2(a) and (b) show the extracted features including vessel diameters, bifurcation points, directional vectors, and vessel centerlines of a left coronary arterial tree.

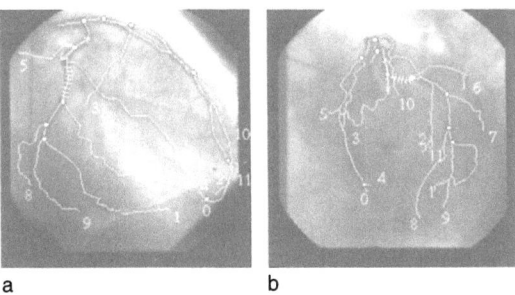

Figure 2. (a)(b) The identified vessel features on the given pair of angiograms including bifurcation points, diameters, directional vectors of bifurcations, and vessel centerlines. Note that only the diameters of an arterial segment and directional vectors at one bifurcation region were demonstrated for each view.

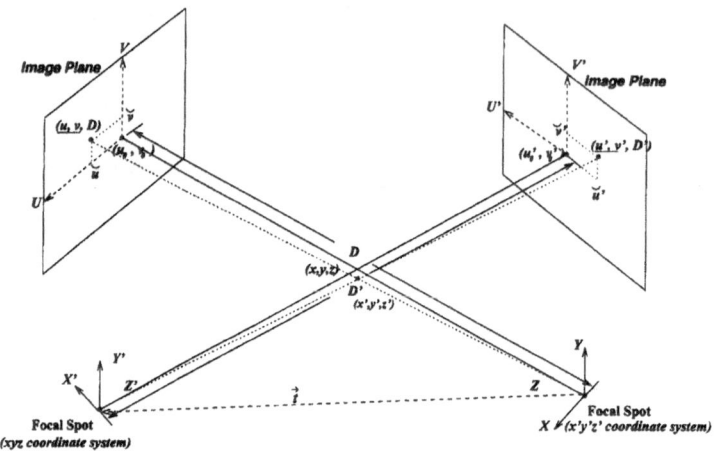

Figure 3. A single-plane imaging system, showing a 3-D object point and its projection in two views characterized by *xyz* and *x'y'z'* coordinate systems, respectively.

Determination of transformation characterizing the two views

By use of a single-plane imaging system for image acquisitions, the spatial relationship between the employed two views can be characterized by a transformation in the forms of a rotation matrix R and a translation vector $\vec{t}$ with the X-ray source (or focal spot) served as the origin of 3-D coordinate space as shown in Figure 3. In the first view, let (u_i, v_i) denote the image coordinates of the i-th object point, located at position (x_i, y_i, z_i). We have $u_i = Dx_i / z_i, v_i = Dy_i / z_i$ where D is the perpendicular distance between the X-ray focal spot and the image plane which is employed during the image acquisition. Let (ξ_i, η_i) denote the scaled image coordinates, defined as $\xi_i = u_i / D = x_i / z_i$, $\eta_i = v_i / D = y_i / z_i$. The second projection view of the employed single-plane imaging system can be described in terms of a second pair of image and object coordinate systems $u' v'$ and $x' y' z'$ defined in an analogous manner. Scaled image coordinates (ξ_i', η_i') in the second view for the i-th object point at position (x_i', y_i', z_i') are given by $\xi_i' = u_i' / D' = x_i' / z_i', \eta_i' = v_i' / D' = y_i' / z_i'$. The geometrical relationship between the two views can be characterized by

$$\begin{bmatrix} x_i' \\ y_i' \\ z_i' \end{bmatrix} = R \cdot \left\{ \begin{bmatrix} x_i \\ y_i \\ z_i \end{bmatrix} - \vec{t} \right\} = \begin{bmatrix} r_{11} & r_{12} & r_{13} \\ r_{21} & r_{22} & r_{23} \\ r_{31} & r_{32} & r_{33} \end{bmatrix} \cdot \begin{bmatrix} x_i - t_x \\ y_i - t_y \\ z_i - t_z \end{bmatrix} \tag{1}$$

In our previously developed technique [33,35], the transformation was calculated based on the identified bifurcation points of the 2-D coronary arterial trees in the two views and can be only effective to the images acquired from the biplane systems or a single-plane system without movement of examination table between the acquisitions.

We have developed a new 3-D reconstruction technique by incorporation of the corresponding bifurcation points and the vessel directional vectors of bifurcations. This new method can also be employed to obtain accurate results of 3-D reconstruction even when the examination table is moving during the injection or with ECG-triggering mode disabled in acquisitions. For performing 3-D reconstruction, the required prior information (*i.e.*, the intrinsic parameters of each single-plane imaging system) include: (1) the distance between each focal spot and its image plane, employed SID (focal-spot to imaging-plane distance) during image acquisition, (2) the pixel size, p_{size} (*e.g.*, 0.3 mm/pixel), (3) the distance ff' between the two focal spots or the known 3-D distance between two points in the projection images, and (4) isocenter distance (with respect to which the rotary motion of the gantry arm rotates) relative to the focal spot.

In single-plane system, gantry angulations associated with different views are always defined based on a unique isocenter as the origin of the spatial coordinate system. However, the transformation calculated by use of gantry angles may not accurately correlate the coronary arterial structures in two different views due to: (1) nonsimultaneously acquired images with heart motion in different cardiac cycles, and (2) movement of examination table between the acquisitions. Although such a calculated transformation can not actually characterize the two views, the estimation is generally good enough to serve as an initial guess to the nonlinear minimization process for obtaining an optimal solution. With the initial solution calculated from gantry angles, the global minimum resulting from the nonlinear optimization can be guaranteed since the initial estimate is close to the actual solution.

To calculate the transformation, the objective function was defined by the minimization of (1) image point errors in term of the square of Euclidean distance between the 2-D input data and the projection of calculated 3-D data points, and (2) directional vector errors between the 2-D vessel directional vectors and the projection of calculated 3-D vessel directional vectors. Given the set of 2-D bifurcation points and directional vectors extracted from the pair of images, an "optimal" estimate of the transformation and 3-D bifurcation points were obtained by minimizing:

$$\min_{P,P',v,v'} F_1(P,P',v,v') = \sum_{i=1}^{n} \left\{ \begin{array}{c} \left(\xi_i - \dfrac{x_i}{z_i}\right)^2 + \left(\eta_i - \dfrac{y_i}{z_i}\right)^2 + \left(\xi_i' - \dfrac{x_i'}{z_i'}\right)^2 + \left(\eta_i' - \dfrac{y_i'}{z_i'}\right)^2 \\ + \left\| \vec{v}_i - [\vec{v}_i]_{xy} \right\|^2 + \left\| \vec{v}_i' - [\vec{v}_i']_{x'y'} \right\|^2 \end{array} \right\} \tag{2}$$

where n denotes the number of pairs of corresponding points extracted from the two images and P and P' denote the sets of 3-D object (*i.e.*, bifurcation point) position vector $\vec{P}_i = (x_i, y_i, z_i)$, and $\vec{P}_i' = (x_i', y_i', z_i')$, respectively, $\vec{v}_i$ and $\vec{v}_i'$, denote the respective 2-D vessel directional vectors of bifurcations in each views, and $v = \{\vec{v}_1, \vec{v}_2, ..., \vec{v}_n\}$ and $v' = \{\vec{v}_1', \vec{v}_2', ..., \vec{v}_n'\}$ denote the calculated 3-D vessel directional vectors of bifurcations in two views, and $[\vec{v}_i]_{xy}$ and $[\vec{v}_i']_{x'y'}$, $i=1,...,n$, denote the calculated 2-D projection vectors of $\vec{v}_i$'s and $\vec{v}_i'$'s on the image planes, respectively. Since the relationship between the two views can be characterized by a rotation matrix R and a translation vector $\vec{t} = [t_x, t_y, t_z]'$ as shown in Eq.(1), Eq.(2) can be expressed as

$$\min_{R,\vec{t},P',v'} F_2(R,\vec{t},P',v') = \sum_{i=1}^{n} \left\{ \begin{array}{c} \left(\xi_i' - \dfrac{x_i'}{z_i'}\right)^2 + \left(\eta_i' - \dfrac{y_i'}{z_i'}\right)^2 + \left(\xi_i - \dfrac{\vec{c}_1 \cdot \vec{P}_i' + t_x}{\vec{c}_3 \cdot \vec{P}_i' + t_z}\right)^2 \\ + \left(\eta_i - \dfrac{\vec{c}_1 \cdot \vec{P}_i' + t_x}{\vec{c}_3 \cdot \vec{P}_i' + t_z}\right)^2 + \left\| \vec{v}_i - [R^{-1} \cdot \vec{v}_i']_{xy} \right\|^2 + \left\| \vec{v}_i' - [\vec{v}_i]_{x'y} \right\|^2 \end{array} \right\} \tag{3}$$

where $\vec{c}_k$ denotes the respective k^{th} column vectors of matrix R, and R^{-1} is the inverse matrix of R.

Recovery of 3-D coronary artery

After the transformation $(R, \vec{t})$ that defines the two views is obtained, this information will be used for establishing the point correspondences on 2-D vessel centerlines in the pair of images and calculating 3-D morphologic structures of coronary arterial tree. The calculated transformation in conjunction with the epipolar constraints were employed as the frame-work for establishing the point correspondences on the vessel centerlines based on the two identified 2-D coronary arterial trees [33]. If the information on relative positions of two cameras is known (*i.e.*, the known locations and orientations of two focal spots F_a and F_b), the correspondences of image points can be solved by use of epipolar constraints" [36]. Let P denote a 3-D point, and let P_a and P_b the projections of P, denote the pair of corresponding points in two images. Such constraints state that these points, F_a, F_b, P_a, P_b, and P, are all on one plane called the *epipolar plane* as shown in Figure 4. The epipolar plane and each image plane intersect along a straight line called the *epipolar line* (see Figure 4). Therefore, the location of point P_b in the second image must lie on the epipolar line resulting from the intersec-

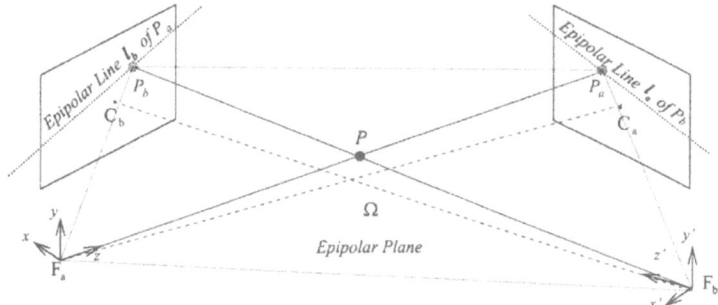

Figure 4. The epipolar geometry where C_a and C_b are centers of imaging planes, F_a and F_b are the focal spots, P_a and P_b are the projections P, Ω denotes the epipolar plane, and l_a and l_b represent the respective epipolar lines.

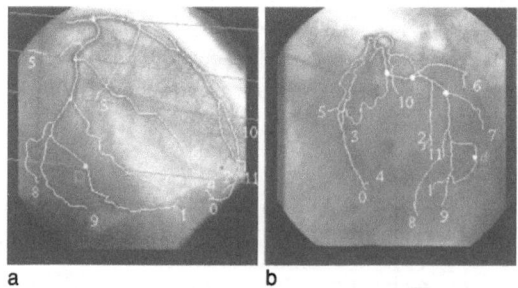

Figure 5. (a) A, B, C, and D are the corresponding points of a, b, c, and d, respectively, which are defined by the intersections between the respective epipolar lines and LCX artery. (b) 4 typical points (a, b, c, d) on the LCX artery employed as examples for correspondence establishment.

tion between the second image plane and the plane defined by point P_a and the two focal spots. Figures 5(a) and (b) show the typical example of correspondence establishment by use of epipolar constraints where points A, B, C, and D at the first view are defined by finding the intersections between the 2-D curve associated with left circumflex artery (LCX) artery and respective epipolar lines defined by a, b, c, and d at the second view.

With the point correspondences on 2-D vessel centerlines (ξ_j, η_j) and (ξ_j', η_j') and the transformation $(R, \vec{t})$, the 3-D vessel centerline points of coronary arteries (x_j, y_j, z_j) can then be calculated based on the following equations:

$$
\begin{bmatrix}
r_{11} - r_{31}\xi_j' & r_{12} - r_{32}\xi_j' & r_{13} - r_{33}\xi_j' \\
r_{21} - r_{31}\eta_j' & r_{22} - r_{32}\eta_j' & r_{23} - r_{33}\eta_j' \\
1 & 0 & -\xi_j \\
0 & 1 & -\eta_j
\end{bmatrix}
\cdot
\begin{bmatrix}
x_j \\
y_j \\
z_j
\end{bmatrix}
=
\begin{bmatrix}
\vec{a} \cdot \vec{t} \\
\vec{b} \cdot \vec{t} \\
0 \\
0
\end{bmatrix},
\tag{4}
$$

where

$$
\vec{a} =
\begin{bmatrix}
r_{11} - r_{31}\xi_j' \\
r_{12} - r_{32}\xi_j' \\
r_{13} - r_{33}\xi_j'
\end{bmatrix},
\vec{b} =
\begin{bmatrix}
r_{21} - r_{31}\eta_j' \\
r_{22} - r_{32}\eta_j' \\
r_{23} - r_{33}\eta_j'
\end{bmatrix}
$$

and r_{ij} denotes the component of the rotational matrix R.

To recover the morphology of the 3-D arterial lumen, the contour points on each circular lumen cross section centered at (x_i, y_i, z_i) are calculated. The normal vector at the plane spanned by the cross section is parallel to the tangent vector at point (x_i, y_i, z_i) on the vessel skeleton (or 3-D vessel centerline). For a local vessel segment, its associated cross section can be modeled as a circular disk centered at (x_i, y_i, z_i) with diameter d_i. Then the 3-D lumen of such a vessel segment can easily be represented by filling up the surfaces between two consecutive circular disks. The 3-D lumen diameter d_i is calculated from the following equation:

$$
d_i = \bar{d}_i \cdot \left(\frac{\sqrt{x_i^2 + y_i^2 + z_i^2}}{\sqrt{\xi_i^2 + \eta_i^2 + D^2}} \right)
\tag{5}
$$

where $\bar{d}_i$ is the extracted 2-D vessel diameter centered at (ξ_i, η_i), and D is the distance between the focal spot and the image intensifier.

Determination of optimal views

When an arbitrary computer-generated image is produced, the gantry information defining the current projection is calculated in the form of left anterior oblique/right anterior oblique (LAO/RAO) and caudal/cranial (CAUD/CRAN). These gantry angles are defined in a spatial coordinate system with the isocenter as the origin (see Figure 6). The LAO/RAO angulation is defined on the y-z plane, while the CAUD/CRAN angulation is defined on the x-z

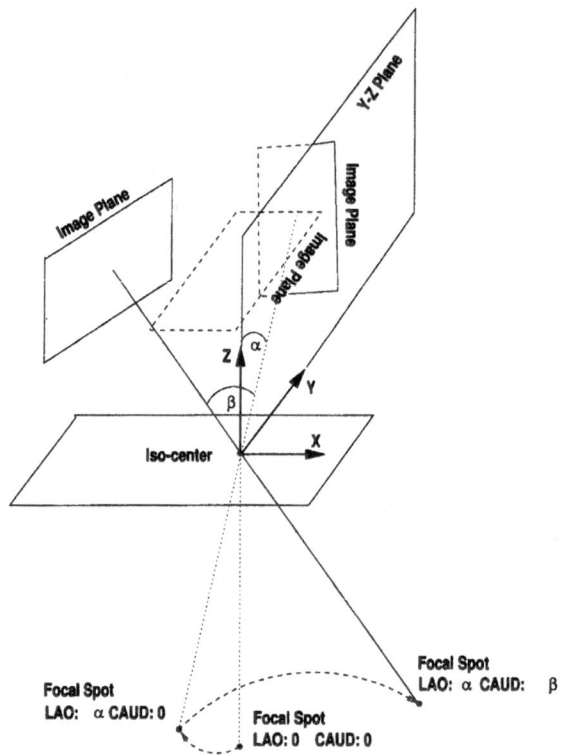

Figure 6. The gantry orientation defined by two angles and in a spatial coordinate system with the isocenter as its origin.

plane. With the spatial coordinates, the position of focal spot (x_f, y_f, z_f) can be formulated by use of two rotations $R_x(\alpha)$ and $R_y(-\beta)$ as,

$$[x_f, y_f, z_f] = [x_n, y_n, z_n] \cdot R_x(\alpha) R_y(-\beta)$$

$$= [x_n, y_n, z_n] \cdot \begin{bmatrix} \cos(-\beta) & 0 & -\sin(-\beta) \\ \sin(\alpha)\cos(-\beta) & \cos(\alpha) & \sin(\alpha)\cos(-\beta) \\ \cos(\alpha)\sin(-\beta) & -\sin(\alpha) & \cos(\alpha)\cos(-\beta) \end{bmatrix}, \quad (6)$$

where $(x_n, y_n, z_n) = (0, 0, D_{fc})$ denotes the neutral position of focal spot (or anterior-posterior (AP) view with 0° LAO and 0° CAUD, D_{fc} is the distance between isocenter and focal spot (which is provided by manufacture), R_x and R_y denotes the rigid rotations with respect to *x*-axis and *y*-axis, and α and β denote the LAO and CAUD angles, respectively.

Given the 3-D character of the coronary artery tree, it is expected that any projection will foreshorten a variety of segments. The visual perception provided by such a projection shows a variety of arterial segments with a degree of foreshortening that may or may not be appreciated. In Figure 7(a), the projected image has 0% degree of foreshortening since the tangential direction of such a line segment is perpendicular to the normal vector of image plane. Note that the projections of different line segments have various magnifications due to the

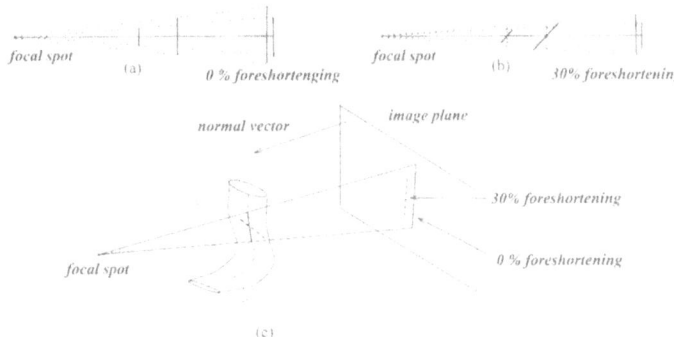

Figure 7. Illustrations of the percentage degree of foreshortening: (a) 0% degree of foreshortening with different magnifications of projected line segment. (b) 30% degree of foreshortening when the tangential direction of line segment is not perpendicular to the normal vector of image plane. (c) 0% and 30% degrees of foreshortening associated the segments of vessel centerline.

different locations relative to the image intensifier. If such a line segment is rotated by an arbitrary angle, *e.g.*, 45 degrees relative to its original orientation in Figure 7(a), there will be 30% degree of foreshortening as shown in Figure 7(b). In Figure 7(c), an example of foreshortening of a typical segment of a curvilinear vessel centerline is illustrated.

Due to the problem of vessel overlap and foreshortening, multiple projections are necessary to adequately evaluate the coronary arterial tree with arteriography. The elimination or at least minimization of foreshortening and overlap is a prerequisite for an accurate quantitative coronary analysis such as determination of intra-coronary lengths in a 2-D display. Hence, the patient might receive additional radiation and contrast material during diagnostic and interventional procedures. This traditional trial-and-error method provides views in which overlapping and foreshortening are minimized, but only in terms of the subjective experience-based judgment of the angiographer. In Figure 8(a) and (b), the same vessel segment between two bifurcation points as marked by two dots at its distal ends depicts 45% and 5% foreshortening in the respective angiograms.

The reconstructed 3-D coronary arterial tree can be rotated to any selected viewing angle yielding multiple computer-generated projections to determine for each patient which standard views are useful and which are of no clinical value due to excessive overlap. Therefore,

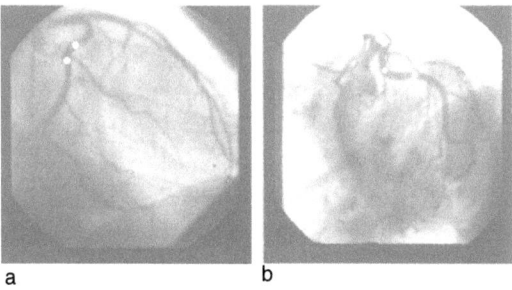

a   b

Figure 8. A typical example of vessel foreshortening where the segment indicated between two dots represents 45% foreshortening in view (a) and 5% foreshortening in view (b).

the 3-D computer assistance provides means to improve the quality and utility of the images subsequently acquired. Let p_i, $i = 0,1,\ldots,m$ denote the points on the centerline of a 3-D vessel. Let $\vec{l}_j = [l_{j_x}, l_{j_y}, l_{j_z}]^t$, $j=1,2,\ldots,m$ denote the vector of vessel segments between p_{j-1} and p_j. The minimal foreshortening of vessel segments can be obtained in term of gantry orientation (α and β angles) by minimizing the objective function as follows:

$$\min_{\alpha,\beta} F_{\{ang\}}(\alpha,\beta) = \sum_{j=1}^{m} \left\| \vec{l}_j \cos(\theta_j) \right\|^2 = \sum_{j=1}^{m} (\vec{l}_j \cdot \vec{z}_p)^2 , \tag{7}$$

subject to the constraints pertinent to the achievable gantry angles of imaging system (which depend on different manufacture designs) $-120° < \alpha < 120°$, $-45° < \beta < 45°$, where "$\cdot$" denotes the inner product and θ_j is the angle between the directional vector $\vec{l}_j$ and projection vector $\vec{z}_p = [-\cos(\alpha)\sin(\beta), -\sin(\alpha), \cos(\alpha)\cos(\beta)]^t$. The gradient of the objective function $F_{\{ang\}}(\alpha,\beta)$ is defined as follows:

$$\frac{\delta F}{\delta \alpha} = \sum_{j=1}^{m} 2\omega_j \cdot (\sin(\alpha)\sin(\beta) \cdot l_{j_z} - \cos(\alpha) \cdot l_{j_y} - \sin(\alpha)\cos(\beta) \cdot l_{j_z}) \tag{8}$$

$$\frac{\delta F}{\delta \beta} = \sum_{j=1}^{m} 2\omega_j \cdot (-\cos(\alpha)\cos(\beta) \cdot l_{j_z} - \cos(\alpha)\sin(\beta) \cdot l_{j_z}) \tag{9}$$

where

$$\omega_j = -\cos(\alpha)\sin(\beta) \cdot l_{j_x} - \sin(\alpha) \cdot l_{j_y} + \cos(\alpha)\cos(\beta) \cdot l_{j_z},$$

By use of Eq. (7), the gantry orientation in terms of $\tilde{\alpha}$ and $\tilde{\beta}$ minimizing the vessel foreshortening will be determined. With the calculated gantry orientation, a sequence of positions of gantry can be obtained each of which lies onto a plane Γ defined by the direction vector of SID at $\tilde{\alpha}$ and $\tilde{\beta}$ angles and the tangential vector of the segment of interest as shown in Figure 9. A series projections of the 3-D coronary model will be produced based on the calculated gantry positions with minimal vessel foreshortening among which the optimal views minimizing vessel overlap can be selected visually to facilitate subsequent image acquisition.

Experimental results

The accuracy of the method described above was evaluated by use of angiograms of a Johnson & Johnson intra-coronary wire with markers of 15 mm inter-distance acquired from Philips Integris H 3000 single-plane imaging system with the movement of table and no ECG-triggering acquisition as shown in Figure 10 (a) and (b). The gantry parameters associated with the two views were 99 cm SID, 57° LAO, 2° CAUD, and 107 cm SID, 5° RAO, 33° CRAN, respectively. Eight markers (in terms of 2-D points) along with the wire (in term of a 2-D curve) were first manually identified on both images. With the identified marker points, the transformation that characterized the two views was calculated. Afterwards, the 3-D intra-coronary guide wire was reconstructed by use of the technique as described in Section 2.4. Based on the calculated 3-D information, the length of intra-coro-

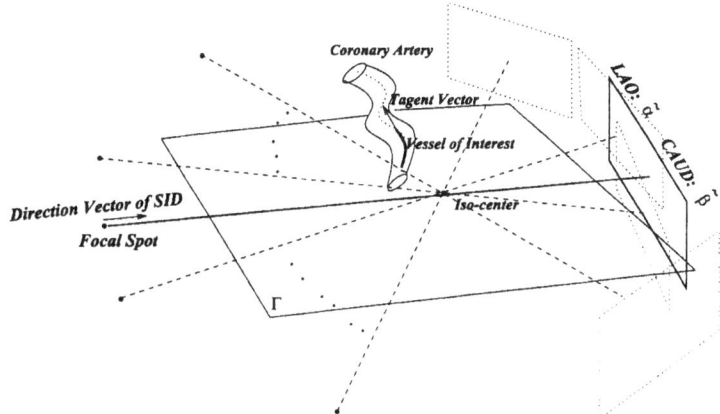

Figure 9. A series projections of 3-D model minimizing foreshortening of vessel of interest and associated gantry orientations are produced for visually selection of optimal views with minimal vessel overlap.

nary guide wire between the *a* and *g* markers was calculated as 102.75 mm resulting in 2.1% error relative to the actual length 105 mm.

Angiograms of more than 120 cases acquired from a single-plane system have been completed for 3-D reconstruction. The transformation were first determined without the need of calibration object, and the 3-D coronary arterial trees were reconstructed including left coronary, right coronary, and bypass graft systems. Among these studies, two typical examples were chosen for demonstration. In Figures 11(a) and 11(b), a pair of right coronary angiograms were employed. The reconstructed 3-D right coronary arterial tree were shown in Figures 11(c)–11(f). The reconstructed 3-D left coronary arterial tree as shown in Figures 12(c)–12(f) were obtained by use of the pair of single-plane angiograms as shown in Figures 12(a) and 12(b).

In Figure 13(a), it shows a selected arterial segment of interest (11.7 mm) on the projection image reproduced from the 3-D coronary model with 19% foreshortening based on the gantry angulations 11.6° RAO and 36.2° CRAN. After the processing of optimal view determination, there will be multiple choices for 0% foreshortening among which 5 views were selected for illustration as shown in Figures 14(b)-(f). The views in Figures 14(b) and

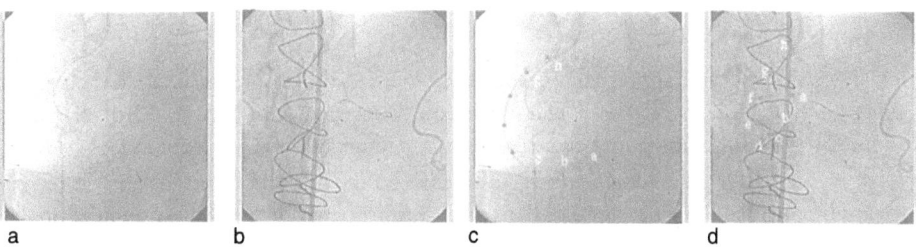

a   b   c   d

Figure 10. (a)(b) The two angiograms of intra-coronary guide wire acquired from a single-plane system based on the angulations 57˚ LAO, 2˚CAUD and 5˚ RAO, 33˚ CRAN. (c)(d) The identified markers a to h and the curve segment of wire.

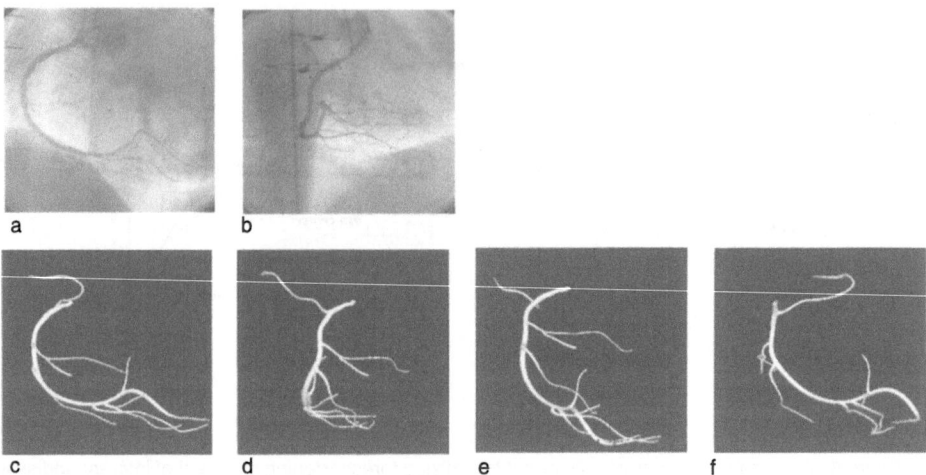

Figure 11. (a)(b) The employed first (48° LAO, 0° CAUD) and second views (15° RAO, 20° CRAN) of right coronary artery angiograms. (c)-(f) The reconstructed RCA coronary tree viewing at 4 different angles.

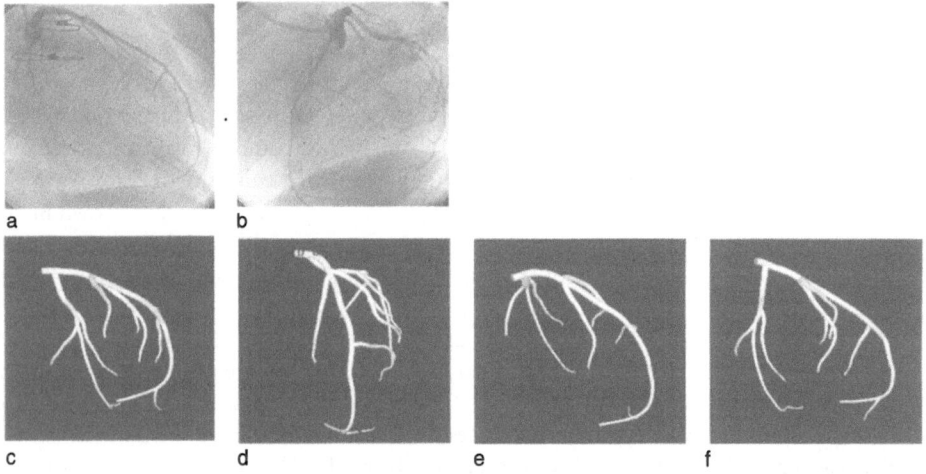

Figure 12. (a)(b) The employed first (36° RAO, 0° CAUD) and second views (89° LAO, 0° CAUD) of left coronary artery angiograms. (c)-(f) The reconstructed LCA coronary tree viewing at 4 different angles.

(c), however, were not appreciated due to excessive vessel overlap and unachievable gantry angle (99.8° LAO), respectively. The projections associated with Figures 13(d)–(f) can be adopted for guiding subsequent acquisitions in the interventional procedure.

In Figure 14(a), the arterial segment of interest on the projection image was selected corresponding to the coronary stenosis (length of 8 mm) based on the gantry angulations 55° RAO and 3.5° CAUD. After the optimal view processing, five views with 0% foreshortening among multiple calculated projections were employed as illustrated in Figures 14(b)–(f). The views associated with Figures 14(b) and (c) will not be adopted for its excessive vessel overlap relative to the segment of interest and unachievable gantry angle at 60.5° CRAN,

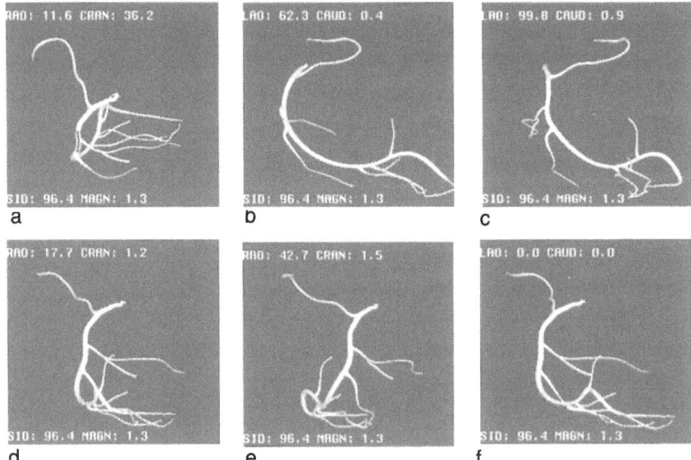

Figure 13. (a) The selected segment of interest (11.7 mm) with 19% foreshortening based on gantry angulation (11.6°RAO, 36.2° CRAN). (b) Unappreciated view with 0% foreshortening due to intensive vessel overlap. (c) Unachievable gantry angle at 99.8°RAO with 0% foreshortening. (d)–(f) Views with 0% foreshortening and minimal vessel overlap adequate to be utilized for subsequent image acquisitions.

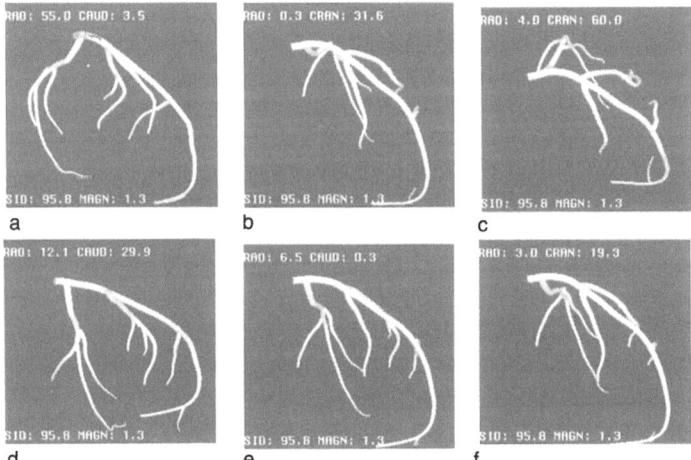

Figure 14. (a) The selected segment of interest (8 mm) with 30% foreshortening based on gantry angulation (55° RAO, 3.5° CAUD). (b) Unappreciated view with 0% foreshortening due to intensive vessel overlap. (c) Unachievable gantry angle at 60.5°CRAN with 0% foreshortening. (d)–(f) Views with 0% foreshortening and minimal vessel overlap adequate to be utilized for subsequent image acquisitions.

respectively. The remaining views demonstrate minimal vessel overlap and 0% foreshortening with respect to the segment of interest as shown in Figures 14(d)–(f) and can be utilized to facilitate further clinical diagnosis.

Concluding remarks

A method has been developed for on-line reconstruction of a patient-specific 3-D coronary arterial tree from routine angiograms acquired at arbitrary angles and without using calibration objects based on single-plane imaging system. More than 120 cases of coronary arterial trees have undergone for 3-D reconstruction including left coronary artery trees, right coronary artery trees, and bypass grafts among which more than 40 cases were performed in-room of our cardiac catheterization laboratory. A validation confirmed the accuracy of 3-D length measurement to within 2.1% error using actual angiograms of intra-coronary guide wire. The length of employed wire is 105 mm with 8 markers of 15 mm inter-distance. The choice of an optimal view of the vasculature of interest can be achieved on the basis of the capability of rotating the reconstructed 3-D coronary arterial tree. Such a unique capability thus provides an optimal visualization strategy that should lead to more efficient and successful diagnostic and therapeutic procedures in assessment of lesion length and diameter narrowing.

Acknowledgment

This project is supported by the Whitaker Foundation. The help of Dr. Bertron M. Groves in providing the angiograms, Keith E. Hellman in implementing the graphical user interface for image transfer, and Dr. Senhu Li in editing this manuscript is greatly appreciated.

References

1.   Kim HC, Min BG, Lee TS *et al.* Three-dimensional digital subtraction angiography. IEEE Trans Med Imaging. 1982;1:152-8.
2.   Parker DL, Pope DL, Van Bree R, Marshall HW. Three-dimensional reconstruction of moving arterial beds from digital subtraction angiography. Comput Biomed Res 1987;20:166-85.
3.   Kitamura K, Tobis JM, Sklansky J. Estimating the three-dimensional skeletons and transverse areas of coronary arteries from biplane angiograms. IEEE Trans Med Imaging 1988;7:173-87.
4.   Saito T, Misaki M, Shirato K, Takishima T. Three-dimensional quantitative coronary angiography. IEEE Trans Biomed Eng 1990;37:768-77.
5.   Pellot CP, Herment A, Sigelle M, Horain P, Maitre H, Peronneau P. A 3D reconstruction of vascular structures from two x-ray angiograms using an adapted simulated annealing algorithm. IEEE Trans Med Imaging 1994;13:48-60.
6.   Guggenheim N, Doriot PA, Dorsaz PA, Descouts P, Rutishauser W. Spatial reconstruction of coronary arteries from angiographic images. Phys Med Biol 1991;36:99-110.
7.   Seiler C, Kirkeeide RL, Gould KL. Basic structure-function relations of the epicardial coronary vascular tree. Basis of quantitative coronary arteriography for diffuse coronary artery disease. Circulation 1991;85:1987-2003.
8.   Coatrieux JL, Rong J, Collorec R. A framework for automatic analysis of the dynamic behaviour of coronary angiograms. Int J Card Imaging 1992;8:1-10.
9.   Yanagihara Y, Hashimoto T, Sugahara T, Sugimoto N. A new method for automatic identification of coronary arteries in standard biplane angiograms. Int J Card Imaging 1994;10:253-61.
10.   Dumay ACM, Reiber JHC, Gerbrands JJ. Determination of optimal angiographic viewing angles: basic principles and evaluation study. IEEE Trans Med Imaging 1994;13:13-24.
11.   Wahle A, Wellnhofer E, Mugaragu I, Sauer HU, Oswald H, Fleck E. Assessment of diffuse coronary artery disease by quantitative analysis of coronary morphology based upon 3-D reconstruction from biplane angiograms. IEEE Trans Med Imaging 1995;14:230-41.

12. Nguyen TV, Sklansky J. Reconstructing the 3-D medial axes of coronary arteries in single-view cineangio-grams. IEEE Trans Med Imaging 1994;13:61-73.

13. Marcus ML, Dellsperger KC. Determinants of systolic and diastolic ventricular function. In: Marcus ML, Skorton DJ, Schelbert HR, Wolf GL, editors. Cardiac imaging. Philadelphia: Saunders; 1991. p. 24-38.

14. Stansfield S. ANGI: A rule based expert system for automatic segmentation of coronary vessels from digital subtracted angiograms. IEEE Trans Pattern Anal Machine Intelligence 1986;8:188-99.

15. Smets C, Van de werf F, Suetens P, Oosterlinck A. An expert system for the labeling and 3D reconstruction of the coronary arteries from two projections. Int J Card Imaging 1990;5:145-54.

16. Garreau M, Coatrieux JL, Collorec R, Chardenon C. A knowledge-based approach for 3-D reconstruction and labeling of vascular networks from biplane angiographic projections. IEEE Trans Med Imaging 1991;10:122-31.

17. Coppini G, Demi M, Mennini R, Valli G. Three-dimensional knowledge driven reconstruction of coronary trees. Med Biol Eng Comput 1991;29:535-42.

18. Delaere D, Smets C, Suetens P, Marchal G, Van de Werf F. Knowledge-based system for the three-dimensional reconstruction of blood vessels from two angiographic projections. Med Biol Eng Comput 1991;29:ns27-36.

19. Fessler JA, Macovski A. Object-based 3-D reconstruction of arterial trees from magnetic resonance angiograms. IEEE Trans Med Imaging 1991;10:25-39.

20. Liu IH, Sun Y. Fully automated reconstruction of 3-dimensional vascular tree structures from two orthogonal views using computational algorithms and production rules. Opt Eng 1992;31:2197-207.

21. Rougee A, Picard C, Sanit-Felix D, Trousset Y, Moll T, Amiel M. Three- dimensional coronary arteriography. Int J Card Imaging 1994;10:67-70.

22. Yen BL, Huang TS. Determining 3-D motion and structure of a rigid body using the spherical projection. Comput Vis Graph Image Processing 1983;21:21-32.

23. Longuet-Higgins HC. A computer algorithm for reconstructing a scene from two projections. Nature 1981;293:133-5.

24. Tsai RY, Huang TS. Uniqueness and estimation of 3-dimensional motion parameters of rigid objects with curved surfaces. IEEE Trans Pattern Anal Machine Intelligence 1984;6:13-27.

25. Fang JQ, Huang TS. Some experiments on estimating the 3-D motion parameters of a rigid body from two consecutive image frames. IEEE Trans Pattern Anal Machine Intelligence 1984;6:545-54.

26. Philip J, Estimation of 3-dimensional motion of rigid objects from noisy observations. IEEE Trans Pattern Anal Machine Intelligence 1991;13:61-6.

27. Metz CE, Fencil LE. Determination of three-dimensional structure in biplane radiography without prior knowledge of the relationship between the two views: theory. Med Phys 1989;16:45-51.

28. Fencil LE, Metz CE. Propagation and reduction of error in three-dimensional structure determined from biplane views of unknown orientation. Med Phys 1990;17:951-61.

29. Weng J, Huang TS, Ahuja N. A two-step approach to optimal motion and structure estimation. In: Proceedings of IEEE Workshop on Computer Vision 1987;355-7.

30. Weng JY, Ahuja N, Huang TS. Closed-form solution and maximum likelihood: a robust approach to motion and structure estimation. In: Proceedings of IEEE Conference on Computer Vision and Pattern Recognition. Washington: IEEE; 1988. p. 381-6.

31. Weng JY, Huang TS, Ahuja N. Motion and structure from two perspective view: algorithms, error analysis and error estimation. IEEE Trans Pattern Anal Machine Intelligence 1989;11:451-76.

32. Weng JY, Ahuja N, Huang TS. Optimal motion and structure estimation. IEEE Trans Pattern Anal Machine Intelligence 1993;15:864-84.

33. Chen SYJ, Hoffmann KR, Carroll JD. Three-dimensional reconstruction of coronary arterial tree based on biplane angiograms. Proc SPIE 1996;2710:103-14.

34. Bartels RH, Beatty JC, Barsky BA. An introduction to splines for use in computer graphics and geometric modeling. Morgan Kaufmann Publishers Inc., Los Altos, California. San Francisco: Morgan Kaufmann; 1996.

35. Chen SYJ, Metz CE. Improved determination of biplane imaging geometry from two projection images and its application to three-dimensional reconstruction of coronary arterial trees. Med Phys 1997;24:633-54.

36. Keating TJ, Wolf PR, Scarpace FL. An improved method of digital image correlation. Photogrammetric Eng Remote Sensing 1975;41:993-1002.

5.　Quantitative coronary ultrasound: state of the art

Jouke Dijkstra, Andreas Wahle, Gerhard Koning, Johan H.C. Reiber & Milan Sonka

Summary

Intravascular Ultrasound (IVUS) provides real-time high resolution images of the arterial wall. By performing a three-dimensional reconstruction, it permits an advanced assessment of the vessel, lumen and wall morphology. Recently, the straight stacking of the IVUS images has been extended by a geometrically correct orientation of the images in 3D space, using biplane angiographic images. Quantification of IVUS images, both in 2D and 3D, requires segmentation of the images. Automated segmentation of IVUS images for quantitative analysis reduces the required time and the subjectivity of boundary tracing. Different segmentation approaches for 2D and 3D IVUS are discussed, including the commercially available packages for analysis of IVUS images. Furthermore different approaches for the 3D reconstruction including the use of biplane angiographic images are discussed. This chapters finishes with a discussion about the future directions of IVUS including the developments in the area of RF-data analysis and the developments of new devices.

Introduction

The assessment of arterial geometry is of paramount importance in the clinical evaluation of patients with ischemic heart disease. For many years, coronary angiography has been a widely accepted method for arterial geometry assessment. Recently, intravascular ultrasound imaging (IVUS) was introduced as a complement to angiography. Conventional angiography-based measurements on single vessel segments (QCA) may not assess the severity of diffuse coronary disease in its early stage [1] and cannot assess plaque composition [2]. In one study of angiographically normal segments, the mean percent area stenosis detected by intravascular ultrasound was $35 \pm 23\%$ [3]. Atherosclerotic plaque is frequently complex and eccentric and the bulk or extent of disease in the vessel cannot be accurately determined from a limited number of angiographic projections. Angiography may overestimate lumen areas after percutaneous coronary angioplasty (PTCA) due to presence of fractured plaque and irregular and rough inside wall surfaces [4], and cannot predict plaque fracture locations which may result from PTCA [5].

IVUS has the additional advantage of permitting assessment of plaque and wall compliance, which may be of importance in assessing the propensity for dissection or in prediction of lesion and wall behavior during balloon stretching. Such information may be particularly useful in choosing which of several available treatment devices would be best suited for a

J.H.C. Reiber and E.E. van der Wall (eds.). What's New in Cardiovascular Imaging, 79–94.
©1998 Kluwer Academic Publishers.

particular vessel and may serve for patient risk assessment and prediction of treatment success. Other, as yet unexplored uses of IVUS are to investigate the disease progression and regression of minimally diseased vessels, the effects of lesion distribution (eccentricity), lesion composition (fibrous, cellular, calcific), and aging on arterial biomechanical properties, and the effects of these properties on the immediate and long-term results of catheter interventions.

Analysis of intravascular ultrasound images is frequently performed by interactive manual measurements of cross-sectional vessel parameters and manual tracing of wall and residual lumen borders. Inter- and intra-observer variability of such measurements is high [6]. IVUS produces a large number of cross-sectional images for the coronary segment of interest. With image locations 0.1 mm apart and just 10 images per cardiac cycle, 1000 images must be analyzed for a 10 mm vessel segment. Manual analysis of these images is tedious, time consuming, and really unpractical for more than a single experiment.

Three-dimensional reconstruction of IVUS [7] permits a more advanced assessment of the vessel, lumen and plaque morphology. Measurement of the plaque area in an entire coronary segment may provide more detail in the complex plaque architecture than in single transversal IVUS images and avoids the difficult mental conception process [8]. Another important limitation of 2D IVUS during studies is the matching of target sites for measurements at the same particular points due to the lack of the third dimension. Recently, the straight stacking of the IVUS images has been extended by a geometrically correct orientation of the images in 3D space, using angiographic images of the catheter during the pullback [9-11]. In this way, volumetric analyses can be performed under consideration of the vessel curvature as well.

Three-dimensional IVUS also permits appropriate sizing of stents (diameter and length), and may help to reduce the frequency of procedural complications of high-pressure stenting [12]. The changes in cross-sectional lumen area in a stent in a pull-back series are often smooth and gradual and may therefore be more difficult to recognize by visual assessment of 2D IVUS images [13]. This explains the overestimation of the minimum in-stent lumen area by 2D IVUS compared with 3D IVUS [14]. By use of 3D IVUS, the spatial geometry of coronary stents can be reconstructed accurately [15], and automated measurement of lumen area by 3D IVUS facilitates the detection of stent under-expansion.

This chapter provides an overview of the current state-of-the-art in intravascular ultrasound image analysis. First the main principles of several existing approaches for automated or semi-automated analysis of 2D and 3D IVUS images and image sequences are discussed. Then, several commercially available IVUS acquisition and analysis systems are described. Next, new approaches to geometrically correct 3D reconstruction are introduced that use data fusion of geometric information from biplane angiography and cross-sectional image data from IVUS pullback sequences. The chapter concludes with a discussion of expected future directions of IVUS research and clinical usage.

Intravascular ultrasound image analysis approaches

Quantification, in 2D and 3D, as well as volume rendering for the visualization of the IVUS images require segmentation of the images. The vessel consists of several layers: the intima, the media and the adventitia as shown in Figure 1. The lumen is identified by the region

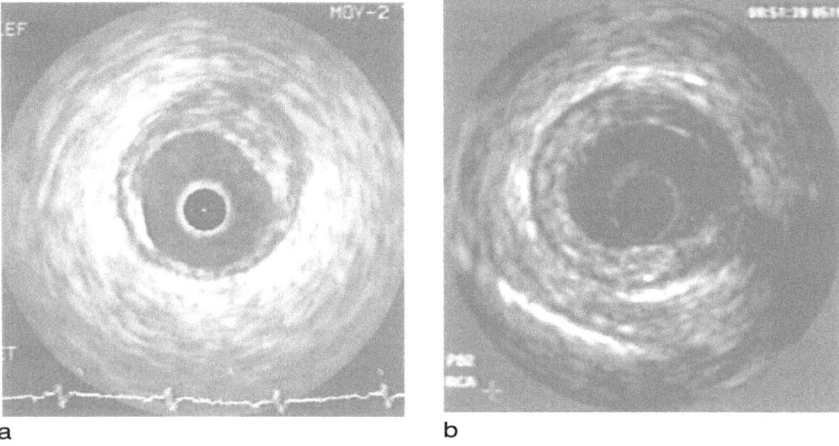

Figure 1. Typical images of the three-layer appearance visualized by a mechanical rotating device (a) and a solid state device (b).

inside the interface between blood and the intima, defined by the leading edge of the lumen-intima interface. The vessel is commonly defined by the region inside the interface between the media and adventitia, defined by the leading edge of the media-adventitia interface.

A potential problem in image segmentation is that features are determined which clinically and ultrasonically do not reflect reality. This can be avoided by keeping in mind the physics of the image formation process and the basics of ultrasound [16]. According to these physics it can be concluded that only leading edges should be used for measurement. Electronically, they correspond to the beginning of the echo pulse. The position of a trailing edge is dependent upon the characteristics of the point spread function (PSF) of the system, since it is convolved with the echo pulse. Any layer of thickness of the order of the wavelength (50 m for 30 MHz transducers) is rendered as wide as the radial resolution, which is three to four times higher. This thickening of any distinct interface is sometimes called the "blooming effect". Due to this artifact, the intima is represented by an overestimated thickness, and consequently the media is represented by a lower thickness than is to be expected from corresponding histologic data. For this reason the plaque is measured by the combination of intima and media, because they often can not be measured separately.

Analysis of two-dimensional IVUS data

Development of computerized techniques for 2D IVUS analysis started in the early nineties. In most cases, single-frame 2D methods became the core of more complex 3D and 4D IVUS analysis methods. These approaches are discussed later on.

Segmentation approaches developed by Herrington et al.

In 1992, Herrington and Snyder of the Bowman Gray School of Medicine developed a segmentation method based on Simulated Annealing. First, the IVUS image is resampled along an interactively marked region of interest (ROI) close to the expected border [17]. The array is filtered by convolution with a 7x7 operator, which combines an unidirectional mean filter in horizontal direction with a unidirectional gradient edge filter in vertical orientation. Thus, the array is smoothed in the horizontal direction while the edges are extracted in the vertical direction. Afterwards, the Simulated Annealing is applied to this array using recirculant multilayer graphs [18]. In their compensated simulated annealing approach, they introduced constraints derived from the a-priori knowledge, e.g. a smoothness of the border as well as the fact that the leading border elements are marked by the brightest pixels. The derived set of optimum points is transformed back from the array into the original image by inverting the resampling function. No validation results have been reported.

Segmentation approaches developed by Meier et al.

Meier *et al.* (Cleveland, Ohio, USA) [19] developed fully automated segmentation of lumen-intima and media-adventitia boundaries in 2D IVUS images of human coronary arteries recorded in-vitro. The methods consisted of three steps:

1. Transforming of the image to the original polar format of the image data. Speckle noise reduction was performed by repeated non-linear filtering, followed by contrast enhancement which was based on local column-wise histogram stretching.
2. Segmentation of the image was carried out using three different methods for comparison: 1) radial scanning for the first occurrence of gray-level gradient values above a fixed threshold; 2) adaptive region growing from luminal seed points; and 3) cost minimization approach which involves an iterative search for connected series of outline points.
3. Filtering of the detected contours to remove dropout sectors, edge pixels values below a selected threshold and guidewire shadows.

For validation purposes, the luminal cross-sectional areas of the manual and the automatically detected lumen contours were computed and compared. Radial scanning showed the best overall agreement (-7.7 ± 11.7%), region growing a tendency towards underestimation (-10.9 ± 9.0%), while dynamic contours showed the highest standard deviation for lumen area (4.1 ± 21.5%). They concluded that computationally intensive concepts such as region growing and dynamic contours for fully automatically contour detection did not perform better than the radial edge scanning technique with a fixed threshold.

ADDER

A fully automatic edge detection technique, based on adaptive active contour models (snakes) was developed by Maurincomme *et al.* (Lyon, France) [20]. It is called ADDER (Adaptive Damping Dependent on Echographic Regions) and allows the quantitation of the vascular lumen area. The system was validated using 53 normal and pathological arterial segments (from coronary, renal, splenic, iliac and carotid arteries). The imaging was done in-vitro using 20 and 30 MHz mechanically rotated transducers. The images were analyzed with ADDER, as well as by two experts who manually traced the luminal contours. The intra-observer variabilities for the lumen areas were -1.7 ± 3.3% for one and 1.3 ± 6.5% for the other expert. The inter-observer variability was 2.1 ± 4.3%. The correlation between the automatically found lumen area and the manual lumen area was r=0.99. They concluded that ADDER was a useful tool in clinical research. However it was evaluated in-vitro and it could only be used for the lumen boundary. The question remains how snakes perform in in-vivo images containing speckle noise and artifacts.

Texture-based IVUS segmentation developed by Mojsilovic et al.

Texture-based IVUS segmentation developed by Mojsilovic *et al.* (University of Belgrade) does not require explicit definition of a region of interest [21]. In contrast to other methods, the IVUS images do not need resampling.

For each pixel in the image, its features are extracted using an area of 0.68 mm in a square surrounding the respective pixel (15x15). The first measure is the horizontal fraction of image in runs value (FOIIR), which indicates the presence of texture in the specific area. The second measure is the mean gray level (MGL) over all pixels of this area. Afterwards, histograms are calculated for both measures. The authors use the FOIIR and MGL distributions to distinguish lumen from plaque and media from the adventitia regions, respectively. For each of the histograms, a threshold is iteratively determined to discriminate the three regions "lumen", "plaque", and "adventitia" best, thus maximizing their interclass variances. The contours of the regions are refined after the segmentation process, closing possible holes using a connectivity constraint, and eliminating rough structures by repeated morphological opening.

The method was validated by comparison of the automatically detected with manually traced borders in 39 in-vivo images of selected patients. Good correlation (r=0.99) was reported for the areas enclosed by the luminal and media-adventitial borders, respectively. However, the authors admit that the horizontal FOIIR and MGL measures result from a compromise of reliability and performance, and that other operators or their combination may yield better results.

Three-dimensional analysis of IVUS image sequences

The basic processing steps to 3D analyze IVUS pullback sequences and obtain a 3D reconstruction from the 2D IVUS images are similar for all systems reported below. The catheter is placed distal to the stenosis and pulled back through the arterial segment of interest, while at the same time images are being digitized and stored in computer memory (pullback series).

The most common approach is the motorized continuous-speed pullback device (common speed is 0.5 to 1.0 mm/sec) and continuous acquisition of IVUS images resulting in an equidistant spacing of adjacent images [22]. Cyclic cardiac motion artifacts (longitudinal and transversal movement), catheter twist (rotational artifacts), arterial deformation (the percent change in lumen cross-sectional area during a cardiac cycle can be up to 14 ± 5%), and differences in slice-orientation are some of the artifacts which affect the quality of the resulting 3D reconstruction as are shown in Figure 2 [23,24]. Another approach uses ECG-triggered IVUS frame marking and acquisition during uniform pullback of the IVUS catheter and is used for off-line 3D reconstruction and quantification. In this way, the influence of the cardiac motion as well as the systolic-diastolic artifacts is minimized.A more complete approach is the ECG-triggered pullback device in combination with an ECG-gated image acquisition system [25] (Echoscan, TomTec, Munich, Germany). A maximum of 25 IVUS images per cardiac cycle can be sampled, after which the catheter is pulled back in constant increments with a stepping motor.

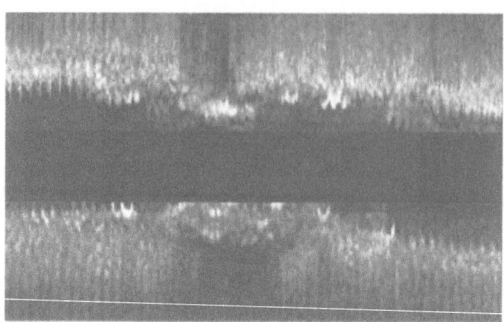

Figure 2. Non-ECG gated pullback series with typical motion artefacts.

Thoraxcenter approach to IVUS data analysis

The Thoraxcenter contour detection system (Rotterdam, The Netherlands) uses a combination of transversal and longitudinal contour detection. The semi-automated contour detection is based on a model of the contours and uses the minimal cost algorithm (MCA) [26]. The semi-automatic contour detection approach consists of three steps:
1. Two perpendicular cut planes through the voxel space are interactively selected which are parallel to the longitudinal axis. The angle and location of the cut planes can be changed by the user to obtain optimal quality of the longitudinal images.
2. Contours of the lumen and plaque in the longitudinal images are determined and manually edited.
3. The transformation of the contours from the two longitudinal planes to the transversal plane results in four pre-defined points for each cross-section. These points indicate the cross-sectional contour positions. Dynamic-programming based border detection is performed in radially-resampled IVUS images.

The in-vitro validation of this method was done in a tubular phantom consisting of four segments with luminal diameters between 2 and 5 mm. A correlation of r=0.99 was found between the 3D lumen area measurements, volume measurements, and the true values. The in-vivo measurements performed in atherosclerotic coronary arteries of 20 patients showed a high correlation with those obtained by the observers (r=0.95-0.98 for areas, r=0.99 for volumes). The standard deviations of the between-measurement differences of the lumen, total vessel, and plaque measurements did not exceed 2.7, 0.7 and 2.8% for the volume and 7.3, 4.4 and 10.8% for the area measurements, respectively [8]. A version of the contour-detection-based analysis software has been customized for use with the EchoScan system (TomTec, Munich, Germany).

Iowa approach to three-dimensional IVUS analysis

The Iowa method [27,28] automatically identifies the plaque/media interface (internal lamina, internal wall border), media/adventitia interface (external lamina, external wall border), and the plaque/lumen interface (plaque border). Due to the use of a priori information about 2D and 3D anatomy of coronary vessels and ultrasound imaging physics, the method can automatically determine vessel wall morphology and plaque volumes (Figure 3). Two key aspects of the approach are:

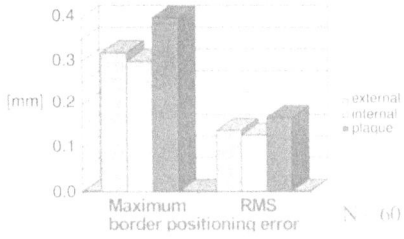 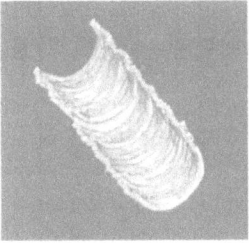 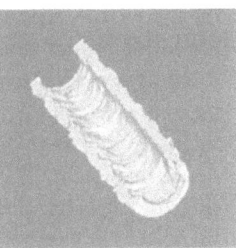

Figure 3. Semi-automated analysis of 3D IVUS pullback sequences. a) Border positioning errors in in-vivo ECG-gated pullback sequences. b) Computer-determined coronary wall in a non-gated in-vivo pullback sequence after atherectomy intervention. c) Computer-identified plaque in the same pullback.

1. Graph searching is utilized to identify globally optimal borders.
2. A priori information is incorporated into the border detection process through the computation of local cost values. In particular, to identify the position of the internal and external wall borders, the method searches for edge triplets representing the leading and trailing edges of the laminae echoes. The interactively defined elliptical shape of the ROI serves as a model of the preferred vessel shape. Knowledge of the vessel wall thickness is also used to constraint the search for the external and internal wall borders.

To facilitate a fully automated 3D analysis of IVUS pullback image sequences, the region of interest in which the borders are determined must be automatically identified after which the 3D border detection is performed. A 3D border detection algorithm was designed that uses contextual information to estimate ROI size and position changes in the successive frames. The general steps of the 3D IVUS segmentation algorithm are as follows: 1) A single elliptic region of interest is interactively identified in the first image of the pullback sequence. 2) Inside the ROI, internal and external wall, and plaque borders are automatically identified using the graph-search based segmentation approach [27]. In subsequent images, current ROIs are automatically determined from the computer-detected borders in the preceding image frames.

Figure 3 shows examples of automated border detection in an IVUS image sequence. The automated method was carefully validated and showed high accuracy in cadaveric and in-vivo IVUS images and image pullback sequences. Lumen and plaque area measurements correlated well with those determined manually by expert observers (r=0.98, y=1.01 x+1.51; r=0.94, y=1.06 x-0.09; respectively). Root-mean-square wall and plaque border positioning errors were under 0.15 mm.

LUMC contour detection system

The Leiden University Medical Center (LUMC, Leiden, The Netherlands) contour detection approach is also based on a combination of transversal and longitudinal contour detection. The (semi-)automated contour detection is based on the model guided contour detection using the minimum cost algorithm (MCA) that allows the detection of not only the leading intimal edge, but also of the external vascular boundary that corresponds to the external elastic lamina [27,29].

The cost values for the lumen-intima interface are produced by a combination of spatial first- and second-derivative gradient filters and local gray value properties. The cost values for the media-adventitia interface is based on the strength of the leading edge of the media-adventitia border and depending on the image quality, the presence of the trailing edges of the intima-media border and media-adventitia border [27]. The contour detection is based on a simultaneous contour detection of the lumen and vessel contours [30]. The basic steps for the (semi-)automatic contour detection are the same as for the Thoraxcenter contour detection system. Major differences are that the number of longitudinal images is not fixed, the cost values are determined in a different way, and the detected contours in the adjacent images are used solely as an indication of the contour location. In order to use all the information provided by the user, the contours which were defined by the user in the transversal images are used to guide the longitudinal contour detection. The complete analysis system will be embedded in a DICOM viewer (CMS-VIEW, MEDIS medical imaging systems, Leiden, the Netherlands). Validation of this method is ongoing.

Commercially available software packages for analysis of IVUS images:

EchoQuant

The acoustic quantification system (EchoQuant, INDEC, Capitola, CA) uses a pattern recognition algorithm to detect the blood-pool inside the lumen followed by 3D segmentation and reconstruction [13,31]. The quality of the automated detection can be corrected manually in the individual cross-sectional images. It requires no geometric assumption of the lumen shape and may therefore provide accurate detection of an irregular shaped lumen. The quality of the original IVUS image can greatly influence the results of the segmentation and it is not capable of detecting the vessel boundary. The system was validated in 29 aortal segments of rabbits [32]. Lumen area measurements by repeated automated analyses, and automated and manual analyses showed a high correlation (r=0.97 for both) and differences of 1 ± 10% and -2 ± 10% respectively. The correlation between the quantitative angiographic measurements and automated 3D IVUS measurements was high (r=0.93). The between-measurements difference was 7 ± 14%.

The validation at the Thoraxcenter in Rotterdam was performed by comparing the 3D IVUS measurements in 38 coronary stents with results obtained by conventional 2D IVUS and both geometric and videodensitometric quantitative coronary angiography [31]. The 3D IVUS measurements resulted in slightly smaller lumen areas than the 2D IVUS measurements (8.1 ± 2.7 mm^2 vs. 8.3 ± 2.5 mm^2, NS); the correlation between the measurements by 3D and 2D IVUS was high (r=0.81). Measurements by 3D IVUS showed a higher correlation with videodensitometry (r=0.70) than with geometric quantitative coronary arteriography (r=0.58).

EchoScan

EchoScan (TomTec, Munich, Germany) uses a combined ECG-gated image acquisition station and a dedicated pullback device (stepping motor). It is a sophisticated and accurate way to overcome the problem of cyclic motion artifacts. The time needed for the image acquisition is somewhat longer than for a continuous pullback acquisition; each time a cycle is stored, the following heart beat is required to perform a pull-back step in order to reach the adjacent scanning site [31]. The ECG-gated system can display the arterial segment in 3D and vascular dimensions can be measured at any point in the cardiac cycle. Up to 25 IVUS images per cardiac cycle can be sampled which permits dynamic visualization of coronary segments during an entire cardiac cycle ('4D IVUS'). The segmentation is based on the definition of gray level thresholds and therefore is affected by the image quality. The 3D reconstruction does not incorporate the vessel curvature.

Oracle imaging system

The Oracle Imaging System and In-vision option (EndoSonics Cooperation, Rancho Cordavo, CA, USA) is capable of processing the information from the Visions 64 electronic imaging catheters [33]. The mobile system consists of a high quality monitor, S-VHS VCR and multi-image display including fluoroscopic images. The images of a pullback series (at the moment a video-loop of one minute) can be stored in digital format onto a CD-Recordable, so they may be played back without loss of image quality. Another feature of the system is the sagittal view and the Chromaflow option for blood flow imaging. The system does not support automated quantification of intravascular ultrasound images.

Galaxy intraluminal ultrasound system

The Boston Scientific Corporation (San Jose, CA) PC-based Intraluminal Ultrasound System *Galaxy* is replacing the previous generation ClearView ULTRA System. It is a console-based mobile unit housing a video monitor, S-VHS VCR, color printer and the necessary electronics to perform real time ultrasound imaging. It presents the following major improvements over the previous generation devices: multiple image displays, longitudinal IVUS view representation, digital image storage and retrieval, patient data base connectivity, angiography video system compatibility, integrated motor drive and automatic pullback system, LAN and Internet interfaces. The system does not support automated quantification of intravascular ultrasound images.

IVUS quantitative analysis software

Technology Solutions Group (Snaker Heights, OH) developed an IVUS analysis package that is available in five options of increasing complexity. The advertised functionality includes semi-automated border detection of the lumen and media-adventitia borders, tissue characterization, catheter motion compensation, pullback visualization, and quantitative volumetric analysis.

Geometrically-correct approaches to 3D IVUS analysis

Commonly used systems for 3D reconstruction of the IVUS images are based on a sequential and straight stacking not considering vessel curvature. Although most algorithms have proven their high accuracy in phantom studies using straight objects [34], they inevitably fail in curved vessels [35]. In particular, there are two effects that have to be handled:
- Due to vessel *curvature*, the IVUS slices are no longer parallel. This distorts a volumetric analysis, because volume fragments at the inner side of the vessel related to its curvature will be overestimated and fragments on the outer side underestimated.

- Due to catheter *torsion*, the axial orientation of an ideal IVUS catheter within the vessel is no longer constant. The torsion is zero only if the vessel lies within a plane (even with curvature present). Whenever the vessel moves outside this plane, the catheter axially twists, and this rotation must be considered in the 3D reconstruction.

The actual vessel course may be determined from the 3D reconstruction of the catheter path, e.g. from biplane angiography that is used for IVUS guidance anyway. At the German Heart Institute of Berlin, a comprehensive reconstruction system has been developed, which provides 3D models of the inner lumen in high accuracy [36]. Among other tasks, this system was applied to extend the Seiler approach for diffuse diseases considerably [37].

For the problem of extracting the IVUS catheter from its biplane projections, it is sufficient to reconstruct a single line in 3D without cross-sectional information. A single point which is visible in both projections can be reconstructed by calculating its projection rays in 3D from the known imaging geometry (Figure 4).

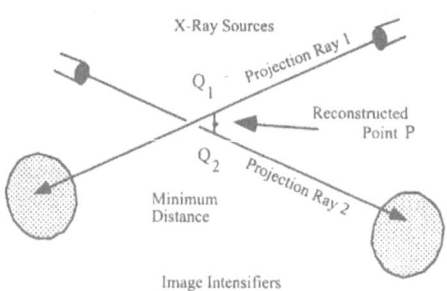

Figure 4. 3D reconstruction of a point P from its 2D projections from the spatial locations of the X-ray sources and the points of impacts on the image intensifiers; the rays are reconstructed for each projection p; the weighted mean of the points Qp on the rays, marking their minimum distance, is the reconstructed 3D point P.

Approaches for IVUS-angiography image fusion

Reconstruction system of Evans et al.

The MacKay approach [38] to reconstruct the location of the IVUS tip from a complete sequence of angiograms taken during the pullback procedure was used by the Evans group (Chicago, IL) [9]. In this way, they could directly match the 3D location of the tip with the IVUS image generated at the same time. While the vessel curvature could be followed accurately, the potential torsion of the vessel has been neglected. The authors describe the twisting by comparing the trajectory within a torsion-free circular and a tortuous spiral phantom.

For the estimation of the actual imaging geometry, a cubic calibration object containing 27 steel markers in known locations is used. This cube is imaged before any other object is examined, and the imaging geometry must be frozen after this calibration step. Two constraints may hamper the clinical application of this method: the need of a calibration cube may disturb the clinical routine, and it may not be acceptable to keep the imaging geometry fixed over a longer period of time; the constant angiographic supervision may not be possible due to physical limitations of the X-ray system, and the additional exposure may not be acceptable for the patient.

The ANGUS system

The approach of the Thoraxcenter in Rotterdam (NL) considers both vessel curvature and torsion, and it only requires a single angiographic pair of images at the start of the pullback [10]. Assuming a constant pullback speed, which can be satisfactorily ensured by an automatic pullback considering both respiration and ECG phases [25], the location of the catheter tip is calculated as the distance along the catheter path from pullback start with respect to the actual time instance.

In contrast to the constant angiographic supervision of the Evans approach, the catheter path has to be reconstructed from a single pair for each time instance. It is assumed that the catheter tip follows the line that is projected at the beginning of the pullback, which is approximately true if a sheathed catheter is used. Here, the corresponding locations are extracted from the bundle of rays reconstructed from the catheter projections. The authors approximate the catheter pullback path by fitting a 3D Fourier function so that its projections onto the angiograms match the extracted 2D projection of the catheter best. The relative axial rotation of the images caused by the vessel torsion is considered analytically by using the 'Frenet frame' to calculate the twist between adjacent time instances. However, the absolute orientation of the IVUS data has to be determined too. This problem is comparable to fitting a sock to a leg: while the leg is fixed in course and orientation, the sock may be arbitrarily rotated around the leg. In the reported work, the absolute orientation was selected interactively using biplane projections of the 3D reconstruction and their comparison with the true angiographic projections.

The Iowa approach

At the University of Iowa, the catheter path is reconstructed from a single pair of angiograms at pullback start [11]. After dewarping of the angiograms and extraction of the catheter path in both projections, the 3D locations are reconstructed [39]. To achieve highest accuracy, the reconstruction is meanwhile performed by the system described in [36,37] . The use of a calibration object is needed only for size calibration. Since modern angiographic devices with digital output deliver most of the geometry parameters along with the images, the imaging geometry is refined from this initial data using a small number (2-5) of uniquely identifiable reference points. The correspondence between the projected elements of the pullback path is determined by a cost matrix approach with dynamic programming, interpolating pairs of 2D elements that are related to the same 3D locations optimally in a least square sense. The path is smoothed afterwards to reflect the stiffness of the catheter and to eliminate remaining small local inaccuracies.

After matching each IVUS frame with its corresponding location in 3D assuming a constant pullback speed, the relative twist is analytically calculated. For each pair of adjacent IVUS images, their tangent vectors are determined using the three surrounding consecutive points along the catheter path. The arc through these three points is a part of the circumscribed circle, whose center is determined as the intersection of the perpendicular bisectors of the tangent vectors. The orientation of image $i+1$ is determined by rotating image i around the normal vector of this triangle. Algorithms to solve the problem of absolute orientation are under development.

The method was validated in phantom studies and in cadaveric pig hearts. For the latter ones, performed in right coronary arteries, a typical pullback length was 100-120 mm, with a manual pullback speed of 0.9-1.3 mm/s. Artificial landmarks like metal clips that show up both in the angiograms and the IVUS images could be matched with an error less than 2.5% relative to the pullback length. The overall twisting range along individual pullbacks was correctly determined as 41.8° in the least tortuous up to 118.1° in the most tortuous vessel. These results show the high clinical significance of the axial twist of the imaging catheter (Figure 5).

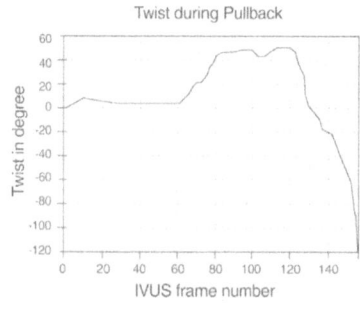
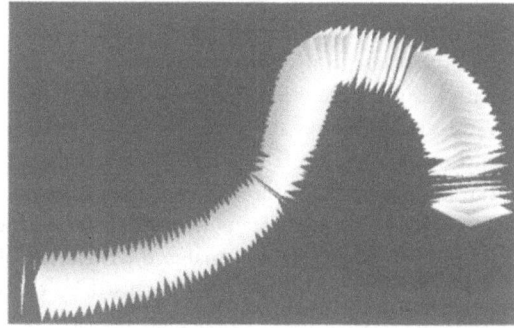

Figure 5. Catheter twisting during IVUS pullback. a) Analytically-determined catheter twist as scalar values along the pullback path. b) Visualization of the orientation of IVUS frames. (For color plate of this figure, see color section)

Future directions of intravascular ultrasound imaging

Despite the relatively recent introduction of intravascular ultrasound imaging, it has quickly become an irreplaceable tool for coronary artery diagnostics and intervention guidance. In the near future, IVUS is expected to be used in a cath lab almost as frequently as contrast angiography for intervention guidance.

In the area of IVUS image sequence acquisition, mechanical pullback devices combined with direct digital image acquisition and facilitating ECG- and respiration-gated 3D and 4D image acquisition will make the transition from a research tool to routine use. Direct digital image acquisition will facilitate more convenient computerized analysis without the need to record image data on videotapes, thus removing the digitization step that is always deteriorating the image quality. As mentioned many times in the earlier sections, image analysis methods frequently resample the image data from the image matrix representation to polar representation that is used for IVUS image segmentation. Ironically, the image matrix is obtained by scan-conversion of original IVUS data that are produced in polar coordinates. Therefore, direct digital image acquisition will likely bypass these two steps (polar - matrix - polar) that also contribute to a decrease of image quality. Additionally, the IVUS acquisition and analysis machines will likely possess networking capabilities. Standardized digital storage media will probably lead to elimination of the analog VCR as a documentation medium.

Together with image data, high frequency radio-frequency (RF) data will be obtained in a digital format and used for more detailed tissue characterization and lumen detection. Currently, image data were shown to provide good distinguishing features between soft and hard plaques. RF data are capable to contribute to much finer analysis of plaque composition including recognition of fixed plaque and thrombus. Potentially, this technique should also be able to detect flow through dissections. One of the current limitations of IVUS imaging is its lack of information about vessel geometry. Methods for combination of vessel geometry information from biplane angiography and information about vessel wall and plaque from automatically-segmented IVUS pullback sequences represent an area of active research and commercial availability of Angio-IVUS image fusion is approaching rapidly.

Advances in automated segmentation of IVUS image sequences, RF-based assessment of plaque composition, and geometrically accurate quantitation of lesion morphology using biplane angiography and IVUS fusion will allow more complex analysis of biomechanical properties of diseased vessels. New research results will likely utilize blood flow analysis and will contribute to assessment of mechanical properties of plaque, especially of unstable and vulnerable plaque that most frequently contributes to clinical events. Biomechanical research may finally work with sufficient information about 3D and 4D geometry, plaque composition and plaque mechanical properties to be able to develop complex models of biomechanical behavior of diseased vessels.

The optimal frequency for intravascular ultrasound has been debated for some time. Frequencies above 40 MHz should provide significant improvement in image quality over the conventional 30 MHz catheters. They should enhance the ability to appreciate plaque structure, to detect subtle dissections and tears, and to visualize more clearly the deployment of stents and the effects of angioplasty. The only problem is the substantial increase of backscatter from blood.

New diagnostic and interventional devices are expected to play an important role in the future of IVUS-based coronary imaging. Catheters combining an IVUS probe and a PTCA balloon have been commercially available for some time. A combination of an IVUS catheter and an atherectomy cutting device is under development and first pilot studies show its good performance. A prototype of a mechanical transducer element mounted on an angioplasty guidewire has been developed that facilitates continuous arterial imaging. Other expected developments include forward-looking IVUS catheters and flow-assessing IVUS catheters that utilize RF signal processing techniques to determine regional blood flow.

Clearly, further increase of intravascular ultrasound imaging performance and its combination with other diagnostic approaches will yield increased usage of IVUS in routine clinical care. Consequently, we are standing on a threshold of rapid development and widespread availability of new highly-computerized commercial IVUS diagnostic machines and novel ultrasound imaging tools.

Acknowledgments

The work performed at the University of Iowa has been supported in part by grants Pr 507/1-2 and Wa 1280/1-1 of the German Research Society (DFG), and by grants IA-94-GS-65 and IA-96-GS-42 of the American Heart Association, Iowa Affiliate. The work at the Leiden University Medical Center has been supported by grant LGN 44.3419 of the Technology Foundation of the Netherlands (STW).

References

1.   Seiler C, Kirkeeide RL, Gould KL. Basic structure-function relations of the epicardial coronary vascular tree. Basics of quantitative coronary arteriography for diffuse coronary artery disease. Circulation 1992;85:1987-2003.

2.   Rasheed Q, Hodgson JM. Applications of intracoronary ultrasonography in the study of coronary artery pathophysiology. J Clin Ultrasound 1993;21:569-78.

3.   Tobis JM. Intravascular ultrasound. A fantastic voyage. Circulation 1991;84:2190- 2.

4.   Mudra H, Blasini R, Klauss V *et al.* Diameter measurements after balloon angioplasty by intravascular ultrasound and quantitative coronary angiography: reasons for discrepancies [abstract]. Circulation 1992;88(Suppl):I411.

5.   Lee RT, Loree HM, Cheng GC, Liegerman EH, Jaramillo N, Schoen FJ. Computational structural analysis based on intravascular ultrasound imaging before in vitro angioplasty: prediction of plaque fracture location. J Am Coll Cardiol 1993;21:777-82.

6.   Potkin BN, Bartorelli AL, Gessert JM *et al.* Coronary artery imaging with intravascular high-frequency ultrasound. Circulation 1990;81:1575-85.

7.   Matar FA, Mintz GS, Douek P *et al.* Coronary artery lumen volume measurement using three-dimensional intravascular ultrasound: validation of a new technique. Cathet Cardiovasc Diagn 1994;33:214-20.

8.   Von Birgelen C, Di Mario C, Wenguang L *et al.* Morphometric analysis in three- dimensional intracoronary ultrasound: an in vitro and in vivo study performed with a novel system for the contour detection of lumen and plaque. Am Heart J 1996;132:516-27.

9.   Evans JL, Ng KH, Wiet SG *et al.* Accurate three-dimensional reconstruction of intravascular ultrasound data. Spatially correct three-dimensional recontruction. Circulation 1996;93:567-76.

10.   Laban M, Oomen JA, Slager CJ *et al.* ANGUS: a new approach to 3-dimensional reconstruction of coronary vessel by combined use of angiography and intravascular ultrasound. Comput Cardiol 1995:325-8.

11.   Prause GPM, DeJong SC, McKay CR, Sonka M. Towards a geometrically correct 3-D reconstruction of tortuous coronary arteries based on biplane angiography and intravascular ultrasound. Int J Card Imaging 1997;13:451-62.

12.   Reimers B, Von Birgelen C, Van der Giessen WJ, Serruys PW. A word of caution on optimizing stent deployment in calcified lesions: acute coronary rupture with cardiac tamponade. Am Heart J 1996;131:192-4.

13.   Gil R, Von Birgelen C, Prati F, Di Mario C, Ligthart J, Serruys PW. Usefulness of three-dimensional reconstruction for interpretation and quantitative analysis of intracoronary ultrasound during stent deployment. Am J Cardiol 1996;77:761-4.

14.   Von Birgelen C, Gil R, Ruygrok P *et al.* Optimized expansion of the Wallstent compared with the Palman-Schatz stent: on-line observations with two- and three-dimensional intracoronary ultrasound after angiographic guidance. Am Heart J 1996;131:1067-75.

15.   Mintz GS, Pichard AD, Satler LF, Popma JJ, Kent KM, Leon MB. Three- dimensional intravascular ultrasonography: reconstruction of endovascular stents in vitro and in vivo. J Clin Ultrasound 1993;21:609-15.

16.   Finet G, Maurincomme E, Douek P, Tabib A, Amiel M, Beaune J. Three-layer appearance of the arterial wall in intravascular ultrasound imaging: artifact or reality? Echocardiography 1994;11:343-63.

17.   Herrington DM, Johnson T, Santago P, Snyder WE. Semi-automated boundary detection for intravascular ultrasound. Comput Cardiol 1992:103-6.

18.   Snyder WE, Johnson T, Herrington D, Bilbro GL. Solution of the recirculent multilayer graph problem using compensated simulated annealing. Proc SPIE 1992;1766:446-53.

19.   Meier DS, Cothren RM, Vince DG, Cornhill JF. Automated morphometry of coronary arteries with digital image analysis of intravascular ultrasound. Am Heart J 1997;133:681-90.

20.   Maurincomme E, Finet G, Reiber JHC, Savalle L, Magnin I. Quantitative intravascular ultrasound imaging: evaluation of an automatic approach [abstract]. J Am Coll Cardiol 1995;25(Suppl):354A.

21.   Mojsilovic A, Popovic M, Amodaj M, Babic R, Ostojic M. Automatic segmentation of intravascular ultrasound images; a texture-based approach. Ann Biomed Eng 1997;25:1059-71.

22.   Fuessl RT, Mintz GS, Pichard AD *et al.* In vivo validation of intravascular ultrasound length measurements using a motorized transducer pullback system. Am J Cardiol 1996;77:1115-8.

23.   Maurincomme E, Finet G. What are the advantages and limitations of three- dimensional intracoronary ultrasound imaging? In: Reiber JHC, van der Wall EE, eds. Cardiovascular imaging. Dordrecht: Kluwer Academic Publishers; 1996. p. 243-55.

24. Roelandt JRTC, Di Mario C, Pandian NG *et al.* Three-dimensional reconstruction of intracoronary ultrasound images. Rationale, approaches, problems, and directions. Circulation 1994;90:1044-55.

25. Bruining N, Von Birgelen C, Mallus MT *et al.* ECG-gated ICUS image acquisition combined with a semi-automated contour-detection provides accurate analysis of vessel dimensions. Comput Cardiol 1996:53-6.

26. Li W, Von Birgelen C, Di Mario C. Semi-automatic contour detection for volumetric quantification of intracoronary ultrasound. Comput Cardiol 1994:277-80.

27. Sonka M, Zhang XM, Siebes M *et al.* Segmentation of intravascular ultrasound images: a knowledge-based approach. IEEE Trans Med Imaging 1995;14:719-32.

28. Sonka M, Liang W, Zhang X, DeJong S, Collins SM, McKay CR. Three- dimensional automated segmentation of coronary wall and plaque from intravascular ultrasound pullback sequences. Comput Cardiol 1995:637-40.

29. Von Birgelen C, Van der Lugt A, Nicosia A *et al.* Computerized assessment of coronary lumen and atherosclerotic plaque dimensions in three-dimensional intravascular ultrasound correlated with histomorphometry. Am J Cardiol 1996;78:1202-9.

30. Sonka M, Winniford MD, Collins SM. Robust simultaneous detection of coronary borders in complex images. IEEE Trans Med Imaging 1995;14:151-61.

31. Von Birgelen C, Mintz GS, De Feyter PJ *et al.* Reconstruction and quantification with three-dimensional intracoronary ultrasound. An update on techniques, challenges, and future directions. Eur Heart J 1997;18:1056-67.

32. Hausman ND, Friedrich G, Sudhir K *et al.* 3D intravascular ultrasound imaging with automated border detection using 2.9F catheters [abstract]. J Am Coll Cardiol 1994;23(Suppl):174A.

33. Erbele MJ. The latest in electronic imaging. Semin Intervent Cardiol 1997;2:19-23.

34. Von Birgelen C, Di Mario C, Wenguang L *et al.* Volumetric quantification by intracoronary ultrasound. In: de Feyter PJ, Di Mario C, Serruys PW, editors. Quantitative coronary imaging. Rotterdam: Barjesteh/Meeuwes; 1995. p. 211-26.

35. Wiet SP, Vonesh MJ, Waligora MJ, Kane BJ, McPherson DD. The effect of vascular curvature on three-dimensional reconstruction of intravascular ultrasound images. Ann Biomed Eng 1996;24:695-701.

36. Wahle A. Präsize Dreidimensionale Rekonstruktion von Gefäßsystemen aus biplanen angiographischen Projektionen und deren klinische Anwendung. Düsseldorf: VDI Verlag; 1997.

37. Wahle A, Wellnhofer E, Mugaragu I, Sauer HU, Oswald H, Fleck E. Assessment of diffuse coronary artery disease by quantitative analysis of coronary morphology based upon 3-d reconstruction from biplane angiograms. IEEE Trans Med Imaging 1995;14:230-41.

38. MacKay SA, Potel MJ, Rubin JM. Graphic methods for tracking heart wall motion. Comput Biomed Res 1982;15:455-73.

39. Prause GPM, DeJong SC, McKay CR, Sonka M. Semi-automated segmentation and 3-D reconstruction of coronary trees: biplane angiography and intravascular ultrasound data fusion. Proc SPIE 1996;2709:82-92.

6.   Genetic factors in the progression of atherosclerosis and response to cholesterol lowering drugs

Peter Paul van Geel, Yigal M. Pinto, Aeilko H. Zwinderman,
J. Wouter Jukema & Wiek H. van Gilst

Summary

Genetic factors play a role in the development of atherosclerosis. While some monogenetic disorders induce premature atherosclerosis, other genetic alterations cooperate in a polygenetic model, modifying the process of atherosclerosis. Genetic alterations can modify disease but can also modify the efficacy of treatment of the disease. An example of such a modifying gene is the deletion polymorphism in the 16th intron of the angiotensin converting enzyme (ACE) gene. This polymorphism is associated with higher ACE activities, and a broad variety of diseases. We assessed in a subset of the REgression GRowth Evaluation Statin Study (REGRESS) whether the ACE gene polymorphism modifies the beneficial effect of pravastatin on the atherosclerotic process. We found that the lipid lowering effect of pravastatin was similar to the three genotype groups. However, the effect of the lipid lowering drug pravastatin on the progression of coronary atherosclerosis was attenuated in the D/D genotype group. This demonstrates that the ACE deletion genotype can modify the response to treatment. Therefore, involvement of genetic alterations in modifying disease and therapy should reserve the treatment of cardiovascular disorders from a population and evidence-based approach, towards an individual-based intervention.

Introduction

Atherosclerosis is encountered in most people of old age, and can almost be regarded as a normal consequence of ageing [1,2]. Therefore, the clinical problem of atherosclerosis is better described by the term 'premature atherosclerosis', which reflects the fact that some patients suffer earlier than average from an accelerated atherosclerotic process. It is this acceleration of an otherwise normal ageing process that is usually the subject of investigation. The question is why some people suffer from atherosclerosis sooner than others, and why some do not suffer from it at all. The progression of atherosclerosis is difficult to measure, so that most of the studies monitor the occurrence of atherosclerotic complications, such as myocardial infarction, cerebrovascular accidents etc., rather than the progression of atherosclerosis itself. Only few studies assess the actual rate of change in atherosclerotic lesions by repeated angiograms.

J.H.C. Reiber and E.E. van der Wall (eds.). What's New in Cardiovascular Imaging, 95–100.
©1998 Kluwer Academic Publishers.

The complications of atherosclerosis are known to be associated with classic risk factors such as hypercholesterolemia, hypertension, smoking etc. Since a positive family history is regarded a risk factor too, it is clear that genetic factors also play a role in the development of complicated atherosclerosis. However, less data is available with regard to the relation between genetic factors and the progression of atherosclerosis itself [3,4].

Genetic risk factors of atherosclerosis: monogenetic versus polygenetic disease

One can discern two types of genetic influence on the atherosclerotic process: a monogenetic disorder in which one single genetic defect induces premature atherosclerotic complications, or a polygenetic model in which genetic alterations cooperate with exogenous factors to accelerate the atherosclerotic process. A clear example of the monogenetic type is atherosclerosis caused by mutations in the LDL receptor [5,6], which results in a clearly inherited form of premature complicated atherosclerotic disease. On the other hand, numerous genetic alterations have been shown to modify the process of atherosclerosis. We will limit this discussion to the genetic polymorphism in genes that encode components of the renin angiotensin system. The renin-angiotensin system is the enzymatic cascade that generates the vasoconstrictor and growth factor angiotensin II. Genetic polymorphism have been described in many components of the cascade: the M235T polymorphism in the gene for angiotensinogen [7], the A1166T polymorphism in the gene for the angiotensin II type 1 receptor [8], and the deletion polymorphism in the gene for ACE [9] have all been linked to cardiovascular risk factors. The deletion polymorphism in the 16th intron of the ACE gene, which is associated with higher ACE activities [10,11], is reported to be a risk factor for myocardial infarction (MI) [9,12-14] and post-MI cardiac dilatation [15], although a prospective study has recently contradicted these findings[16].

Although the ACE gene polymorphism has been related to many different manifestations of cardiac disease [9,12-15], few studies relate it to the direct progression of atherosclerosis: and some report a relation with post PTCA restenosis [17].

Can genetic variations alter treatment efficacy?

The relation between genetic variations as disease modifiers is well established: as with the polymorphism in the gene for ACE, this has been associated with an unanticipated broad variety of diseases (Table 1).

However, it is unknown whether disease modifying genes also modify the efficacy of treatment of the disease. Therefore, we assessed in a subset of the REGRESS study [18] whether the ACE gene polymorphism modifies the beneficial effect of pravastatin on the atherosclerotic process.

The genotype for ACE was determined in patients included in the REGRESS trial [18]. In short, REGRESS is a double blind, placebo controlled multicenter study to assess the effect of two years of treatment with the 3-hydroxy-3-methylglutaryl- coenzyme A (HMG-CoA) reductase inhibitor pravastatin 40 mg on angiographically documented coronary atherosclerosis, in 885 male coronary artery disease (CAD) patients with a serum cholesterol between 4 and 8 mmol/l and triglycerides < 4.0 mmol/l.

Table 1: Diseases related to the ACE gene polymorphism

Myocardial infarction

Left ventricular hypertrophy

Exercise-related left ventricular growth

Hypertrophic cardiomyopathy

Ischemic and idiopathic dilated cardiomyopathy

Post myocardial infarction cardiac dilatation

restenosis after PTCA and /or stenting

Coronary artery spasm

Ischemic stroke in hypertensives

IgA nephropathy

Diabetic nephropathy (IDDM/NIDDM)

Carotid arterial wall thickness in NIDDM

Coronary heart disease in NIDDM

Carotid intima-media thickening

Features of the ACE gene polymorphism

Higher plasma ACE concentrations

Higher cardiac and T-lymphocyte ACE concentrations

Clinical events were analyzed during the study, and serial coronary angiograms at baseline and after 2 years were analyzed quantitatively using the Cardiovascular Measurement System (MEDIS medical imaging systems, Leiden, the Netherlands).

Genotyping was possible in 782 patients; 399 of these patients received pravastatin and 383 placebo. In total 206 of 782 patients were genotyped as D/D: 107 in the placebo group (13.7%) and 99 in the pravastatin group (12.7%) (p=NS). No significant differences were observed with respect to extent and severity of coronary disease, or with respect to the bio-chemical parameters.

The lipid lowering effect of pravastatin was similar in the three genotype groups. Table 2 shows the clinical events, subdivided by treatment and genotype, that occurred during the trial. Taking the whole study group into account, these events occurred more often in the group of patients with D/D genotype (18%) than in the other two genotype groups (I/I; 11 and I/D; 14%), p=0.038 by the Mantel-Haenszel test for linear association. However, in the pravastatin group, coronary atherosclerosis progressed differently in patients genotyped as D/D compared to I/I and I/D patients. Table 3 summarizes the changes in minimum obstruction diameter (MOD) and mean segment diameter (MSD) in the three genotype groups, both in the whole (overall) study group, and stratified by treatment. As previously documented [18], pravastatin attenuated the progression of disease, as measured by the MOD, but failed to do so in the D/D genotype group. This effect on outcome measures was not caused by a lack of response to the lipid lowering effects of the drug.

Table 2: Clinical events during the two year REGRESS study

	placebo			pravastatin		
ACE[a] genotype	I/I	I/D	D/D	I/I	I/D	D/D
Number of patients	79	197	107	109	191	99
Nonfatal myocardial infarction	2	6	2	2	2	0
Fatal myocardial infarction	0	1	0	0	0	0
Coronary heart disease death	0	1	1	0	0	0
Death due to unknown cause	0	0	1	0	0	0
Nonscheduled PTCA[a]	6	20	12	1	8	10
Nonscheduled CABG[a]	6	8	6	5	11	6
Stroke and TIA[a]	1	0	3	0	0	3
Total	15	36	25	8	21	19

a. ACE= angiotensin converting enzyme; PTCA= percutaneous transluminal coronary angioplasty;
    CABG= coronary artery bypass graft surgery; TIA= transient ischemic attack.

Table 3: Change in angiographic outcome measures in all patients and in patients randomized to placebo or pravastatin

	overall	placebo	pravastatin	p[*]
	(n[a]=605)	(n=305)	(n=300)	
MSD (mm): mean (SD):				
I/I	0.09 (0.21)	0.12 (0.22)	0.06 (0.20)	0.11
I/D	0.09 (0.20)	0.10 (0.22)	0.07 (0.18)	0.28
D/D	0.08 (0.17)	0.09 (0.18)	0.07 (0.21)	0.31
p †	0.89	0.77	0.93	
MOD (mm): median (IQR):				
I/I	0.05 (0.26)	0.10 (0.31)	0.03 (0.23)	0.06
I/D	0.07 (0.19)	0.09 (0.19)	0.03 (0.19)	0.0075
D/D	0.06 (0.21)	0.06 (0.22)	0.06 (0.20)	0.54
p †	0.92	0.79	0.54	

a. n= number of patients; SD=standard deviation; IQR= interquartile range. MSD= mean segment
    diameter; MOD= minimum obstruction diameter. Change was defined as the baseline minus the
    follow-up measurement. p-values were determined using covariance analysis of ACE genotypes with
    baseline measures as covariates, or chi-square test, where appropriate. p = p-value between placebo
    versus pravastatin within genotypic classes. p †= p-value between genotypic classes in the whole
    (overall) and treatment groups.

This demonstrates again that the D/D genotype is associated with an increased risk for recurrent ischemic events. Furthermore, this genotype also seems to modify the response to treatment. This study suggests that a decrease LDL cholesterol is mainly anti-atherosclerotic when the RAS is not activated. When there is an increased RAS activity as in D/D genotype patients, LDL lowering is not as effective in reducing risk in patients not carrying this marker. In accordance, Talmud et al. [19] showed that in D/D patients cholesterol lowering treatment could not prevent progression of angiographically defined coronary atherosclerosis.

Conclusions

In this short description we have presented an example of the complicated way by which genetic differences can influence the outcome of coronary atherosclerosis, other than in the monogenetic disorders that directly cause complicated atherosclerosis, genetic polymorphisms that activate the renin-angiotensin system (such as the DD type gene for ACE) modulate the progression of atherosclerosis in a subtle way. The risk of complications ('events') is increased without an apparent acceleration of the atherosclerotic process itself. Moreover, this polymorphism seems to be associated with a decreased efficacy of lipid-lowering therapy. Therefore, genetic factors in atherosclerosis can be viewed to act on three different levels:
1. directly causing disease
2. modifying disease
3. modifying therapy.
The dissection of the rapidly growing number of genetic variations will thereby surely reverse the treatment of cardiovascular disorders from a population and evidence-based approach, towards a tailored therapy to fit individual risk profiles.

References

1. White NK, Edwards JE, Dry TJ. Relationship of degree of coronary atherosclerosis with age, in men. Circulation 1950;1:645-54.
2. Holman RL, McGill HC Jr, Strong JP, Geer JC. The natural history of atherosclerosis: the early aortic lesions as seen in New Orleans in the middle of the 20th century. Am J Pathol 1958;34:209-35.
3. Neufeld HN, Goldbourt U. Coronary heart disease: genetic aspects. Circulation 1983;67:943-54.
4. Goldbourt U, Neufeld HN. Genetic aspects of arteriosclerosis. Arteriosclerosis 1986;6:357-77.
5. Langer T, Strober W, Levy RI. The metabolism of low density lipoprotein in familial type II hyperlipoproteinemia. J Clin Invest 1972;51:1528-36.
6. Brown MS, Goldstein JL. A receptor-mediated pathway for cholesterol homeostasis. Science 1986;232:34-47.
7. Jeunemaitre X, Soubrier F, Kotelevstev YV *et al.* Molecular basis of human hypertension: role of angiotensinogen. Cell 1992;71:169-80.
8. Bonnardeaux A, Davies E, Jeunemaitre X *et al.* Angiotensin II type 1 receptor gene polymorphism in human essential hypertension. Hypertension 1994;24:63-9.
9. Cambien F, Poirier O, Lecerf L *et al.* Deletion polymorphism in the gene for angiotensin-converting enzyme is a potent risk factor for myocardial infarction. Nature 1992;359:641-4.
10. Rigat B, Hubert C, Alhenc-Gelas F, Cambien F, Corvol P, Soubrier F. An insertion/deletion polymorphism in the angiotensin I-converting enzyme gene accounting for half the variance of serum enzyme levels. J Clin Invest 1990;86:1343-6.

11. Tiret L, Rigat B, Visvikis S *et al.* Evidence, from combined segregation and linkage analysis, that a variant of the angiotensin I-converting enzyme (ACE) gene controls plasma ACE levels. Am J Hum Genet 1992;51:197-205.

12. Tiret L, Kee F, Poirier O *et al.* Deletion polymorphism in angiotensin- converting enzyme gene is associated with a parental history of myocardial infarction. Lancet 1993;341:991-2.

13. Arbustini E, Grasso M, Fasani R *et al.* Angiotensin converting enzyme gene deletion allele is independently and strongly associated with coronary atherosclerosis and myocardial infarction. Br Heart J 1995;74:584-91.

14. Ludwig E, Corneli PS, Anderson JL, Marshall HW, Lalouel JM, Ward RH. Angiotensin-converting enzyme gene polymorphism is associated with myocardial infarction but not with development of coronary stenosis. Circulation 1995;91:2120-4.

15. Pinto YM, Van Gilst WH, Kingma JH, Schunkert H. Deletion-type allele of the angiotensin converting enzyme gene is associated with progressive ventricular dilation after anterior myocardial infarction. Captopril and Thombolysis Study Investigators. J Am Coll Cardiol 1995;25:1622-6.

16. Lindpaintner K, Pfeffer MA, Kreutz R *et al.* A prospective evaluation of an angiotensin-converting-enzyme gene polymorphism and the risk of ischemic heart disease. N Engl J Med 1995;332:706-11.

17. Ohishi M, Fujii K, Minamino T *et al.* A potent genetic risk factor for restenosis. Nat Genet 1993;5:324-5.

18. Jukema JW, Bruschke AVG, Van Boven AJ *et al.* Effects of lipid lowering by pravastatin on progression and regression of coronary artery disease in symptomatic men with normal to moderately elevated serum cholesterol levels. The Regression Gowth Evaluation Statin Study" (REGRESS). Circulation 1995;91:2528-40.

19. Talmud PJ, Watts GF, McBride S *et al.* Angiotensin converting enzyme gene polymorphism and the course of angiographically defined coronary artery disease. Atherosclerosis 1995;114:133-5.

7.

Effect of lipid lowering therapy on myocardial perfusion; results from REGRESS and LAARS

Wim R.M. Aengevaeren, Gerard J.H. Uijen,
Anton F.H. Stalenhoef & Tjeerd van der Werf

Summary

In patients with coronary artery disease, lipid lowering therapy during 2-5 years is associated with less progression of coronary atherosclerosis in comparison to placebo [1-6]. The effect of lipid lowering therapy on regional myocardial perfusion is less well known. We evaluated the effect of lipid lowering therapy during 2 years on myocardial perfusion by assessment of the hyperemic mean transit time (HMTT) of contrast passage by means of digital subtraction angiography [7,8]. This effect was studied in patients with coronary artery disease with normal to moderately elevated cholesterol levels within a substudy of the REgression GRowth Evaluation Statin Study (REGRESS), and in patients with extensive coronary artery disease and severe hypercholesterolemia in the LDL-Apheresis Atherosclerosis Regression Study (LAARS) [7,9]. The methodologic issues and results of both studies are summarized, and discussed in relation to each other.

Introduction

An elevated cholesterol level is one of the causal factors in the pathogenesis of coronary atherosclerosis. Treatment of elevated cholesterol levels has a beneficial effect on the incidence of cardiovascular events and development of coronary atherosclerosis [1-6]. Despite diet and lipid lowering drugs, cholesterol levels remain often elevated in patients with familial hypercholesterolemia. High LDL-cholesterol levels are strongly associated with premature development of coronary artery disease especially in males [10]. In several angiographic trials the reduction of clinical events was more pronounced than would be expected by the modest influence of lipid lowering on progression of atherosclerosis, which suggests the possibility of a plaque stabilizing effect [11,12]. In normal coronary arteries the endothelium produces nitric oxide, which protects the vessel wall by inhibiting platelet adhesion and aggregation, smooth muscle cell proliferation and smooth muscle cell contraction. Atherosclerosis and hypercholesterolemia have a detrimental effect on endothelial function in both the epicardial coronary arteries and the resistance vessels [13,14]. Endothelial dysfunction leads to paradoxical vasoconstriction with impairment of myocardial perfusion and contributes to the pathogenesis of myocardial ischemia. Lipid lowering therapy improves the endothelium

J.H.C. Reiber and E.E. van der Wall (eds.). What's New in Cardiovascular Imaging, 101–112.
©1998 Kluwer Academic Publishers.

mediated vasomotion after relative short periods of time [15,16]. The functional improvement of the coronary circulation precedes structural improvement [17]. The cumulative effects of all anatomical and functional abnormalities of the epicardial coronary arteries in combination with possible dysfunction of conduit and resistance vessels are responsible for the ultimate effect of atherosclerosis on myocardial perfusion. In this scope it should be emphasized that minor changes in severe coronary artery stenosis have a major effect on vascular resistance, according to Poisseuille's law.

Lipid lowering strategies

The introduction of the HMG-CoA reductase inhibitors was an enormous stimulus for the treatment of patients with elevated cholesterol levels. Drugs as lovastatin, simvastatin and pravastatin were able to lower LDL-cholesterol levels with 25-40%, with only few side-effects. Intervention studies with HMG-CoA reductase inhibitors showed a favorable effect of lipid lowering treatment on survival, cardiovascular events and on progression of coronary atherosclerosis in different patient populations [1-6,18-20]. However, in patients with homozygous familial hypercholesterolemia, and in some patients with primary hyperlipidemia and very high cholesterol levels, drug treatment was less satisfactory. Already in the mid seventies plasmapheresis was introduced as an alternative approach for cholesterol lowering in these patients and proved to be effective [21]. Improved methods for removal of LDL-cholesterol from plasma became available with selective precipitation of LDL-cholesterol by heparin (HELP apheresis) and later by selective absorption of LDL-cholesterol by dextran sulfate cellulose columns [22,23]. One single session of LDL-apheresis lowers LDL-cholesterol acutely to a low level, which gradually increases over days to weeks [24]. Biweekly LDL-apheresis can induce time averaged LDL-cholesterol levels well below the range obtained with lipid lowering drugs. LDL-apheresis is considered a valuable therapeutic option for patients with homozygous familial hypercholesterolemia and for patients with coronary artery disease and hypercholesterolemia refractory to diet and drugs [25-27]. In the FHRS trial, a randomized trial in patients with familial hypercholesterolemia, biweekly LDL-apheresis versus drug therapy during two years showed, however, no difference in coronary anatomy as measured by quantitative coronary angiography (QCA) [28]. In the LAARS trial, there also was no difference in quantitatively assessed coronary anatomy but patients on LDL-apheresis had a significant improvement in exercise parameters versus patients on drug therapy alone [9].

Functional methods for assessment of the effect of lipid lowering therapy

At the moment the most popular method for functional evaluation of lipid lowering therapy is the angiographic evaluation of coronary vasomotion after intracoronary infusions of acetylcholine for assessment of endothelial function [13-16]. However, a rather broad spectrum of methods can be used for functional assessment of lipid lowering therapy with assessment of more diverse aspects of the pathophysiology of coronary artery disease. Among the methods are evaluation of angina pectoris complaints, as used in trials with lifestyle modification and lipid lowering [2,29,30]. Although the reliability of this kind of examination is improved by the use of standardized questionnaires and double blind assessment, it remains difficult to assess because of the large variability in the natural occurrence of angina pectoris and because of the poor relation to the amount of myocardial ischemia during daily life [31,32]. Exercise testing is well validated for the assessment of myocardial ischemia, and is considered as a valuable and inexpensive tool [33,34]. However, the application of this test for the evaluation of lipid lowering therapy is very limited until now. Ambulatory ECG monitoring is able to demonstrate periods of ST-segment depression during daily life [35]. Ischemia at ambulatory ECG monitoring occurs in general at lower heart rates than during exercise testing. Not only increased oxygen demand, but also a decrease in supply is suspected to be the mechanism of transient ischemia at low heart rate [36]. Endothelial dependent increase in vasomotor tone in both the epicardial vessels as well as in the microcirculation might be the responsible mechanism for this type of transient ischemia. Cholesterol lowering improves endothelial dysfunction and thus may have a beneficial effect on transient ischemia. In two studies with ambulatory ECG monitoring in patients with coronary artery disease and normal to moderately elevated cholesterol levels, transient ischemia was indeed reduced in the patients with lipid lowering therapy [37,38]. Stress testing with Thallium-201 scintigraphy and positron emission tomography are validated techniques for the functional assessment of coronary artery disease. Recently, these tests have been used for the evaluation of lipid lowering therapy [39-41]. Intensive lipid lowering during 3 months showed a decrease in perfusion defects by positron emission tomography, which returned to the original level after discontinuation of therapy [42]. It was concluded that this short-term change in perfusion defects is not due to anatomic changes, but rather to recovery of endothelial dysfunction. Digital subtraction angiography (DSA) with assessment of the HMTT of contrast passage, as used in our studies, reveals a time parameter that is proportionally related to the vascular volume and inversely to flow. HMTT is a relative measure of flow, that is affected by changes in the resistance to flow at the level of the epicardial vessels as well as the microcirculation.

Assessment of regional myocardial perfusion

We used the method of DSA, followed by densitometry and calculation of the hyperemic mean transit time (HMTT) of contrast to compare the maximal regional myocardial perfusion in the areas of the left anterior descending artery (LAD), circumflex artery (Cx) and right coronary artery (RCA) at baseline and at follow-up. This method has been developed in our laboratory and has been validated in model studies, animal experiments and in humans [43-45]. In short, before cardiac catheterization patients were trained to hold their breath, with use of a nose clamp at maximal inspiration during 15-20 seconds. During DSA the heart was triggered in synchrony with the radiographic pulses, slightly above its inherent rate, to provide a strictly regular heart rhythm. One image per heart cycle was obtained just before the onset of the QRS complex after administration of 8-12 mg papaverine. Images were generated with the automatic brightness control switched off after the fourth image in every study to enable density calculation. Subsequently, the images were digitized in a 512 x 512 matrix with 1,024 density levels. Image and data processing were performed off-line using a Sun SPARC station 10 (Sun Microsystems Inc., Mountain View, USA) with programmed Khoros software. Figure 1 is an example of 6 subtracted images out of a series of 20-25 images with a region of interest (ROI) at the injection site and 2 ROI's at the myocardial level. Time-density curves were generated by sampling the averaged pixel density within

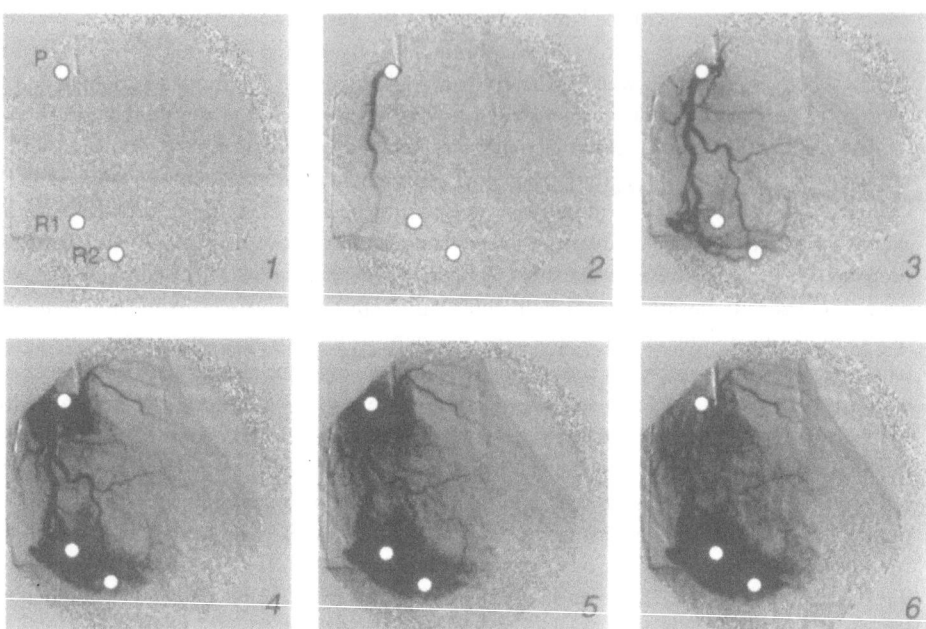

Figure 1. An example of 6 subtracted images out of a series of 20-25 images with a region of interest (P ROI) at the injection site and 2 ROI's R1-2 at the myocardial level.

a region of interest (ROI) in consecutive images and subsequently, these curves were fitted with a gamma-variate function (Figure 2). The HMTT is the difference of the mean transit time of the myocardial ROI and the mean injection time at the injection site (P ROI). Because of the pressure dependency of flow during maximal hyperemia, HMTT's were corrected for a normalized mean aortic blood pressure of 100 mmHg for comparison between the two studies. Regional myocardial perfusion was assessed by averaging the comparative HMTT's (1-2 ROI's) in the area supplied by the LAD, the RCx and the RCA to one value per perfusion area per session. In LAARS also perfusion areas supplied by bypass grafts were

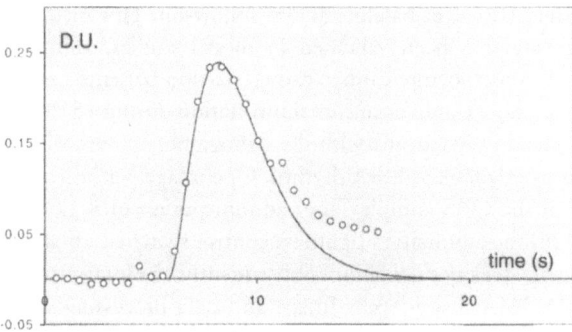

Figure 2. An example of a time-density curve of a region of interest (ROI) at the myocardial level. The line represents the curves with the gamma-variate fit. From these curves together with the mean injection time at the injection site the hyperemic transit time (HMTT) is calculated.

imaged by the DSA protocol, carefully avoiding evaluation of perfusion areas with competitive flow through native coronary artery and the bypass. Effect analysis of both lipid lowering treatments was calculated on a regional-based and a patient-based assessment of HMTT. The patient-based evaluation was performed by averaging the regional HMTT values to one value per patient as a global estimate of myocardial perfusion.

Results

The change in mean lipid levels between baseline and during follow-up of both studies are depicted in Figure 3. In the medical management stratum of the REGRESS substudy 32 patients completed the study according to the protocol. Comparative baseline and follow-up DSA's were available of 15 patients in the pravastatin group and of 10 patients in the placebo group. Regional myocardial perfusion was assessed in 31 regions in the pravastatin group and in 25 regions in the placebo group. The mean change in HMTT in the pravastatin group was -0.18 s (-5%) and in the placebo group +0.52 s (+18%), respectively, difference 0.70 s (p = 0.004). In the patient- based comparison the mean change in HMTT was -0.10 s, -3% (p = 0.75) in the pravastatin group and +0.48 s, +16% (p=0.01) in the placebo group, respectively. The difference in change between the pravastatin and placebo groups was 0.58 seconds (p=0.45). In LAARS, 42 male patients were randomized into two groups of 21 patients. In 18 patients of the LDL-apheresis group and in 17 patients of the simvastatin only group, comparative data of the first study and subsequent follow-up were available. Paired HMTT measurements were assessed in 43 regions in the LDL-apheresis group and 35 regions in the simvastatin only group. In the LDL-apheresis group regional HMTT decreased over 2 years from 3.35 ± 1.18 (mean ± 1 SD) to 2.87 ± 0.82 s, -14% (p = 0.001), whereas no change in the simvastatin only group was observed: 2.95 ± 1.06 to 2.96 ± 0.90 s (NS). In the patient-based comparison the mean change in HMTT was -0.45 s, -14% (p = 0.01) in the LDL-apheresis group and -0.05 s, -2% (NS) in the simvastatin only group, respectively. The relative changes in HMTT of both studies are shown in Figure 4.

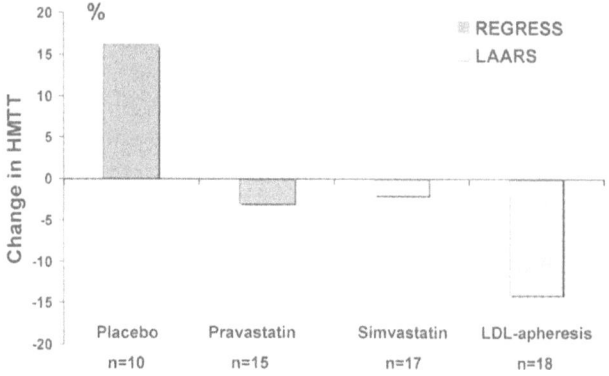

Figure 3. This graph shows the relative changes in LDL- and HDL- cholesterol during the lipid-lowering interventions.

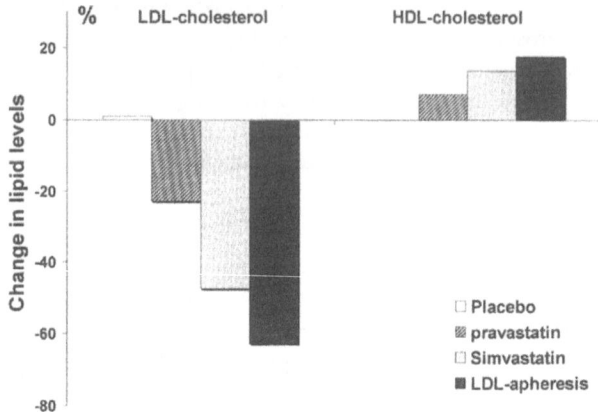

Figure 4. Change in myocardial perfusion after 2 years of therapy in REGRESS and LAARS. Myocardial perfusion is assessed by the hyperemic mean transit time (HMTT), patient based. In the LDL-apheresis group all patients used simvastatin.

Discussion

Because the differences in patient characteristics and in design between REGRESS and LAARS, comparative evaluation of both studies should be interpreted with caution. In general it seems obvious that placebo therapy leads to deterioration of regional myocardial perfusion, whereas therapy with pravastatin or simvastatin results in a preserved or even a little improved regional myocardial perfusion. Biweekly LDL-apheresis during 2 years is able to induce an improvement in regional myocardial perfusion, even after one month after the last LDL-apheresis. Because bypass grafts and PTCA's may have a major impact on flow and distribution of flow, patients who underwent these procedures were excluded from functional evaluation of the effect of lipid lowering therapy. In REGRESS, only patients in the medical management group were included in the final effect analysis of lipid lowering therapy. When not-affected vessels from the PTCA group were included in this analysis, the results were nearly identical. The results of myocardial perfusion assessment in both REGRESS and LAARS were in accordance with the results of exercise testing [7-9]. In REGRESS, patients on pravastatin showed a trend to less ischemia, and a better preserved exercise tolerance in comparison to the placebo group. In LAARS, the group of patients on LDL-apheresis had an improved ischemic threshold and a trend to an improved exercise capacity. The results of the various therapeutic interventions on myocardial perfusion in REGRESS and LAARS are not fully elucidated. Suggested mechanisms are: improved endothelium dependent vasodilatation, improved collateral circulation, and change in blood viscosity. We will discuss these potential mechanism successively.

Endothelial function

Maximal myocardial perfusion is determined by both the resistance in the conductance vessels and in the microcirculation. Coronary resistance vessels are spared from the development of overt atherosclerosis, but the endothelial function of the microcirculation can be disturbed in the presence of hypercholesterolemia [12]. Due to the method of assessment of the HMTT (isosorbide dinitrate sublingually before the coronary angiography and papaverine intracoronary during the image acquisition), the hyperemia is induced by an endothelial independent vasodilatation of the resistance vessels and a flow mediated vasodilatation of the epicardial vessels. The flow mediated response is endothelium dependent [46]. The difference in myocardial perfusion between the pravastatin and the placebo group might be induced by an impaired flow mediated vasodilatation in the epicardial vessels in response to the induced hyperemia in the resistance vessels in the placebo group. This hypothesis is adapted from Gould et al. who described this phenomenon in relation to dipyridamole infusion intravenously during positron emission tomography (PET) for flow assessment in lipid lowering therapy by diet [40]. Acute cholesterol lowering with LDL-apheresis directly improves endothelium dependent relaxation of the epicardial coronary arteries, suggesting a direct effect of LDL-cholesterol [47]. Thus, the more pronounced lipid lowering in the group of patients with LDL-apheresis may result in a better recovery of endothelial function.

Collateral circulation

Whether collateral circulation has an effect on regional myocardial perfusion in these studies is very doubtful. In the first days after myocardial infarction collateral circulation will develop and gradually increase over months. In both these studies, patients with myocardial infarction within 3 months prior to randomization were excluded. Furthermore, collateral circulation often is present in perfusion areas with occluded or severely stenosed vessels. DSA with assessment of HMTT was only performed in vessel territories with open arteries and the number of vessel territories with a combination of anterograde and collateral flow was very limited in both studies. So a direct effect of collateral circulation on our results is unlikely.

Blood viscosity

The data of the effect of HMG-CoA reductase inhibitors on blood viscosity are conflicting [48-50]. In studies with lovastatin and simvastatin no effect on blood viscosity was observed, so it is unlikely that change in blood viscosity caused the changes in myocardial perfusion in the pravastatin and simvastatin group. Improved myocardial perfusion might be due to changes in blood rheology as a result of repeated LDL-apheresis [51,52]. Due to this observation the assessment of HMTT in this study was performed about one month after the last LDL-apheresis to avoid a direct effect of LDL-apheresis on viscosity. In LDL-apheresis over dextran sulfate cellulose columns plasma fibrinogen, a determinant of viscosity, returns to pretreatment levels between 2 and 7 days [9]. During the LAARS study there was a small decrease in hematocrit level in the group of patients on LDL-apheresis but at cardiac catheterization the hematocrit levels were not significantly different in and between both groups.

Comparison with other studies

The number of studies evaluating lipid lowering therapy with assessment of myocardial perfusion is limited [39-42]. Thallium-201 scintigraphy and PET were used for semi-quantitative evaluation. In these studies myocardial perfusion defects improved in the actively treated patient groups, without significant changes in coronary anatomy, as measured or supposed. In the "long-term intense risk factor modification study", the change in dipyridamole PET images of normalized counts worsened in controls by 13.5 % and improved in the experimental group by 4.2%, numbers that correspond very well with our results [40]. In some studies, patients in the active treatment group were subjected to a regular exercise program. The effect of training precludes a direct comparison of the effect of lipid lowering therapy on the exercise parameters [39]. In the short-term lipid lowering study with fluvastatin the improvement of perfusion defects is established after only 12 weeks of therapy. The improvement was especially found in areas of ischemia [41].

Conclusions

In symptomatic men with coronary artery disease and normal to moderately raised cholesterol levels, pravastatin therapy during 2 years resulted in a preserved regional myocardial perfusion, whereas this parameter deteriorated in patients on placebo. In symptomatic men with extensive coronary artery disease and severe hypercholesterolemia, biweekly LDL-apheresis plus simvastatin improved regional myocardial perfusion whereas in the group of patients on simvastatin only, regional myocardial perfusion remained stable. The additional decrease in LDL-cholesterol levels due to LDL-apheresis may be one of the explanations for the functional improvement of the coronary circulation although rheologic changes can not be fully ruled out. The functional improvement may be due to endothelium dependent changes in the coronary circulation. Assessment of regional myocardial perfusion in lipid lowering studies is feasible and has the benefit of a combined evaluation of the epicardial coronary tree as well as the microcirculation.

References

1.   Blankenhorn DH, Azen SP, Kramsch DM *et al.* Coronary angiographic changes with lovastatin therapy: the Monitored Atherosclerosis Regression Study (MARS). The MARS Research Group. Ann Intern Med 1993;119:969-76.
2.   Waters D, Higginson L, Gladstone P *et al.* Effects of monotherapy with an HMG- CoA reductase inhibitor on the progression of coronary atherosclerosis as assessed by serial quantitative arteriography. The Canadian Coronary Atherosclerosis Intervention Trial. Circulation 1994;89:959-68.
3.   Effect of simvastatin on coronary atheroma: the Multicentre Anti-Atheroma Study (MAAS) [published erratum appears in Lancet 1994;344:762]. Lancet 1994;344:633-8. [Erratum, Lancet.1994;344:762].
4.   Sacks FM, Pasternak RC, Gibson CM, Rosner B, Stone PH. Effect of coronary atherosclerosis of decrease in plasma cholesterol concentrations in normocholesterolaemic patients. Harvard Atherosclerosis Reversibility Project (HARP)Group. Lancet 1994;344:1182-6.
5.   Jukema JW, Bruschke AVG, Van Boven AJ *et al.* Effects of lipid lowering by pravastatin on progression and regression of coronary artery disease in symptomatic men with normal to moderately elevated serum cholesterol levels. The Regression Growth Evaluation Statin Study (REGRESS). Circulation 1995;91:2528-40.
6.   Pitt B, Mancini GB, Ellis SG, Rosman HS, Park JS, McGovern ME. Pravastatin limitation of atherosclerosis in the coronary arteries (PLAC I): reduction in atherosclerosis progression and clinical events. PLAC I investigation. J Am Coll Cardiol 1995;26:1133-9.
7.   Aengevaeren WRM, Kroon AA, Stalenhoef AFH, Uijen GJH, van der Werf T. Low density lipoprotein-apheresis improves regional myocardial perfusion in patients with hypercholesterolemia and extensive coronary artery disease. LDL-Apheresis Atherosclerosis Regression Study (LAARS). J Am Coll Cardiol 1996;28:1696-704.

8.   Aengevaeren WRM, Uijen GJH, Jukema JW, Bruschke AVG, van der Werf T. Functional evaluation of lipid-lowering therapy by pravastatin in the Regression Growth Evaluation Statin Study (REGRESS). Circulation 1997;96:429-35.

9.   Kroon AA, Aengevaeren WRM, Van der Werf T *et al.* LDL-Apheresis Atherosclerosis Regression Study (LAARS). Effect of agressive versus conventional lipid lowering treatment on coronary atherosclerosis. Circulation 1996;93:1826-35.

10.   Mabuchi H, Koizumi J, Shimizu M, Takeda R. Development of coronary heart disease in familial hypercholesterolemia. Circulation 1989;79:225-32.

11.   Brown BG, Zhao XQ, Sacco DE, Albers JJ. Lipid lowering and plaque regression. New insights into prevention of plaque disruption and clinical events in coronary disease. Circulation 1993;87:1781-91.

12.   Sellke FW, Armstrong ML, Harrison DG. Endothelium-dependent vascular relaxation is abnormal in the coronary microcirculation of atherosclerotic primates. Circulation 1990;81:1586-93.

13.   Zeiher AM, Drexler H, Sauerbier B, Just H. Endothelium-mediated coronary flow modulation in humans. Effects of age, atherosclerosis, hypercholesterolemia, and hypertension. J Clin Invest 1993; 92:652-62.

14.   Gilligan DM, Guetta V, Panza JA, García CE, Quyyumi AA, Cannon RO 3rd. Selective loss of microvascular endothelial function in human hypercholesterolemia. Circulation 1994;90:35-41.

15.   Egashira K, Hirooka Y, Kai H, Sugimachi M, Suzuki S, Inou T, Takeshita A. Reduction of serum cholesterol with pravastatin improves endothelium-dependent coronary vasomotion in patients with hypercholesterolemia. Circulation 1994;89:2519-24.

16.   Treasure CB, Klein JL, Weintraub WS *et al.* Beneficial effects of cholesterol- lowering therapy on the coronary endothelium in patients with coronary artery disease. N Engl J Med 1995;332:481-7.

17.   Benzuly KH, Padgett RC, Kaul S, Piegors DJ, Armstrong ML, Heistad DD. Functional improvement precedes structural regression of atherosclerosis. Circulation 1994;89:1810-8.

18.   Kane JP, Malloy MJ, Ports TA, Phillips NR, Diehl JC, Havel RJ. Regression of coronary atherosclerosis during treatment of familial hypercholesterolemia with combined drug regimens. JAMA 1990;264:3007-12.

19.   Randomised trial of cholesterol lowering in 4444 patients with coronary heart disease: The Scandinavian Simvastatin Survival Study (4S). Lancet 1994;344:1383-9.

20.   Shepherd J, Cobbe SM, Ford I *et al.* Prevention of coronary heart disease with pravastatin in men with hypercholesterolemia. West of Scotland Coronary Prevention Study Group. N Engl J Med 1995;333:1301-7.

21.   Thompson GR, Miller JP, Breslow JL. Improved survival of patients with homozygous familial hypercholesterolaemia treated by plasma exchange. Br Med J 1985;291:1671-3.

22.   Fuchs C, Windisch M, Wieland H *et al.* Selective continuous extracorporal elimination of low-density lipoproteins from plasma by heparin precipitation without cations. In: Lysaght MJ, Gurland HJ, editors. Plasma separation and plasma fractionation. Basel: Karger; 1983. p. 272-80.

23.   Mabuchi H, Michishita I, Takeda M *et al.* A new low density lipoprotein apheresis system using two dextran sulfate cellulose columns in an automated column regenerating unit (LDL continuous apheresis). Atherosclerosis 1987;68:19-25.

24.   Kroon AA, van 't Hof MA, Stalenhoef AFH. Assessment of time-averaged levels in treatment of hypercholesterolemia by LDL-apheresis (LA) [abstract]. Neth J Med 1992;40:A50-1.

25.   Tatami R, Inoue N, Itoh H *et al.* Regression of coronary atherosclerosis by combined LDL-apheresis and lipid-lowering drug therapy in patients with familial hypercholesterolemia: a multicenter study. The LARS Investigators. Atherosclerosis 1992;95:1-13.

26.   Gordon BR, Kelsey SF, Bilheimer DW *et al.* Treatment of refractory familial hypercholesterolemia by low-density lipoprotein apheresis using an automated dextran sulfate cellulose adsorption system. The Liposorber Study Group. Am J Cardiol 1992;70:1010-6.

27.   Gordon BR, Stein E, Jones, P, Illingworth DR. Indications for low-density lipoprotein apheresis. Am J Cardiol 1994;74:1109-12.

28.   Thompson GR, Maher VM, Matthews S *et al.* Familial Hypercholesterolaemia Regression Study: a randomised trial of low-density-lipoprotein apheresis. Lancet 1995;345:811-6.

29.   Ornish D, Brown SE, Scherwitz LW *et al.* Can lifestyle changes reverse coronary heart disease? The Lifestyle Heart Trial. Lancet 1990;336:129-33.

30.   Schuler G, Hambrecht R, Schlierf G *et al.* Regular physical exercise and low-fat diet. Effects on progression of coronary artery disease. Circulation 1992;86:1-11.

31.   Cox JL, Naylor CD, Johnstone DE. Limitations of Canadian Cardiovascular Society classification of angina pectoris. Am J Cardiol 1994;74:276-7.

32.   Deanfield JE, Maseri A, Selwyn AP *et al.* Myocardial ischaemia during daily life in patients with stable angina: its relation to symptoms and heart rate changes. Lancet 1983;2:753-8.

33.   Gibbons RJ, Balady GJ, Beasley JW *et al.* ACC/AHA Guidelines for Exercise Testing. A report of the American College of Cardiology/American Heart Association Task Force on Practice Guidelines (Committee on Exercise Testing). J Am Coll Cardiol 1997;30:260-311.

34.   Froelicher VF. The standard exercise test is still the most cost-effective. J Am Coll Cardiol 1995;25:1477.

35.   Stern S, Tzivoni D. Early detection of silent ischaemic heart disease by 24-hour electrocardiographic monitoring of active subjects. Br Heart J 1974;36:481-6.

36.   Cohn PF. Silent myocardial ischemia and infarction. 3rd ed. New York: Marcel Dekker; 1993.

37.   Van Boven AJ, Jukema JW, Zwinderman AH, Crijns HJ, Lie KI, Bruschke AV. Reduction of transient myocardial ischemia with pravastatin in addition to the convential treatment in patients with angina pectoris. REGRESS Study Group. Circulation 1996;94:1503-5.

38.   Andrews TC, Raby K, Barry J *et al.* Effect of cholesterol reduction on myocardial ischemia in patients with coronary disease. Circulation 1997;95:324-8.

39.   Schuler G, Hambrecht R, Schlierf G *et al.* Myocardial perfusion and regression of coronary artery disease in patients on a regimen of intensive physical exercise and low fat diet. J Am Coll Cardiol 1992;19:34-42.

40.   Gould KL, Martucci JP, Goldberg DI *et al.* Short-term cholesterol lowering decreases size and severity of perfusion abnormalities by positron emission tomography after dipyridamole in patients with coronary artery disease. A potential noninvasive marker of healing coronary endothelium. Circulation 1994;89:1530-8.

41.   Eichstädt HW, Eskötter H, Hoffman I, Amthauer HW, Weidinger G. Improvement of myocardial perfusion by short-term fluvastatin therapy in coronary artery disease. Am J Cardiol 1995; 76:122A-125A.

42.   Hasdai D, Gibbons RJ, Holmes DR Jr, Higano ST, Lerman A. Coronary endothelial dysfunction in humans is associated with myocardial perfusion defects. Circulation 1997;96:3390-5.

43.   Van der Werf T, Heethaar RM, Stegehuis H, Meijler FL. The concept of apparent cardiac arrest as a prerequisite for coronary digital subtraction angiography. J Am Coll Cardiol 1984;4:239-44.

44.   Pijls NHJ, Uijen GJH, Hoevelaken A *et al.* Mean transit time for the assessment of myocardial perfusion by videodensitometry. Circulation 1990;81:1331-40.

45.   Pijls NHJ, Uijen GJH, Pijnenburg T *et al.* Reproducibility of the mean transit time for maximal myocardial flow assessment by videodensitometry. Int J Card Imaging 1990-1991;6:101-8.

46.   Cox DA, Vita JA, Treasure CB *et al.* Atherosclerosis impairs flow-mediated dilation of coronary arteries in humans. Circulation 1989;80:458-65.

47.   Tamai O, Matsuoka H, Itabe H, Wada Y, Kohno K, Imaizumi T. Single LDL apheresis improves endothelial-dependent vasodilatation in hypercholesterolemic humans. Circulation 1997;95:76-82.

48.   Fawcett JP, Menkes DB. Does cholesterol depletion have adverse effects on blood rheology? Angiology 1994; 45:199-206.

49.   Tsuda Y, Satoh K, Takahashi T *et al.* Effect of medication with pravastatin sodium on hemorheological parameters in patients with hyperlipoproteinemia. Int Angiol 1993;12:360-4.

50.   Mcdowell IF, Smye M, Trinick T *et al.* Simvastatin in severe hypercholesterolaemia: a placebo controlled trial. Br J Clin Pharmacol 1991;31:340-3.

51.   Schuff-Werner P, Schutz E, Seyde WC *et al.* Improved haemorheology associated with a reduction in plasma fibrinogen and LDL in patients being treated by heparin-induced extracorporeal LDL precipitation (HELP). Eur J Clin Invest 1989;19:30-7.

52.   Rubba P, Iannuzzi A, Postiglione A *et al.* Hemodynamic changes in the peripheral circulation after repeat low density lipoprotein apheresis in familial hypercholesterolemia. Circulation 1990;81:610-6.

8. How well does angiographic progression correlate with clinical events?

Linda Cashin-Hemphill

Summary

An understanding of how angiographic progression correlates with events is useful at this time for two reasons. First, to more fully comprehend the contribution of these trials in the past and second, to interpret trials which are currently underway or in the planning stages. A grave disservice has been done to the angiographic trials by introduction of the concept of "small angiographic change" leading to a "large reduction in events". The former is due solely to the denominator effect and the latter was not generally seen, at lest in terms of the traditional endpoint of death from coronary disease plus non-fatal myocardial infarction. The predictive power of angiographic progression of *future* clinical events (its ability to serve as a "surrogate") has been demonstrated during long term follow-up of three major angiographic trials. The success of sequential angiography to serve as a surrogate is probably based on the fact that angiography can detect plaque rupture. Thus angiographic trials could best be referred to as "plaque repture trails".

Introduction

An understanding of how angiographic progression correlates with events is useful at this time for two reasons. First, to more fully comprehend the contribution of these trials in the past and second, to interpret trials which are currently underway or in the planning stages. Hormone therapy in women is being tested in the WellHeart study at the University of Southern California and the NIH has undertaken the Womens Angiographic Vitamin and Estrogen trial ("WAVE"). A study in diabetics is underway [1] as is an NIH study in patients with low HDL. The primary results of the NIH post CABG study (response to moderate vs aggressive lipid lowering in bypass grafts) are published [2] but analysis of native vessels is underway.

Historical rationale for angiographic trials

Very early after the development of coronary angiography, it was recognized that coronary artery disease risk factors correlate with the extent and severity of disease on a single angiogram as well as with progression of disease on sequential angiograms [3]. Use of sequential angiography (femoral) as a means to investigate the effectiveness of various risk factor inter-

J.H.C. Reiber and E.E. van der Wall (eds.). What's New in Cardiovascular Imaging, 113–118.
©1998 Kluwer Academic Publishers.

ventions was first suggested by Ost and Stenson in 1967 [4]. Further angiographic investigation in the femoral arteries was undertaken at the University of Southern California [5,6] with the addition of computerized edge detection. The first prospective randomized angiographic trial in the coronary arteries was the NHLBI Type II Coronary Intervention Study [7]. The primary angiographic endpoint (a human panel analysis) in this trial of modest LDL reduction with cholestyramine was negative. It is interesting to note, however, that even in this early trial the incidence of progression from visually normal segment to $\geq 50\%$ diameter stenosis (likely to represent plaque rupture) was halved in the cholestyramine treated group (n=6, cholestyramine vs n=11, placebo, p=ns).

The lipid-lowering angiographic trials

Numerous angiographic trials investigating lipid lowering by diet and/or drugs followed [2, 8-23]. All of these trials demonstrated statistically significant reduction in progression of disease, whether assessed by human panel or by quantitative coronary angiography (QCA). Using a strict definition of coronary events as death from coronary disease plus non-fatal myocardial infarction, only two of these trials showed a statistically significant reduction (POSCH and PLAC I), although there was often a trend in favor of the treated group. Angiographic trials, being small and generally of short duration, are not designed to provide data regarding reduction in events on-trial.

"Small angiographic change"

With the introduction of QCA as a method of analyzing sequential coronary angiograms came the concept of the "per patient mean change". Thus a highly quantitated number replaced the qualitative visual assessment of progression provided by human panels. Whereas human panel assessment gives results in terms of clinical "mild, moderate and severe" overall progression on a per patient basis, QCA gives a precise number which is derived from an average of changes measured in all the lesions within a patient. It is important to recognize that there is very little change either visually or by QCA *on a per lesion basis*, over the two to four years of these trials. Thus, even a patient with a cardiac event will have only a small per patient mean QCA change if other lesions within the patient remain stable. For example, a patient who experiences an anterior myocardial infarction has a lesion in the left anterior descending which progresses from 30 to 100% diameter stenosis (a dramatic change likely representing plaque rupture). Nine other lesions within the patient, however, remain stable. The per patient mean change in % diameter stenosis for this patient is 7. Thus, the "small change" in angiographic QCA trials is due solely to the denominator effect and the rarity of plaque rupture. As an aside, it is unfortunate, that the "small angiographic change" in QCA trials has been coupled with the trend to reduced events and used as evidence of improvement in endothelial function with cholesterol lowering therapy. Standard angiographic trials cannot, in fact, provide information regarding endothelial function which can only be evaluated by pre and post challenge (flow or acetycholine) measurements.

Angiographic progression and events

The question remains, how does angiographic progression correlate with clinical events? Although the term "surrogate endpoint" should probably be dropped [24], it should be clear that angiography is the closest thing we have to a surrogate. This is because angiography not only demonstrates the plaque ruptures associated with on trial events (which are small in number in these small trials) but also demonstrates silent plaque ruptures. What have been called "new lesions" in the past are likely plaque ruptures of the diffuse atherosclerotic substrate which appears smooth and "normal" by angiography at baseline [25]. These changes from 0% to 20 or 30% diameter stenosis are "diluted" by the denominator effect to per patient mean changes of 2-3%. In addition there are silent plaque ruptures of lesions which are evident on baseline angiography (for example, a change from 20 to 40% diameter stenosis).

Patients who experience silent plaque rupture(s) in the two to four year interval of an angiographic trial are the ones who are at risk of a "noisy" plaque rupture in the future. All that is needed is a slightly deeper fissure and/or change in the thrombotic milieu. There is ample evidence in the literature of the predictive power of angiographic progression for future events. Moise et al. in a retrospective study demonstrated that progression on sequential coronary angiograms added to the predictive power for acute MI over that of baseline status of the coronary anatomy and left ventricular function [26]. The Program on the Surgical Control of the Hyperlipidemias (POSCH), which demonstrated benefit on coronary artery lesions with cholesterol lowering by partial ileal bypass surgery, performed long term follow-up and demonstrated that the 3-year human panel-based "global change score (GCS)" was predictive of subsequent clinical coronary events, fatal coronary events and all-cause mortality [27]. Waters et al. also performed long term follow-up of the nicardipine angiographic trial [28]. Angiographic progression, defined as a 2-year increase of at least 15% diameter stenosis in at least one coronary segment, predicted coronary events and coronary death over a subsequent 4.5 year period. Finally, the two year Cholesterol Lowering Atherosclerosis Study (CLAS) cohort was followed for an average of 7 years after follow-up angiography. Both GCS and the two patient-averaged QCA endpoints (mean per patient change in minimum lumen diameter and % diameter stenosis) were predictive of clinical coronary events during follow-up [29]. The relative risk for any coronary event (nonfatal MI, cardiac death, PTCA/CABG) was 2.2 (CI: 1.4, 3.5, p<0.001) per 10% increase in diameter stenosis and 2.0 (CI:1.1, 3.5, p=0.03) for new lesions.

"Regression trials"

It is unfortunate that angiographic trials were ever labeled "regression" trials. When these trials were formulated in the late 1970's and early 1980's, our understanding of what we would see on angiography was based on experimental models of atherosclerosis induction/regression where lipid content of lesions was affected by diet and drugs. It was felt that angiographic progression represented swelling of lesions with "lipid insudation". Conversely, regression was felt to be shrinkage due to lipid extraction. Since large lipid cores in human coronary arteries can reach one to two millimeters in diameter, it *would* be possible to detect an increase/reduction in lipid core size by serial angiography. Nonetheless, other processes are more likely to occur within the resolution of angiography. Since neither CLAS [9,10] nor FATS [12] required nitroglycerin administration, some "regression" in these trials may well represent resolution of vascular spasm, which may be related to cholesterol level, in treated subjects. Clearly, the most dramatic angiographic change is induced by plaque rupture with superimposed thrombosis. It is interesting that a focal ≥ 15% diameter stenosis progression was predictive of long term coronary morbidity and mortality after the Montreal nicardipine study [28]. A 15% diameter stenosis change in a 3 mm vessel is 450 microns-almost a half millimeter progression in 2 years. This is not likely to represent lipid insudation. Thus, although many factors could contribute to angiographic change, it is probably best to think of angiographic trials as "plaque rupture" trials.

In conclusion, plaque rupture is the final common pathway to most cardiac events. Therapies may provide benefit in terms of reduced plaque rupture by changing the structure (lipid content, fibrous cap) and/or function (thrombotic, inflammatory, vasomotor state [30]) of the vessel. Angiography, by documenting both "silent" and "noisy" (associated with a clinical event) plaque rupture, can tell us benefit has occurred, but not the mechanism.

References

1.   Steiner G. The Diabetes Atherosclerosis Intervention Study (DAIS): a study conducted in cooperation with the World Health Organization. The DAIS Project Group. Diabetologia 1996;39:1655-61.

2.   The effect of aggressive lowering of low-density lipoprotein cholesterol levels and low-dose anticoagulation on obstructive changes in saphenous-vein coronary artery bypass grafts. The Post Coronary Artery Bypass Graft Trial Investigators. N Engl J Med 1997;336:153-62.

3.   Bemis CE, Gorlin R, Kemp HG, Herman MV. Progression of coronary artery disease. A clinical arteriographic study. Circulation 1973;47:455-64.

4.   Ost CR, Stenson S. Regression of peripheral atherosclerosis during therapy with high doses of nicotinic acid. Scand J Clin Lab Invest Suppl 1967;99:241-5.

5.   Barndt R Jr, Blankenhorn DH, Crawford DW, Brooks SH. Regression and progression of early femoral atherosclerosis in treated hyperlipoproteinemic patients. Ann Intern Med 1977;86:139-46.

6.   Blankenhorn DH, Brooks SH, Selzer RH, Barndt R Jr. The rate of atherosclerosis change during treatment of hyperlipoproteinemia. Circulation 1978;57:355-61.

7.   Brensike JF, Levy RI, Kelsey SF *et al.* Effects of therapy with cholestyramine on progression of coronary arteriosclerosis: results of the NHLBI Type II Coronary Intervention Study. Circulation 1984;69:313-24.

8.   Arntzenius AC, Kromhout D, Barth JD *et al.* Diet, lipoproteins, and the progression of coronary atherosclerosis: The Leiden Intervention Trial. N Engl J Med 1985;312:805-11.

9.   Blankenhorn DH, Nessim SA, Johnson RL, Sanmarco ME, Azen SP, Cashin- Hemphill L. Beneficial effects of combined colestipol-niacin therapy on coronary atheroclerosis and coronary venous bypass grafts [published erratum appears in JAMA 1988;259:2698]. JAMA 1987;257:3233-40.

10.   Cashin-Hemphill L, Mack WJ, Pogoda J, Sanmarco ME, Azen SP, Blankenhorn DH. Beneficial effects of colestipol-niacin on coronary atherosclerosis. A 4-year follow-up. JAMA 1990;264:3013-7.

11.   Buchwald H, Varco RL, Matts JP *et al.* Effect of partial ileal bypass surgery on mortality and morbidity from coronary heart disease in patients with hypercholesterolemia. Report of the Program on the Surgical Control of the Hyperlipidemias (POSCH). N Engl J Med 1990;323:946-55.

12.   Brown G, Albers JJ, Fisher LD *et al.* Regression of coronary artery disease as a result of intensive lipid-lowering therapy in men with high levels of apolipoprotein B. N Engl J Med 1990;323:1289-98.

13.   Watts GF, Lewis B, Brunt JNH et al. Effects on coronary artery disease of lipid- lowering diet, or diet plus cholestyramine, in the St Thomas' Atherosclerosis Regression Study (STARS). Lancet 1992;339:563-9.

14.   Blankenhorn DH, Azen SP, Kramsch DM *et al.* Coronary angiographic changes with lovastatin therapy. The Monitored Atherosclerosis Regression Study (MARS). The MARS Research Group. Ann Intern Med 1993;119:969-76.

15.   Effect of simvastatin on coronary atheroma: the Multicentre Anti-Atheroma Study (MAAS) [published erratum appears in Lancet 1994;344:762]. Lancet 1994;344:633-8.

16.   Haskell WL, Alderman EL, Fair JM *et al.* Effects of intensive multiple risk factor reduction on coronary ath-erosclerosis and clinical cardiac events in men and women with coronary artery disease. The Stanford Coronary Risk Intervention Project (SCRIP). Circulation 1994;89:975-90.

17.   Waters D, Higginson L, Gladstone P *et al.* Effects of monotherapy with an HMG-CoA reductase inhibitor on the progression of coronary atherosclerosis as assessed by serial quantitative arteriography. The Canadian Coronary Atherosclerosis Intervention Trial. Circulation 1995;89:959-68.

18.   Pitt B, Mancini GBJ, Ellis SG, Rosman HS, Park JS, McGovern ME. Pravastatin limitation of atherosclero-sis in the coronary arteries (PLAC I): reduction in atherosclerosis progression and clinical events. PLAC I investigation. J Am Coll Cardiol 1995;26:1133-9.

19.   Jukema JW, Bruschke AVG, Van Boven AJ *et al.* Effects of lipid lowering by pravastatin on progression and regression of coronary artery disease in symptomatic men wtih normal to moderately elevated serum choles-terol levels. The Regression Growth Evaluation Statin Study (REGRESS). Circulation 1995;91:2528-40.

20.   Ericsson CG, Hamsten A, Nilsson J, Grip L, Svane B, De Faire U. Angiographic assessment of effects of bezafibrate on progression of coronary artery disease in young male postinfarction patients. Lancet 1996;347:849-53.

21.   Niebauer J, Hambrecht R, Velich T *et al.* Attenuated progression of coronary artery disease after 6 years of multifactorial risk intervention: role of physical exercise. Circulation 1997;96:2534-41.

22.   Frick MH, Syvanne M, Nieminen MS *et al.*Prevention of the angiographic progression of coronary and vein-graft atherosclerosis by gemfibrozil after coronary bypass surgery in men with low levels of HDL cho-lesterol. Lopid Coronary Angiography Trial (LOCAT) Study Group. Circulation 1997;96:2137-43.

23.   Herd JA, Ballantyne CM, Farmer JA *et al.* Effects of fluvastatin on coronary atherosclerosis in patients with mild to moderate cholesterol elevations (Lipoprotein and Coronary Atherosclerosis Study [LCAS]). Am J Cardiol 1997;80:278-86.

24.   Sobel BE, Furberg CD. Surrogates, semantics, and sensible public policy. Circulation 1997;95:1661-3.

25.   Leung WH, Alderman EL, Lee TC, Stadius ML. Quantitative arteriography of apparently normal coronary segments with nearby or distant disease suggests presence of occult, nonvisualized atherosclerosis. J Am Coll Cardiol 1995;25:311-7.

26.   Moise A, Bourassa MG, Theroux P *et al.* Prognostic significance of progression of coronary artery disease. Am J Cardiol 1985;55:941-6.

27.   Buchwald H, Matts JP, Fitch LL *et al.* Changes in sequential coronary arteriograms and subsequent coro-nary events. Surgical Control of the Hyperlipidemias (POSCH) Group. JAMA 1992;268:1429-33.

28.   Waters D, Craven TE, Lesperance J. Prognostic significance of progression of coronary atherosclerosis. Cir-culation 1993;87:1067-75.

29.   Azen SP, Mack WJ, Cashin-Hemphill L *et al.* Progression of coronary artery disease predicts clinical coro-nary events. Long-term follow-up from the Cholesterol Lowering Atherosclerosis Study. Circulation 1996;93:34-41.

30.   Harrison DG. Endothelial dysfunction in atherosclerosis. Basic Res Cardiol 1994;89(Suppl 1):87-102.

9.   How should future angiographic trials be designed?

Albert V.G. Bruschke, J. Wouter Jukema & Johan H.C. Reiber

Summary

As compared to ischemic events-based studies, angiographic trials have the advantage that the effect of therapeutic interventions can be assessed in relatively short periods of time in patient populations of modest size. They also provide insight into the mechanisms of action of mechanical (e.g. PTCA and stent implantations) and other (e.g. pharmacological) interventions. On the other hand angiographic studies cannot replace events-based studies; both approaches should be considered mutually supplementary.

Angiographic trails have been used extensively to determine the efficacy of lipid lowering therapy, particularly of HMG Co-A reductase inhibitors. In spite of differences in patient selection and methods used (including angiographic endpoints) the main results of these studies are remarkably similar, that is, progression of coronary atherosclerosis is significantly reduced but not completely abolished by lipid lowering. Studies which included a large number of patients like REGRESS (n=884) have provided a wealth of useful additional data such as the significance of genetic factors in the atherosclerotic process.

We anticipate that angiographic trails will continue to play an essential role in the study of coronary artery disease, in particular in the evaluation of mechanical revascularization procedures and in studies assessing the effect of pharmacological anti-atherosclerotic treatment. In future there will probably be a growing need for more extensive angiographic evaluations including studies of endothelial function and coronary perfusion.

Introduction

Indisputably coronary angiography is still the most convenient and most extensively tested method to assess the effect of coronary mechanical revascularization procedures such as coronary bypass surgery, percutaneous transluminal coronary angioplasty (PTCA), and stent implantations. Until a few years ago angiography was also frequently used to determine the effect of medical interventions. However, the spectacular results of some recently completed clinical trials, beginning with the Scandinavian Simvastatin Survival Study (4S) [1], have raised the question whether angiographic trials may still be considered adequate to assess the efficacy of medical interventions in patients with coronary artery disease. We will therefore first discuss the specific merits and limitations of each approach and then focus on the potential of coronary angiographic trials and how these may be fully exploited.

J.H.C. Reiber and E.E. van der Wall (eds.). What's New in Cardiovascular Imaging, 119–132.
©*1998 Kluwer Academic Publishers.*

Clinical events studies

Studies which use the occurrence of ischemic cardiac events to assess the effect of therapeutic interventions we will call clinical events studies. The endpoints always include cardiac death and nonfatal myocardial infarction but in addition a variety of other events have been used as primary or secondary endpoints. The latter group includes the occurrence of unstable angina pectoris, life threatening arrhythmias, heart failure, and percutaneous transluminal coronary angiography (PTCA) or coronary bypass surgery (CABG). The design of these studies is usually fairly straightforward, that is, patients with proven coronary atherosclerosis or subjects at increased risk for the development of coronary artery disease are randomized to receive a certain type of therapy or placebo and are subsequently followed for the occurrence of coronary events. The great strength of these studies lies in the fact that the occurrence of events is the main factor which is clinically relevant. Another advantage is the patient friendliness because patients participating in these trails usually do not have to undergo invasive investigations, more specifically, they do not have to undergo cardiac catheterization which may influence favourably patient compliance. Another advantage of this approach is its suitability for primary as well as secondary prevention studies.

However, clinical events studies also have limitations which are in the first place related to diagnostic problems. For a better understanding of the supposed beneficial effects of the therapy under study it is desirable if not mandatory to obtain sufficient certainly about the presence (in secondary prevention studies) or absence (in primary prevention studies) of coronary atherosclerosis. This diagnostic certainly cannot be obtained without coronary angiography unless patients are selected who have either unequivocal clinical evidence of coronary artery disease or, conversely, on clinical grounds may be considered free from coronary atherosclerosis. This may easily lead to a selection bias in that only high risk patients with coronary artery disease or low risk subjects are included whereas the large and clinically highly relevant group of patients belonging to an intermediate risk category (patients with relatively benign forms of coronary atherosclerosis) is under represented. This effect may be demonstrated by the earlier mentioned 4S trial [1]. This study included 4444 patients with unequivocal clinical evidence of coronary atherosclerosis and a baseline serum cholesterol between 5.5 and 8.0 mmol/l. It appeared that 79% of the selected patients had a previous history of acute myocardial infarction. The patients were randomized to receive simvastatin or placebo. After a median follow-up of 5.4 years, 28% of the patients in the placebo group and 19% of the patients in the simvastatin group had experienced a major coronary event (cardiac death or myocardial infarction) which corresponds with yearly event rates of respectively about 5.2 and 3.5 percent. This is markedly higher than was found in angiographic trials which were designed to test the efficacy of treatment by statins (Tables 1 and 2). Also in comparison to another clinical events trial which studied the effect of a statin, that is the Cholesterol And Recurrent Events trial (CARE) [2], the major coronary event rates are high. CARE included 4159 patients with myocardial infarction who had plasma total cholesterol levels below 6.2 mmol/l and LDL-cholesterol levels below 4.5 mmol/l. The primary endpoint was a fatal coronary event or a nonfatal myocardial infarction and this occurred in 2.6% per year in the placebo group and in 2.0% in the pravastatin treatment group. This

Table 1: Overview of angiographic lipid lowering drug trials

Acronym	Reference	Number of pts included	Number of pts completed	Drugs used	First publication (yr)
NHLBI					
Type II	6	143	116	cholestyramine	1984
CLAS	7	188	162	colestipol HCL 30 g niacin 3-12 g	1987
SCOR	8	97	72	colestipol, niacin, lovastatin	1990
FATS	9	146	120	lovastatin, colesti-pol, niacin	1990
STARS	10	90	74	cholestyramine	1992
MARS	11	270	246	lovastatin 80 mg	1993
CCAIT	12	331	299	lovastatin 40-80 mg	1994
MAAS	13	381	345	simvastatin 20 mg	1994
HARP	14	91	79	pravastatin, niacin, cholestyramine, gemfibrosil	1994
REGRESS	15	885	778	pravastatin 40 mg	1995
PLAC 1	16	408	320	pravastatin 40 mg	1995
BECAIT	17	92	81	bezafibrate 600 mg	1996
CIS	18	254	203	simvastatin 20-40 mg	1997
CARS	19	90	80	pravastatin 10 mg	1997
LCAS	20	429	340	fluvastatin 40 mg (+cholestyramine)	1997

Table 2: Lipid lowering drug trials. Primary angiographic endpoints

Acronym	Interval (mos)	Primary angiographic endpoints
NHLBI	60	categorical assessment by panel
CLAS	24+48	global change score (panel assessment)
SCOR	26	mean difference in % area stenosis of all lesions per patient
FATS	30	mean change in % stenosis proximal segments; averaged change in minimum lumen diameter
STARS	39	change in mean absolute width of the coronary segments per patient and per segment (categorical interpretation)
MARS	26	change in mean % stenosis per patient of lesions causing >20% narrowing
CCAIT	24	Coronary change score (change of minimum lumen diameter narrowings)
MAAS	24+48	change in mean segment diameter per patient; change in minimum lumen diameter of lesions causing 20% or more narrowing
HARP	27	change minimum diameter on a per lesion basis
REGRESS	24	change average mean segment diameter; change average minimum obstruction diameter
PLAC 1	36	change in mean coronary artery diameter
BECAIT	24+60	changes in mean segment diameter and minimum lumen diameter; % stenosis; categorical classification
CIS	28	Change minimum lumen diameter and global change score
CARS	24	Change of 15% or more narrowing or new lesion 15% or more
LCAS	30	within-patient per-lesion change in minimum lumen diameter of qualifying lesions

indicates that in 4S a relatively high risk population was selected while perhaps in CARE low-risk myocardial infarction patients were selected.

Perhaps the selection problem is less important if only the modification of risk factors (e.g. hypercholesterolemia) is studied, however, even then it is desirable to know the prevalence of coronary artery disease at baseline. The West of Scotland (WOS) study [3] may serve as an example in this regard. This study was designed to determine whether the administration of pravastatin to men with hypercholesterolemia and no history of myocardial infarction reduced the incidence of major coronary events. Of the 6595 men included 338 were categorized as having angina pectoris, however, the true prevalence of coronary atherosclerosis cannot be determined and therefore it cannot be accurately assessed to what extent the beneficial treatment effect (31% reduction of nonfatal myocardial infarction or death from coronary artery disease) is in fact retardation of progression of coronary atherosclerosis.

It may be emphasized that these limitations do not detract from the great value of these three well-designed studies, however, each approach has specific merits and limitations.

A practical problem in clinical events studies is related to the current low mortality and morbidity for patients with coronary artery disease. Consequently, to demonstrate statistically significant therapeutic effects large populations should be followed over long periods of time. This also makes it difficult to study the effect of therapy in subgroups for which the study originally was not specifically designed.

Angiographic trials in comparison to clinical events trials

In (coronary) angiographic trials morphology of the coronary arteries is documented by coronary angiography at one point in time and this is repeated after a certain interval, which allows assessment of progression or regression of atherosclerotic changes. One of the obvious advantages of angiographic trials is the fact that in all patients a baseline coronary angiogram is available which provides certainty about the presence of coronary atherosclerosis, to a certain extent irrespective of clinical manifestations. This allows the inclusion of a diversity of patients encompassing a wide range in severity of coronary atherosclerotic changes. Consequently it is possible to include patients with relatively mild or aspecific symptoms of coronary artery disease. Because angiographic trials by definition show changes over time in the coronary arteries, they provide insight into the effect of interventions on progression or regression of coronary artery disease which cannot be obtained by studies focusing on clinical events. Since progression (and to a lesser extent regression) is a time related phenomenon which sooner or later occurs in most patients [4], it is usually possible to assess the efficacy of interventions in a relatively short period of time in populations of modest size. For the same reason angiographic trials are better suited than clinical events trials to determine therapeutic effects in subgroups of patients.

In view of the invasive nature of coronary angiography and the related risks it is ethically not justifiable to study in this manner large populations of asymptomatic subjects in whom on clinical grounds no indication for coronary angiography is present. Consequently, angiographic trials are not suitable for primary prevention studies. Likewise, patients at increased risk for the occurrence of complications of coronary angiography (e.g. elderly patients) and in whom it is unlikely that coronary angiography will have direct therapeutic consequences, should in general not be included. This leads to a selection bias which favors inclusion of middle aged patients with moderately severe coronary artery disease and well preserved left ventricular function. The invasive nature of coronary angiography also makes it ethically unjustifiable to perform the examinations at regular intervals. Thus the assessment of progression and regression is in all studies limited to one interval or (rarely) to two intervals (Table 2). Since there are indications that the progression of coronary atherosclerosis is a discontinuous process [4], one may wonder if patients who have no or retarded progression over a certain period of time will continue to show the same over more prolonged periods of time. Likewise the absence of progression over a certain period of time does not exclude the possibility of (accelerated) progression later. Furthermore, if a patient experiences an ischemic event during the scheduled interval between angiographic studies it may be impossible to perform a follow-up coronary angiogram; this is obviously the case if the patient dies but this may also happen if a nonfatal event leads to marked deterioration of the patient's clinical condition. Presumably these patients have more than average progression and therefore angiographic trials tend to underestimate the true rate of progression.

Examples of angiographic trials

Angiographic trials have been used to assess the efficacy of a variety of life style or medical interventions, in particular that of lipid lowering therapy with or without life-style changes. One of the first studies in this field was the Leiden Intervention Trial [5] which was also the first study that made use of sophisticated computer-assisted quantitative coronary angiography. Although not designed as a randomized trial the Leiden Intervention Study may still be considered a landmark study.

Table 1 lists the lipid-lowering drug trials published to date (studies in which lipid lowering is only part of the intervention or in which other lipid-lowering modalities like LDL-apheresis [21,22] or ilial bypass surgery [23] have been used are not included here). Since this is a fairly straightforward and uniform goal we will compare the design and outcome of these studies and endeavour to establish guidelines for future trials.

General design features

All studies listed were designed as randomized trials to determine the effect of one drug or a combination of drugs. In some studies a fixed dosage was used whereas in other studies the dosage or combination of drugs was adjusted to achieve predefined serum lipid levels. In the Coronary Artery Regression Study (CARS [19]) an unusual low fixed dosage of pravastatin (10 mg) proved to be effective. As might be expected the more recently published studies were mainly designed to assess the therapeutic effect of HMG-CoA reductase inhibitors.

Basically all trials were designed as secondary prevention trials, that is, only patients who had atherosclerotic lesions at baseline coronary angiography were included. However, in some studies not all patients had clinical evidence of coronary artery disease; e.g. in the Specialized Center of Research Intervention Trials (SCOR [8]) this was the case in less than 5 of the 72 patients who completed the study. One study, the Cholesterol-Lowering Atherosclerosis Study (CLAS [7]) selected exclusively patients who had a history of coronary bypass surgery, whereas for instance in the Canadian Coronary Intervention Trial (CCAIT [12]) these patients were excluded. Likewise, some studies included a high proportion of patients who had a history of percutaneous transluminal coronary angiography (PTCA) whereas these were excluded in some other studies; about half of the patients included in the Multicentre Anti-Atheroma Study (MAAS [13]) and in the Pravastatin Limitation of Atherosclerosis in the Coronary Arteries study (PLAC 1 [16]) had prior PTCA whereas in the REgression GRowth Evaluation Statin Study (REGRESS [15]) only 6% of the patients had previous PTCA.

There is also a great diversity in the baseline lipid levels. The earlier studies were mainly designed to determine whether lipid lowering therapy in patients with markedly disturbed lipid metabolism has a beneficial effect on progression of coronary lesions. Later studies have tried to assess the effect of lipid lowering in patients with only moderately elevated serum lipid levels. However, only REGRESS and CARS included patients with baseline total cholesterol below 4.5 mmol/l.

Angiographic techniques

Although there is undeniably merit in visual interpretation of coronary angiograms and the changes over time, especially if panels of experienced angiographers are used as was done in CLAS, automated quantitative interpretation should be considered mandatory for modern trials. Indeed, all trials published in the nineties have used this technique, however, there are significant differences between trials with regard to technique and quality control. Earlier we presented a critical review on these issues and pointed out that some trials did not or not entirely fulfill strict criteria for quality assurance which were discussed in detail [24]. Apart from technical aspects there has been a great deal of discussion about the advisability to use vasodilators before the angiographic recordings. After it was demonstrated that lipid lowering may restore endothelial function and thus lead to vasodilation [25,26], the use of endothelium independent vasodilation like nitroglycerin appeared to be mandatory.

In fact, it is conceivable that the observed beneficial effect of lipid lowering in trials which did not use vasodilators (e.g. the St.Thomas Atherosclerosis Regression Study (STARS [10]) was in part only a vasodilatory effect. Although it should be recognized that orally or sublingually administered vasodilators may not fully abolish the effect of vasomotor tone this reduces the influence of this confounding factor to a minimum.

Angiographic endpoints

In principle, in all trials primary angiographic endpoints were defined (Table 2). In many studies also secondary endpoints were defined; however, this distinction appears to be of little consequence because several studies (e.g. MARS and PLAC 1) were considered to be strongly "positive" in favour of the treatment group although there was no significant difference between placebo and treatment groups for the primary angiographic endpoints. The diversity of angiographic endpoints and differences in methodology of interpreting angiograms makes comparison of angiographic trials cumbersome and to a certain extent impossible. We will briefly discuss angiographic endpoints; more details may be found elsewhere [27,28]. The first choice which has to be made is whether the angiographic data will be treated as categorical or continuous variables. If a categorical approach is elected patients or segments are categorized as progressing, unchanged, regressing and sometime as showing a mixed reaction. This approach is particularly suitable for visual interpretation of coronary angiograms and it has the advantage that the angiographic findings are classified in an easy to understand and clinically relevant manner. If this type of division is made in quantitative analysis of coronary angiogram it requires that threshold values be adopted for the classification, e.g. progression or regression may be considered to be present if the changes over time exceed two times the standard deviation of measurements. Thus smaller changes, which may be numerous, are not included in the final analysis. Treating the coronary arterial dimensions as continuous variables has the advantage that it allows a certain grading of progression and regression in an objective manner.

Some angiographic endpoints relate primarily to narrowing lesions whereas other endpoints relate to the average width of an artery or a segment. The first category includes percentage stenosis and parameters like "minimum lumen diameter" or "minimum obstruction diameter"; the second category has been termed "mean absolute width", "mean segment diameter" and "mean coronary artery diameter". Obviously (changes of) the average lumen diameter can only be adequately assessed by quantitative analysis. It is conceivable that some interventions affect mainly focal changes whereas other interventions affect mainly global changes and therefore we recommend the use of two angiographic endpoints reflecting both aspects. The possibility of a differential effect is corroborated by studies using clinical endpoints which showed specific effects on different endpoints by certain drugs on nutriments [29].

The development of new lesions has gained a certain popularity as an angiographic endpoint after this appeared to be the only positive angiographic effect in a trial using a calcium channel blocker [30]. There is no harm in using this terminology as long as it is well defined; however, it should be realized that it is a misnomer. It has been known for a very long time that normal looking segments in patients with significant coronary artery disease in fact often show pathological changes at autopsy. Furthermore, quantitative coronary angiography, which is based on single frames, is not a suitable technique to detect minor irregularities which can only be detected on the moving cine angiogram.

There is also some controversy about the use of absolute versus relative measurements. The use of relative measurements (percentage obstruction) has the advantage that most clinicians are used to characterizing narrowing lesions by percentage lumen narrowing; however, in some cases the seemingly normal portion of the artery used as reference may not be normal and change over time. In principle it is even possible that the percentage narrowing seems to decrease solely because the reference diameter decreases. We therefore prefer absolute measures although this has the disadvantage that it requires calibration of the radiographic system, for which purpose usually the catheter tip is used [31], which introduces a potential source of error or inaccuracy.

Number of patients and duration of follow-up

As shown in Table 1 there is a wide range in numbers of patients included per trial. In general, a relatively small number of patients is adequate in studies which comprise high risk patients whereas large numbers of patients are required if the patients show little progression. A longer follow-up may compensate for a smaller number of patients as was shown in the MAAS trial, which showed no significant treatment effect after two years but became "positive" after four years [13]. Inclusion of a large number of patients may allow a meaningful analysis of subgroups. This is clearly demonstrated by the largest angiographic trial published to date, that is REGRESS, which has provided useful data on a number of subjects such as the combination of pravastatin with calcium channel blockers and the significance of various genetic characteristics [32-36].

Outcome of lipid lowering angiographic trials

In spite of the diversity in number and type of patients included, medication used, and angiographic techniques and endpoints there is a remarkable consistency in the outcome of these trials. Practically all studies have shown that lipid lowering significantly retards progression of coronary atherosclerosis. Progression is not abolished and on average there is no regression. However, if a categorical classification is used most studies show that in both the placebo and the treatment group there are individual patients who show regression while the number of "regressors" is highest in the treatment group. In only one study, the Harvard Atherosclerosis Reversibility Project (HARP [14]) there was no beneficial treatment effect. However, HARP included only 79 patients who finished the study of whom 31 had a history of coronary bypass surgery which makes the interpretation of the angiographic findings cumbersome. An important finding is the absence of a correlation between baseline lipid levels and treatment effect. This aspect was extensively analyzed in REGRESS and FATS [15,37]. In practice this means that baseline lipid levels should not be regarded as the only, and perhaps not even an important, criterion upon which a decision to treat patients with HMG Co-A reductase inhibitors should be based. Of course this in only true for patients with proven coronary artery disease. If the disease had developed in the presence of normal or only mildly elevated serum lipid levels we surmise that in these patients the vascular wall is more susceptible to atherosclerosis causing agents, including lipids, than is normally the case, which may explain the beneficial effect of lipid lowering. It may also be an indication that HMG Co-A reductase inhibitors have an effect beyond lipid lowering by a direct influence on atherosclerotic plaques. This discussion, however, is beyond the scope of this chapter.

Is there still a place for angiographic trials and if so, for what purpose?

Apart from the considerations in favor of clinical events studies mentioned earlier, several arguments have been brought forward to question the usefulness of angiographic studies. This concerns particularly trials which are designed to assess the anti-atherosclerotic properties of drugs. It has been stated that the effect of certain drugs on clinical events is so much greater than the effect on angiographically determined progression that it may be concluded that progression is not a good indication of the efficacy of drugs. There is some truth in this statement; however, apparently some investigators do not understand the meaning of averaged changes. If, for instance, a patient has 2 mm progression of a narrowing lesion in one segment and 12 segments are analyzed then the average progression for that patient is only 0.17 mm. The situation becomes even more complex if other lesions in the same patient show some regression or if other patients belonging to the same randomization group show no change or regression. In this context it is reassuring that a good correlation between angiographic progression and the future occurrence of clinical events has been demonstrated [38,39] as is more extensively discussed elsewhere in this volume.

Another criticism concerns the accuracy of angiographic findings, particularly of complex lesions [40]. It is true that the ability of angiography to depict irregularly shaped luminal narrowings is very limited. It is also true that quantitative analysis of coronary angiograms is hampered by the fact that the analyses are based upon single frames and that information provided by integration of the moving images, as is automatically done by experienced angiographers, is lost. However, the question is how important these limitations are considering the objectives of a specific study. If changes over time are the primary focus of attention, as is the case in progression studies, then the accurate delineation of complex luminal narrowings may not be of crucial importance. Likewise, analysis of single frames is entirely adequate if the proper conditions for quality assurance, including standardization, are fulfilled and only lesions exceeding a certain threshold (e.g. 20% luminal narrowing) are included. In comparison to other imaging modalities, especially in comparison to intravascular ultrasound, (quantitative) coronary angiography has the advantages that extensive experience in many trials and continuing research have led to perfection of the method and a thorough insight into the potential and limitations of the method has been obtained. Furthermore, it is the only method which enables visualization of the entire coronary arterial tree, down to vessels of 0.5 to 0.1 mm diameter, in a standardized manner at minimal risk to the patients. Apart from providing valid "surrogate" endpoints for the clinical effect of various therapeutic modalities, angiographic trials also have merits in their own right in that they provide a certain insight into the mechanism of action.

How should future angiographic trials be designed?

The strength of angiographic trials lies in their potential to demonstrate therapeutic effects in a relatively short period of time in relatively small numbers of patients. Therefore they are particularly suited to assess effects of interventions in patients exhibiting specific characteristics (e.g. genetic characteristics) or in groups of patients in whom the clinical event rate is low which makes clinical studies cumbersome. On the other hand it should be recognized that angiographic studies can never replace clinical events based studies and therefore both methodologies should be considered mutually supplementary. Some angiographic studies also show a significant effect on the occurrence of clinical events (e.g. REGRESS [15] and PLAC1 [16]); however, the effect on clinical events can more adequately and easier be assessed by studies designed for this purpose and it makes angiographic trials unnecessarily unwieldy if they are powered to demonstrate these effects. For the assessment of mechanical revascularization procedures angiography is commonly considered a gold standard. Intravascular ultrasound studies may provide useful additional information but still lack the standardization and easy applicability of angiography. For non-mechanical interventions (particularly evaluation of drugs) there is a trend towards event driven trials. However, as pointed out earlier, for specific purposes angiographic trials will remain highly suitable. Angiography also makes it possible to study mechanisms which cannot properly be assessed by other methods, such as influence on endothelial function [41] or change of coronary flow or flow reserve [42,43]. This requires that during angiography special tests be performed and specific analyses be carried out.

In future there may be a greater need for these extensive angiographic assessments in small numbers of patients than for traditional angiographic trials involving very large numbers of patients. In either case, angiographic trials will continue to play an essential role in the evaluation of drugs and will provide insight into the mechanisms involved in the action of anti-atherosclerotic drugs.

References

1.   Randomised trial of cholesterol lowering in 4444 patients with coronary heart disease: the Scandinavian Simvastatin Survival Study (4S). Lancet 1994;344:1383-9.
2.   Sacks FM, Pfeffer MA, Moye LA *et al.* The effect of pravastatin on coronary events after myocardial infarction in patients with average cholesterol levels. Cholesterol and Recurrent Events Trial investigators. N Engl J Med 1996;335:1001-9.

3.   Shepherd J, Cobbe SM, Ford I *et al.* Prevention of coronary heart disease with pravastatin in men with hypercholesterolemia. West of Scotland Coronary Prevention Study Group. N Engl J Med 1995;333:1301-7.

4.   Bruschke AVG, Kramer JR Jr, Bal ET, Haque IU, Detrano RC, Goormastic M. The dynamics of progression of coronary atherosclerosis studied in 168 medically treated patients who underwent coronary arteriography three times. Am Heart J 1989;117:296-305.

5.   Arntzenius AC, Kromhout D, Barth JD *et al.* Diet, lipoproteins, and the progression of coronary atherosclerosis. The Leiden Intervention Trial. N Engl J Med 1985;312:805-11.

6.   Brensike JF, Levy RI, Kelsey SF *et al.* Effects of therapy with cholestyramine on progression of coronary arteriosclerosis: results of the NHLBI Type II Coronary Intervention Study. Circulation 1984;69:313-24.

7.   Blankenhorn DH, Nessim SA, Johnson RL, Sanmarco ME, Azen SP, Cashin-Hemphill L. Beneficial effects of combined colestipol-niacin therapy on coronary atherosclerosis and coronary venous bypass grafts [published erratum appears in JAMA 1988;259:2698]. JAMA 1987;257:3233-40.

9.   Brown G, Albers JJ, Fisher LD *et al.* Regression of coronary artery disease as a result of intensive lipid-lowering therapy in men with high levels of apolipoprotein B. N Engl J Med 1990;323:1289-98.

10. Watts GF, Lewis B, Brunt JNH *et al.* Effects on coronary artery disease of lipid-lowering diet, or diet plus cholestyramine, in the St Thomas' Atherosclerosis Regression Study (STARS). Lancet 1992;339:563-9.

11. Blankenhorn DH, Azen SP, Kramsch DM *et al.* Coronary angiographic changes with lovastatin therapy. The Monitored Atherosclerosis Regression Study (MARS). The MARS Research Group. Ann Intern Med 1993;119:969-76.

12. Waters D, Higginson L, Gladstone P *et al.* Effects of monotherapy with an HMG-CoA reductase inhibitor on the progression of coronary atherosclerosis as assessed by serial quantitative arteriography. The Canadian Coronary Atherosclerosis Intervention Trial. Circulation 1994;89:959-68.

13. Effect of simvastatin on coronary atheroma: the Multicentre Anti-Atheroma Study (MAAS) [published erratum appears in Lancet 1994;344:762]. Lancet 1994;344:633-8.

14. Sacks FM, Pasternak RC, Gibson CM, Rosner B, Stone PH. Effect on coronary atherosclerosis of decrease in plasma cholesterol concentrations in normocholesterolaemic patients. Harvard Atherosclerosis Reversibility Project (HARP) Group. Lancet 1994;344:1182-6.

15. Jukema JW, Bruschke AVG, Van Boven AJ *et al.* Effects of lipid lowering by pravastatin on progression and regression of coronary artery disease in symptomatic men with normal to moderately elevated serum cholesterol levels. The Regression Growth Evaluation Statin Study (REGRESS). Circulation 1995;91:2528-40.

16. Pitt B, Mancini GBJ, Ellis SG, Rosman HS, Park JS, McGovern ME. Pravastatin limitation of atherosclerosis in the coronary arteries (PLAC I): reduction in atherosclerosis progression and clinical events. PLAC I investigation. J Am Coll Cardiol 1995;26:1133-9.

17. Ericsson CG, Hamsten A, Nilsson J, Grip L, Svane B, de Faire U. Angiographic assessment of effects of bezafibrate on progression of coronary artery disease in young male postinfarction patients. Lancet 1996;347:849-53.

18. Bestehorn HP, Rensing UFE, Roskamm H *et al.* The effect of simvastatin on progression of coronary artery disease. The Multicenter Coronary Intervention Study (CIS). Eur Heart J 1997;18:226-34.

19. Tamura A, Mikuriya Y, Nasu M. Effect of pravastatin (10 mg/day) on progression of coronary atherosclerosis in patients with serum total cholesterol levels from 160 to 220 mg/dl and angiographically documented coronary artery disease. Coronary Artery Regression Study (CARS) Group. Am J Cardiol 1997;79:893-6.

20. Herd JA, Ballantyne CM, Farmer JA *et al.* Effects of fluvastatin on coronary atherosclerosis in patients with mild to moderate cholesterol elevations (Lipoprotein and Coronary Atherosclerosis Study [LCAS]). Am J Cardiol 1997;80:278-86.

21. Kroon AA, Aengevaeren RM, Van der Werf T *et al.* LDL- Apheresis Atherosclerosis Regression Study (LAARS). Effect of aggressive versus conventional lipid lowering treatment on coronary atherosclerosis. Circulation 1996;93:1826-35.

22. Waidner T, Franzen D, Voelker W *et al.* The effect of LDL apheresis on progression of coronary artery disease in patients with familial hypercholesterolemia. Results of a multicenter LDL apheresis study. Clin Investig 1994;72:858-63.

23. Buchwald H, Varco RL, Matts JP *et al.* Effect of partial ileal bypass surgery on mortality and morbidity from coronary heart disease in patients with hypercholesterolemia. Report of the Program on the Surgical Control of the Hyperlipidemias (POSCH). N Engl J Med 1990;323:946-55.

24. Reiber JHC, Jukema JW, Koning G, Bruschkle AVG. Quality control in quantitative coronary arteriography. In: Bruschke AVG, Reiber JHC, Lie KI, Wellens HJ, editors. Lipid-lowering therapy and progression of coronary atherosclerosis. Dordrecht: Kluwer Academic Publishers; 1996. p. 45-63.

25. Gould KL, Martucci JP, Goldberg DI *et al.* Short-term cholesterol lowering decreases size and severity of perfusion abnormalities by positron emission tomography after dipyridamole in patients with coronary artery disease. A potential noninvasive marker of healing coronary endothelium. Circulation 1994;89:1530-8.

26. Vogel RA. Coronary risk factors, endothelial function, and atherosclerosis: a review. Clin Cardiol 1997;20:426-32.

27. Jukema JW, Van Boven AJ, Zwinderman AH, Bal ET, Reiber JHC, Bruschke AVG. The influence of angiographic endpoints on the outcome of lipid intervention studies. A proposal for standardization. REGRESS Study Group. Angiology 1996;47:633-42.

28. Bruschke AVG, Jukema JW, Van Boven AJ, Bal ET, Reiber JHC, Zwinderman AH. Angiographic endpoints in progression trials. In: Bruschke AVG, Reiber JHC, Lie KI, Wellens HJ, editors. Lipid-lowering therapy and progression of coronary atherosclerosis. Dordrecht: Kluwer Academic Publishers; 1996. p. 71-7.

29. De Lorgeril M, Salen P, Martin JL *et al.* Effect of a mediterranean type of diet on the rate of cardiovascular complications in patients with coronary artery disease. Insights into the cardioprotective effect of certain nutriments. J Am Coll Cardiol 1996;28:1103-8.

30. Lichtlen PR, Hugenholtz PG, Rafflenbeul W, Hecker H, Jost S, Deckers JW. Retardation of angiographic progression of coronary artery disease by nifedipine. Results of the International Nifedipine Trial on Antiatherosclerotic Therapy (INTACT). INTACT Group Investigators. Lancet 1990;335:1109-13.

31. Reiber JHC, Jukema W, Van Boven A, Van Houdt RM, Lie KI, Bruschke AVG. Catheter sizes for quantitative coronary arteriography. Cathet Cardiovasc Diagn 1994;33:153-5.

32. Jukema JW, Zwinderman AH, Van Boven AJ *et al.* Evidence for a synergistic effect of calcium channel blockers with lipid-lowering therapy in retarding progression of coronary atherosclerosis in symptomatic patients with normal to moderetaly raised cholesterol levels. The REGRESS Study Group. Arterioscler Thromb Vasc Biol 1996;16:425-30.

33. Groenemeijer BE, Hallman MD, Reymer PWA *et al.* Genetic variant showing a positive interaction with beta-blocking agents with a beneficial influence on lipoprotein lipase activity, HDL cholesterol, and triglyceride levels in coronary artery disease patients. The Ser447-stop substitution in the lipoprotein lipase gene. REGRESS Study Group. Circulation 1997;95:2628-35.

34. Jukema JW, Van Boven AJ, Groenemeijer B *et al.* The Asp9 Asn mutation in the lipoprotein lipase gene is associated with increased progression of coronary atherosclerosis. REGRESS Study Group, Interuniversity Cardiology Institute, Utrecht, The Netherlands. Regression Growth Evaluation Statin Study. Circulation 1996;94:1913-8.

35. Kuivenhoven JA, Jukema JW, Zwinderman AH *et al.* The role of a common variant of the cholesterol ester transfer protein gene in the progression of coronary atherosclerosis. Regression Growth Evaluation Statin Study (REGRESS) Study Group. N Engl J Med 1998;338:86-93.

36. Cobbaert C, Jukema JW, Zwinderman AH, Withagen AJAM, Lindemans J, Bruschke AVG. Modulation of lipoprotein(a) atherogenicity by high density lipoprotein cholesterol levels in middle-aged men with symptomatic coronary artery disease and normal to moderately elevated serum cholesterol. Regression Growth Evaluation Statin Study (REGRESS) Study Group. J Am Coll Cardiol 1997;30:1491-9.

37. Stewart BF, Brown BG, Zhoa XQ *et al.* Benefits of lipid-lowering therapy in men with elevated apolipoprotein B are not confined to those with very high low density lipoprotein cholesterol. J Am Coll Cardiol 1994;23:899-906.

38. Waters D, Craven TE, Lesperance J. Prognostic significance of progression of coronary atherosclerosis. Circulation 1993;87:1067-75.

39. Azen SP, Mack WJ, Cashin-Hemphill L *et al.* Progression of coronary artery disease predicts clinical coronary events. Long-term follow-up from the Cholesterol Lowering Atherosclerosis Study. Circulation 1996;93:34-41.

40. Topol EJ, Nissen SJ. Our preoccupation with coronary luminology. The dissociation between clinical and angiographic findings in ischemic heart disease. Circulation 1995;92:2333-42.

41. Mancini GBJ, Henry GC, Macaya C *et al.* Angiotensin-converting enzyme inhibition with quinapril improves endothelial vasomotor dysfunction in patients with coronary artery disease. The TREND (Trial on Reversing ENdothelial Dysfunction) Study [published erratum appears in Circulation 1996;94:1490]. Circulation 1996;94:258-65.

42. Geldof MJA, Schalij MJ, Manger Cats V *et al.* Comparison between regional myocardial perfusion reserve and coronary flow reserve in the canine heart. Eur Heart J 1995;16:1860-71.

43. Aengevaeren WRM, Uijen GJH, Jukema JW, Bruschke AVG, Van der Werf T. Functional evaluation of lipid-lowering therapy by pravastatin in the Regression Growth Evaluation Statin Study (REGRESS). Circulation 1997;96:429-35.

10.

Applications of intravascular ultrasound in cardiology

Jean-Claude Tardif & Hai Shiang Lee

Summary

Intravascular ultrasound (IVUS) is a clinically useful tool that provides cross-sectional images of the coronary arterial lumen and wall. Diagnostic applications of IVUS include the evaluation of left main coronary artery disease and of other ambiguous lesions on angiography particularly at bifurcations. IVUS is extremely useful for the assessment of coronary vasculopathy in cardiac transplant recipients, and it can also help to characterize other abnormalities such as syndrome-X, myocardial bridging and coronary artery spasm. Used as a complement to angiography, IVUS can optimize the monitoring of percutaneous coronary interventions and lead to a smaller residual plaque burden. It is also the best tool to assess stent deployment. IVUS allows the precise evaluation of the effects of approaches such as antioxidation or brachytherapy for the prevention of restenosis. It also represents the ideal tool for assessing regression of atherosclerosis. Three-dimensional reconstruction, elastography and imaging guidewires are some of the recent advances in the field of intravascular ultrasound.

Introduction

Intravascular ultrasound (IVUS) imaging uses miniaturized transducers at the tip of catheters to provide cross-sectional images of coronary and other arteries [1,2]. IVUS was developed to supply detailed information not only on arterial stenosis, but also on atherosclerotic lesions and on the vessel wall [3] (Figure 1). Coronary angiography, the traditional approach used to evaluate coronary artery disease, has well-known limitations. One shortcoming is that angiography only provides a planar perspective of the coronary arterial lumen. Depiction of the coronary lumen, and not the wall, is another important limitation of angiography, atherosclerosis being primarily a disease of the arterial wall. The severity of stenosis may be underestimated by angiography because the reference segment used to quantitate the lesion is involved in the diffuse atherosclerotic process. In addition, the composition and morphology of atherosclerotic lesions, which can not be assessed with angiography, are major determinants of the clinical expression of coronary atherosclerosis and of the response to percutaneous interventions.

J.H.C. Reiber and E.E. van der Wall (eds.). What's New in Cardiovascular Imaging, 133–148.
©*1998 Kluwer Academic Publishers.*

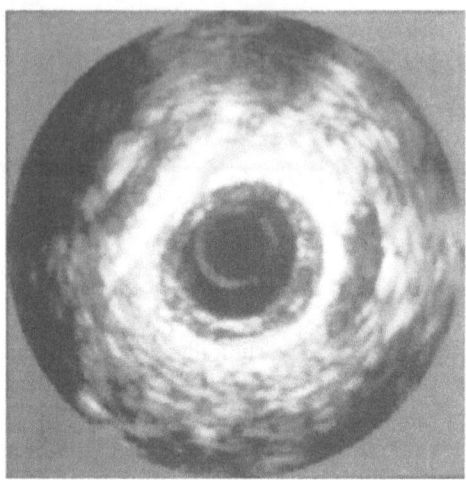

Figure 1. IVUS image showing intimal thickening in a coronary artery. The IVUS catheter is in the center of the coronary lumen. A vein is seen at 3 to 4 o'clock.

Intravascular ultrasound imaging instrumentation

Because high-frequency ultrasound transducers have greater resolution but a smaller depth of field, 20-50 MHz transducers (with 2.9 to 3.5 French catheters) are employed for IVUS imaging. These catheters use either mechanical or solid state (multi-element) designs. Several types of mechanical instruments exist, but they basically rely on a shaft which is connected to a motor that rotates a single, small ultrasound element. In contrast, solid-state catheters use up to 64 elements activated in sequence. Dynamic focusing is achieved electronically in a solid-state system to create a synthetic aperture resulting in optimal focus in both the near and far fields. Since a drive shaft is not required with a multi-element system, the central lumen can be used for other purposes. In addition, the absence of a rotating component in a solid-state system prevents potential artefacts due to nonuniform rotational distortion (NURD) that may occur with mechanical systems. On the other hand, the acoustic power of older multi-element systems was limited and the central ringdown artifact used to be large. However, manufacturers have improved both types of designs and they are now relatively equivalent both for clinical and research purposes [4] (Figure 2). Instruments that combine ultrasound with other capabilities such as a balloon angioplasty catheter or an atherectomy device have been developed to facilitate guidance of interventions [5,6]. Interestingly, an imaging guidewire has also been produced by one manufacturer [7]. A limitation common to all these instruments is the lack of forward-viewing capability. A prototype catheter that allows visualization beyond the catheter tip has recently been developed [8].

Mild Atherosclerotic Plaque

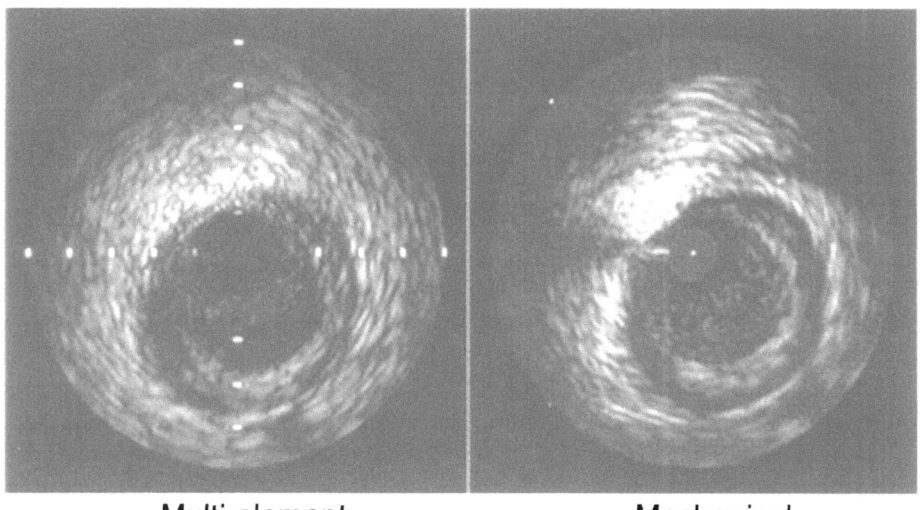

Multi-element   Mechanical

Figure 2. IVUS images of the same cross-section using multi-element and mechanical designs.

Intravascular ultrasound examination

The IVUS procedure is performed by advancing the catheter distal to the site of interest to an easily recognizable landmark, most often a side branch, using a 0.014 or 0.018 inch coronary angioplasty guidewire. Intracoronary nitroglycerin is administered (200-300 µg) before IVUS examination. The most distal position of the IVUS catheter is noted and used for follow-up IVUS examinations. It is recommended that the guiding catheter be disengaged to ensure visualization of the aorto-ostial junction by IVUS imaging. The transducer is then pullbacked automatically at a speed of 0.5 (or 1.0) mm/sec up to the guiding catheter. The use of reproducible landmarks and a known pullback speed facilitates comparison of identical cross-sectional images on serial studies and permits volumetric (three-dimensional) analysis. Alternatively, slow manual pullbacks (approximately 0.5 mm/sec) can be performed up to the guiding catheter. A detailed running audio commentary describing the location of the ongoing IVUS interrogation and of areas of interest is extremely useful with either type of pullback. Simultaneous high-resolution fluoroscopic images can also be recorded on the IVUS imaging screen during pullbacks to constantly know the location of the IVUS transducer. IVUS images are usually recorded only during transducer pullback and not during transducer advancement to ease off-line image interpretation.

For safe imaging of coronary arteries, the catheter must be small and flexible enough to allow passage in tortuous vessels. Although miniaturization of catheters has taken place in the past years (2.9-3.5 French, 0.9-1.1 mm), it occasionally remains not possible to cross severe narrowings before angioplasty. Major complications are rare despite increasing clinical use of IVUS imaging [9]. Most major and acute procedural complications associated with (but not necessarily caused by) IVUS imaging occur during interventional cases. Coronary spasm occurs in approximately 2-3% of patients during interventional and diagnostic catheterization but it usually can be reversed rapidly by the administration of nitroglycerin. Importantly, heparin (5,000 to 10,000 units) should be administered before IVUS examination even for diagnostic imaging. The 1-year safety of intracoronary ultrasound imaging has been assessed by serial quantitative coronary angiography in 38 cardiac transplant recipients [10]. There was no significant difference between instrumented and noninstrumented vessels in percentage or absolute change in diameter 1 year after the initial IVUS examination.

Intravascular assessment of arterial anatomy and pathology

IVUS measurements of arterial dimensions have been shown by several investigators to correlate closely with histologic measurements [11]. When an internal layer is visualized with IVUS, its normal thickness does not exceed 0.20 mm. An intermediate echolucent zone is observed in 60 to 70% of patients. When present, its thickness also is 0.20 mm or less. A third layer, outside the external elastic membrane (junction of media and adventitia), is present but its thickness can rarely be defined in native vessels because of surrounding tissues. Abnormalities of the arterial lumen and wall are depicted in details by IVUS [12] (Figure 3). Histologically, progressive accumulation of plaque in the intima is often associated

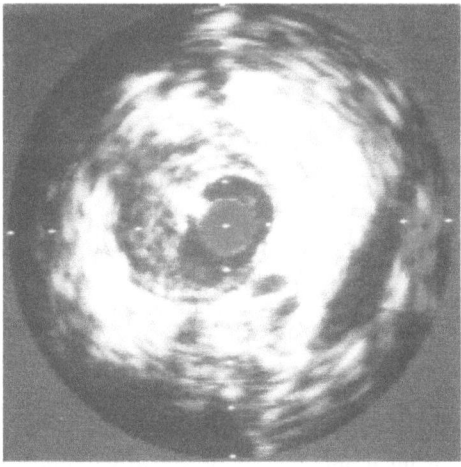

Figure 3. Severe, eccentric atherosclerotic plaque seen with IVUS. The guidewire is seen at 10 o'clock.

with disruption of the internal elastic lamina and increased collagen content in the media. The resulting modifications in the echogenicity of these structures may render difficult the identification of the intimal-medial border [13]. The interface between lumen and intima and the border between media and adventitia (the external elastic membrane) however remain easily discernable and reliable. For these reasons, quantitative analysis on IVUS cross-sections consists in measurements of lumen area and of the area circumscribed by the external elastic membrane (Figure 4). The difference between these 2 areas is the intima + plaque area, i.e. the wall area apart from the surrounding adventitia.

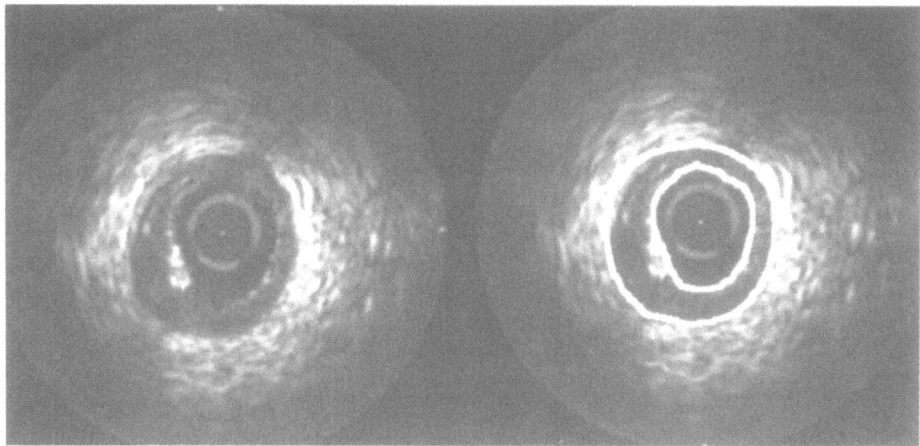

Figure 4. Illustration of IVUS measurements. The inner and outer white lines indicate lumen and external elastic membrane areas, respectively.

IVUS imaging provides characterization of the vessel wall based on tissue reflectivity and not on histology per se. Depending of the composition of the atheroma and of the changes in the vascular wall, different patterns will be observed. Calcium causes the greatest impedance to transmission of ultrasound, resulting in considerable reflection with minimal penetration of ultrasound signals. Calcium deposits in atherosclerotic plaques are very bright and cause acoustic shadowing (Figures 5A and B). Fibrous plaques are bright but do not cause acoustic shadowing. Atheroma rich in lipids ("soft plaque") and lesions composed of proliferating smooth muscle cells and extracellular matrix are less echogenic than the surrounding

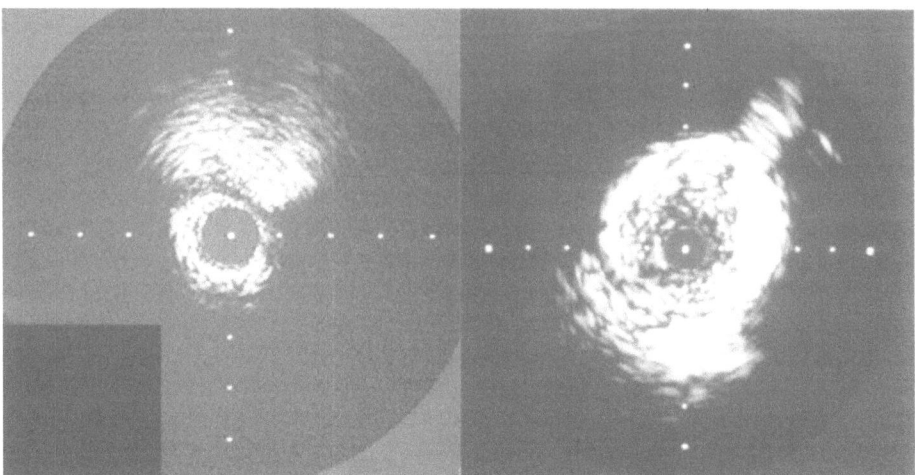

Figure 5. Coronary artery calcifications on IVUS. A- Severe coronary stenosis with superficial calcium causing acoustic shadowing from 2 to 10 o'clock . B- Deep calcifications located in the plaque away from the lumen.

adventitia and less than fibrous or calcified plaque. An heterogeneous appearance is frequently present in atheromatous arteries, because they often contain the combination of lipid-laden, fibrous and calcified plaques. IVUS also allows the identification of necrotic debris and lipid lakes. Arterial thrombus can be noted, but distinction between soft plaque and thrombus can be difficult. Interestingly, one study has shown that this classification of plaque morphology by IVUS correlated very well with the clinical angina syndrome, but not with the angiographic lesion descriptors [14]. In that study, patients with unstable angina had more soft plaques and less fibrous and calcified plaques.

IVUS versus coronary angiography

The limitations of coronary arteriography are now well known [2,15]. The planar, two-dimensional silhouette of the arterial lumen provided by coronary angiography and the lack of depiction of the arterial wall are the most important limitations. Because the lesion is assessed by comparing the lumen of the narrowed and "normal" segments, disease of the reference segment and compensatory enlargement (arterial remodeling or Glagov phenomenon [16]) of the stenosed segment frequently lead to angiographic underestimation of the extent and severity of coronary artery disease. Study of angiographically mildly diseased coronary arteries has revealed that 50% of these patients have narrowings of 50% or more with IVUS [17]. Moreover, the majority of angiographically normal reference segments are involved in the atherosclerotic process on IVUS imaging [18].

Visual interpretation of arteriograms is associated with significant intra-observer and inter-observer variability. The advent of quantitative coronary angiography has reduced this variability, but it has not improved the ability of the radiographic two-dimensional silhouette of the arterial lumen to accurately depict complex tridimensional coronary anatomy. Correlations between IVUS and angiographic measurements vary depending on the presence or absence of atherosclerotic disease, the eccentricity of lesions, the performance of an

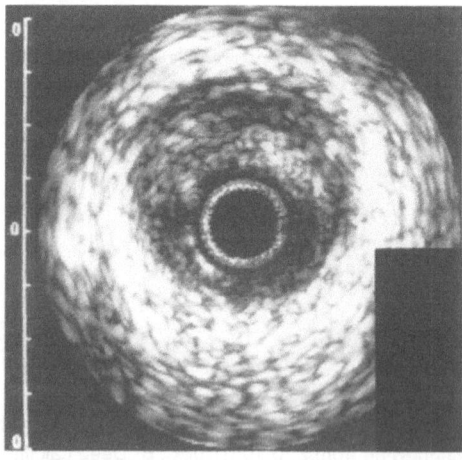

Figure 6. Severe residual plaque burden on IVUS, despite "good" angiographic results of balloon angioplasty.

interventional procedure, and the index measured [2,19,20]. In normal subjects, the correlations between angiographic and ultrasound diameters are excellent. However, the correlations are not as good in patients with atheromatous vessels. The presence of tortuous arteries, vessel overlap, stenoses at bifurcations and eccentric lesion morphology compound the problem of reliable depiction of the coronary lumen.

An imperfect correlation is noted between IVUS and angiography in the evaluation of residual stenosis and luminal areas after angioplasty [21]. These differences are probably due to the larger angiographic diameters caused by the presence of contrast in fissures in the arterial wall, whereas the tomographic sections on IVUS precisely depict the architecture and dimensions of the arterial lumen. Serious underestimation of residual plaque burden after a percutaneous intervention frequently occurs when only angiographic monitoring is used, with cross-sectional area narrowings of 60% or significantly more being commonly present on IVUS [22] (Figure 6).

Diagnostic applications of intracoronary ultrasound

Clinical indications for IVUS are evolving. One extremely important application of IVUS during diagnostic catheterization is for the evaluation of left main coronary artery disease when doubts persist after angiography [23]. This particularly occurs when a diagnostic catheter repetitively wedges in the left coronary artery, when the left main trunk is diffusely small without any discrete lesion or when an ostial lesion or a stenosis at the bifurcation is suspected (Figures 7A and B). In order to assess the left main coronary artery adequately, the IVUS catheter is first advanced in the left anterior descending or circumflex artery, the guiding catheter is disengaged and IVUS imaging is performed up to the guiding catheter to ensure visualization of the aorto-ostial junction. If a significant lesion is not observed in the left main artery in this fashion, we frequently instrument the other major coronary branch (i.e. the circumflex artery if the guidewire was initially introduced in the left anterior

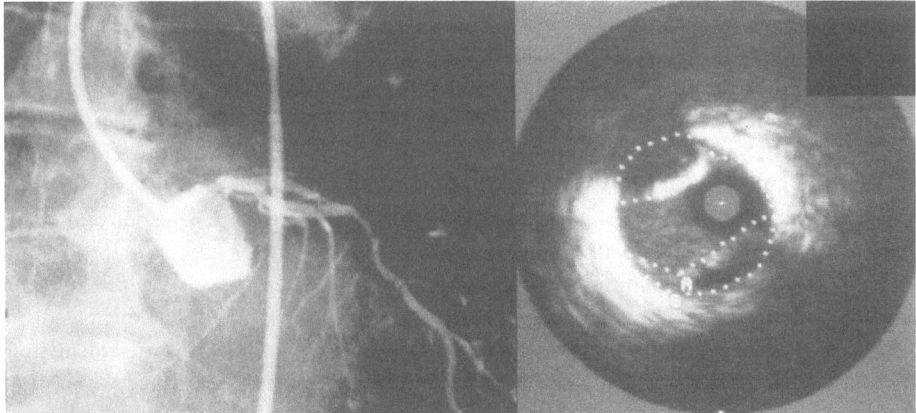

Figure 7. A) Angiogram in which severe stenosis of the proximal left main coronary artery is suspected. B) Lumen and external elastic membrane areas were 12.1 mm² and 23.0 mm² on IVUS, respectively. Cross-sectional area narrowing was only 47.6%. IVUS examination thus excluded a critical stenosis of the left main coronary artery.

descending artery) and image its proximal portion to rule out the presence of a left main equivalent disease (severe ostial narrowings of circumflex and LAD). Although IVUS provides anatomic depiction of narrowings and not a physiologic assessment, it nevertheless clarifies the vast majority of problematic angiographic images of the left main artery. Indeed, IVUS imaging in this context will often show minimal plaque accumulation or very severe narrowing. In intermediate cases with at least moderate disease, we rely on several off-line ultrasound measurements performed immediately after imaging is completed. We first require the presence of a cross-sectional area narrowing greater than 75% before considering a lesion as "significant". We also measure the true minimal lumen diameter (MLD) and divide it by the lumen diameter of a normal left main segment if present, to obtain a percent diameter stenosis. This is particularly useful in ostial lesions and in heavily calcified arteries (causing shadowing of the external elastic membrane area). In diffusely diseased left main coronary arteries, we also divide the MLD by the expected normal dimension of the left main artery (based on autopsy series and angiographic studies of normal patients). A greater than 50% diameter stenosis is taken to represent a significant stenosis. It is important to stress that these values have not been specifically validated for use in this context. Nevertheless, experimental obstruction to coronary flow in animals has shown that coronary flow reserve begins to be significantly limited with a cross-sectional area narrowing of 75% [24], which roughly corresponds to a 50% diameter stenosis. We have also recently demonstrated that a 75% or greater cross-sectional area narrowing in a coronary artery on IVUS correlates very well with the presence of ST segment depression during treadmill testing [25].

Other ambiguous lesions on angiography can also be clarified with IVUS [26]. The value of angiography is more limited at coronary bifurcations. Unfortunately, atherosclerotic plaques preferentially accumulate at bifurcation points, where turbulence is more important. Bifurcation lesions of uncertain severity thus represent another diagnostic application of IVUS. Intracoronary ultrasound imaging can also provide valuable information for the problematic lesions visualized well in only a single angiographic projection. We have also found that IVUS is helpful in patients with chest pain in the first 6 months after angioplasty to determine whether a severe narrowing is present despite the absence of significant angiographic restenosis [25]. Because IVUS imaging does not provide functional assessment of lesions, the narrowings of truly intermediate severity however can benefit from Doppler assessment of the flow reserve [27].

Coronary vasculopathy is the leading cause of late mortality following cardiac transplantation. A high prevalence of false negative coronary arteriograms has been documented with the use of IVUS during routine serial catheterization in cardiac transplant recipients [28]. Concentric intimal thickening is often not detected by angiography because of the diffuse nature of this immune process. In contrast, IVUS imaging offers early detection and quantitation of coronary vasculopathy in patients who have undergone cardiac transplantation [29]. The presence of significant intimal thickening on IVUS has been shown to be predictive of survival in these patients, even in the absence of angiographically apparent disease [30]. The use of IVUS may therefore allow the early use of more effective treatment strategies in cardiac transplant recipients. Interestingly, IVUS imaging performed within a few weeks of transplantation has revealed the presence of angiographically silent focal atherosclerotic plaques in 25 to 30% of patients, which most likely represent disease transferred from the donor [31].

IVUS can also help to characterize other coronary syndromes (syndrome-X, myocardial bridging, coronary artery spasm). The majority of patients with syndrome-X have abnormal coronary arteries (atheroma or marked intimal thickening) by IVUS imaging, despite the absence of angiographic abnormalities [32]. Similarly, a very high incidence of atherosclerotic plaque is detected proximal to bridging segments with the use of IVUS [33]. Occasionally, these plaques are sufficiently important to justify angioplasty. Controversy however persists concerning the clinical significance of myocardial bridging. Finally, marked atherosclerotic thickening is generally demonstrated by IVUS at the site of focal coronary vasospasm in the absence of angiographically significant disease [34].

Applications of IVUS during coronary interventions

IVUS has been extremely useful to understand the mechanisms of lumen enlargement with different percutaneous coronary interventions (Figure 8). We have learned that the improvement in lumen dimensions after balloon angioplasty was predominantly the result of both vascular expansion (increase in the area circumscribed by the external elastic membrane, particularly for compliant non-calcified plaques), and dissection [35]. We have also realized that plaque could be redistributed along the long-axis of the vessel. On the other hand, IVUS has shown that extraction of plaque is the principal mechanism for lumen enlargement after atherectomy [36].

IVUS is a more sensitive tool than fluoroscopy to detect coronary calcifications in patients in whom angioplasty is required (75% vs 48% in one study) [37]. The extent (number of quadrants, axial length) and localization (superficial or deep) of these calcifications can be precisely defined with IVUS (Figure 5). Calcification of the culprit coronary lesion is

Mechanisms of PTCA

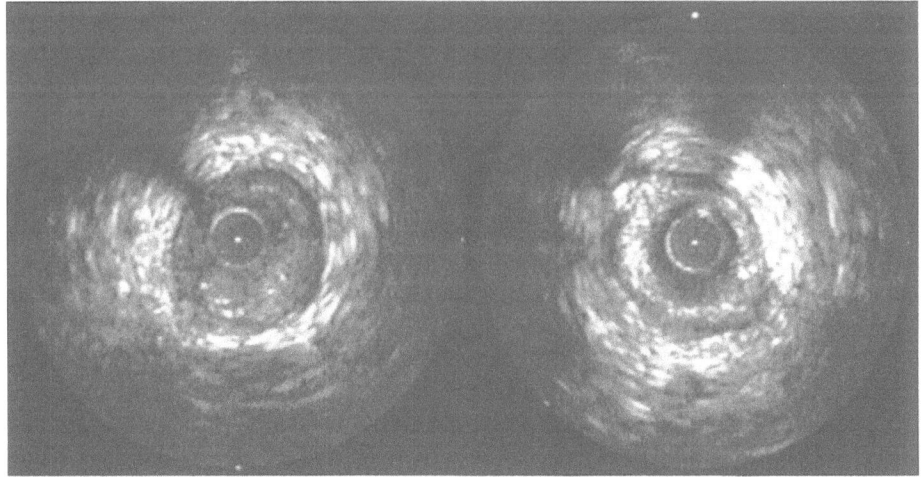

Lumen (mm²)	2.37	3.66
EEM (mm²)	10.11	10.92

Figure 8. IVUS images before (left) and after (right) angioplasty. Lumen enlargement was predominantly obtained by vessel expansion (increase in the area circumscribed by the external elastic membrane).

a determinant of the response to interventions [38]. Directional atherectomy does not remove calcium very well and the presence of more than mild calcification represents a contraindication to its use. In contrast, rotational atherectomy results in preferential ablation of calcified lesions. Balloon angioplasty may cause dissection at calcified lesions, particularly at the junction with a more normal wall. IVUS can also depict plaque eccentricity at the stenosis site more reliably than angiography [39] (Figure 9). Although the GUIDE trial investigators have reported that such IVUS findings (calcifications, plaque eccentricity) have resulted in changes in therapy in approximately 50% of their patients [40], reductions in restenosis rates have unfortunately not been reported.

Sizing of instruments is usually based on the dimensions of the reference segments. The indiscriminate use of balloons larger than the angiographic reference segment lumen has resulted in a high rate of complications after balloon angioplasty. However, it has been demonstrated that angiography significantly underestimates plaque burden of the reference segment because of adaptive vascular remodeling, the process whereby compensatory vessel enlargement develops to preserve the arterial lumen. There is, on average, approximately 50% cross-sectional area narrowing at "reference" segments [18]. The CLOUT Pilot Trial investigators have shown that remodeled arteries (as shown by IVUS) can safely accommodate oversized balloons [41]. In that study, balloons sized halfway between the lumen and external elastic membrane resulted in upsizing in 73% of cases, by an average of 0.5 mm compared to angiographically guided angioplasty. This increased the nominal balloon-to-artery ratio from 1.12 to 1.30 and the minimal lumen diameter on IVUS from 1.75 to 2.10 mm, without increased rates of complications. Whether this strategy will result in lower restenosis rates and improved long-term outcomes is not known. However, phase 2 of the GUIDE Trial has shown that a residual plaque area of less than 65% and a minimal lumen diameter of more than 2.0 mm on IVUS were associated with a low likelihood of restenosis [42]. Given the strong predictive value of post-procedural plaque area on IVUS, it is tempting to speculate that IVUS-guidance during interventions to reduce residual atheroma will translate into better long-term outcome. Data supporting this hypothesis is now emerging. Careful IVUS guidance of directional atherectomy and adjunct PTCA in the ABACAS trial resulted in a residual plaque area of 42%, and a restenosis rate of 14% (at 3 months) [43]. In

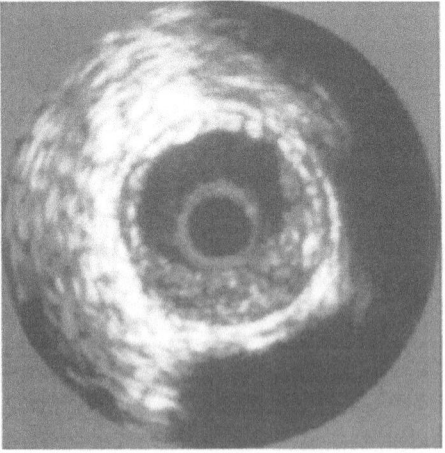

Figure 9. Eccentric atherosclerotic plaque depicted by IVUS.

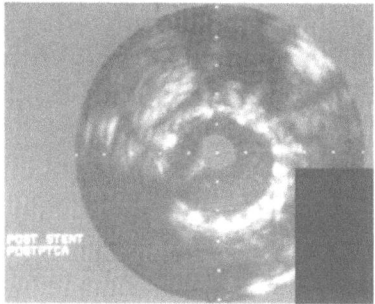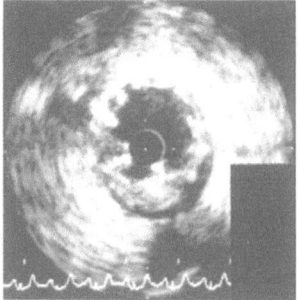

Figure 10. Stent deployment assessed by IVUS. A- Adequate expansion. B- Inadequate apposition of the stent to the coronary wall (from 6 to 8 o'clock) demonstrated by IVUS.

comparison, final plaque burden was 58% in the Optimal Atherectomy Restenosis Study, and the restenosis rate was 29% [44]. Thus, lowering residual plaque burden by using IVUS guidance may have been responsible for the decrease in restenosis rate in the ABACAS trial.

True lumen dimensions at the dilated site are more accurately defined with the tomographic images obtained with IVUS than with angiography, particularly when there is non-homogeneous contrast density or when vessel borders are indistinct. The causes of angiographic haziness are usually identified with IVUS. Surface ulcerations and dissections are detected more frequently with IVUS than with angiography. However, there are presently no criteria to distinguish useful from pathologic dissection with IVUS.

IVUS has dramatically changed the world of coronary artery stenting. Colombo et al. initially demonstrated that stent deployment was commonly sub-optimal on IVUS despite an apparently adequate expansion on angiography [45] (Figures 10A and B). It was then shown that oral anticoagulation was not necessary to prevent subacute thrombosis when deployment was optimized using strict IVUS criteria [46]. Optimization of stent deployment according to IVUS criteria usually involved the aggressive use of high-pressure balloon inflations. Building on the knowledge acquired with IVUS, other investigators then obtained favorable results with systematic high-pressure inflations, without using IVUS or coumadin [47,48]. This led to a controversy regarding the need for and cost-effectiveness of the continued use of IVUS during stenting. However, angiographic criteria predicting adequate stent expansion on IVUS have not been developed [49]. In addition, some investigators argue that IVUS has demonstrated that inflations at very high pressures are not always necessary to obtain adequate stent deployment and sometimes may only lead to injury at stent edges. Such injuries in turn will often require the use of additional balloon inflations or the deployment of one or more additional stents. Randomized, multicenter clinical trials are currently underway to reassess the role of IVUS in coronary stenting (AVID, OPTICUS).

Full apposition of the stent to the arterial wall represents one of the most important IVUS criterion of adequate deployment (Figure 11). Experienced observers also visually assess the relationship between the proximal and distal portions of the stent and their adjacent reference segments. Quantitative criteria usually involve a symmetry index (ratio of minimal to maximal lumen diameters on the same cross-section greater than 0.7) and ratios of the minimal intra-stent luminal area and lumen areas of the reference segments. For example, the criteria used in MUSIC were rigid and required that the smallest lumen area in the stent was both 100% or more of the lumen area of the smallest reference segment (90%

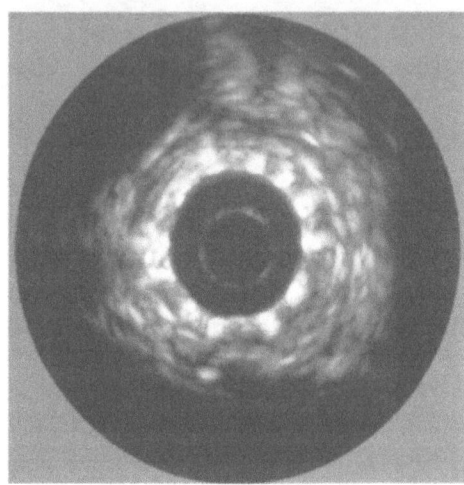

Figure 11. Adequate stent deployment as assessed by IVUS. The stent is well apposed to the arterial wall, its expansion is symmetric, and coronary lumen is large.

if minimal intra-stent luminal area ≥ 9 mm^2) and 90% of the average of the lumen areas of the references (80% if minimal intra-stent luminal area ≥ 9 mm^2) [50]. Most investigators presently use quantitative criteria that are slightly less stringent.

Several pharmacologic approaches have failed to modify the high incidence of restenosis after balloon coronary angioplasty. This inability to alter the restenosis process was in part caused by our incomplete understanding of its pathophysiology. It was assumed for several years that restenosis was solely caused by intimal hyperplasia. IVUS has allowed for a better understanding of the mechanisms responsible for restenosis after angioplasty in humans (Figure 12). Several groups of investigators including our team at the Montreal Heart Institute have shown using serial IVUS examinations that lumen loss after balloon angioplasty is caused by the combination of inadequate or deleterious vessel remodeling and tissue hyperplasia [51-53]. Vascular remodeling is defined in this context as the change in external elastic membrane area. Importantly, IVUS has also taught us that an important residual plaque burden after angioplasty is an important contributor to restenosis in patients. In contrast, Hoffmann et al. have shown that the difficult problem of in-stent restenosis is caused by tissue hyperplasia [54] and that there is no significant chronic stent recoil at follow-up IVUS examination (Figure 13).

The emerging role of vascular remodeling in the pathophysiology of restenosis after coronary interventions not involving stents has created a new target for its prevention [55]. Indeed, we recently demonstrated that the antioxidant probucol prevents restenosis after coronary angioplasty by improving vascular remodeling [52,56]. The exciting concept of a "vessel remodeler" has thus largely arisen because of IVUS imaging. In comparison, brachytherapy does not appear to improve adaptive vessel enlargement but rather seems to be effective at inhibiting tissue proliferation [57,58].

Mechanisms of restenosis

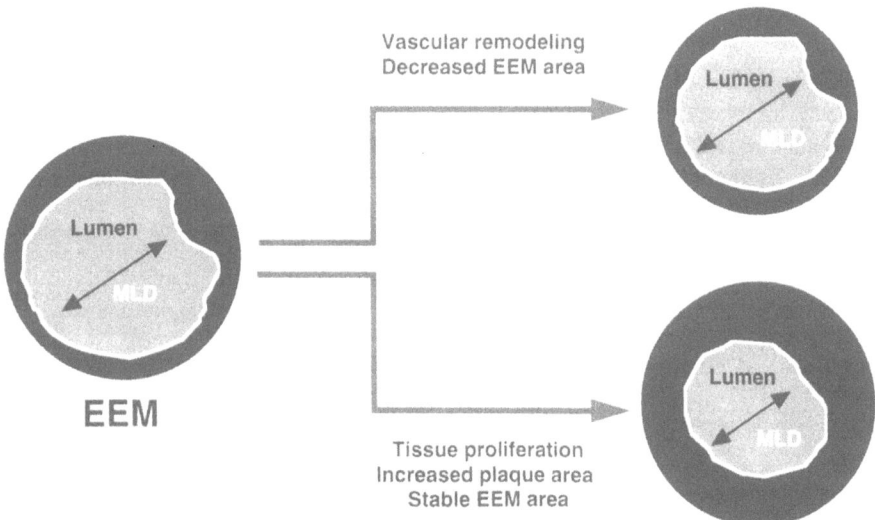

Figure 12. Mechanisms of lumen loss and restenosis after angioplasty. These processes can be assessed by serial IVUS examinations in patients. EEM: external elastic membrane; MLD: minimal lumen diameter.

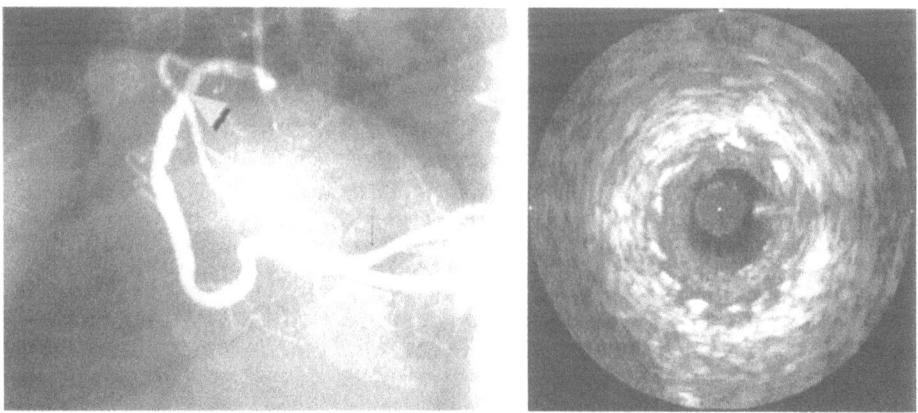

Figure 13. Angiographic and IVUS images of a Wallstent at follow-up. IVUS shows tissue proliferation within the stent at follow-up.

Research applications of intravascular ultrasound and technical developments

The precise assessment of the extent of plaque burden by IVUS makes it the ideal tool for clinical trials of regression of atherosclerosis [59]. Clinical studies with lipid-lowering agents have resulted in small angiographic improvement but drastic reductions in clinical events [60]. This apparent paradox may be due, in addition to improvement of endothelial function, to the poor sensitivity of arteriography to detect changes in plaque burden in the presence of bidirectional remodeling. Quantitative analysis of two-dimensional IVUS images in future regression trials will require the selection of several cross-sections which needs to be carefully matched at baseline and at follow-up. Three-dimensional reconstruction of IVUS images using dedicated systems and software will also be used to derive the changes in plaque volume over time in coronary segments measuring 20 to 40 mm [61]. Three-dimensional analysis is also being used for the assessment of in-stent restenosis [54] and of its prevention. Technical requirements and present limitations of three-dimensional IVUS are beyond the scope of this chapter [62].

Other interesting technical advances in the field of IVUS include development of imaging guidewires and color flow mapping. The elastic properties of the coronary arterial wall can also be assessed with IVUS. This method called elastography uses computer processing of the radiofrequency signals. Finally, although this chapter has dealt with spatial information provided by IVUS, temporal correlation of ultrasound images can provide information on blood velocity and on actual volume flow.

References

1. Tardif JC, Pandian NG. Intravascular and intracardiac ultrasound. Coron Artery Dis 1995;6:35-41.
2. Tardif JC, Pandian NG. Intravascular ultrasound imaging in peripheral arterial and coronary artery disease. Curr Opin Cardiol 1994;9:627-33.
3. Pandian NG, Kreis A, Weintraub A *et al.* Real-time intravascular ultrasound imaging in humans. Am J Cardiol 1990;65:1392-6.
4. Tardif JC, Bilodeau L, Doucet S, Bonan R, Cote G. Comparison between mechanical and phased-array designs for intravascular ulrasound in stented and non-stented coronary arteries: animal studies. Circulation 1995;92(Suppl 1):I600-1.
5. Mudra H, Klauss V, Blasini R *et al.* Ultrasound guidance of Palmaz-Schatz intracoronary stenting with a combined intravascular ultrasound balloon catheter. Circulation 1994;90:1252-61.
6. Fitzgerald PJ, Belef M, Connolly AJ, Sudhir K, Yock PG. Design and initial testing of an ultrasound-guided directional atherectomy device. Am Heart J 1995; 129: 593-8.
7. Moussa I, Di Mario C, Moses J *et al.* Coronary stenting after rotational atherectomy in calcified and complex lesions. Angiographic and clinical follow-up results. Circulation 1997;96:128-36.
8. Evans JL, Ng KH, Vonesh MJ *et al.* Arterial imaging with a new forward-viewing intravascular ultrasound catheter, I. Initial Studies. Circulation 1994;89:712-7.
9. Hausmann D, Erbel R, Alibelli-Chemarin MJ *et al.* The safety of intracoronary ultrasound. A multicenter survey of 2207 examinations. Circulation 1995;91:623-30.
10. Pinto FJ, St. Goar FG, Gao SZ *et al.* Immediate and one-year safety of intracoronary ultrasonic imaging. Evaluation with serial quantitative angiography. Circulation 1993; 88:1709-14.
11. Liebson PR, Klein LW. Intravascular ultrasound in coronary atherosclerosis: a new approach to clinical assessment. Am Heart J 1992;123:1643-60.
12. Waller BF, Pinkerton CA, Slack JD. Intravascular ultrasound: a histological study of vessels during life. The new 'gold standard' for vascular imaging. Circulation 1992; 85:2305-10.
13. Porter TR, Radio SJ, Anderson JA, Michels A, Xie F. Composition of coronary atherosclerotic plaque in the intima and media affects intravascular ultrasound measurements of intimal thickness. J Am Coll Cardiol 1994;23:1079-84.
14. Hodgson JM, Reddy KG, Suneja R, Nair RN, Lesnefsky EJ, Sheehan HM. Intracoronary ultrasound imaging: correlation of plaque morphology with angiography, clinical syndrome and procedural results in patients undergoing coronary angioplasty. J Am Coll Cardiol 1993;21:35-44.

15. Vlodaver Z, Frech R, van Tassel RA, Edwards JE. Correlation of the antemortem coronary angiogram and the postmortem specimen. Circulation 1973;47:162-9.

16. Glagov S, Weisenberg E, Zarins CK, Stankunavicius R, Kalettis GJ. Compensatory enlargement of human atherosclerotic coronary arteries. N Engl J Med 1987;316:1371-5.

17. Porter TR, Sears T, Xie F *et al.* Intravascular ultrasound study of angiographically mildly diseased coronary arteries. J Am Coll Cardiol 1993;22:1858-65.

18. Mintz GS, Painter JA, Pichard AD *et al.* Atherosclerosis in angiographically "normal" coronary artery reference segments: an intravascular ultrasound study with clinical correlations. J Am Coll Cardiol 1995;25:1479-85.

19. De Scheerder I, De Man F, Herregods MC *et al.* Intravascular ultrasound versus angiography for measurement of luminal diameters in normal and diseased coronary arteries. Am Heart J 1994;127:243-51.

20. Nissen SE, Gurley JC, Grines CL *et al.* Intravascular ultrasound assessment of lumen size and wall morphology in normal subjects and patients with coronary artery disease. Circulation 1991;84:1087-99.

21. Nakamura S, Mahon DJ, Maheswaran B, Gutfinger DE, Colombo A, Tobis JM. An explanation for discrepancy between angiographic and intravascular ultrasound measurements after percutaneous transluminal coronary angioplasty. J Am Coll Cardiol 1995;25:633-9.

22. Tobis JM, Mallery J, Mahon D *et al.* Intravascular ultrasound imaging of human coronary arteries in vivo. Analysis of tissue characterizations with comparison to in vitro histological specimens. Circulation 1991;83:913-26.

23. Pande AK, Tardif JC, Doucet S, De Guise PD, Pasternac A. Intravascular ultrasound for diagnosis of left main coronary artery stenosis. Can J Cardiol 1996;12:757-9.

24. Wilson RF. Assessing the severity of coronary-artery stenoses. N Engl J Med 1996; 334:1735-7.

25. Rodes J, Malekianpour M, Juneau M, Cote G, Dupont C, Tardif JC. Exercise electrocardiography for the detection of restenosis after coronary angioplasty: insights from intravascular ultrasound [abstract]. Circulation 1997;96(Suppl 1):I462.

26. White CJ, Ramee SR, Collins TJ, Jain A, Mesa JE. Ambiguous coronary angiography: clinical utility of intravascular ultrasound. Cathet Cardiovasc Diagn 1992;26:200-3.

27. Miller DD, Donohue TJ, Younis LT *et al.* Correlation of pharmacological 99m- Tc-sestamibi myocardial perfusion imaging with poststenotic coronary flow reserve in patients with angiographically intermediate coronary artery stenoses. Circulation 1994; 89:2150-60.

28. St Goar FG, Pinto FJ, Alderman EL *et al.* Intracoronary ultrasound in cardiac transplant recipients. In vivo evidence of "angiographically silent" intimal thickening. Circulation 1992;85:979-87.

29. Pinto FJ, Chenzbraun A, Botas J *et al.* Feasibility of serial intracoronary ultrasound imaging for assessment of progression of intimal proliferation in cardiac transplant recipients. Circulation 1994;90:2348-55.

30. Rickenbacher PR, Pinto FJ, Lewis NP *et al.* Prognostic importance of intimal thickness as measured by intracoronary ultrasound after cardiac transplantation. Circulation 1995; 92:3445-52.

31. Tuzcu EM, Hobbs RE, Rincon G *et al.* Occult and frequent transmission of atherosclerotic coronary disease with cardiac transplantation. Insights from intravascular ultrasound. Circulation 1995; 91:1706-13.

32. Wiedermann JG, Schwartz A, Apfelbaum M. Anatomic and physiologic heterogeneity in patients with syndrome X: an intravascular ultrasound study. J Am Coll Cardiol 1995;25:1310-7.

33. Ge J, Erbel R, Rupprecht HJ *et al.* Comparison of intravascular ultrasound and angiography in the assessment of myocardial bridging. Circulation 1994;89:1725-32.

34. Yamagishi M, Miyatake K, Tamai J, Nakatani S, Koyama J, Nissen SE. Intravascular ultrasound detection of atherosclerosis at the site of focal vasospasm in angiographically normal or minimally narrowed coronary segments. J Am Coll Cardiol 1994;23:352-7.

35. Tenaglia AN, Buller CE, Kisslo KB, Stack RS, Davidson CJ. Mechanisms of balloon angioplasty and directional coronary atherectomy as assessed by intracoronary ultrasound. J Am Coll Cardiol 1992;20:685-91.

36. Braden GA, Herrington DM, Downes TR, Kutcher MA, Little WC. Qualitative and quantitative contrasts in the mechanisms of lumen enlargement by coronary balloon angioplasty and directional coronary atherectomy. J Am Coll Cardiol 1994;23:40-8.

37. Mintz GS, Douek P, Pichard AD *et al.* Target lesion calcification in coronary artery disease: an intravascular ultrasound study. J Am Coll Cardiol 1992;20:1149-55.

38. Mintz GS, Pichard AD, Kovach JA *et al.* Impact of preintervention intravascular ultrasound imaging on transcatheter treatment strategies in coronary artery disease. Am J Cardiol 1994;73:423-30.

39. Mintz GS, Popma JJ, Pichard AD *et al.* Limitations of angiography in the assessment of plaque distribution in coronary artery disease: a systematic study of target lesion eccentricity in 1446 lesions. Circulation 1996;93:924-31.

40. Impact of intravascular ultrasound on device selection and end-point assessment of interventions: phase I of the GUIDE trial. The GUIDE trial Investigators [abstract]. J Am Coll Cardiol 1993;21(Suppl A):134A.

41. Stone GW, Hodgson JM, St Goar FG *et al.* Improved procedural results of coronary angioplasty with intravascular ultrasound-guided balloon sizing. the CLOUT pilot trial. Clinical Outcomes with Ultrasound Trial (CLOUT) Inverstigators. Circulation 1997;95:2044-52.

42. IVUS-determined predictors of restenosis in PTCA and DCA: final report from the GUIDE trial, Phase II [abstract]. The GUIDE Trial Investigators. J Am Coll Cardiol 1996;27(Suppl A):156A

43. Hosokawa H, Suzuki T, Ueno K *et al.* Clinical and angiographic follow-up of adjunctive balloon angioplasty following coronary atherectomy study (ABACAS) [abstract]. Circulation 1996;94(Suppl 1):I318.

44. Simonton CA, Leon MB, Baim DS *et al.* 'Optimal' directional coronary atherectomy. Final results of the Optimal Atherectomy Restenosis Study (OARS). Circulation 1998;97:332-9.

45. Nakamura S, Colombo A, Gaglione A *et al.* Intracoronary ultrasound observations during stent implantation. Circulation 1994;89:2026-34.

46. Colombo A, Hall P, Nakamura S *et al.* Intracoronary stenting without anticoagulation accomplished with intravascular ultrasound guidance. Circulation 1995; 91:1676-88.

47. Karrillon GJ, Morice MC, Benveniste E *et al.* Intracoronary stent implantation without ultrasound guidance and with replacement of conventional anticoagulation by antiplatelet therapy. 30-day clinical outcome of the French Multicenter Registry. Circulation 1996;94:1519-27.

48. Goods CM, Al-Shaibi KF, Yadav SS *et al.* Utilization of the coronary balloon- expandable coil stent without anticoagulation or intravascular ultrasound. Circulation 1996;93:1803-8.

49. Bilodeau L, Doucet S, Cote G, Tardif JC, Olivier RB, Bertrand F. Can quantitative coronary analysis replace intravascular ultrasound to assess optimal stent deployment [abstract]. J Am Coll Cardiol 1996;27(Suppl A):305A.

50. De Jaegere P, Mudra H, Almagor Y *et al.* In-hospital and 1-month clinical results of an international study testing the concept of IVUS guided optimized stent expansion alleviating the need of systemic anticoagulation [abstract]. J Am Coll Cardiol 1996;27(Suppl A):137A-138A.

51. Mintz GS, Popma JJ, Pichard AD *et al.* Arterial remodeling after coronary angioplasty: a serial intravascular ultrasound study. Circulation 1996;94:35-43.

52. Tardif JC, Cote G, Lesperance J *et al.* Effect of probucol on vascular remodeling and tissue hyperplasia after coronary angioplasty: intravascular ultrasound results from the MVP randomized trial [abstract]. Circulation 1997;96(Suppl 1):I154.

53. Di Mario C, Gil R, Camenzind E *et al.* Quantitative assessment with intracoronary ultrasound of the mechanisms of restenosis after percutaneous transluminal coronary angioplasty and directional coronary atherectomy. Am J Cardiol 1995;75:722-7.

54. Hoffmann R, Mintz GS, Dussaillant GR *et al.* Patterns and mechanisms of in-stent restenosis. A serial intravascular ultrasound study. Circulation 1996;94:1247-54.

55. Libby P, Ganz P. Restenosis revisited - new targets, new therapies. N Engl J Med 1997;337:418-9.

56. Tardif JC, Cote G, Lesperance J *et al.* Probucol and multivitamins in the prevention of restenosis after coronary angioplasty. Multivitamins and Probucol Study Group. N Engl J Med 1997;337:365-72.

57. Teirstein PS, Massullo V, Jani S *et al.* Catheter-based radiotherapy to inhibit restenosis after coronary stenting. N Engl J Med 1997;336:1697-703.

58. Bonan R, Arsenault A, Tardif JC *et al.* Beta energy restenosis trial, Canadian arm [abstract]. Circulation 1997;96(Suppl 1):I219.

59. Takagi T, Yoshida K, Akasaka T, Hozumi T, Morioka S, Yoshikawa J. Intravascular ultrasound analysis of reduction in progression of coronary narrowing by treatment with pravastatin. Am J Cardiol 1997;79:1673-6.

60. Brown G, Albers JJ, Fisher LD *et al.* Regression of coronary artery disease as a result of intensive lipid-lowering therapy in men with high levels of apolipoprotein B. N Engl J Med 1990;323:1289-98.

61. Evans JL, Ng KH, Wiet SG *et al.* Accurate three-dimensional reconstruction of intravascular ultrasound data. Spatially correct three-dimensional reconstructions. Circulation 1996;93:567-76.

62. Roelandt JRTC, di Mario C, Pandian NG *et al.* Three-dimensional reconstruction of intracoronary ultrasound images. Rationale, approaches, problems, and directions. Circulation 1994;90:1044-55.

11. Cardiovascular flow measurements with IVUS

Nicolaas Bom, Wenguang Li, Stéphane Carlier,
Ignacio Céspedes & Antonius F.W. van der Steen

Summary

Current intravascular ultrasound techniques produce real-time imaging of a vessel cross-section with a scan plane normal to blood flow. When randomly distributed blood particles travel through this ultrasound imaging plane, the received echo signals decorrelate as a function of time. The speed of such a decorrelation procedure is proportional to the flow velocity. This phenomenon provides a potential to estimate blood velocities by means of decorrelation analysis.

In this paper, we present a method for measuring local blood velocity and quantifying volume flow directly from cross-sectional intravascular ultrasound data. This method is based on multiple decorrelation assessments with a sequence of radio frequency echo signals. The velocity measurement is obtained by comparing the measured decorrelation value with the prior knowledge of the beam characteristics of an intravascular ultrasound transducer. Volume flow is derived by integrating the cross-sectional area and its corresponding velocity vector over the vessel lumen.

In vivo validation results obtained in various flow conditions and preliminary patient studies indicate that the proposed decorrelation-based method is able to provide an accurate and reproducible measure of blood volume flow rate, offering a unique opportunity to simultaneously assess physiologic and anatomic parameters in human.

Introduction

Quantitative measurement of blood flow is of important diagnostic value for functional assessment of a vascular stenosis. Development of the miniaturized Doppler transducer mounted on a guide wire has made it possible to measure coronary blood velocities with minimal hemodynamic perturbation [1,2]. Intracoronary Doppler has been applied in the assessment of coronary flow reserve [3,4] and of the severity of coronary lesion [5]. The use of Doppler velocimetry alone, however, does not allow direct measurement of flow volume. For the purpose of measuring volumetric flow, the cross-sectional area and the velocity component of the flow normal (perpendicular) to the measurement plane must be assessed. Quantitative angiography may be used to estimate the cross-sectional area at the site of the Doppler sample volume, but the silhouette nature of angiography techniques limits the accuracy of the area estimate, especially in the presence of an eccentric lesion.

J.H.C. Reiber and E.E. van der Wall (eds.). What's New in Cardiovascular Imaging, 149–158.
©1998 Kluwer Academic Publishers.

Intravascular ultrasound (IVUS) techniques provide tomographic imaging of a vessel in real-time, allowing accurate measurement of the cross-sectional area irrespective of vessel geometry [6-8]. Thus, the combined/simultaneous use of intracoronary Doppler for velocity measurement and IVUS imaging for area measurement may potentially improve the accuracy of volumetric flow quantitation [9-13]. Despite the improved accuracy in dimensional assessment by IVUS, the measurement of volume flow using the Doppler approach is still indirect. The mean cross-sectional velocity is derived from the peak Doppler velocity under the assumption of a parabolic velocity profile, while studies show a plug-like profile for most practical situations [14]. The accuracy of the estimated mean velocity highly depends on the position of a Doppler transducer within the lumen. The Doppler guide wire, therefore, must be carefully positioned to record the maximum velocity along the centreline of the flow stream. Another potential limitation of these multiple catheter approaches is the Doppler sample volume and the imaging plane can not be obtained coincidentally in time and space. Rapid changes in the luminal dimension over time (e.g. arterial wall compliance) and space (e.g. heavily diseased artery) may induce errors in integration of the velocity and area measurements. Additionally, the simultaneous use of multiple ultrasound transducers could cause possible interference between devices: for example, the Doppler transducer creates interference that presents as cross-talk on the IVUS image [13].

A new method for volumetric flow quantitation has been developed that extracts local blood velocity directly from IVUS data by means of decorrelation analysis of radio frequency (RF) echo signals [15-16]. This method provides two-dimensional velocity information that can be color-mapped and displayed simultaneously with the ultrasound image. A true measure of the volumetric blood flow is obtained by integrating all IVUS area elements with their corresponding velocity measurements over a complete lumen cross-section.

Decorrelation of blood echoes

The displacement of an ultrasound-scattering material such as blood moving through the beam of an ultrasound transducer results in concomitant changes (decorrelation) in the received echo signal. The decorrelation phenomenon can be clearly observed in the intravascular environment in which the ultrasound beam is transmitted perpendicularly to the arterial tissue and blood flow (Figure 1). In IVUS, it is commonly observed from real-time display that the scattering pattern of flowing blood varies rapidly over time. This is due to the fact that the flow stream drives the randomly distributed blood particles constantly washing in/out of the image plane, causing the received echo signals to decorrelate as a function of time delay. Two important characteristics in decorrelation of blood scattering signals should be addressed. First, because the flow usually has a higher velocity than wall motion, blood echo signals decorrelate significantly faster than those of tissues. The different correlation time in the received RF signals between blood and tissue has been documented in vivo in our earlier studies [17]. The time in which the blood RF signals remains correlated is approximately 1 ms, which is significantly shorter than that measured in wall echoes (>> 6 ms). Based on these observations, an RF processing technique has been developed for automated detection of the arterial lumen boundary [18]. Several research groups have also demonstrated that methods based on either video or RF processing can take advantages of the time-varying feature of blood echoes to improve the image quality [17,19-22].

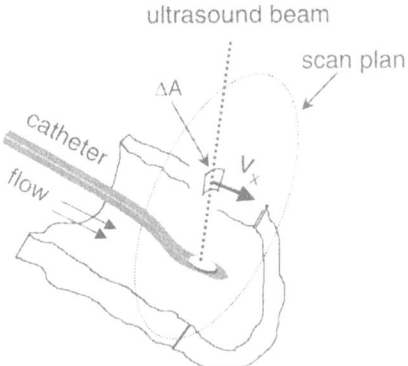

Figure 1. The coordinate of the IVUS imaging setup. The scanning plane is perpendicular to the direction of blood flow. The product of *A* and V_x yields a small flow element at each point, which can be summed over the complete cross-section for volumetric flow measurement.

Secondly, it is a reasonable hypothesis that the speed of the blood decorrelation process should be related to the flow velocity. In other words, the faster blood particles move across the ultrasound beam, the higher the decorrelation rate of the received signals will be. This hypothesis was tested with an in vitro experimental setup where the echo correlation of a blood mimicking phantom was measured at various flow velocities. Figure 2 clearly depicts that the decorrelation rate of RF signals increases with an increase of the flow rate. The relationship between echo decorrelation and flow velocity is approximately linear. This result suggests that if the velocity-correlation relation is pre-quantified for the type of transducers used, the measured decorrelation value from blood scattering signals can be converted into flow velocity.

Other applications of decorrelation have been described, which utilize the decorrelation due to in-plane motion. Measurements of echo decorrelation have been reported in application of tissue motion detection [23] and in the estimation of the beam-flow angle in order to retrieve the true blood velocity vector [24,25].

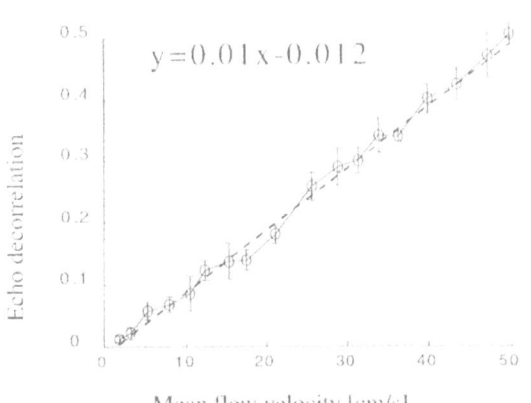

Figure 2. Plot of the measured echo decorrelation versus the flow velocity showing a linear relation. The linear fit is plotted as a dotted line.

$$y = 0.01x - 0.012$$

Decorrelation-to-flow quantification

The proposed method is based on decorrelation processing of a series of RF signals (time RF sequence) acquired approximately at the same transmission angle.

Spatial decorrelation model

Unlike most other medical imaging techniques, the majority of IVUS signals is acquired in the near field of the ultrasound beam (0.1–4 mm). As discussed above, the relationship between the correlation of echo signals and the scatterer motion across the ultrasound beam (lateral decorrelation) can be approximated with a linear model:

$$\rho_i = 1 - \alpha_i^x \Delta x, \tag{1}$$

where ρ_i is the correlation output at the ith window position and Δx is the lateral displacement of the blood scatterers. The slope α_i^x, termed the displacement decorrelation slope [mm^{-1}], is characterized by the beam pattern. As demonstrated in Figure 2, the linear dependence of signal correlation upon the scatterer lateral displacement has been validated in both computer simulation and in vitro with a flow phantom. Our results show that, because the beam pattern may change significantly in the near field, α_i^x is a beam dependent factor that requires to be calibrated for the type of transducer used [26,27].

Time decorrelation measurement

At each transmission angle, a sequence of N RF traces $(S_1 ... S_N)$ separated by a fixed time interval T, is acquired at a high pulse repetition rate. The decorrelation rate of the range-gated echo signals at ith depth window is evaluated in two steps:
1. align RF trace $S_2 ... S_N$ with S_1 by determining the time lag δT where the cross- correlation function reaches maximum. This is a phase matching procedure that removes the decorrelation due to the axial displacement (along the ultrasound beam) of blood scatterers.
2. calculate the correlation coefficient $\rho_{n,m}$ between pairs of traces S_n and S_m in the aligned RF windows. A slope α_i^t is obtained by fitting $\rho_{n,m}$ with a linear model:

$$\rho_i' = 1 - \alpha_i^t \Delta t, \tag{2}$$

where ρ_i' is the decorrelation output estimated in the ith window position and Δt is time delay. The slope α_i^t, termed the time decorrelation slope [s^{-1}], is related to the transverse blood velocity (normal to the ultrasound beam) for a given beam position.

Velocity estimation

When only the lateral decorrelation effect is considered, ρ_i in (1) and ρ_i' in (2) are identical. Equating (1) and (2), the transverse velocity is derived by:

$$v_x(i) = \Delta x / \Delta t = \alpha_i^t / \alpha_i^x, \tag{3}$$

Thus, the transverse velocity can be estimated at each window position from the ratio between the *calibrated* decorrelation function and the *measured* decorrelation slope from a time RF sequence. Note that the calibration procedure in equation (1) needs to be carried out only once for a specific type of transducer.

Volume flow integration

The local velocity measurement in a number of small, consecutive range windows can be repeated over the lumen cross-section to provide two-dimensional flow mapping. As illustrated in Figure 1, the volume flow is calculated by integrating the local transverse velocity with its corresponding area element over the complete imaging plane:

$$Q = \Delta r \Delta \theta \sum_{\theta} \sum_{R} v_x(\theta, r) r, \qquad (4)$$

where $v_x(\theta, r)$ is the local transverse velocity measured at angle θ and radial distance r. The resolution of the flow mapping is determined by $\Delta\theta$ and Δr, which are the scanning step sizes in the angular and radial measurements, respectively. Because the lateral motion of wall tissues has a much lower velocity ($v_x(\theta, r) \approx 0$) than blood, the contribution of tissue velocities in (4) can be automatically removed by setting a threshold. Thus, no contour tracing of the arterial lumen is needed.

Animal validation study

The above-described method was validated in vivo in pig experiments. The experimental procedures were approved by the Committee on Animal Experiments of the Erasmus University Rotterdam. After an overnight fast, 2 Yorkshire pigs were sedated and subsequently intubated and mechanically ventilated. Under sterile conditions, a femoral artery and vein were cannulated for infusion of drugs and blood pressure (BP) monitoring. One pacemaker lead was advanced in the right atrium via a jugular vein. An electromagnetic (EM) flow probe was placed around the contralateral common carotid artery after dissection. Via a sheath introduced in the free femoral artery, a guiding catheter was advanced under fluoroscopy up to this carotid artery root. A Princeps 4.3F IVUS catheter was than advanced 5 cm proximally to the EM probe. Zatebradine (UL-FS 49) 0.5 mg/kg was given to produce complete AV block, and the pacemaker was set at different heart rates. Simultaneous recordings of RF signals, BP and ECG were performed for different position of the IVUS catheter in baseline conditions. Adenosine (0.5 mg/kg/min, IV) was administered to produce hyperemic flow, and new RF and physiological signals were recorded. Finally, in order to lower the flow, ergotamine (20 g/kg) was infused.

Data acquisition

A single-element 30 MHz IVUS imaging system (Du-Med, The Netherlands) was used. The received RF echo signals were digitized at 200 MHz sampling frequency using a DA500A waveform digitizer and a MEM500 memory board (Signatec, USA), which enables real-time acquisition of 60 cross-sectional RF frames. Cross-sectional data were scanned at 16 frames per second with 100 angles per frame. Eight RF traces were acquired at each angle at 15.6 KHz pulse repetition rate (Ts=64 μs).

For each flow condition, a series of 60 consecutive RF frames was acquired over a period of 3.75 seconds, resulting in a time flow curve of 60 measurements. A total of 5 flow curves with 300 individual flow measurements (phasic flow data) was obtained in two pig experiments (hyperemic flow condition did not occur in one pig). EM flow signals were sampled at 4.4 kHz synchronously with the ultrasound transmission pulse.

Validation results

The volume flow data are in the range of 20–557 cc/min with mean values of 175.8 cc/min and 181.7 cc/min for EM and IVUS, respectively. The range of the mean cross-sectional velocities is between 3–79 cm/s, derived from the mean measured vessel diameter of 4.3 mm. As shown in the scatter plot (Figure 3), IVUS- and EM-flow data are in good agreement for low, basal and high flow conditions. The regression results between the two methods are: [IVUS] = 1.00 x [EM] + 5.72, r=0.98, p<<0.0001 and SEE=25.2 cc/min.

The paired comparison of the mean EM- and IVUS-flow values of the 5 time flow curves shows that no significant differences were found between the two methods (Mean ± SD: 5.9 ± 11.7 cc/min, p=ns). The SD of the paired differences is approximately 7% of the mean flow range measured.

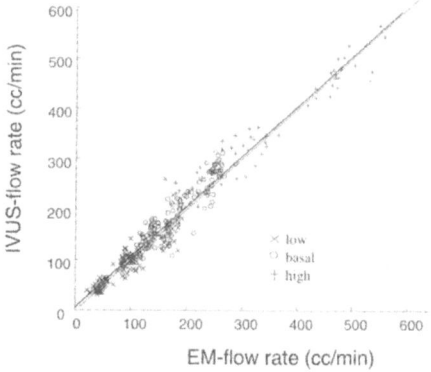

Figure 3. Scatter plot of EM and IVUS phasic flow data depicting a high correlation between the two methods. Data obtained under low flow, baseline and hyperemic condition are plotted with different symbols.

The upper panel of Figure 4 illustrates two color velocity mappings superimposed on the original IVUS echograms obtained in low and high flow rates during the cardiac cycle. The EM and IVUS volume flow curves in one serial measurement is plotted on the lower panel, demonstrating a reproducible cyclic change of the flow rate and excellent phase matching between the data obtained with the two methods.

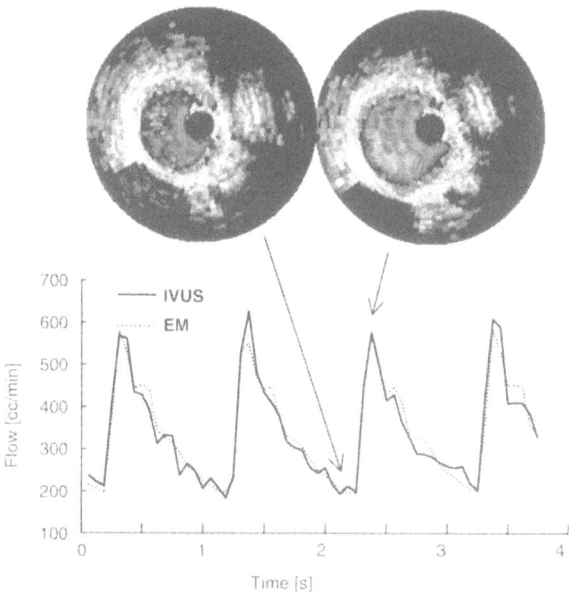

Figure 4. Upper panel: *In vivo* color flow mapping images obtained at low (left) and high (right) velocity settings. Lower panel: Flow curves of phasic EM-flow (dotted line) and IVUS-flow (solid line) showing an almost identical beat-to-beat change in blood flow volume.

Patient study

A series of patient studies was carried out to test the feasibility of using the decorrelation method under the clinical settings. The IVUS flow measurements were applied to several patients in peripheral and coronary arteries. If possible, volume flow data were measured in both basal and hyperemic flow conditions to assess the coronary flow reserve (a ratio between hyperemic and basal flows).

Results of the patient studies show that flow data with corresponding phasic changes during the cardiac cycle (systolic flow in peripheral arteries and diastolic flow in coronary arteries) were obtained in most of the studies. Increases of volume flow during the induced hyperemic condition were observed in more than half of the cases. In the study of a renal artery, a good agreement between the IVUS flow measurement and the flow estimated from the product of the mean Doppler peak velocity and the angiographic luminal area was reported [28]. Figure 5 shows an example of the IVUS flow measurements in a coronary artery during the hyperemic flow condition.

Discussion and summary

We have demonstrated the potentials of a new ultrasound method for measuring local blood velocities and volumetric blood flow with the same transducer that produces cross-sectional

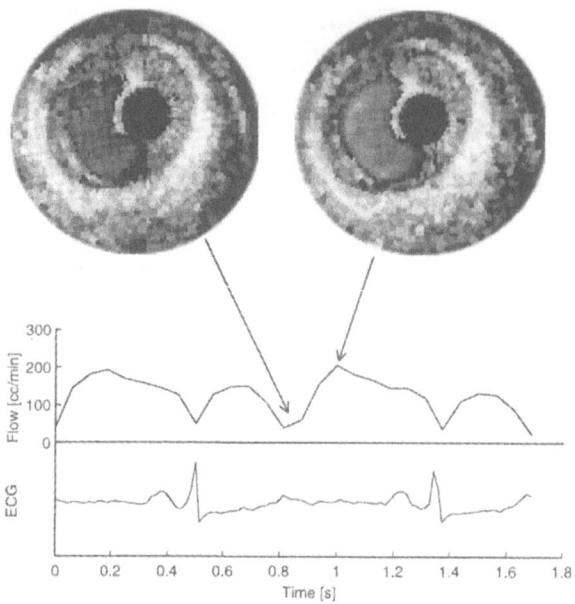

Figure 5. Upper panel: Coronary flow mappings obtained in patient for low (left) and high (right) flow rates during the cardiac cycle. Lower panel: IVUS-flow curve showing a typical 2-phasic diastolic flow pattern of a coronary artery in synchronization with the ECG signal.

image. Unlike Doppler velocimeter based approaches where flow is derived from the maximum/mean velocities and assumed flow profiles, the flow measurement by our method is calculated from all points in a cross-sectional velocity distribution. Thus, no assumptions are made concerning the shape of the lumen area or prior knowledge of velocity profiles. The accuracy of the volumetric flow measurement may also be improved by the fact that the area of integration and the flow velocity are computed from the same signals, which warrants that the area and velocity are obtained simultaneously and in place. Moreover, this single catheter approach should potentially provide a simpler and less expensive means to combine morphologic data and functional assessment of atherosclerotic lesions.

Doppler processing and time domain correlation techniques are the two most common methods for measurements of blood velocity [29,30]. In general, both techniques are used to measure the axial velocity component (velocity along the ultrasound beam) of the blood flow, which requires that the ultrasound beam has a beam-flow angle << 90°. The right angle between the flow direction and the scanning plane in IVUS imaging, on one hand, limits straightforward application of these conventional ultrasonic methods for velocity estimates. On the other hand, this unique geometric configuration allows assessment of blood volume flowing through the imaging plane using decorrelation techniques. The relatively fixed spatial relationship between blood flow and the ultrasound beam minimizes errors caused by an undetermined beam-flow angle encountered in many clinical applications.

One error source concerning this method is the measurement variation due to the use of a small window in the decorrelation-velocity estimation. Since the flow volume is derived from the velocity data over the entire cross-section, one may expect that variations of each individual velocity measurement will be generally averaged out by the integration procedure.

In vivo validation results obtained in various flow conditions indicate that the proposed IVUS flow quantitation method is able to provide accurate and reproducible measure of blood volume flow rate. Evaluation in the cathlab has shown its capability to measure volume flow in human, offering a unique opportunity to simultaneously assess physiologic and anatomic parameters with the same device. This enhances the diagnostic capability of the intravascular ultrasound imaging technique and will have significant impact on clinical decision making.

References

1. Doucette JW, Corl PD, Payne HM *et al.* Validation of a Doppler guide wire for intravascular measurement of coronary artery flow velocity. Circulation 1992;85:1899-911.
2. Porenta G, Schima H, Turalic F *et al.* Distortion of coronary flow profiles by Doppler wires: impact of pulsatility [abstract]. Circulation 1996;94(Suppl 1):I560.
3. Wilson RF, Laughlin DE, Ackell PH *et al.* Transluminal, subselective measurement of coronary artery blood flow velocity and vasodilator reserve in man. Circulation 1985;72:82-92.
4. Serruys PW, Zijlstra F, Laarman GJ, Reiber HH, Beatt K, Roelandt J. A comparison of two methods to measure coronary flow reserve in the setting of coronary angioplasty: intracoronary blood flow velocity measurements with a Doppler catheter, and digital subtraction cineangiography. Eur Heart J 1989;10:725-36.
5. Johnson EL, Yock PG, Hargrave VK *et al.* Assessment of severity of coronary stenoses using a Doppler catheter. Validation of a method based on the continuity equation. Circulation 1989;80:625-35.
6. Bom N, Ten Hoff H, Lancée CT, Gussenhoven WJ, Bosch JG. Early and recent intraluminal ultrasound devices. Int J Card Imaging 1989;4:79-88.
7. Yock PG, Linker DT. Intravascular ultrasound. Looking below the surface of vascular disease. Circulation 1990;81:1715-8.
8. Nissen SE, Gurley JC, Grines CL *et al.* Intravascular ultrasound assessment of lumen size and wall morphology in normal subjects and patients with coronary artery disease. Circulation 1991;84:1087-99.
9. Eichhorn EJ, Alvarez LG, Jessen MF *et al.* Measurement of coronary and peripheral artery flow by intravascular ultrasound and pulsed Doppler velocimetry. Am J Cardiol 1992;70:542-5.
10. Grayburn PA, Willard JE, Haagen DR, Brickner ME, Alvarez LG, Eichhorn EJ. Measurement of coronary flow using high-frequency intravascular ultrasound imaging and pulsed Doppler velocimetry: in vitro feasibility studies. J Am Soc Echocardiogr 1992;5:5-12.
11. Sudhir K, Maccgregor JS, Barbant SD *et al.* Assessment of coronary conductance and resistance vessel reactivity in response to nitroglycerin, ergonovine and adenosine: in vivo studies with simultaneous intravascular two-dimensional and Doppler ultrasound. J Am Coll Cardiol 1993;21:1261-8.
12. Chou TM, Sudhir K, Iwanaga S, Chatterjee K, Yock PG. Measurement of volumetric coronary blood flow by simultaneous intravascular two-dimensional and Doppler ultrasound: validation in an animal mode. Am Heart J 1993; 2:237-43.
13. Isner JM, Kaufman J, Rosenfield K *et al.* Combined physiologic and anatomic assessment of percutaneous revascularization using a Doppler guidewire and ultrasound catheter. Am J Cardiol 1993;71:70D-86D.
14. Asakura T, Karino T. Flow patterns and spatial distribution of atherosclerotic lesions in human coronary arteries. Circ Res 1990;66:1045-66.
15. Li W, Lancée CT, Van der Steen AFW, Gussenhoven EJ, Bom N. Blood velocity estimation with high-frequency intravascular ultrasound. Proc IEEE Ultrason Symp 1996:1485-8.
16. Li W, Van der Steen AFW, Lancée CT, Gussenhoven EJ, Bom N. Automated lumen detection and flow estimation with radio frequency intravascular ultrasound: in vitro and in vivo feasibility studies [abstract]. Circulation 1996;94(Suppl 1):I-603.
17. Li W, Van der Steen AFW, Lancée CT, Honkoop J, Gussenhoven EJ, Bom N. Temporal correlation of blood scattering signals in vivo from radiofrequency intravascular ultrasound. Ultrasound Med Biol 1996;22:583-90.
18. Li W, Van der Steen AFW, Lancée CT, Gussenhoven EJ, Bom N. Lumen enhancement and flow estimation by temporal correlation of radio frequency intravascular ultrasound. Proc IEEE EMBS 1996;18:838.

19.   Pasterkamp G, Van der Heiden MS, Post MJ, Ter Haar Romeny B, Mali WPTM, Borst, C. Discrimination of the intravascular lumen and dissections in a single 30-MHz US image: use of 'confounding' blood back-scatter to advantage. Radiology 1993;187:871-2.

20.   Li W, Gussenhoven, EJ, Zhong Y *et al.* Temporal averaging for quantification of lumen dimensions in intra-vascular ultrasound images. Ultrasound Med Biol 1994;20:117-22.

21.   Gronningsaeter A, Angelsen BA, Gresli A, Torp H, Linker DT. Blood noise reduction in intravascular ultra-sound imaging. IEEE Trans Ultrason Ferroelectr Freq Contr 1995;42:200-9.

22.   Gronningsaeter A, Angelsen BAJ, Heimdal A, Torp HG. Vessel wall detection and blood noise reduction in intravascular ultrasound imaging. IEEE Trans Ultrason Ferroelectr Freq Contr 1996;43:359-69.

23.   Dickinson RJ, Hill CR. Measurement of soft tissue motion using correlation between A-scans. Ultrasound Med Biol 1982;8:263-71.

24.   Zhang X, Shikutani M, Yamamoto K. Measurement of displacement and flow vectors with a single ultra-sound beam using a correlation technique (II) - Computer simulation and basic experiments. Techn Report IEICE 1995;35:23-30.

25.   Dotti D, Lombardi R. Estimation of the angle between ultrasound beam and blood velocity through corre-lation functions. IEEE Trans Ultrason. Ferroelectr Freq Cont 1996;43:864-9.

26.   Li W, Lancée CT, Céspedes EI, van der Steen AFW, Bom N. Decorrelation of intravascular echo signals: potentials for blood velocity estimation. J Acoust Soc Am 1997;102:3785-94.

27.   Li W, Van der Steen AFW, Lancée CT, Céspedes EI, Bom N. Blood flow imaging and volume flow quanti-tation with intravascular ultrasound. Ultrasound Med Biol. In press 1998.

28.   Carlier S, Li W, Céspedes EI *et al.* Simultaneous morphological and functional assessment of a renal artery stenting with intravascular ultrasound. Circulation. In press 1998.

29.   Hoeks APG, Arts TGJ, Brands PJ, Reneman RS. Comparison of the performance of the RF cross correla-tion and Doppler autocorrelation technique to estimate the mean velocity of simulated ultrasound signals. Ultrasound Med Biol 1993;19:727-40.

30.   Jensen JA. Estimation of blood velocities using ultrasound: a signal processing approach. New York: Univer-sity Press;1996.

12.

Optimal ultrasound guided balloon angioplasty

Carlo Di Mario, Joseph De Gregorio, Issam Moussa, Remo Albiero,
Nobuyoshi Kobayashi, Marco Vaghetti & Antonio Colombo

Summary

In the early '90ies an important discrepancy has been shown between angiographic and ultrasound findings after balloon angioplasty, but only in the last years, new strategies of aggressive balloon dilatation based on the ultrasound measurements have been applied. In the CLOUT study, upsizing of the balloon based on the ultrasound measurements was required in 73% of the lesions, ranging from 0.25 mm to 1.25 mm. An even more aggressive strategy was allowed by the availability of coronary stents, allowing focal treatment of the segments of residual lumen narrowing or severe dissection. The balloon was further upsized, matching the media-to-media diameter and, at least in the Milan and Washington experience, high inflation pressures were used. In the Tubingen study, the additional dilatation induced an increase in minimal lumen diameter from 1.95 ± 0.49 mm to 2.21 ± 0.47 mm and a decrease in residual diameter stenosis from 28.3 ± 14.9% to 18.1 ±14.4%, both p<0.0001. In Washington, ultrasound was used before treatment to select the appropriate balloon and the result was accepted only if the lumen area in the treated segment was ≥ 70% of the reference lumen area and no flow limiting dissections were observed. In 94/242 lesions (39%) these criteria were fulfilled, with a minimal lumen area of 6.0 ± 2.8 mm^2 and a residual plaque burden of 54 ± 16%. No procedural coronary ruptures or abrupt vessel closure were observed. At a mean follow-up of 8 months, target lesion revascularization was lower in the group treated with PTCA only (7.8%) than in the group crossed-over to stent implantation (12.9%, p<0.08). In Milan, the IVUS guided PTCA strategy was addressed primarily to long lesions (>15 mm) and to lesions located in small vessels (<3.0 mm reference diameter). Balloon angioplasty was initially performed using an angiographically oversized balloon inflated until full balloon expansion was achieved and then an IVUS examination was performed. IVUS success criteria were defined as the presence of a true minimal lumen area ≥ 5.5 mm^2 or of a minimal lumen cross-sectional area ≥ 50% of the vessel cross-sectional area at the lesion site. In this unfavourable lesion subset, at 5 months clinical follow-up, the cumulative incidence of major adverse cardiac events (death, Q-wave myocardial infarction, target lesion revascularization) was 28%, with an angiographic restenosis rate (≥50% diameter stenosis) of 27%.

These preliminary results from different centers suggest that the procedural success is higher than the success obtained with conventional PTCA in similar lesion subsets and, with the application of stents when needed, similar to the success of elective stenting. Randomized trials are required to establish whether this strategy can improve immediate and long-term results of percutaneous coronary revascularization procedures.

J.H.C. Reiber and E.E. van der Wall (eds.), What's New in Cardiovascular Imaging, 159–170.
©1998 Kluwer Academic Publishers.

ICUS during balloon angioplasty: observational studies

The first clinical applications of intracoronary ultrasound were performed during and after balloon angioplasty. The detection of large dissection flaps, of severe residual plaque burden, of discrepancy between angiographic and ultrasound measurements of lumen dimensions were the first elements which convinced the pioneers of intracoronary ultrasound that this technique had a real usefulness for guidance of coronary interventions [1-5]. The first studies in this field aimed at the classification of the vessel changes and wall disruption observed after PTCA and to the assessment of the prognostic value of the ultrasound observations after PTCA [6-7]. The most complete classifications of the ultrasound findings after PTCA were proposed by the groups of Irvine and Mainz/Essen, identifying several classes based on presence, radial and longitudinal extension of wall disruptions. Plaque tears or dissections were observed in the majority of the patients treated in both studies (63% and 83%, respectively) but the two groups observed opposite differences in long-term outcome. In the Irvine study [6] the highest incidence of restenosis was observed in the absence of plaque tears, suggesting that plaque compression and wall stretch are quickly reversible after PTCA, at high risk of early recoil. This observation is confirmed by the study of the mechanisms of PTCA, showing that plaque fracture with exposure of the elastic vessel adventitia to the intraluminal pressure is an essential component of the PTCA success [8]. In the German study [7], circumferential dissections extending to the media showed the highest incidence of restenosis (59%), suggesting early obliteration of the neolumen.

These initial observations outlined the advantage of ultrasound versus angiography during balloon angioplasty. The haziness and intraluminal defects frequently observed after PTCA with angiography reflect the irregular contours of the vessel neolumen but a planar technique such as angiography cannot identify and measure the complex wall changes occurring during balloon angioplasty. A new definition ("pseudo restenosis") was introduced by Steve Nissen to indicate the false perception of a successful angiographic result after PTCA generated by the presence of circumferential dissection around a persistently small true lumen [9]. The high incidence of this phenomenon was confirmed by intracoronary Doppler studies revealing that inadequate improvement of distal coronary flow reserve is observed in patients with early recurrence of symptoms after PTCA [10]. Ultrasound provides tomographic images of the vessel lumen and wall, ideal for the assessment of these complex wall disruptions. Only if superficial calcium is present, a condition associated with a higher incidence of dissections [11], the detection of wall dissections around the calcified plaque is more difficult because of calcium induced shadowing. Since the angiographic parameters, including quantitative angiographic measurements, are poor predictors of the long-term result after balloon angioplasty [12], the best application of ICUS after balloon angioplasty was felt to be the detection of lesions at high-risk of development of restenosis at the time of the initial procedure. This would allow the operator to immediately perform further interventions to improve the long-term outcome.

In 1993, the Interuniversity Cardiology Institute of the Netherlands (ICIN) promoted the first large prospective multicenter trial (PICTURE, Post IntraCoronary Treatment Ultrasound Restenosis Evaluation) to identify the ultrasound predictors of restenosis after PTCA. The seven participating centers performed analyzable ultrasound studies after PTCA in 170 lesions in 154 patients, and 82% of these patients returned for follow-up angiography. The qualitative analysis in this study simplified the classification of wall disruptions after PTCA and distinguished them into rupture, defined as a tear perpendicular to the vessel wall and dissection, parallel to the vessel wall, indicating their depth (within the plaque or involving the adventitia) and circumferential extension (in degrees) (Figure 1) [13]. This qualitative

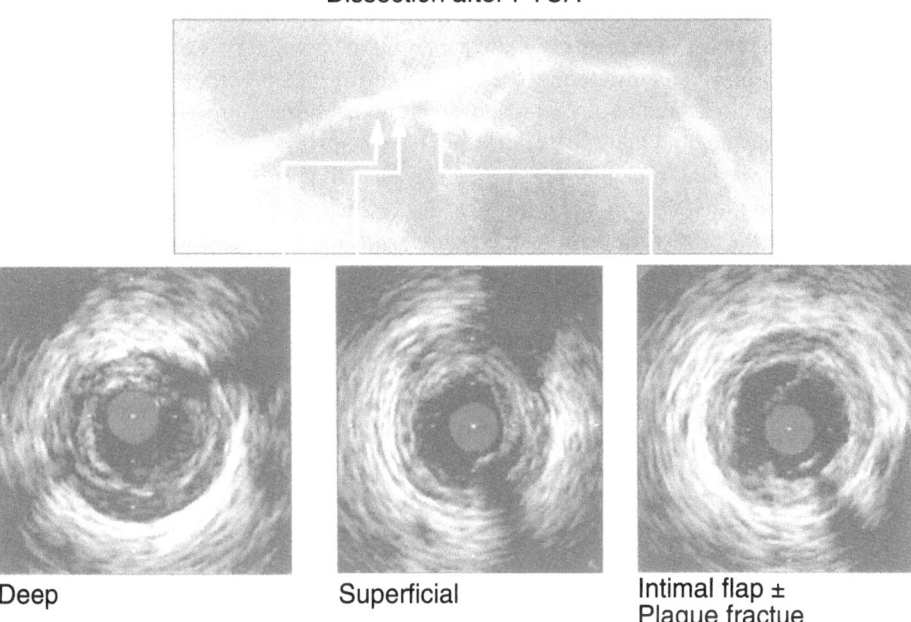

Figure 1. Upper panel: Angiogram after balloon dilatation of a long lesion in the proximal left anterior descending coronary artery. Lower panels: ultrasound cross-sections in the mid-distal segment of the lesion treated. A small true lumen and a large residual plaque is observed at the more proximal location (left panel), with a deep dissection between 2:00 and 7:00 o'clock explaining the apparently satisfactory angiographic result. More distal (right panels), at sites with less plaque, a superficial dissection (entry at 6:00 o'clock) and a plaque fracture (7:00 o'clock) with a small intimal flap are observed (1:00 o'clock). Ultracross 30 MHz, Boston-Scientific-Cvis, Mountain View, CA

classification, endorsed by the Study Groups on Intracoronary Ultrasound within the European Society of Cardiology [14], is now universally accepted. The correct methodology to perform measurements of lumen area after PTCA is more controversial. In the PICTURE study, all the surface occupied by blood was measured as lumen area, with the risk that functionally ineffective dissection planes are included in the final lumen area measurement inducing an overestimation of the true lumen open for blood passage. As in previous studies of mechanisms of PTCA [15,16], the PICTURE study observed that calcified plaques and hard fibrous plaques and, among these plaques, number of vessel quadrants with calcium were associated with a smaller minimal lumen diameter at the end of the procedure but no correlation was observed between plaque characteristics and minimal lumen diameter at follow-up. Presence of dissection at the narrowest site was the only predictor of MLD at follow-up (1.81 ± 0.54 mm in the group with ICUS visible dissections, 1.60 ± 0.60 mm in the group without, p< 0.02). The quantitative measurements of final lumen area and vessel area were positively correlated with the final MLD at follow-up while residual plaque area and percent obstruction was negatively correlated. These last two parameters, however, had a weak nonsignificant correlation with restenosis if a categorical 50% criterion was used.

Improvements in catheter design and image quality as well as the enrolment of a larger patient population may explain the different results observed in the more recent trials conducted at Washington Heart Center [17] and at Stanford, coordinating center of the GUIDE II Study (Guidance by Ultrasound Imaging for Decision Endpoints) [18]. This last study, not yet published, has enrolled 500 patients undergoing PTCA or directional atherectomy (DCA) and used ultrasound only at the end of the procedure, with the operator blinded to the ultrasound results. This approach, similar to the approach used in PICTURE, differs from the method used in Washington [17] where, in 351 consecutive patients, ultrasound was performed throughout the procedure, including a pre-intervention study in most cases and used to select the most appropriate device, including Rotablator and excimer laser, and optimize the final result. Despite these differences, the two studies yielded similar results in the identification of ultrasound parameters predictive of long-term angiographic and clinical outcome. In the GUIDE II trial the only post-procedural parameters predictive of recurrence of symptoms, major adverse clinical events (most often re-PTCA) and angiographic restenosis after PTCA and DCA were ultrasound-based measurements. In particular, residual plaque burden, expressed as the ratio between plaque area and total vessel area after the procedure, showed the highest relative risk of recurrence of symptoms (RR=1.68). The other ultrasound predictors included post-procedure minimal lumen diameter, calculated from the planimetric measurement of true lumen area (dissections excluded), and reference lumen area. A curvilinear relation was found between angiographic restenosis (50% criterion) and residual plaque burden, with a steep slope in the range of plaque burden between 60% or above, associated with a restenosis rate of 50% or higher, and 50% or below, associated with a restenosis rate of 25% or lower. The importance of residual plaque burden has been more recently confirmed by the results of ultrasound guided directional atherectomy trials which showed a progressive decrease in restenosis rate according to the final percent plaque burden (58% in the OARS trial (Optimal Atherectomy Restenosis Trial) [19], with a restenosis rate of 29%, 43% in ABACAS (Adjunct Balloon Angioplasty Coronary Atherectomy Study) with a restenosis rate of 21%) [20].

Also in the Washington experience residual percent plaque burden was the most consistent predictor of follow-up angiographic results (dichotomic restenosis, follow-up diameter stenosis and late lumen loss). In this study, however, the highest correlation (r= 0.58) was achieved by a measurement not performed at the treated site, ultrasound reference lumen area, highlighting the importance of vessel size. An original contribution to understand why residual plaque area is so important in determining the long-term lumen patency came from a serial ultrasound study by the same group, comparing lumen and vessel changes immediately after the procedure and at follow-up in 212 lesions [21]. Contrary to the common belief that intimal thickening was the sole responsible of restenosis, a reduction in the total vessel area (chronic recoil or wall shrinkage) was the main mechanism of restenosis, responsible of 73% of the late lumen loss and of almost all cases of >50% angiographic restenosis. Other studies have confirmed this initial observation [22], showing that recoil is a late phenomenon after PTCA [23]. In lesions with a severe residual plaque at the end of the procedure a moderate percent reduction in total vessel area can dramatically impair lumen patency while the same percent change will have little impact on the lumen dimension if a low residual plaque burden was present immediately after treatment. The prevalence of wall recoil as the main mechanism of restenosis also explains the efficacy of the stent, an intraluminal mechanical scaffold preventing wall recoil, for restenosis prevention.

From observational ultrasound studies to active ultrasound guidance of PTCA

The diffuse nature of the atherosclerotic vascular involvement and the presence of compensatory enlargement in the early phases of atherosclerosis [24-27] explain the discrepancy between angiography and ultrasound, with the detection of moderate to severe intimal thickening also in angiographically normal vessel segments. Ultrasound, moreover, does not require calibration, a necessary step with quantitative angiography which is mostly performed using the guiding catheter with frequent underestimation of the true lumen dimensions [28]. Modifications of the dilatation strategy based on ICUS results include changes in balloon size, length and inflation pressure. If the ultrasound assessment is performed before interventions, the use of alternative treatment modalities (Rotablator for severely calcified lesions, directional atherectomy for large bulky soft plaques), can facilitate subsequent expansion with the PTCA balloon [29,30]. Although various reports suggested the use of ultrasound for optimal device selection and to judge and eventually improve the final PTCA result, a standardized protocol of PTCA based on ultrasound measurements was only recently proposed and tested in a pilot series in the CLOUT study (CLinical Outcomes with intracoronary Ultrasound Trial) [31]. In this study intracoronary ultrasound was used to guide the balloon selection, with a predefined strategy of balloon oversizing based on the amount of plaque burden. In this protocol ultrasound was performed only after an initial dilatation with a balloon sized on the angiographic reference diameter. The operator was then required to use a second balloon if the initial balloon diameter was smaller than the average of the mean lumen and mean vessel diameter of the proximal or distal reference segment. Quarter-size balloons were used routinely for accurate sizing. Upsizing of the balloon was required in 73% of the lesions, ranging from 0.25 mm to 1.25 mm and with a median increase of 0.50 mm, with a balloon-to-vessel ratio measured with quantitative angiography which increased from 1:1 to1:1.12. After balloon upsizing, no increase in incidence and severity of dissections was observed with a low incidence of abrupt vessel closure (2 patients, 1.9%, in 1 patient after recanalization of a recently occluded artery 4 days after myocardial infarction). The additional dilatation induced an increase in minimal lumen diameter from 1.95 ± 0.49 mm to 2.21 ± 0.47 mm and a decrease in residual diameter stenosis from 28.3 ± 14.9% to 18.1 ± 14.4%, both p<0.0001. Parallel changes were observed in the ultrasound measurements after standard balloon angioplasty and after IVUS based balloon upsizing, with an increase in lumen area from 3.16 ± 1.05 mm^2 to 4.56 ± 1.14 mm^2, p<0.0001. Interestingly, a large residual plaque burden was still observed at the end of the procedure (reduced from 77.6 ± 6.9% to 69.1 ± 7.5%, p<0.0001), with a high potential risk of restenosis based on the previously quoted ultrasound observations. Although the CLOUT pilot study demonstrated the safety of IVUS guidance for balloon selection during PTCA, the clinical efficacy of this strategy for restenosis prevention was not directly tested since no long-term angiographic or clinical results were available. Furthermore, based on the ultrasound observations after stent implantation [32-34], at the low nominal pressure used in the study (7.3 ± 2.3 Atm) it is unlikely that a full balloon expansion was achieved in all lesions because of the resistance of the fibrotic/calcified vessel wall.

In the same years important observations were made using ultrasound for a different type of intervention, stent implantation. The detection of incomplete stent expansion as a major determinant of subacute stent thrombosis was established by the pilot work of the Milan group [32-34] and contributed, with the use of the more effective antiplatelet agent ticlopidine [35,36], to a major reduction of this dramatic complication and, consequently, to the rapid growth of the stent implantation procedures. After the initial enthusiasm for the technique, it was soon apparent that stent implantation has clear limitations when not used for ideal indications (> 3 mm vessels, short lesions), because of a high risk of restenosis [37-41]. These limitations determined a revival in the interest for the "old plain balloon angioplasty", not seen as a cheap second rank alternative to stenting but approached with a new strategy based on the lesson learned from stenting. Appropriate balloon sizing and high pressure became an essential part of the procedure and the availability of stents as easy bail-out in case of dissection encouraged the interventionalists to try more aggressive approaches to exploit the full potential of lumen enlargement with balloon dilatation before stenting. Abizaid et al. reported the pilot experience of the Washington group, with significant methodological differences from the CLOUT approach [42]. Ultrasound was used before treatment to select the appropriate balloon based on the ultrasound measurements of the media-to-media proximal reference diameter. The large balloons selected (3.5 ± 0.6 mm) were then inflated at high pressure (>10 Atm, mean 13.5 ± 3.3 Atm) and ultrasound was used to measure the lumen enlargement. The result was accepted only if the lumen area in the treated segment was ≥ 60% of the reference lumen area and no flow limiting dissections were observed. In 94/242 lesions (39%) these criteria were fulfilled, with a minimal lumen area of 6.0 ± 2.8 mm^2 and a residual plaque burden of 54 ± 16%. No procedural coronary ruptures or abrupt vessel closure were observed in this group. At a mean follow-up of 8 months, target lesion revascularization was lower in the group treated with PTCA only (7.8%) than in the group crossed-over to stent implantation (12.9%, p<0.08). The group of Tubingen [43] has used an aggressive approach to balloon angioplasty with some similarities to the Washington study. The balloon was sized on the media-to-media diameter but the minimal pressure required for full balloon expansion was used (7 ± 2 Atm) and no predefined end-points were required, with stents used as bail-out only in a small minority of patients. With a 78% angiographic follow-up at one year, restenosis was observed in 19% of lesions.

Especially considering the unfavourable lesion length and vessel size in the Washington study, the incidence of late recurrence appears low. The main limitation of these studies is the absence of a control group so that the real usefulness of the ultrasound guidance cannot de determined.

The SIPS trial (Strategy of ICUS-guided PTCA and Stenting) was a prospective randomized comparison of immediate and long-term results of interventional procedures (PTCA/ stenting) guided by angiography or by intracoronary ultrasound [44]. Because of the broad inclusion criteria, vessels with reference diameter between 2.2 and 4.6 mm were included. Among the 286 procedures, stenting was performed in 48% of cases, with exactly the same incidence in the group with and without ultrasound guidance. Despite the additional cost of the ultrasound catheter, the cost of treatment was lower in the ultrasound arm because IVUS guidance was associated with a better clinical and angiographic outcome. In particular, in the lesions treated with PTCA only, the restenosis rate in the ICUS guided group was 24% vs 45% in the angiographically guided group, p<0.05.

Our experience in Milan uses some of the guidelines and end-points defined by the previous studies but differed because the IVUS guided PTCA strategy was addressed primarily to long lesions (>15 mm) and to lesions located in small vessels (<3.0 mm reference diameter). Balloon angioplasty was initially performed using an angiographically oversized balloon inflated until full balloon expansion was achieved and then an IVUS examination was performed. IVUS success criteria were defined as the presence of a true minimal lumen area ≥5.5 mm^2 or of a minimal lumen cross- sectional area ≥ 50% of the vessel cross-sectional area at the lesion site. Dissections were not considered a reason to cross-over to stenting as long as the previous two criteria were fulfilled and TIMI 3 flow was present. If the criteria were not met, upsizing of the PTCA balloon was performed by selecting a balloon with a diameter, taking into account balloon compliance, equal to the lesion media-to-media diameter. Regular (20 mm) or short balloons were used to avoid overstretching of the distal vessel in case of vessel tapering. If after high pressure dilatation (14.5 ± 3.8 Atm) with oversized balloon (balloon-to-vessel ratio= 1.29 ± 0.23) the lumen gain was still insufficient and the ultrasound criteria of optimal PTCA were not met, stent implantation was performed using a slotted-tube or modular stent implanted focally at the site where IVUS showed focal recoil (Figure 2). A total of 54 lesions underwent balloon angioplasty alone, while 55 lesions underwent balloon angioplasty and spot stenting. The operator was required to select the shortest stent necessary to cover the segment of severe residual lumen narrowing but still a total stent length of 19 mm was used. Type B2 and C lesions were present in 75 cases (58% of the total cohort) but type C lesions were more common in the group requiring stent implantation (49% vs 26%, p<0.04). Fluoroscopically visible calcification, present in 33 lesions, were also more common in the group undergoing spot stenting (p<0.03). The final percent diameter stenosis was 19 ± 14% in the PTCA group and 2 ± 13% in the spot stenting group (p<0.01), with angiographically visible dissections in 55% of the lesions, without differences in the two groups. Clinical success was achieved in 68/71 patients (96%), with procedural complications observed in 5 patients (1 vessel rupture after high pressure stent implantation, requiring open heart surgery, 2 patients with Q wave and 2 patients with non-Q wave myocardial infarction). One patient in the spot stenting group had subacute thrombosis and one patient in the optimal PTCA group had sudden death 2 weeks after treatment. At 5 months clinical follow-up, the cumulative incidence of major cardiac events (death, Q-wave myocardial infarction, target lesion revascularization) was 28%, with an angiographic restenosis rate (≥ 50% diameter stenosis) of 27%.

A common limitation of all these studies is the absence of a control group treated with conventional stenting (lesion covered from proximal normal to distal normal reference segment). These preliminary results from different centers, however, suggest that the procedural success is higher than the success obtained with PTCA in similar lesion subsets [45-46] and, with the application of stents when needed, similar to the success of elective stenting. The fear of an increased risk of acute complications due to the oversized balloons was not confirmed by these initial observations. More difficult is the assessment of the adequacy of medium-term results and especially of the need for target lesion revascularization and of the angiographic restenosis. Although the percentages in the IVUS guided PTCA patients may appear quite high at first glance, in small vessels and long lesions poor results were observed also after elective ultrasound guided stent implantation. The additional cost and duration of the procedure is a potential concern which can be solved with the development of combined ultrasound-balloon catheters and of ultrasound imaging wires [47].

Conclusions

Intracoronary ultrasound has gained widespread acceptance as the optimal method to detect stent malapposition and incomplete expansion. During balloon angioplasty, the use of IVUS has been limited to the detection of suboptimal results and angiographically silent dissections. The unique information on plaque composition and true vessel dimensions provided

Before procedure

Angiography

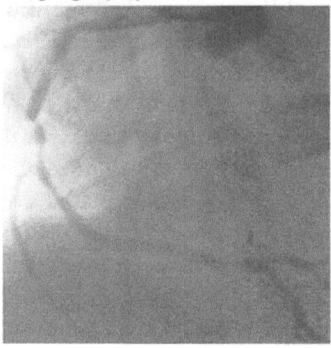

QCA

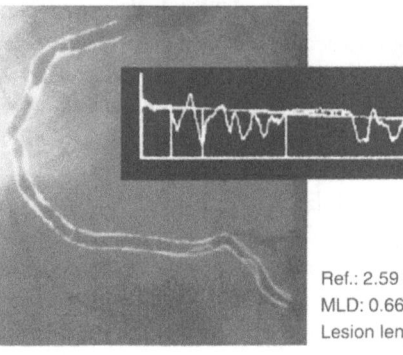

Ref.: 2.59 mm
MLD: 0.66 mm
Lesion length: 41.33 mm

IVUS findings after balloon angioplasty

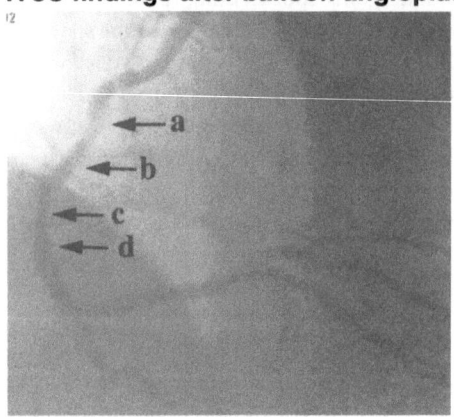

VOYAGER-C: 3.0 mm 20 mm 8 atm
b*: Media to media = 4.2 mm

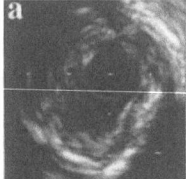
LCSA = 3.2 mm²

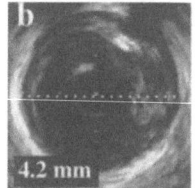
LCSA = 8.8 mm²

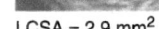
LCSA = 2.9 mm²

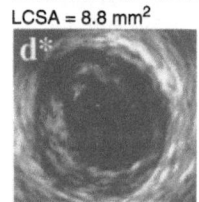
LCSA = 5.2 mm²

Final result

Angiography

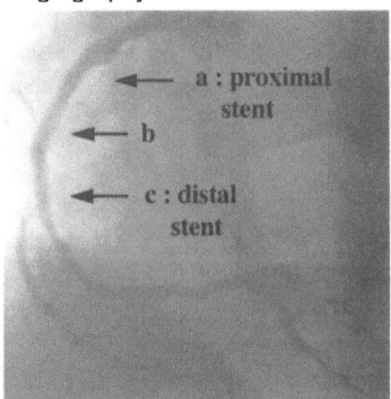

IVUS finding

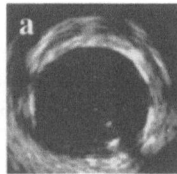
LCSA = 11.2 mm²
DART stent 16 mm

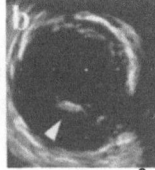
LCSA = 9.8 mm²
(arrowhead: flap)

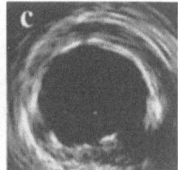
LCSA = 9.9 mm²
DART stent 16 mm

post dilatation
VOYAGER-C: 4.0 mm 20 mm 8 atm

Figure 2. Upper panel: angiogram showing a long tandem lesion of the mid-segment of the right coronary artery and a distal stenosis at the crux cordis. Note the measurements of reference diameter and lesion length with quantitative angiography, using catheter calibration (8 Fr). QCA-CMS, Leiden, The Netherlands.
Middle panels: After balloon dilatation (3.0 mm balloon, inflation pressure of 8 Atm) a dissection and severe residual narrowing of the proximal and distal lesions is observed, confirmed by ultrasound (Panels "a" and "c"). Note that the vessel diameter in the reference segment is much larger than expected from angiography, with a media-to-media diameter of 4.2 mm.
Lower panel: based on these ultrasound findings a 4.0 mm balloon is used and two stents, much shorter than the initial lesion length, are expanded at the sites of most severe residual narrowing and plaque accumulation. Note that a large lumen is measured with intracoronary ultrasound both within the proximal (Panel "a") and distal stent (Panel "c") and in a segment not covered by stents where a small flap is observed (Panel "b").

by ultrasound can offer much more for guidance of PTCA. Selection of balloon diameters matching the true vessel diameter improves the results obtained with balloons selected with angiography without increasing the risk of complications. Full metal coverage with long stents is not the answer in the treatment of complex lesions because a high risk of developing aggressive malignant hyperplastic responses is present. Learning the application of an interactive strategy in which ablation techniques, stenting and high-pressure balloon angioplasty are used if and when needed is the new challenge for the interventionalist with the potential of improving immediate and long-term results of percutaneous coronary revascularization procedures.

References

1. Nissen SE, Gurley JC, Grines CL *et al.* Intravascular ultrasound assessment of lumen size and wall morphology in normal subjects and patients with coronary artery disease. Circulation 1991;84:1087-99.
2. Tenaglia AN, Buller CE, Kisslo KB, Stack RS, Davidson CJ. Mechanisms of balloon angioplasty and directional coronary atherectomy as assessed by intracoronary ultrasound. J Am Coll Cardiol 1992;20:685-91.
3. Honye J, Mahon DJ, Jain A *et al.* Morphological effects of coronary balloon angioplasty in vivo assessed by intravascular ultrasound imaging. Circulation 1992;85:1012-25.
4. Hodgson JM, Reddy KG, Suneja R, Nair RN, Lesnefsky EJ, Sheehan HM. Intracoronary ultrasound imaging: correlation of plaque morphology with angiography, clinical syndrome and procedural results in patients undergoing coronary angioplasty. J Am Coll Cardiol 1993;21:35-44.
5. Discrepancies between angiographic and intravascular ultrasound appearance of coronary lesions undergoing intervention. A report of phase I of the 'GUIDE' trial. The GUIDE trial Investigators [abstract]. J Am Coll Cardiol 1993;21(Suppl A):118A.
6. Honye J, Mahon DJ, Jain A *et al.* Morphological effects of coronary balloon angioplasty in vivo assessed by intravascular ultrasound imaging. Circulation 1992;85:1012-25.
7. Gerber TC, Erbel R, Gorge G, Ge J. Rupprecht HJ, Meyer J. Classification of morphologic effects of percutaneous transluminal coronary angioplasty assessed by intravascular ultrasound. Am J Cardiol 1992;70:1546-54.
8. Botas J, Clark DA, Pinto F, Chenzbraun A, Fischell TA. Balloon angioplasty results in increased segmental coronary distensibility: a likely mechanism of percutaneous transluminal coronary angioplasty. J Am Coll Cardiol 1994;23:1043-52.
9. Nissen SE, Di Mario C, Murat Tuzcu E. Intravascular ultrasound, angioscopy, Doppler and pressure measurements. In: Topol EJ, editor. Textbook of cardiovascular medicine. Philadelphia: Lippincott-Raven; 1997. p. 2119-54.
10. Serruys PW, Di Mario C, Piek J *et al.* Prognostic value of intracoronary flow velocity and diameter stenosis in assessing the short- and long-term outcomes of coronary balloon angioplasty: the DEBATE Study (Doppler Endpoints Balloon Angioplasty Trial Europe). Circulation 1997;96:3369-77.

11. Fitzgerald PJ, Ports TA, Yock PG. Contribution of localized calcium deposits to dissection after angioplasty. An observational study using intravascular ultrasound. Circulation 1992;86:64-70.

12. Rensing BJ, Hermans WRM, Vos J *et al*. Luminal narrowing after percutaneous transluminal coronary angioplasty. A study of clinical, procedural, and lesional factors related to long-term angiographic outcome. Coronary Artery Restenosis Prevention on Repeated Thromboxane Antagonism (CARPORT) Study Group. Circulation 1993;88:975-85.

13. Di Mario C, Gorge G, Peters R *et al*. Clinical application and image interpretation in intracoronary ultrasound. Eur Heart J 1998;19:207-29.

14. Peters RJG, Kok WEM, Di Mario C *et al*. Prediction of restenosis after coronary balloon angioplasty. Results of PICTURE (Post-IntraCoronary Treatment Ultrasound Result Evaluation), a prospective multicenter intracoronary ultrasound imaging study. Circulation 1997;95:2254-61.

15. Gil R, Di Mario C, Prati F *et al*. Influence of plaque composition on mechanisms of percutaneous transluminal coronary balloon angioplasty assessed by ultrasound imaging. Am Heart J 1996;131:591-7.

16. Baptista J, Di Mario C, Ozaki Y *et al*. Impact of plaque morphology and composition on the mechanisms of lumen enlargement using intracoronary ultrasound and quantitative angiography after balloon angioplasty. Am J Cardiol 1996;77:115-21.

17. Mintz GS, Popma JJ, Pichard AD *et al*. Arterial remodeling after coronary angioplasty: a serial intravascular ultrasound study. Circulation 1996;94:35-43.

18. IVUS-determined predictors of restenosis in PTCA and DCA: an interim report from the GUIDE Trial, phase II The GUIDE Trial Investigators [abstract]. Circulation 1994;90(2 Suppl);I23.

19. Baim DS, Popma JJ, Sharma SK *et al*. Final results in the balloon vs optimal atherectomy trial (BOAT): 6 month angiography anf 1 year clinical follow-up. [abstract]. Circulation 1996;94(8 Suppl):I436.

20. Sumitsuij S, Suzuki T, Hosokawa H, Aizawa T, Tsuchikane E. Vessel and plaque changes in 3 and 6 months follow-up after aggressive directional coronary atherectomy in adjunctive balloon angioplasty following coronary atherectomy study (ABACAS) [abstract]. Circulation 1997:96(8 Suppl):I408.

21. Mintz GS, Popma JJ, Pichard AD *et al*. Arterial remodeling after coronary angioplasty: a serial intravascular ultrasound study. Circulation 1996;94:35-43.

22. Di Mario C, Gil R, Camenzind E *et al*. Quantitative assessment with intracoronary ultrasound of the mechanism of restenosis after percutaneous transluminal balloon angioplasty and directional coronary atherectomy. Am J Cardiol 1995;75:772-7.

23. Kimura T, Kaburagi S, Tamura T *et al*. Remodeling of human coronary arteries undergoing coronary angioplasty or atherectomy. Circulation 1997;96:475-83.

24. Glagov S, Weisenberg E, Zarins CK, Stankunaricius R, Kolettis GJ. Compensatory enlargement of human atherosclerotic coronary arteries. N Engl J Med 1987;316:1371-5.

25. Ge J, Erbel R., Zamorano J *et al*. Coronary artery remodeling in atherosclerotic disease: an intravascular ultrasonic study in vivo. Coron Artery Dis 1993;4:981-6.

26. Hermiller JB, Tenaglia AN, Kisslo KB *et al*. In vivo validation of compensatory enlargement of atherosclerotic coronary arteries Am J Cardiol 1993;71:665-8.

27. Gerber TC, Erbel R, George G, Ge J, Rupprecht HJ, Meyer J. Extent of atherosclerosis and remodeling of the left main coronary artery determined by intravascular ultrasound. Am J Cardiol 1993;73:666-71.

28. Di Mario C, Hermans WR, Rensing BJ, Serruys PW. Calibration using angiographic the catheters as scaling devices: importance of filming the catheter not filled with contrast medium. Am J Cardiol 1992;69:1377-8.

29. Lee DY, Eigler N, Luo H, *et al*. Effect of intracoronary imaging on clinical decision making. Am Heart J 1995;129:1084-93.

30. Mintz GS, Pichard AD, Kovach JA *et al*. Impact of preintervention intravascular ultrasound imaging on transcatheter treatment strategies in coronary artery disease. Am J Cardiol 1994;73:423-30.

31. Stone GW, Hodgson JM, St.Goar FG *et al*. Improved procedural results of coronary angioplasty with intravascular ultrasound-guided balloon sizing: the CLOUT Pilot Trial. Clinical Outcomes With Ultrasound Trial (CLOUT) Investigators. Circulation 1997;95:2044-52.

32. Nakamura S, Colombo A, Gaglione A *et al*. Intracoronary ultrasound observations during stent implantation. Circulation 1994;89:2026-34.

33. Goldberg SL, Colombo A, Nakamura S, Almagon Y, Maiello L, Tobis JM. Benefit of intracoronary ultrasound in the deployment of Palmaz-Schatz stents. J Am Coll Cardiol 1994;24:996-1003.

34. Colombo A, Hall P, Nakamura S *et al*. Intracoronary stenting without anticoagulation accomplished with intravascular ultrasound guidance. Circulation 1995;91:1676-88.

35.   Karrillon GJ, Morice MC, Benveniste E *et al.* Intracoronary stent implantation without ultrasound guidance and with replacement of conventional anticoagulation by antiplatelet therapy. 30 day clinical outcome of the French Multicenter Registry. Circulation 1996;94:1519-27.

36.   Schomig A, Neumann FJ, Kastratie A *et al.* A randomized comparison of antiplatelet and anticoagulant treatment therapy after placement of coronary-artery stents. N Engl J Med 1996;334:1084-9.

37.   Kobayashi Y, Di Mario C. Immediate and follow-up results following single long coronary stent implantation [abstract]. Circulation 1997;96(8 Suppl):I472.

38.   Saucedo JF, Abizaid AS, Kennard ED *et al.* Vessel size is an independent predictor of 1 year clinical events after new device angioplasty: a NACI Registry report [abstract]. Circulation 1997;96(8 Suppl):I23.

39.   Kawagishi N, Tsurumi Y, Ishii Y, Tanino S, Kawaguchi M, Magosaki N. Palmaz- Schatz stenting in ultra small coronary arteries (<2.5 mm) [abstract]. Circulation 1997;96(8 Suppl):I274.

40.   Fernandez-Ortiz A, Perez-Vizcayno MJ, Goicolea J *et al.* Should we stent small coronary vessels? Comparison with balloon angioplasty [abstract]. Circulation 1997;96(8 Suppl):I274.

41.   Akiyama T, Goldberg SL, Di Mario C *et al.* Stenting small vessels [abstract]. Eur Heart J 1997;18(abstract suppl):381.

42.   Abizaid A, Pichard AD, Calabuig JN *et al.* Can aggressive ultrasound-guided balloon angioplasty produce 'stent-like' clinical results? [abstract] Circulation 1997;96(8 Suppl):I582.

43.   Haase KK, Athanasiadis A, Mahrholdt H *et al.* Acute and one year follow-up results after vessel size adapted PTCA using intracoronary ultrasound [abstract]. Circulation 1997;96(8 Suppl):I194.

44.   Hodgson MJ, Roskamm H, Frey AW. Target lesion revascularization reduced after ultrasound guided interventions: findings after 6-month follow-up from the Strategy of ICUS guided PTCA and Stenting (SIPS) trial [abstract]. Circulation 1997;96(8 Suppl):I582.

45.   Reifart N, Vandormael M, Krajcar M *et al.* Randomized comparison of angioplasty of complex coronary lesions at a single center. Excimer Laser, Rotational Atherectomy and Balloon Angioplasty Comparison (ERBAC) study. Circulation 1997;96:91-8.

46.   Erbel R, Dill T, Dietz U *et al.* A randomized study of high speed rotational atherectomy and percutaneous transluminal coronary angioplasty in patients with complex coronary artery stenoses (COBRA study) [abstract]. Circulation 1997;96(8 Suppl):I80.

47.   Di Mario C, Fitzgerald PJ, Colombo A. New developments in intracoronary ultrasound. In: Reiber JHC, van der Wall EE, editors. Cardiovascular Imaging. Dordrecht: Kluwer Academic Publishers; 1996. p. 257-75.

13.   Prediction of restenosis by IVUS

Junbo Ge, Fengqi Liu, Rahul Bhate, Raimund Erbel

Summary

Restenosis after coronary interventions remains to be an unsolved problem of the transcatheter therapy. Recently, intravascular ultrasound has been considered as the current "gold standard" for precise diagnosis and quantification of coronary artery disease. It is a complementary technique to optimize the results of mechanical revascularization. The Guide Trial has shown that residual stenosis after coronary intervention is a strong predictor of restenosis. In addition, the CLOUT trial has shown approximately a 30% improvement in lesion lumen area after intravascular ultrasound guided balloon sizing. The final stenosis severity was similar to that achieved by coronary stenting in the Benestent and STRESS trials. The mechanism of stent restenosis is not very well understood. Intimal hyperplasia seems to be the main reason. However, how to prevent intimal hyperplasia, whether stent deployment using ultrasound guidance is superior to using angiography alone, or symmetric deployment using high pressure inflation is superior to appropriate pressure inflation, continues to be an unresolved issue. The ongoing trails such as MUSIC, OPTICUS, and RAVES may probably give us a clear answer. It is very clear today that intravascular ultrasound guided coronary intervention is able to adequately remove the amount of plaque and therefore reduce the restenosis rate.

Introduction

Sones performed the first coronary angiography in 1959 [1] and a new "gold standard" test became available for the evaluation of the coronary artery disease. The traditional approach for transcatheter coronary revascularization since the introduction PTCA by Gruentzig in September 1977 had been visual assessment of the lesion as well as the results of the intervention by coronary angiography [2]. Refinements in the technology and techniques for mechanical revascularization in the decade of 1980 lead to explosion of "new devices" mainly in an attempt to attenuate the major limitation of PTCA, restenosis. Various pharmacological agents have shown promising results in reducing the rate of restenosis, including monoclonal antibodies against the Glycoprotein receptors on platelet cells surface [3]. Yet restenosis continues to be the "Achilles heel" of transcatheter interventions. Restenosis occurs in 30% to 50% of transcatheter coronary procedures; however, the natural history and pathophysiology of restenosis are still incompletely understood [4]. Certain clinical, angiographic and procedure related variables have been identified as risk factors for restenosis [5,6].

J.H.C. Reiber and E.E. van der Wall (eds.). What's New in Cardiovascular Imaging, 171–182.
©1998 Kluwer Academic Publishers.

Restenosis after PTCA

In aiming to reduce the restenosis rate, one must understand the mechanism of lumen enlargement by PTCA as well as the limitations of coronary angiography which had been the traditional "guide" to PTCA. In the early 1970's, investigators challenged the accuracy and the reproducibility of coronary angiograms, especially inter- and intra-observer variability [7]. Comparative studies of angiography and pathology have shown the inaccuracy of angiography for evaluation of the extent as well as severity of coronary obstruction [8]. Angiography has limitations in assessing stenosis severity and morphologic characteristics of coronary atherosclerosis since it depicts complex coronary anatomy as two-dimensional silhouette. This "lumenography" is hardly of use in assessing the vessel wall.

IVUS appeared on the screen of interventional cardiology in the mid-1980's [9]. In it's early days IVUS had limited application because of too large size of the catheter. Miniatur-

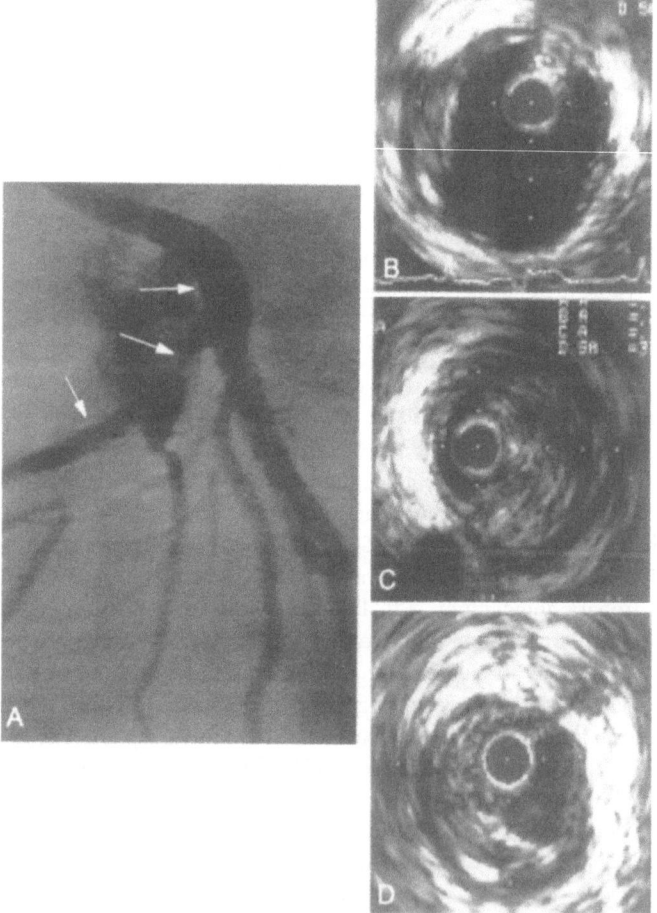

Figure 1.   Comparison of coronary angiogram (A) and intravascular ultrasound images (B-D). A severe stenosis is seen in the proximal LAD (A, middle arrow). Coronary arterial remodeling exists in the lesion segment (C). In addition, the angiographic reference segments (B and D) are also involved with atherosclerotic plaques.

ization of the IVUS catheter size (1mm diameter) revolutionized the field of interventional cardiology [10]. IVUS imaging provides cross sections of the coronary artery with high spatial resolution and within a few years of its introduction, IVUS has emerged from a research tool into an intrinsic part of modern invasive cardiology, mainly because histology can be obtained "in-vivo". For the first time in invasive cardiology it is possible to base decisions not only on "lumenograms" but also on vessel wall assessment [11]. The sensitivity and accuracy of IVUS technique for qualitative and quantitative study have been well validated; including validation of normal coronary anatomy, plaque composition and morphology measurements of vessel area, lumen area and plaque area [12-14]. Quantitative coronary angiography (QCA) had improved the reproducibility of angiogram and is often used to determine balloon sizing in relation with a "normal" reference segment as well as to calculate minimal lumen diameter and percent diameter stenosis and subsequent assessment of the intervention. IVUS has shown fallacies of QCA (Figure 1) by demonstrating compensatory enlargement of the diseased coronary artery in response to atherosclerosis (adaptive remodeling), presence of significant "silent" atherosclerosis in the so called "normal" reference segment [15]. Hence, QCA actually underestimates the balloon sizing. Also QCA often overestimates results of "successful" PTCA. It is because of frequent fissures and dissections, angiographically apparent lumen diameter appears increased. In reality, 60% to 70% of the vessel cross section within the lesion remains occupied by plaque (i.e. residual plaque burden) which

Table 1: Qualitative characteristics of the lesions in the target segments, and the proximal and distal nontreated segments before intervention[a]

	Proximal segments (n=27)		Target segments (n=30)		Distal segments (n=25)	
	No	*%*	*No*	*%*	*No*	*%*
Echo signal intensity categories						
Type A	15	56	6	20	14	56
Type B	8	30	4	13	4	16
Type C	4	14	20	67	7	28
Plaque eccentricity						
Concentric lesion	7	26	16	53	3	12
Eccentric lesion	20	74	14	47	22	88
Eccentric lesion type I	16	59	3	10	16	64
Eccentric lesion type II	4	15	11	37	6	24

a. Echo signal intensity type A plaques were defined as plaques whose echo signals were weaker than those of the reference adventitia. Plaques of this type contain mainly lipid, loose connective tissue or intimal hyperplasia. Echo signal intensity type B plaques were defined as plaques that had bright echo signals without acoustic shadowing. The echo signals were as bright as the adventitia or higher. Plaques of this type have been shown to be of dense fibrous tissue. Echo signal intensity type C plaques were defined as plaques with bright echoes (brighter than the adventitia with acoustic shadowing).

Table 2: Qualitative results of the target segments in the subgroup with IVUS examinations pre-, post-PTCA and at follow-up (n=30) [a]

	Before PTCA		After PTCA		Follow-up	
	No	*%*	*No*	*%*	*No*	*%*
Echo signal intensity categories						
Type A	8	27	8	27	5	17
Type B	4	13	4	13	6	20
Type C	18	60	18	60	19	63
Plaque eccentricity						
Concentric lesion	17	57	10	33	14	47
Eccentric lesion	13	43	20	67	16	53
Eccentric lesion type I	4	31	4	20	4	25
Eccentric lesion type II	9	69	16	80	12	75

a. Echo signal intensity type see Table 1.
   Eccentric lesion Type I: Eccentric plaque with still plaque-free wall on IVUS image (Figure 1C).
   Eccentric lesion Type II: Eccentric lesion with the whole vessel circumference occupied by plaque.

goes undetected by angiography [16]. Also fissures and dissections are much more frequently seen by IVUS than angiography.

If IVUS is considered as the current "gold standard" for precise diagnosis and quantification of coronary artery disease as well as for optimizing the results of mechanical revascularization, can certain morphometric and quantitative variables by IVUS imaging then predict restenosis following transcatheter revascularization?

We evaluated the mechanism of "successful" PTCA and late luminal loss by IVUS imaging. The study group included patients undergoing only PTCA for native coronary atherosclerotic lesions. A sub-group of patients were serially examined three times by IVUS: pre- and post-PTCA as well as at follow-up after 6 months. A total of 30 lesions could be successfully followed-up out of the 59 balloon dilations. The lesion characteristics at baseline, post-dilation and at 6 months follow-up are shown in Tables 1 and 2. The type C lesions [17] were the majority accounting for 64% lesions.

Plaque fracture and non-flow limiting dissections were the major mechanisms of the acute luminal gain (Figure 2). Dissections occurred in 80% of calcified lesions (calcium arc >90%), compared with 29% dissections in lesions without calcification or with <90% calcium arc. Axial redistribution of the plaque (i.e. concentric lesions changing into eccentric after PTCA and visa-versa) was more important than plaque compression. This was mainly due the advanced nature of the lesions rich in fibrosis and calcification.

Elastic recoil was noted in 35% of lesions on immediate post–balloon dilation IVUS imaging. After PTCA, there was a significant decrease in the cross-sectional plaque area from 14.5 ± 5.7 mm^2 to 11.7 ± 3.7 mm^2 (Figure 3). This accounted for the increase in lumen area although vessel area did not increase significantly. Six months later, the plaque area increased significantly and induced an increase in the percent area stenosis from 58.7% to 64.7%. But

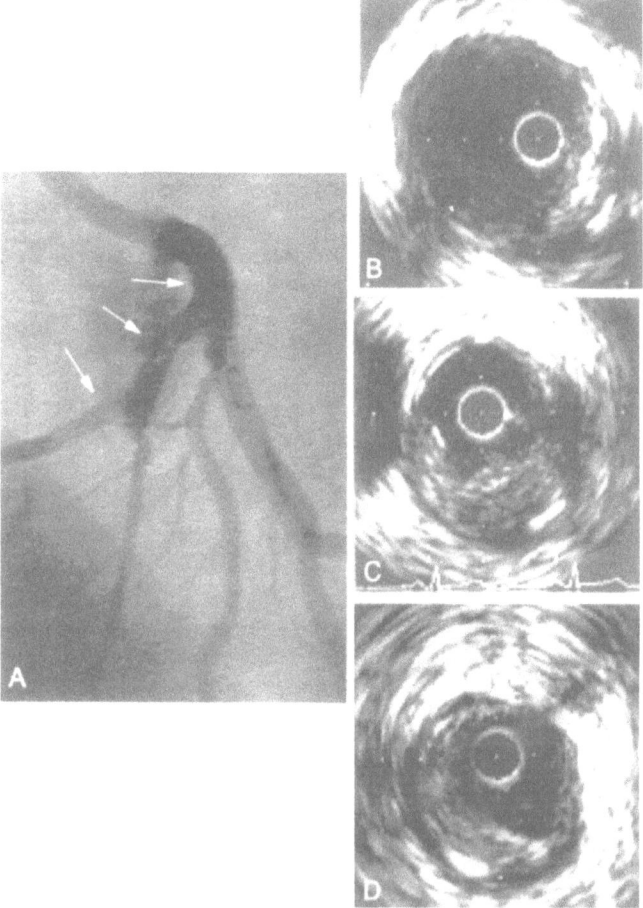

Figure 2. The same patient as in Figure 1 at corresponding sites post-PTCA. A sub-medial dissection can be seen on IVUS image (C). Coronary angiogram shows a good result (middle arrow).

the vessel area showed only a slight decrease (Figure 4). After PTCA there were more concentric lesions in the restenosis group than in the non-restenosis group (53% vs. 25%). The
residual plaque area was larger in the restenosis group than in the non-restenosis group, 12.0
± 4.7mm² to 15.4 ± 5.0mm². Thus intimal hyperproliferation is a major cause of late restenosis rather than chronic arterial remodeling (Figure 5).

The CLOUT Pilot Trial [18] has shown approximately a 30% improvement in lesion
lumen area after IVUS-guided balloon upsizing. This improvement was observed without
any significant change in dissection rate. The final stenosis severity after IVUS-guided
PTCA in this trial was similar to that achieved by coronary stenting in the Benestent [19]
and STRESS [20] trials. Thus, insufficient angioplasty can be considered as an additional
mechanism of restenosis following PTCA which only IVUS can detect and not the QCA.
Seo et al. [21] performed IVUS imaging immediately after PTCA to determine the need for
additional interventions and their effectiveness to prevent restenosis. The restenosis rate was

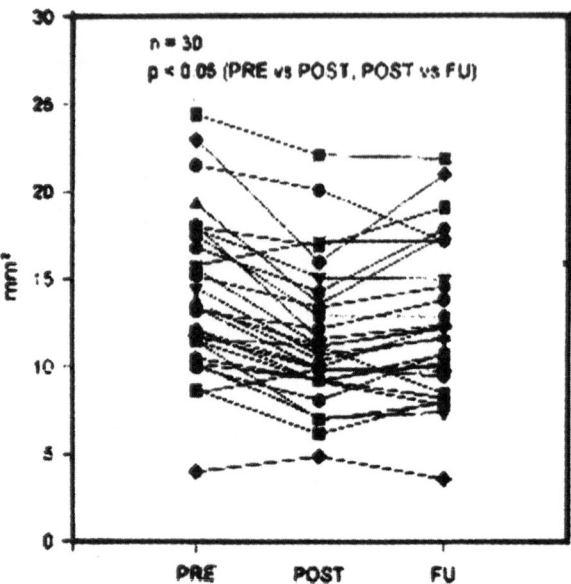

Figure 3. Comparison of the vessel areas pre-, post-PTCA and at 6-month follow-up in lesions with pre-interventional IVUS examination. There were no significant changes. FU: follow-up.

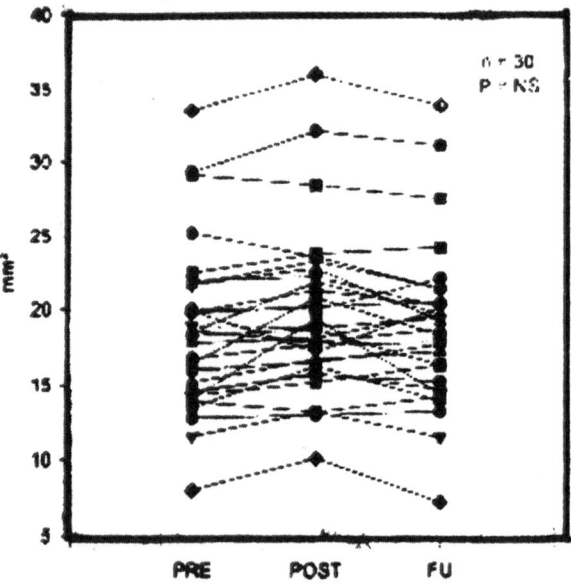

Figure 4. Comparison of the plaque areas pre-, post-PTCA and at 6-month follow-up in lesions with pre-interventional IVUS examination. The plaque area decreased post-PTCA and increased at follow-up, both statistically significant. FU: follow-up.

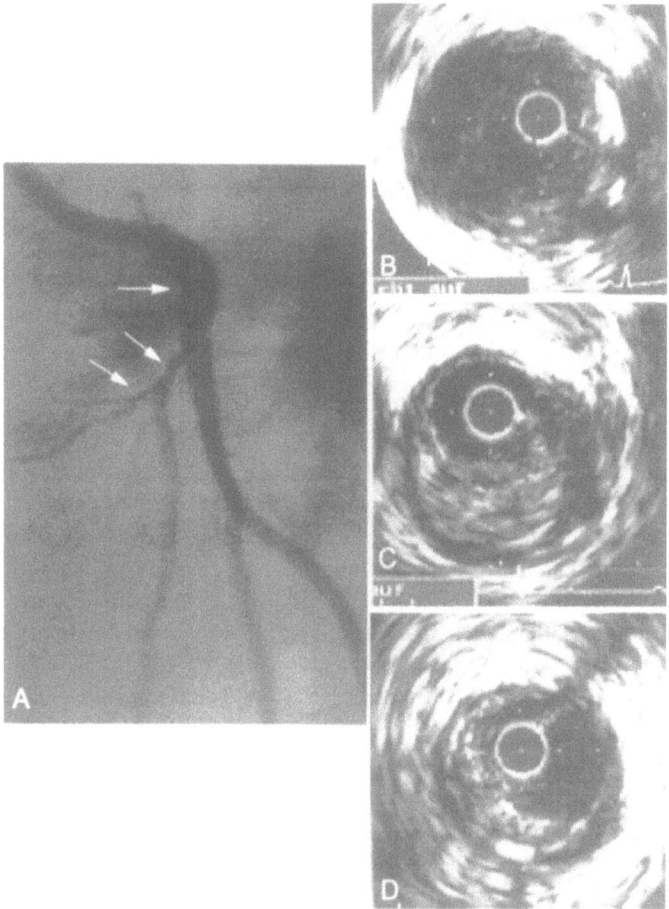

Figure 5. Coronary angiogram (A) and IVUS images of the same patient as in Figure 1 and Figure 2 at 6-month follow-up. Restenosis occurs at the PTCA site.

42% in patients who underwent PTCA without IVUS imaging and was 25% in those who underwent "sufficient" dilatation as guided by IVUS. The insufficient dilatation group exhibited hard plaque and calcification more frequently (58%) than in the other group.

Mintz et al. [22] used IVUS imaging for pre- and post-coronary intervention to assess restenosis rate using IVUS predictors. In particular, the IVUS post-intervention cross-sectional narrowing predicted the primary end point (restenosis) and two of the other three secondary end points (follow-up diameter stenosis and late lumen loss) and was therefore the most consistent predictor of restenosis than currently accepted clinical or angiographic risk factors.

In an "angiographic restenosis" study, Jain et al. [23] reported that the absence of plaque fracture, the existence of major dissection, and greater plaque burden as assessed by immediate IVUS study after coronary intervention were associated with increased incidence of restenosis. Tanaglia et al. [24] in a "angiographic" as well as "clinical" restenosis study noted by IVUS imaging immediately after successful coronary intervention, that the incidence of dissection detected by IVUS imaging after an intervention was significantly greater in patients than in those without a subsequent adverse event (63% vs. 53%, p<0.05). The severity of dissection also appeared to be related to outcome (p<0.05). Honye et al. [25] assessed morphological effects of PTCA by immediate post-PTCA IVUS imaging and reported that restenosis was more likely to occur when the original dilation left a concentric plaque without a fracture or dissection.

The angiographic assessment of lesion characteristics for transcatheter intervention is subjective and can be misleading. Assessment of lesion calcification by angiography and IVUS revealed only moderate sensitivity of angiography for detecting extensive calcification and 11% of lesions with angiographic calcification failed to show calcium by IVUS, i.e. false positives [26].

Restenosis in newer devices

At the moment IVUS is the only method for analyzing plaque distribution and composition in-vivo. IVUS imaging before intervention allows a plaque specific approach. PTCA of calcified lesions is often associated with dissection at the interface between calcified plaque and normal vessel wall. The presence of calcium is highly predictive of dissections after balloon dilatation and subsequent high restenosis rate [27]. Rotational atherectomy effectively pulverizes superficial calcium. In an IVUS study [28] of Rotablator followed by PTCA, DCA (Directional Coronary Atherectomy) or stents, Rotablator + stent achieved the largest lumen and smallest residual stenosis (Rotablator + PTCA = 24%, Rotablator + DCA = 16%, Rotablator + stent = 12%, p<0.0001). Lesions with deep calcification are more suitable for DCA. However, tissue removal is incomplete, since 40% to 60% of the cross-sectional area of the target lesion is still occupied by plaque [29]. This may be the reason for discouraging results of DCA in the CAVEAT-I [30] and CCAT [31] trials. But the Optimal Atherectomy Restenosis Study (OARS) utilized the spatial guidance by IVUS to detect residual plaque burden and better orienting the Atherocath with subsequent achievement of optimal results [32].

Honye et al. [33] used IVUS imaging to elucidate the mechanism of Eximer LASER Coronary Angioplasty (ELCA). No difference was found in lumen cross sectional area or plaque cross sectional area in the group treated with ELCA plus PTCA versus these measurements in the group treated with PTCA alone. Thus ELCA does not ablate a large amount of atheroma (9% reduction), but creates a pathway to permit easier passage of a PTCA balloon. These quantitative and morphological results may help to explain similar restenosis rate of ELCA plus PTCA and PTCA alone.

Benestent [19] and STRESS [20] trials have clearly shown that stenting by effectively tackling elastic recoil and chronic arterial remodeling, reduces the restenosis rate of transcatheter interventions. But adequate stent deployment is mandatory. Although IVUS may add cost and time, routine use of high pressure PTCA does not ensure optimal stent implantation by IVUS criteria [34]. Also edges of the stent struts often interfere with the edge-detection logarithm of QCA and this may lead to incomplete expansion of the stent with subsequent restenosis. Use of IVUS imaging to detect optimal stent deployment and for post-deployment high-pressure balloon has already relaxed intensive anticoagulation protocols, as well as reduced subacute thrombosis [35]. The mechanism of stent restenosis remains not well understood, some of the findings are even controversial. Some studies have indicated that in-stent restenosis uniformly distributes over the length of the stent [36]. However, coverage of the whole atherosclerotic lesion is a important factor for preventing

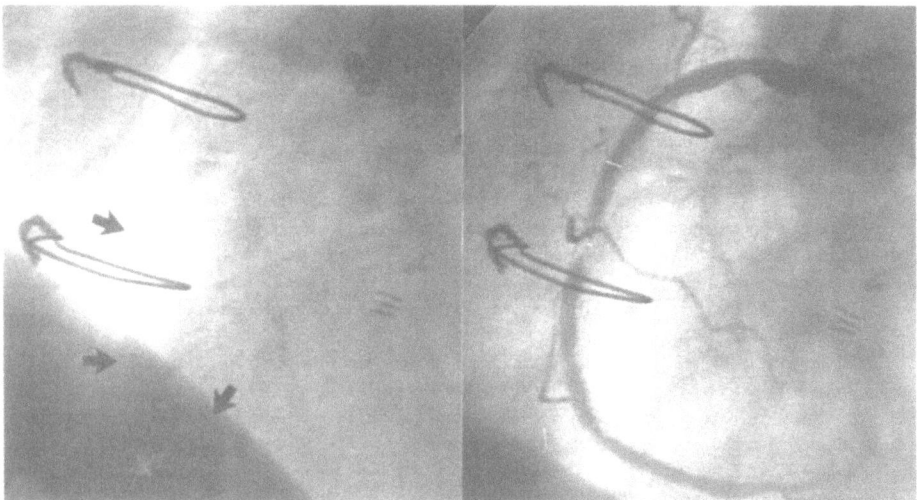

Figure 6. A patient after successful multiple stent implantation in the right coronary artery (left). Arrows indicate the junction between stents. Restenosis (right) occurs at 6-month follow-up. Renarowing occurs exact at the junction sites.

restenosis [37]. Our preliminary observation demonstrates that restenosis seems to involve more frequently the junction area in multiple stenting (Figure 6). The MUSIC, RAVES [38] and OPTICUS [39] studies are evaluating the role of IVUS guidance in further reducing stent restenosis rate.

Conclusion

In conclusion, IVUS can be considered as a gold standard for assessment of lumen size, plaque geometry and composition. Morphometric and quantitative variables on IVUS imaging can identify a subset of patients in whom restenosis is likely to develop. IVUS imaging is a valuable tool in modern coronary interventions for plaque specific interventional strategy which can optimize lumen size and possibly reduce the restenosis rate. But the cost effectiveness of IVUS in its clinical application should be determined by prospective studies. Residual stenosis after coronary intervention seems to be a strong predictor of restenosis. Therefore, IVUS guided effective removal of plaque may reduce restenosis rate. It remains unclear, whether using IVUS-guided stent implantation with high pressure inflation to achieve a symmetric deployment is able to reducing restenosis and if ever, to what extent. A newer stent material that could prevent intima hyplasia may solve this problem in interventional cardiology. IVUS may contribute in the future monitoring of the mechanism of restenosis.

References

1.   Sones FM, Shirey EK, Prondfit WL *et al.* Cine coronary angiography. Circulation 1959;20(Suppl):773.

2.   Gruntzig AR. Transluminal dilatation of coronary artery stenosis. Lancet 1978;1:263.

3.   Use of a monoclonal antibody directed against the platelet glycoprotein IIb/IIIa receptor in high-risk coronary angioplasty. The EPIC Investigation. N Engl J Med 1994;330:956-61.

4.   Mintz GS, Popma JJ, Pichard AD *et al.* Arterial remodeling after coronary angioplasty: a serial intravascular ultrasound study. Circulation 1996;94:35-43.

5.   Popma JJ, Topol EJ. Factors influencing restenosis after coronary angioplasty. Am J Med 1990;88:16N-24N.

6.   Glazier JJ, Varricchione TR, Ryan TJ, Ruocco NA, Jacobs AK, Faxon DP. Factors predicting recurrent restenosis after percutaneous transluminal coronary balloon angioplasty. Am J Cardiol 1989;63:902-5.

7.   Zir LM, Miller SW, Dinsmore RE, Gilbert JP, Harthorne JW. Interobserver variability in coronary angiography. Circulation 1976;53:627-32.

8.   Vlodaver Z, Frech R, van Tassel RA, Edwards JE. Correlation of the antemortem coronary arteriogram and the postmortem specimen. Circulation 1973;47:162-9.

9.   Hodgson JM, Eberle MJ, Savakus AD. Validation of a new real time percutaneous intravascular ultrasound imaging catheter [abstract]. Circulation 1988;78(4 Suppl):II21.

10.   Pandian NG, Kreis A, Brockway B *et al.* Ultrasound angioscopy: real-time, two- dimensional, intraluminal ultrasound imaging of blood vessels. Am J Cardiol 1988;62:493-4.

11.   Görge G, Ge J, Haude M *et al.* Intravascular ultrasound: a guide for management of complications during intervention? Eur Heart J 1995;16(Suppl L):86-92.

12.   Ge J, Erbel R, Seidel I *et al.* Experimentelle Überprüfung der Genauigkeit und Sicherheit des intraluminalen Ultraschalls. Z Kardiol 1991;80:595-601.

13.   Nishimura RA, Edwards WD, Warnes CA *et al.* Intravascular ultrasound imaging: in vitro validation and pathologic correlation. J Am Coll Cardiol 1990;16:145-54.

14.   Ge J, Erbel R, Gerber T *et al.* Intravascular ultrasound imaging of angiographically normal coronary arteries: a prospective study in vivo. Br Heart J 1994;71:572-8.

15.   Ge J, Liu F, Görge G, Haude M, Baumgart D, Erbel R. Angiographically "silent" plaque in the left main coronary artery detected by intravascular ultrasound. Coron Artery Dis 1995;6:805-10.

16.   Gorge G, Erbel R, Gerber T, Ge J, Trauth B, Meyer J. Morphological findings by intravascular ultrasound and clinical outcome after PTCA [abstract]. Circulation 1992;86(4 Suppl):I518.

17.   Guidelines for percutaneous transluminal coronary angioplasty. A report from the American College of Cardiology/American Heart Association Task Force on Assessment of Diagnostic and Therapeutic Cardiovascular Procedures (Subcommittee on Percutaneous Transluminal Coronary Angioplasty). J Am Coll Cardiol 1988;12:529-45.

18.   Hodgson LM, Stone GW, St Goar FG, Linnemaier T, Sheenan H. Can intracoronary ultrasound improve PTCA results? Preliminary core lab ultrasound analysis from the CLOUT pilot study [abstract]. J Am Coll Cardiol 1995;25(Suppl):143A.

19.   Serruys PW, de Jaegere P, Kiemeneij F *et al.* A comparison of balloon- expandable-stent implantation with balloon angioplasty in patients with coronary artery disease. Benestent Study Group. N Engl J Med 1994;331:489-95.

20.   Fischman DL, Leon MB, Baim DS *et al.* A randomized comparison of coronary- stent placement and balloon angioplasty in the treatment of coronary artery disease.Stent Restenosis Investigators. N Engl J Med 1994;331:496-501.

21.   Seo T, Yamao K, Hayashi T *et al.* Intravascular ultrasound in determining the end point of percutaneous transluminal coronary angioplasty [Japanese]. J Cardiol 1996;28:183-9.

22.   Mintz GS, Popma JJ, Pichard AD *et al.* Intravascular ultrasound predictors of restenosis after percutaneous transcatheter coronary revascularization. J Am Coll Cardiol 1996;27:1678-87

23.   Jain SP, Jain A, Collins TJ, Ramee SR, White CJ. Predictors of restenosis: a morphometric and quantitative evaluation by intravascular ultrasound. Am Heart J 1994;128:664-73.

24.   Tenaglia AN, Buller CE, Kisslo KB, Phillips HR, Stack RS, Davidson CJ. Intracoronary ultrasound predictors of adverse outcomes after coronary artery interventions. J Am Coll Cardiol 1992;20:1385-90.

25.   Honye J, Mahon DJ, Jain A *et al.* Morphological effects of coronary balloon angioplasty in vivo assessed by intravascular ultrasound imaging. Circulation 1992;85:1012-25.

26.   Mintz GS, Popma JJ, Pichard AD *et al.* Patterns of calcification in coronary artery disease. A statistical analysis of intravascular ultrasound and coronary angiography in 1155 lesions. Circulation 1995;91:1959-65.

27.   Fitzgerald PJ, Ports TA, York PG. Contribution of localized calcium deposits to dissection after angioplasty. An observational study using intravascular ultrasound. Circulation 1992;86:64-70.

28. Mintz GS, Dussaillant GR, Wong SC *et al.* Rotational atherectomy followed by adjunct stents: the preferred therapy for calcified lesions in large vessels ? [abstract]. Circulation 1995;92(8 Suppl):I329-30.

29. DeFranco AC, Tuzcu EM, Moliterno DJ *et al.* "Directional" coronary atherectomy removes atheroma more effectively from concentric than eccentric lesions: intravascular ultrasound predictors of lesional success [abstract]. J Am Coll Cardiol 1995;25(4 Suppl):137A.

30. Topol EJ, Leya F, Pinkerton CA *et al.* A comparison of directional atherectomy with coronary angioplasty in patients with coronary artery disease. The CAVEAT Study Group. N Engl J Med 1993;329:221-7.

31. Adelman AG, Cohen EA, Kimball BP *et al.* A comparison of directional atherectomy with balloon angioplasty for lesions of the left anterior descending coronary artery. N Engl J Med 1993;329:228-33.

32. Dussaillant GR, Mintz GS, Poppa JJ *et al.* Intravascular ultrasound, directional coronary atherectomy, and the Optimal Atherectomy Restenosis Study (OARS). Coron Artery Dis 1996;7:294-8.

33. Honye J, Mahon DJ, Nakamura S *et al.* Intravascular ultrasound imaging after eximer laser angioplasty. Cathet Cardiovasc Diagn 1994;32:213-22.

34. Gorge G, Haude M, Ge J *et al.* Intravascular ultrasound after low and high inflation pressure coronary artery stent implantation. J Am Coll Cardiol 1995;26:725-30.

35. Nakamura S, Colombo A, Gaglione A *et al.* Intracoronary ultrasound observations during stent implantation. Circulation 1994;89:2026-34.

36. Hoffmann R, Mintz GS, Dussaillant GR *et al.* Patterns and mechanisms of in-stent restenosis. A serial intravascular ultrasound study. Circulation 1996;94:1247-54.

37. Malik N, Gunn J, Shepherd L *et al.* In-stent restenosis: quantitative analysis in the porcine coronary model [abstract]. Eur Heart J 1997;18(Abstract Suppl):451.

38. Wong SC, Popma J, Mintz G *et al.* Preliminary results from the Reduced Anticoagulation in Saphenous VEin Graft Stent (RAVES) trial [abstract]. Circulation 1994;90(4 Suppl):I125.

39. Mudra H, Henneke KH, Kanig A, Zeiher AM, De Jaegere P, Di Mario C. Interim results of the OPTICUS randomized stent restenosis study [abstract]. Circulation 1997;96(8 Suppl):I582-3.

14. Assessment of plaque composition using intravascular ultrasound

Milan Sonka & Xiangmin Zhang

Summary

The structure and composition of atherosclerotic plaque play important roles in coronary artery disease and in the outcomes of coronary interventions. The ability to visually identify the morphology and composition of atherosclerotic plaque has increased the usage of intravascular ultrasound during and/or after therapeutic interventions. However, visual evaluation and characterization of plaque requires integration of complex information form a large number of images and suffers from substantial inter- and intra-observer variability. Automated analysis is needed to bring quantitative three-dimensional analysis of IVUS pullback image data to routine clinical utility.

This chapter gives an overview of existing approaches to characterization of plaque composition, describes image-based ultrasonic appearance of wall and plaque as provided by the intravascular ultrasound, presents an automated method for plaque characterization, proposes several quantitative indices of plaque composition, and discusses the method's initial validation. The reported plaque characterization method produced good assessment of soft and hard plaque composition in the analyzed IVUS images and image sequences. The method itself is not limited to classification of soft and hard plaque but is in general also applicable to more detailed plaque characterization.

Introduction

Growing evidence exists suggesting that the structure and composition of atherosclerotic plaque play important roles in coronary artery disease and in the outcomes of coronary interventions. The ability to visually identify the morphology and composition of atherosclerotic plaque has increased the usage of intravascular ultrasound during and/or after therapeutic interventions such as balloon angioplasty, directional atherectomy and stent placement. Intravascular ultrasound findings may give rise to a modification of the treatment strategy. Lesion eccentricity and the presence or absence of calcium and its superficial or deep location in the atherosclerotic plaque demonstrated by IVUS imaging have major implications in the choice of an intervention device [1,2].

However, visual evaluation and characterization of plaque requires integration of complex information from a large number of images and suffers from substantial inter- and intra-observer variability. Improvements in intravascular ultrasound imaging have increased the clinical utility and feasibility of the three-dimensional quantitative analysis of the coronary

J.H.C. Reiber and E.E. van der Wall (eds.). What's New in Cardiovascular Imaging, 183–196.
©1998 Kluwer Academic Publishers.

wall and plaque. Three-dimensional (3-D) analysis requires processing of long image sequences acquired during catheter pullback. The pullback sequence consists of a series of cross-sectional images acquired by manually or mechanically pulling the catheter back along the vessel segment. With 30 frames/s, pullback image sequences consist of hundreds of IVUS frames. Manual border identification in such image sequences is tedious and impractical for clinical use. Automated analysis is needed to bring quantitative three-dimensional analysis of IVUS pullback image data to routine clinical utility [3-11].

Several techniques for three-dimensional segmentation of coronary wall and plaque from IVUS image sequences are discussed in other chapters of this book [12]. Recently, the importance of geometrically correct 3-D reconstruction of coronary vessels and the associated plaque morphology was addressed [13]. IVUS reconstruction methods that use fusion of image data from biplane angiography and intravascular ultrasound are beginning to appear [14-17].

Approaches to plaque composition assessment

In addition to plaque morphology, plaque composition was shown to correlate with clinical variables in atherosclerotic coronary artery disease [18,19]. Mintz studied the role of calcium within the plaque burden [18]. Rasheed classified plaque regions as soft or hard and studied their relationship with patient-related clinical variables [19]; quantitative gray-level statistics were used for computer-assisted assessment of plaque characterization [20]. It was demonstrated in comparison with histology that IVUS images can be used for reliable visual assessment of plaque composition in regions of soft (cellular), hard (fibrocalcific), and calcified plaque [20-24].

Direct estimation of the acoustic parameters of the microscopic anatomy of plaques using ultrasound radiofrequency signal analysis represents another very promising approach to assessment of plaque composition. Using frequency-domain signal processing techniques, it is possible to compute the average scatterer size, scatterer density, and tissue echogenicity that can serve for tissue characterization in vivo [25]. Wilson and later Bridal demonstrated that there is correlation between ultrasonic attenuation and constituents of atherosclerotic plaque [26,27]. Wilson *et al*. used radiofrequency signal recorded during 20 MHz intravascular imaging to calculate local values of attenuation slope throughout the tissue [26]. They showed that high attenuation slope corresponded to locations of degenerative plaque. Wickline *et al*. analyzed acoustic properties of fatty plaques in cholesterol-fed rabbits to distinguish plaque composition change from fatty to fibrous [28]. Analyzing backscattered radiofrequency data using an acoustic microscope operated at 50 MHz, they found clear differences among normal vessel wall, fibrous lesions, or fatty lesions. The radiofrequency approach to tissue characterization is an active and very challenging area of atherosclerosis research. Examples include ultrasonic studies of plaque morphology and composition in carotid arteries [29-32].

Despite the unquestionable clinical utility of IVUS imaging, estimates of vessel morphology and plaque characteristics continue to be made visually. Such estimates are often based on an arbitrary selected IVUS frame representing a single vessel cross section. Only a limited number of computer-aided plaque characterization methods have been published. Picano *et al*. showed that biochemical plaque composition can be determined from ultrasound images in conventional video-format [23]. Rasheed *et al*. developed a computerized method for two-dimensional (single-frame) plaque classification in vivo and validated the method against histologic analysis of tissue from coronary atherectomy [20]. While the approach showed good agreement with visual and histologic assessment of plaque composition, plaque characterization was based exclusively on gray level distribution of the IVUS images and did not offer any volumetric information. As stated in [33], analysis of the composition rather than the luminal encroachment of an atheroma is a new avenue of research available to intravascular ultrasound techniques with potential revolutionary repercussions.

Tissue characterization in IVUS images

Assuming that the IVUS pullback image sequence has been segmented, three-dimensional plaque morphology can be determined since the ultrasonic appearance of the atherosclerotic plaque depends on its composition [20,24,33]. The following sections describe a newly developed automated texture-based method for plaque composition assessment.

Ultrasonic appearance of wall and plaque

High-frequency (20 to 30 MHz) ultrasonography allows imaging of relatively small structures (< 0.2 mm). The bright reflection of ultrasound at any tissue interface depends on the angle of the beam to the reflector and the relative stiffness differences between the bordering substances. In general, the structural components of the elastic artery consist of a highly organized arrangement of lamellae. The lamellae consist of repeating modules of elastin, collagen, and smooth muscle cells, which obscure reflections from any discrete internal and external elastic layers. An overview of the potential utility and limitations of IVUS for quantitative characterization of vascular tissue can be found in [34].

Among all the components, the adventitia normally produces the highest gray level intensity. Characteristic gray level appearances of other tissue types have been defined with their relative brightness compared to that of the adventitia:

- Hard plaques are composed of fibrous tissue often in complex layers and may include areas of dense calcium. In IVUS images, hard plaques are highly reflective of ultrasound and produce bright echoes similar to the adventitia (Figure 1). Calcified hard plaque regions are typically identified by high-amplitude echo signals with complete distal shadowing. Consequently, hard plaque regions are characterized in IVUS images as heterogeneous, high contrast regions located inside of thick plaque that contain very bright echoes and are often trailed by shadowed areas.
- Soft plaques usually consist of highly cellular areas of intimal hyperplasia and often contain cholesterol, thrombus, and loose connective tissue types. Ultrasound images of soft plaque are characterized by weaker and more homogeneous echoes and show low contrast (Figure 1).

If the hard plaque is calcified, the composition of the shadowed region behind the calcified plaque is not depicted on the IVUS image. Therefore, shadows behind the calcified hard plaque form a third class. An example of observer-defined plaque composition is given in Figure 2.

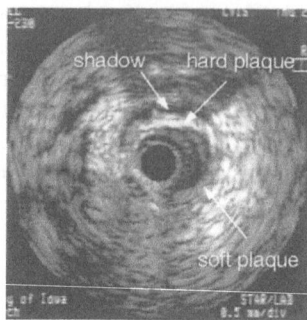

Figure 1. Ultrasonic appearance of wall and plaque.

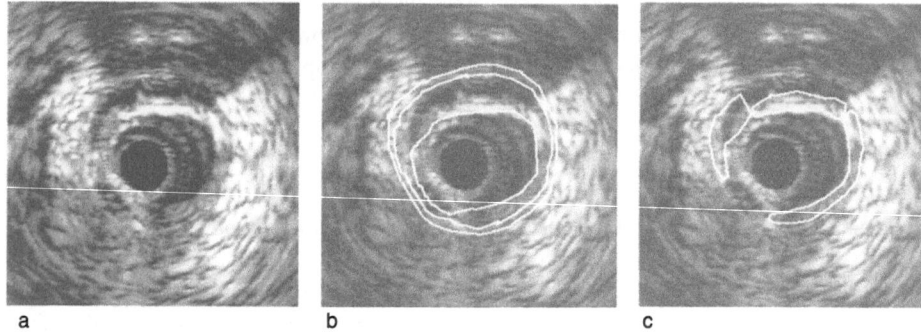

Figure 2. Observer-defined plaque composition. (a) Original intravascular ultrasound image. (b) Manual segmentation of the IVUS frame. (c) Manual plaque classification; soft plaque (two side regions) and hard plaque (top region)..

Plaque description in elementary regions

In general, texture appearance of soft and hard plaque regions is different in IVUS images (Figure 3). To determine plaque composition, plaque type is determined in narrow plaque

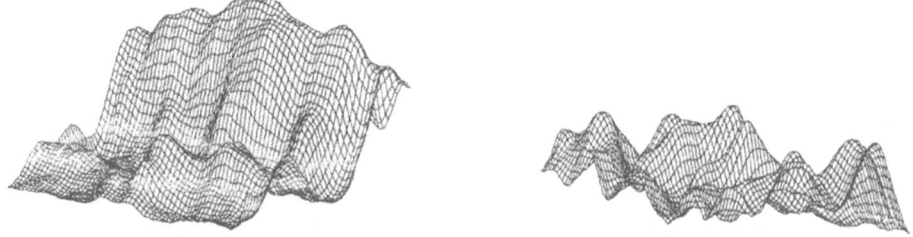

Figure 3. Gray-level profile plots. (left) hard plaque regions; (right) soft plaque regions.

wedges called elementary regions. Classification labels are assigned to the pixel of interest (POI) associated with each elementary region. Prior to defining the elementary regions, the entire plaque region A is straightened into a rectangular region B of a constant height H along the plaque/lumen interface (Figure 4). The width W of the straightened region B is equal to the lengths of the plaque/lumen border.

In order for B to contain all elementary regions in the radial direction, maximum thickness t_{max} of the plaque region A is computed first. Then, the height of the region B is determined as

$$H = t_{max} + h$$

where h is the constant height of all elementary regions. The straightened rectangular region B thus contains all plaque, and may include some portions of the wall and adventitia. Each pixel in B is a POI candidate and one and only one POI is selected in each column (along direction y in Figure 4). To become a POI, the candidate pixel must belong to the plaque region and have the highest intensity level of the plaque region in this column as described below.

The elementary region associated with the point of interest $P(x,y)$ is defined as a wedge (a rectangle in the straightened image), the upper left and lower right corners of which are ($x-w/2,y$) and ($x+w/2,y+h$), where w and h are the width and height of the elementary region, respectively (Figure 4). Only one elementary region is defined for every column in the

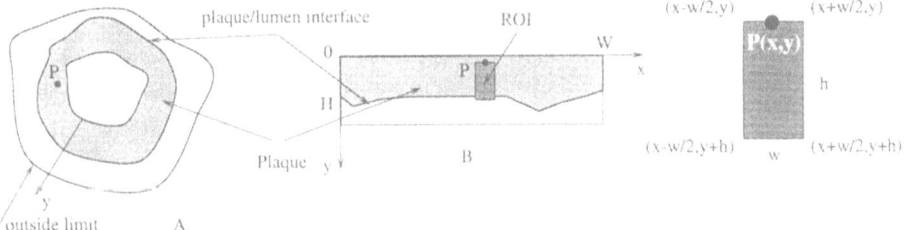

Figure 4. Plaque region straightened along the plaque border. Original plaque region A, straightened plaque region B, point of interest P and its elementary region (bottom, enlarged).

straightened rectangular region. Adjacent elementary regions overlap by $w-1$ pixels.

Plaque wedges may contain a mixture of soft and hard plaque. Consequently, for each wedge containing hard plaque, the plaque wedge may appear as a two- or three-layered structure along the y direction: hard plaque/shadow, or soft plaque/hard plaque/shadow. The rationale for defining the point of interest as the pixel associated with the brightest plaque location along the y direction is to maximize the homogeneity of the elementary plaque region. Thus, soft plaque tissue located closer to the lumen/plaque border than the hard plaque is excluded from the elementary region since it does not belong to hard plaque region and consequently has different texture appearance. Therefore, elementary regions are positioned in the plaque wedge along the y axis to start at the point with the maximum gray level of the plaque in order to enhance sensitivity of the employed texture descriptors.

To determine the POI and the elementary region for each plaque wedge, a horizontal line segment L of the same width w as the elementary regions is moving inside of the region B (Figure 5). When searching for the elementary region at column x_1 the line segment L is initially placed centered at ($x_1,0$) and moves vertically along the y direction. Gray levels of pixels are averaged along the line segment L, $M(x_1,y)$ represents the mean gray values:

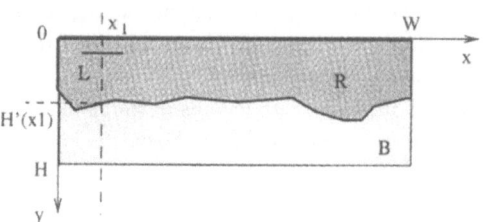

Figure 5. Searching for elementary regions inside of the plaque region.

$$M(x_1, y) = (1/w) \sum_{i=-w/2}^{w/2} I(x_1 + i, y)$$

Then, the y_1 coordinate of the point of interest $P(x_1, y_1)$ associated with the column x_1 is determined to satisfy the following equation:

$$E(x_1, y_1) = \max_{0 \le y \le H'x_1} M(x_1, y)$$

where $H'(x_1)$ is the thickness of the plaque at column x_1. The region between the plaque/lumen interface ($y=0$) and the POI row ($y=y_1-1$) is excluded from the elementary region and is not used for determining quantitative plaque descriptions.

Texture measurements

In the elementary regions, the following texture measures are computed to serve as features distinguishing between the hard and soft plaque. The texture descriptors were selected since they have proved useful in a variety of medical and non-medical applications in the past [35].

   Gray-level-based texture descriptors included standard features of *histogram contrast, skewness, kurtosis, dispersion,* and *variance*. In addition, a property describing the *radial profile* was designed to reflect the different gray level profile characteristics of the hard and soft plaque. For an elementary region with the POI at (x,y) (Figure 4), the *radial profile* property can be determined as

$$radial\_profile = \frac{E(x, y)}{\max_{\Delta y} E(x, y + \Delta y)}$$

where $\Delta y = 10, ..., h$.

   Co-occurrence matrices describe repeated occurrences of some gray level configurations in the plaque texture classes. An occurrence of some gray level configuration may be described by a matrix of relative frequencies $F_{\phi,d}(a,b)$, describing how frequently two pixels with the gray levels a,b appear in the texture separated by a distance d in direction Φ [35]. The features *energy, entropy, maximum probability, contrast,* and *inverse difference moment* were computed.

   Run-length measures describe the maximum contiguous set of constant gray level pixels located at a specified direction. A large number of neighboring pixels of the same gray level represents a coarse texture, a small number of these pixels represents a fine texture and the lengths of texture primitives at different directions can serve as texture descriptors. Two run-length features were computed: *short primitives emphasis and long primitives emphasis*.

Fractal-based measures are calculated through the transformation of image space to fractal dimension, *Brownian fractal dimension* was computed [36].

Plaque recognition

From the large number of calculated features, correlated ones were removed. Then, features with the highest discrimination power were identified using the inter-class distance search criterion and the Euclidean metric. The following three descriptors were identified as providing the best features for soft/hard plaque classification in IVUS images: Radial profile, long run emphasis, and the fractal dimension. A classifier with piecewise linear discrimination functions was trained using the three selected features and used for classification. The number of exemplars defining the piecewise linear discrimination function results from the learning process. This is an iterative learning process. Initially, a small number of exemplars, possibly one, is given to each class by grouping the training samples. An exemplar is computed as the center of each group. The training set is then classified using the exemplars. If the classification is not correct, the number of exemplars is increased and the training samples re-grouped. New exemplars are derived. This process is repeated until specified criteria are satisfied.

In the testing set of IVUS images, each elementary region was classified as containing soft or hard plaque. The elementary regions labelled as hard plaque were further divided into hard plaque and shadow subregions based on their gray level intensities. This was done using gray level thresholding along each row.

To suppress classification artifacts that are present in the shadow region, a 7×7 median filter is applied to the entire region.

After the plaque type classification was performed in pullback sequences, a post-processing method was included that considered three-dimensional contextual information. After the classification of individual elementary regions was completed in the entire sequence, the plaque type of each pixel was determined as the majority type among the pixels of the same spatial location in the preceding 3 frames, the current frame, and the successive 3 frames.

Experimental methods

Image acquisition

Intravascular ultrasound images were obtained from coronary arteries in vivo and in vitro, using 2.9 and/or 4.3 French intracoronary ultrasound imaging catheters (CVIS, Sunnyvale, CA). IVUS images were recorded on S-VHS video tapes and digitized using a high-end commercially-available digitizer (Parallax Xvideo 700) at image resolution of 640×480 pixels, 0.03 mm/pixel, digitization rate up to 30 frames/second.

Single-frame images were stored as JFIF format and later converted to 8-bit gray level raw data format. Image sequences were digitized using JPEG standard with highest quality provided by the digitizer and later decompressed into the raw data format.

Experimental data

To validate our segmentation method in IVUS pullback image sequences, six in vivo IVUS pullback sequences were acquired. The speed of the catheter pullback was approximately 1 mm/s and the images were digitized at a frame rate of 30 frames/s. Each pullback sequence depicted 5-11 mm of the left anterior descending coronary artery (LAD) and contained between 150 and 330 video frames. The IVUS pullback images were acquired from patients undergoing interventional coronary treatment. Pullbacks were acquired after directional coronary atherectomy. In one of the six sequences, calcified plaque did not permit ultrasound visualization of the wall in a large portion of the sequence and this sequence was excluded from further experiments.

In the digitized in vivo pullback sequences, systolic and mid-diastolic frames were selected to form ECG-gated pullback sequences. The frame selection was performed according to the accompanying ECG signal available on the IVUS frames. The ECG-gated sequences contained 5-11 frames each and were analyzed in both directions (distal to proximal and proximal to distal). Thus, the total of 20 ECG-gated IVUS pullback sequences were available for the validation experiments.

To validate our plaque characterization method, 12 IVUS images from 8 diseased cadaveric human hearts were digitized from video tapes. Each image contained both soft and hard plaque regions and consisted of 150-300 elementary regions per image. First, the plaque regions in all 12 images were segmented using our border detection approach. Then, each elementary plaque region was labelled as containing soft or hard plaque. The classifier was trained on manually-determined patterns of soft and hard plaque elementary regions. Non-homogeneous elementary regions, containing a mixture of soft and hard plaque tissues, were excluded from the training set.

Due to the limited data set that was available for validation, we used the *leave-one-out*, or *Jackknife*, approach to assess classification correctness. First, 11 of the 12 images were selected to train the classifier. The remaining image was then used for testing the resulting classifier. The process was repeated 12 times, always using 11 images to train the classifier and the remaining image to test the classifier. This is a standard process used in pattern recognition when limited numbers of training/testing data are available. Note that the classifier did not produce a single decision per training session. Rather, 200–300 decisions were made each time since each elementary region was classified.

To demonstrate the feasibility of three-dimensional analysis of plaque morphology and composition in IVUS pullback sequences, a 14 mm pullback sequence was acquired from a diseased cadaveric human heart. This IVUS pullback sequence contained 425 frames.

Independent standards

To assess performance of our segmentation method in IVUS image sequences, we compared the automatically detected borders with the manually identified borders defined by an expert observer in a blinded fashion. The observer-defined borders served as an independent standard. In each IVUS sequence, the first, middle, and last frames of each ECG-gated IVUS sequence were manually traced to define the independent standard for coronary wall and plaque borders. Unlimited amount of tracing and editing was allowed.

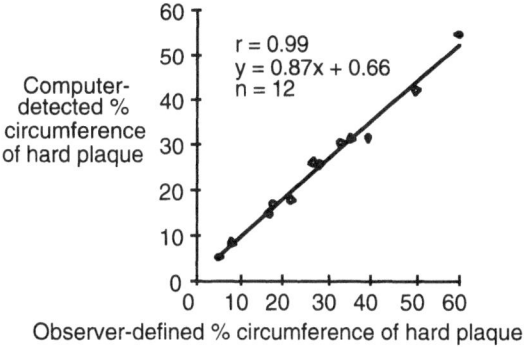

Figure 6. Comparison of computer-detected and observer-defined percent circumference of hard plaque.

To assess the correctness of plaque characterization, the automatically classified plaque regions were compared with the manual classification of plaque composition. Soft and hard plaque regions were carefully outlined by an expert observer in a blinded fashion.

Quantitative indices

To evaluate the accuracy of a clinically important measure of plaque composition, the *percent circumference of hard plaque* was defined as

$$\frac{circumference\_of\_hard\_plaque}{circumference\_of\_plaque} \times 100\%$$

where *circumference_of_hard_plaque* was expressed in degrees. The error of percent circumference of hard plaque was defined as the difference between observer-defined and computer-detected percent circumference of hard plaque.

All errors are expressed as mean ± standard deviation. Regression equations were compared to the equation of the line of identity using t-statistic for the slope and intercept.

Tissue characterization results

Plaque composition in the 12 images was automatically determined with classification correctness of 89.9% overall. Hard plaque was correctly classified in 89.2% of elementary regions (653/732) and soft plaque classification correctness was 90.2% (1805/2001).

A good correlation was found between the computer-detected and observer-defined percent circumference of hard plaque ($y=0.87x+0.66$, $r=0.99$) (Figure 6). The average error of percent circumference of hard plaque was 3.2 ± 2.7%. An example of automated plaque classification is given in Figure 7.

To explore the feasibility of 3-D plaque characterization, the 14 mm cadaveric pullback sequence was first segmented using our 3-D segmentation approach. Then, plaque characterization was performed. Each frame was classified using the classifier previously trained in the 12 IVUS images used for quantitative validation for which the training set was available. Vessel wall and lumen borders of the diseased cadaveric coronary artery were detected and

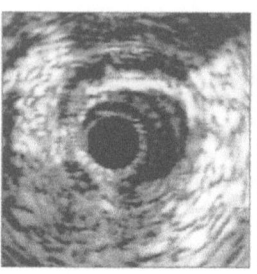 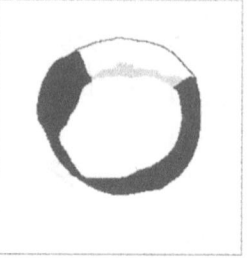 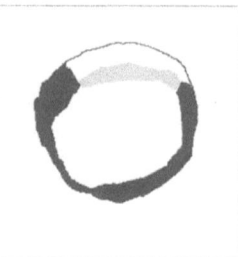

Figure 7. Automated plaque characterization. (left) Original image. (middle) Computer-detected soft (black), hard (gray) plaque, and shadow (white) regions, plaque borders were determined automatically. (right) Observer-identified soft, hard, and shadow plaque regions.

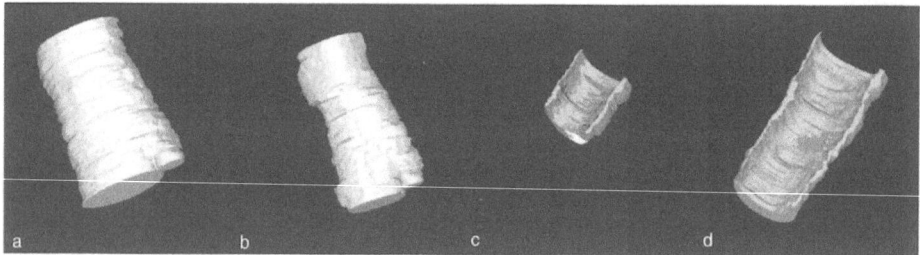

Figure 8. A 3-D reconstruction of a coronary vessel from a 14 mm pullback sequence. (a) Coronary wall reconstruction. (b) Lumen reconstruction. (c) Plaque composition within hard plaque. Hard plaque regions is dark and soft plaque regions are gray. (d) Plaque composition of the entire pullback sequence (For color plate of this figure, see color section).

the plaque characterized. The 3D reconstruction of the entire pullback is shown in Figures 8a,b. In both pictures, a vessel branch is clearly shown at the lower section of the artery. Plaque characterization within the region of hard plaque is shown in Figure 8c and the reconstruction of the entire pullback is given in Figure 8d.

Utility of plaque composition assessment

The method for automated plaque characterization presented here was developed and validated in individual IVUS image frames and its applicability was demonstrated in a 3-D pullback sequence. We expect that by combining our 3-D IVUS image segmentation method [37] and our plaque characterization approach [38], we will be able to develop and fully validate a method for truly three-dimensional plaque characterization. Additional contextual information, such as 3-D connectivity, should further improve the plaque classification results.

Using the currently available IVUS images, even quantitation of the total amount of vessel calcification or hard plaque volume has its limitations. Total calcium burden often cannot be estimated, because deeper structures that may or may not be calcified are hidden in the shadow of more superficially calcified regions. At the same time, brightness of the initial bright echo does not indicate the total depth or amount of calcification. Therefore quantification of calcification by intravascular ultrasound can be expressed only as the arc length [33,39-41].

On the other hand, intravascular ultrasound images provide detailed morphology of atherosclerotic lesions and can be used to differentiate tissue characteristics and to evaluate plaque composition. In agreement with our previous studies comparing visual analysis of plaque composition from cross-sectional IVUS images and histology [42], plaque was classified in three classes - soft, hard, and shadow in the presented study. Visual assessment of plaque type is limiting the number of classes that can be reliably distinguished by a human observer. However, plaque characterization may not necessarily be limited to classification of soft and hard plaques especially if RF data are available for computerized image analysis. Ultrasonic methods for more detailed plaque characterization can be expected in the future.

Several limitations of our work are worth noting. First, observer identification of wall and lumen morphology inevitably suffers from inter- and intra-observer variability and may not represent an ideal independent standard. Similarly, expert definition of plaque composition from IVUS images is irreproducible and only quantitative histology can provide an alternative independent standard. Unfortunately, when used for validation purposes, histology has associated problems with shrinkage and geometric distortions that make direct comparison of IVUS and histology a non-trivial task.

Automated determination of coronary wall and plaque borders plays a very important role in visualization and quantitation of three-dimensional volumetric data from IVUS pullback image sequences. Although additional validation is needed in slower pullback sequences that offer larger numbers of ECG-gated images from each pullback, the presented method holds great promise for reliable, robust, and clinically applicable segmentation of IVUS pullback image sequences.

The automated plaque characterization method reported here produced good assessment of plaque composition in the analyzed IVUS images. The method itself is not limited to classification of soft and hard plaque but is in general also applicable to more detailed plaque characterization.

Although truly accurate assessment of vessel morphology and plaque composition can currently only be obtained using quantitative histology, our results clearly demonstrate the feasibility of automated segmentation and plaque classification in intravascular ultrasound data. The presented method holds substantial promise for segmentation and tissue characterization in 2-D and 3-D IVUS images when applied in clinical setting.

Acknowledgment

The work was supported in part by the American Heart Association, Iowa Affiliate (IA-94-GS-65 and IA-96-GS-42).

References

1.   Mintz GS, Popma JJ, Ditrano CJ, Mackenzie J, Satler LF. Intravascular ultrasound vs quantitative coronary angiography: a statistical comparison of 538 consecutive target lesions [abstract]. Circulation 1993;88(4 suppl):I411.

2.   Mintz GS, Pichard AD, Kovach JA *et al.* Impact of preintervention intravascular ultrasound imaging on transcatheter treatment strategies in coronary artery disease. Am J Cardiol 1994;73:423-30.

3.   Rosenfield K, Losordo DW, Ramaswamy K *et al.*. Three-dimensional reconstruction of human coronary and peripheral arteries from images recorded during two-dimensional intravascular ultrasound examination. Circulation 1991;84:1938-56.

4.   Hermiller JB, Buller CE, Tenaglia AN *et al.*. Unrecognized left main coronary artery disease in patients undergoing interventional procedures. Am J Cardiol 1993;71:173-6.

5.   Roelandt JRTC, Ten Cate FJ, Vletter WB, Taams MA. Ultrasonic dynamic three-dimensional visualization of the heart with a multi-plane transesophageal imaging transducer. J Am Soc Echocardiogr 1994;7:217-29.

6.   Dhawale PJ, Wilson DL, Hodgson JM. Volumetric intracoronary ultrasound: methods and validation. Cathet Cardiovasc Diagn 1994;33:296-307.

7.   Reid DB, Douglas M, Diethrich EB. The clinical value of three-dimensional intravascular ultrasound imaging. J Endovasc Surg 1995;2:356-64.

8.   Von Birgelen C, Di Mario C, Li W *et al.*. Morphometric analysis in three- dimensional intracoronary ultrasound: an in vitro and in vivo study performed with a novel system for the contour detection of lumen and plaque. Am Heart J 1996;132:516-27.

9.   Gil R, Von Birgelen C, Prati F, Di Mario C, Ligthart J, Serruys PW. Usefulness of three-dimensional reconstruction for interpretation and quantitative analysis of intracoronary ultrasound during stent deployment. Am J Cardiol 1996;77:761-4.

10. Reiber JHC, Van der Wall EE, editors. Cardiovascular imaging. Dordrecht: Kluwer Academic Publisher; 1996.

11. Meier DS, Cothren RM, Vince DG, Cornhill JF. Automated morphometry of coronary arteries with digital image analysis of intravascular ultrasound. Am Heart J 1997;133:681-90.

12. Dijkstra J, Wahle A, Koning G, Reiber JHC, Sonka M. Quantitative coronary ultrasound: State of the art. Reiber JHC, van der Wall EE, eds. In What's New in Cardiovascular Imaging. Dordrecht: Kluwer Academic Publishers, 1998;79-93

13. Wiet SP, Vonesh MJ, Waligora MJ, Kane BJ, McPherson DD. The effect of vascular curvature on three-dimensional reconstruction of intravascular ultrasound images. Ann Biomed Eng 1996;24:695-701.

14. Prause GPM, DeJong SC, McKay CR, Sonka M. Geometrically correct 3-D reconstruction of tortuous coronary arteries: fusion of biplane coronary angiography and intravascular ultrasound pullback imaging [abstract]. Circulation 1996;94(8 suppl):I255.

15. Baumgart D, Haude M, Ge J *et al.*. Online integration of intravascular ultrasound images into angiographic images. Cathet Cardiovasc Diagn 1996;39:328-9.

16. Pellot C, Bloch I, Herment A, Sureda F. An attempt to 3D reconstruct vessel morphology from X-ray projections and intravascular ultrasounds modeling and fusion. Comput Med Imaging Graph 1996;20:141-51.

17. Prause GPM, DeJong S, McKay CR, Sonka M. Towards a geometrically correct 3-D reconstruction of tortuous coronary arteries based on biplane angiography and intravascular ultrasound. Int J Card Imaging 1997;13:451-62.

18. Mintz GS, Pichard AD, Popma JJ *et al.*. Determinants and correlates of target lesion calcium in coronary artery disease: a clinical, angiographic and intravascular ultrasound study. J Am Coll Cardiol 1997;29:268-74.

19. Rasheed Q, Nair R, Sheehan H, Hodgson JM. Correlation of intracoronary ultrasound plaque characteristics in atherosclerotic coronary artery disease patients with clinical variables. Am J Cardiol 1994;73:753-8.

20. Rasheed Q, Dhawale PJ, Anderson J, Hodgson JM. Intracoronary ultrasound-defined plaque composition: computer-aided plaque characterization and correlation with histologic samples obtained during directional coronary atherectomy. Am Heart J 1995;129:631-7.

21. Liebson PR, Klein LW. Intravascular ultrasound in coronary atherosclerosis: a new approach to clinical assessment. Am Heart J 1991;123:1643-60.

22. Di Mario C, The SHK, Madretsma S *et al.*. Detection and characterization of vascular lesions by intravascular ultrasound: an in vitro study correlated with histology. J Am Soc Echocardiogr 1992;5:135-46.

23. Picano E, Landini L, Urbani MP, Mazzarisi A, Paterni M, Mazzone AM. Ultrasound tissue characterization techniques in evaluating plaque structure. Am J Card Imaging 1994;8:123-8.

24. De Feyter PJ, Di Mario C, Serruys PW. Quantitative coronary imaging. Rotterdam: Barjesteh, Meeuwes & Co.; 1995.

25. Insana MF. Ultrasonic imaging of microscopic structures in living organs. Int Rev Exp Pathol 1996;36:73-92.

26. Wilson LS, Neale ML, Talhami HE, Appleberg M. Preliminary results from attenuation-slope mapping of plaque using intravascular ultrasound. Ultrasound Med Biol 1994;20:529-42.

27. Bridal SL, Fornes P, Bruneval P, Berger G. Correlation of ultrasonic attenuation (30 to 50 MHz and constituents of atherosclerotic plaque. Ultrasound Med Biol 1997;23:691-703.

28. Wickline SA, Shepard RK, Daugherty A. Quantitative ultrasonic characterization of lesion composition and remodeling in atherosclerotic rabbit aorta. Arterioscler Thromb 1993;13:1543-50.

29. Belcaro G, Laurora G, Cesarone MR *et al.*. Ultrasonic classification of carotid plaques causing less than 60% stenosis according to ultrasound morphology and events. J Cardiovasc Surg (Torino) 1993;34:287-94.

30. Mazzone AM, Urbani MP, Picano E *et al.*. In vivo ultrasonic parametric imaging of carotid atherosclerotic plaque by videodensitometric technique. Angiology 1995;46:663-72.

31. Griewing B, Schminke U, Morgenstern C, Walker ML, Kessler C. Three- dimensional ultrasound angiography (power mode) for the quantification of carotid artery atherosclerosis. J Neuroimaging 1997;7:40-5.

32. Noritomi T, Sigel B, Swami V *et al.*. Carotid plaque typing by multiple- parameter ultrasonic tissue characterization. Ultrasound Med Biol 1997;23:643-50.

33. Kimura BJ, Bhargava V, DeMaria AN. Value and limitations of intravascular ultrasound imaging in characterizing coronary atherosclerotic plaque. Am Heart J 1995;130:386-96.

34. Wickline SA, Miller JG, Rechia D, Sharkey AM, Bridal SL, Christy DH. Beyond intravascular imaging: quantitative ultrasonic tissue characterization of vascular pathology. In: Levy M, Schneider SC, McAvoy BR, editors. Ultrasonic symposium. New York: EIII; 1994. p. 1589-97.

35. Sonka M, Hlavac V, Boyle R. Image processing, analysis and machine vision. London: Chapman and Hall; 1993.

36. Wu CM, Chen YC, Hsieh KS. Texture features for classification of ultrasonic liver images. IEEE Trans Med Imaging 1992;11:141-52.

37. Sonka M, Liang W, Zhang X, DeJong S, Collins SM, McKay CR. Three- dimensional automated segmentation of coronary wall and plaque from intravascular ultrasound pullback sequences. Comput Cardiol 1995;637-40.

38. Zhang X, DeJong SC, McKay CR, Collins SM, Sonka M. Automated characterization of plaque composition from intravascular ultrasound images. Comput Cardiol 1996;649-52.

39. Fitzgerald PJ, Ports TA, Yock PG. Contribution of localized calcium deposits to dissection after angioplasty. An observational study using intravascular ultrasound. Circulation 1992;86:64-70.

40. Mintz GS, Potkin BN, Keren G *et al.*. Intravascular ultrasound evaluation of the effect of rotational atherectomy in obstructive atherosclerotic coronary artery disease. Circulation 1992;86:1383-93.

41. Honye J, Mahon DJ, Jain A *et al.*. Morphological effects of coronary balloon angioplasty in vivo assessed by intravascular ultrasound imaging. Circulation 1992;85:1012-25.

42. Bissing M, DeJong S, Thomas P, Spencer K, McKay C. Identification of eccentric lesions and lipid laden plaques by IVUS: validation by quantitative histology in fresh cadaveric hearts [abstract]. Circulation 1994;90(4 suppl):I551.

15. Magnetic resonance in cardiology: which clinical questions can be answered now and in the near future?

Ernst E. van der Wall

Summary

Magnetic resonance (MR) techniques are increasingly being used in clinical cardiology because they offer unique noninvasive information of the heart. MR techniques provide high-resolution images of the heart and great vessels without the use of ionizing radiation. In recent years the availability of MR systems has increased enormously and MR techniques can be effectively used in the clinical evaluation of a variety of cardiovascular diseases. Currently, primary indications for MR imaging are great vessel disease (aortic dissection, aortic aneurysm), complex congenital heart disease, para- and intracardiac masses, and pericardial disease. Secondary applications are valvular heart disease, cardiomyopathies, congestive heart failure, and myocardial tissue abnormalities. Ischemic heart disease forms a relative new area of interest for MR imaging, which allows already the evaluation of myocardial perfusion and function. Major developments in MR coronary angiography suggest an important future role for cardiac MR imaging in daily clinical cardiology practice.

Introduction

MR techniques may increasingly contribute to the management of clinical cardiology problems. For several manifestations of cardiac disease, the MR techniques are already being used as a first imaging modality of choice (Table 1). The currently used MR techniques can be

Table 1: Current indications for cardiac MR imaging

Primary indications	Secondary indications	Research applications
Congenital heart disease	Congestive heart failure	Aortocoronary bypass
Great vessel disease	Myocardial tissue abnormalities	angiography
(Para)cardiac masses	Valvular heart disease	Coronary angiography
Pericardial processes		Ischaemic heart disease

grossly divided into MR imaging, MR angiography, and MR spectroscopy. MR *imaging* provides detailed anatomical and functional images of the cardiovascular system in any desired

J.H.C. Reiber and E.E. van der Wall (eds.). What's New in Cardiovascular Imaging, 197–206.
©1998 Kluwer Academic Publishers.

imaging plane without the limitations inherent to more traditional techniques like echocardiography, nuclear imaging, cine computed tomography (CT), and X-ray ventriculography. MR imaging techniques reveal three-dimensional information on anatomy, function and flow [1,2]. Also regional as well as global heart function can be evaluated both at rest and under pharmacologic stress [3-5]. High-speed MR imaging techniques allow the assessment of myocardial perfusion [6]. MR tagging is an imaging method that uses a myocardial grid to allow the monitoring of progressive distortion of the myocardium during the cardiac cycle. Specialized MR techniques, such as MR *angiography*, are available to visualize the proximal coronary arteries [7] and to quantitate blood flow velocity and volume [8]. MR *spectroscopy* offers unique information on cardiac metabolism in a variety of cardiac diseases [9].

The integration of all this information from one single examination requires the availability of dedicated software to extract and display the plethora of information potentially present in the MR images. Further development includes the improvement of rapid imaging sequences that allow real-time image acquisition. The challenge therefore is to develop MR techniques into a cost-effective method for evaluating cardiovascular anatomy, function, flow, myocardial perfusion, and cardiac metabolism in a single diagnostic MR study. The replacement of multiple diagnostic tests with one single MR test will have major effects on cardiovascular health care economics. This chapter describes the currently accepted indications and potential future applications of the MR techniques in clinical cardiology. Very recently, the clinical role of magnetic resonance in cardiovascular disease has been defined and laid down in a Task Force Report instituted by a Task Force of the European Society of Cardiology, in Collaboration with the Association of European Paediatric Cardiologists [10].

Technical aspects of MR techniques

For a better understanding of the MR techniques, the most important techniques are briefly described.

Spin-echo MR imaging

Multislice spin-echo MR imaging, with triggering of the image acquisition to the R-wave of the electrocardiogram, is the most commonly used strategy for defining the morphology of the heart and great vessels [11]. The flowing blood provides natural contrast, thereby allowing anatomical evaluation of cardiovascular pathology. Slice thickness, image orientation and image contrast can be selected by the operator, depending on the anatomical structures under investigation. The MR imaging approach provides unlimited access to the chest without the problems of obtaining adequate imaging windows inherent to echocardiography. Spin-echo MR images, however, provide only static information, require relatively long acquisition times, and may be degraded by motion or flow artefacts.

Gradient-echo MR imaging

In contrast to spin-echo sequences, gradient-echo MR imaging provides dynamic information on blood flow and cardiac function [12]. Gradient-echo images display blood flow as a bright signal, whereas spin-echo images show blood flow generally as a dark signal or no signal. Flow disturbances, like those associated with valvular stenoses and insufficiencies, are visualized because of low-signal turbulent jet effects contrasting with the bright signal of normal flowing blood. The images are acquired with high temporal resolution with 20 or more phases per cardiac cycle. They can be displayed in a pseudo-real-time movie loop format to provide a dynamic impression of flow and function. However, gradient-echo acquisitions require electrocardiographical gating and are not real time.

High-speed MR imaging

Ultrafast MR imaging techniques and real-time echo-planar techniques have recently become available. High-speed MR imaging will reduce image degradation from physiological motion effects such as respiration. Echo-planar imaging operates in a single-shot or multi-shot format, allowing the reduction of acquisition times to 50 ms or less per image [13]. It may become clinically useful in imaging the entire heart with multiple imaging sections within a single breathhold. These fast techniques may be particularly useful in assessing function, flow and myocardial perfusion. However, echo-planar technology places heavy demands on the MR gradient system and the radiofrequency receiver of the MR imaging machine.

MR angiography

MR angiography is based on gradient-echo sequences that allow visualization and quantification of blood flow non-invasively without the use of contrast agents [14]. Such techniques are categorized as time-of-flight or phase-contrast methods. In the resulting angiographic image the vessels are depicted as a bright signal against a dark background because of the phenomenon of 'flow-related enhancement'. The phase-contrast method is based on velocity-induced phase shifts of spins in blood flow in the presence of a magnetic field gradient. The measured phase shift is proportional to flow velocity, which allows the extraction of quantitative data on flow velocity and volume. MR flow mapping is widely used to measure blood flow in the aorta, pulmonary circulation, intracardiac flow, native coronary vessels and coronary artery bypass grafts, as well as a number of other vascular areas throughout the body.

MR spectroscopy

MR spectroscopy is an exciting tool for evaluation of cardiac metabolism by direct measurement of changes in high-energy phosphates using surface coils directly applied to the surface of the heart. Quantification of metabolism however is difficult because volumes of interest are relatively large as compared to myocardial wall thickness (minimal sample volume 5 cm^3). Successful preliminary studies have been carried out in normal individuals and in patients with coronary artery disease, congestive heart failure, heart transplantation, cardiomyopathy, and left ventricular hypertrophy [15-18]. In our institution, we have focused on the various manifestations of left ventricular hypertrophy such as occurring in patients with hypertension and aortic valve disease, and in highly trained athletes [19]. The long-term clinical value of MR spectroscopy, however, remains to be proven.

Safety of MR techniques

MR techniques appear to be without hazard and no long-term ill effects have been described. Approximately 2-5% of patients complain of claustrophobia which may be avoided by administration of the appropriate anxiolytic therapy. Absolute and relative contraindications are given in Table 2. In particular, patients with pacemakers cannot be studied

Table 2: Safety evaluations of MR techiques

Absolute contra-indications
Cerebral aneurysm clips
Cochlear implants
Contrast agents during pregnancy
Intraocular metal implants
Pacemakers
Relative contra-indications
Artificial heart valves
Vascular clips other than for cerebral aneurysms
Vena cava filters

because of the risk of fibrillation from potentials induced in the endocardial wire and the rapid rhythms that some pulse generators develop in a rapidly changing magnetic environment. Patients with mechanical heart valves and sternal sutures are only relative contraindications as the materials used are usually not ferromagnetic; these materials may however result in large MR image artefacts.

Congenital heart disease

MR imaging has proven to be a useful tool in pre-operative planning of complex cardiovascular malformations and may provide information that can not be obtained by echocardiography or cardiac catheterization [20]. Its value has been established in the follow-up of patients with a variety of congenital heart disease and great vessel abnormalities [21]. This is partly due to the complexity of the postoperative anatomy and function of the right ventricle in this category of patients. MR imaging is especially well suited to assessing right ventricular morphology and function. Left and right ventricular volumetrics can be derived from the MR images, without the need for geometrical assumptions. This may especially hold for patients with arrhythmogenic right ventricular dysplasia [22]. Moreover, ventricular volume measurements with MR imaging appear to be more reproducible than those obtained with other imaging modalities. In addition, MR imaging proves to be a useful technique for assessing anatomy and flow of the pulmonary circulation in patients who have undergone surgical procedures to improve pulmonary blood flow [23]. It appears to offer advantages over echocardiography for determining the presence or absence of a confluence of the pulmonary arteries in patients with pulmonary atresia. Obtaining an accurate diagnosis of obstruction in extracardiac conduits, e.g. in patients following Fontan operation [24], is also possible with MR techniques. MR flow mapping can be used to quantitate pulmonary regurgitation after surgical correction of tetralogy of Fallot [25,26]. In addition, MR flow imaging techniques allow the assessment of diastolic function of the right ventricle after Mustard or Senning repair for transposition of the great arteries [27].

The use of MR imaging to diagnose vascular rings and other arch anomalies, Marfan's disease [28], pulmonary artery malformations, patency of postoperative shunts and conduits has also been well demonstrated. MR imaging can reveal the site and functional severity of narrowing of the distal aortic arch i.e. coarctation of the aorta [29]. MR flow mapping of collateral flow below the coarctation provides direct assessment of the haemodynamic significance of the narrowing, which is critical in planning the surgical procedure.

To summarize, MR imaging is generally superior to other imaging modalities in congenital heart disease, particularly in complex congenital lesions. MR imaging is developing into a complete tool for the evaluation of postsurgical sequelae in patients with congenital heart disease.

Acquired heart disease

Cardiac masses

Acquired heart disease such as paracardiac masses, intracardiac masses, and pericardial disease, are very well depicted by MR imaging and they are considered to be primary indications for MR imaging [30]. In particular, the use of paramagnetic contrast agents allows the distinction between a cardiac thrombus and a tumour.

Great vessel disease

A number of large vessel abnormalities can be assessed in considerable detail using computerized CT as well as MR imaging. A comparison of the diagnostic yield of CT, transthoracic and transesophageal echocardiography (TEE), angiography, and MR imaging in patients with suspected aortic dissection has shown that MR imaging provides the most reliable information as to the presence and extent of dissection [31]. Currently, TEE and fast CT are the methods of choice in the (hyper)acute phase of aortic dissection, and MR imaging is the preferred tool for diagnosis and follow-up of aortic dissection in more stable patients. Other acquired abnormalities of the aorta such as aneurysms can be well defined and followed over time using MR imaging. The size and extent of aortic aneurysms can be measured in this way and may in time obviate the need for CT or contrast angiography. In summary, great vessel disease is nowadays accepted as a primary indication for MR imaging, and a combination of echocardiography (acute phase) and MR imaging (subacute phase) may well eliminate the need for invasive aortography.

Coronary artery disease

Many efforts have been undertaken to evaluate the various aspects of coronary artery disease using MR imaging technology. Abnormalities in regional contraction and perfusion of the heart are early and sensitive markers for the presence of ischemic heart disease which are nicely visualized by MR imaging. In particular, MR imaging enables the quantitative evaluation of regional and global heart function using our home-made MR Analytical Software System (MASS 3.0), which is a dedicated software package for automatic delineation of the subepicardial and subendocardial borders [32,33]. Wall motion abnormalities, either induced by pharmacological stress [34] or following myocardial infarction [35], can be accurately and reliably assessed using the MASS-derived centerline method. MR perfusion imaging, with the aid of contrast agents for MR imaging, may be used to assess the functional significance of coronary artery stenoses by demonstrating perfusion defects in the myocardial bed distal to the stenoses [6,36]. Currently, one of the most clinically useful approaches of MR imaging in coronary artery disease is the assessment of myocardial viability (Table 3). Absence of wall motion or reduced end-diastolic wall thickness may be unique MR hallmarks to demonstrate lack of myocardial viability [37,38]. Comparative studies with radionuclide markers have shown excellent correlations between MR imaging techniques and scintigraphic modalities such as positron emission tomography (PET) [39] and single photon emission tomography (SPECT) [40].

MR coronary angiography may become a useful screening tool for imaging the main coronary arteries for detecting significant stenoses [7,41-44], and the abnormal origin and course of the coronary arteries [45,46]. In addition, the evaluation of coronary bypass patency by MR flow measurements is an important step forward [47]. To summarize, the value of MR techniques in coronary artery disease for daily clinical practice remains to be established, but developments such as high-speed imaging, improved surface coils, and real time tracking of diaphragmatic motion to avoid the need for breath-holding indicate a major role for MR coronary artery imaging in the near future.

Future perspectives

Currently, MR techniques provide useful information that is not readily available from other non-invasive modalities such as echocardiography, radionuclide imaging techniques, and CT. The superb resolution, the inherent contrast, the three-dimensional nature, and its morphological and functional imaging capabilities justify the application of MR imaging in clinical cardiology. The development of one single comprehensive procedure to study cardiovascular anatomy, function, flow, coronary angiography, myocardial perfusion, and cardiac metabolism will be a major challenge for cardiovascular MR techniques [48]. Although the number of MR machines are explosively increasing (>1 per 100.000 inhabitants in the USA and Japan, >1 per 200.000 inhabitants in Switzerland and in The Netherlands, 1998), very fast real-time MR imaging is only possible using specially designed dedicated imagers. At present, the use of these imaging systems is largely restricted to research centres. Technological improvements in both the hardware - for example, to allow rapid switching of magnetic field gradients - and software is therefore still required to enable

Table 3: Indications for magnetic resonance imaging in patients with coronary artery disease[a]

Indication	Class
Assessment of myocardial function	III
Detection of coronary artery disease	
Analysis of regional left ventricular function during stress	III
Assessment of myocardial perfusion	Inv
Coronary angiography	Inv
Bypass graft angiography	III
Assessment of coronary flow	Inv
Detection and quantification of acute myocardial infarcts	IV
Sequelae of myocardial infarction	
Myocardial Viability	II
Ventricular septal defect	III
Mitral regurgitation	III
Intraventricular thrombus	II

Class I	provides clinically relevant information and is usually apropriate ; may be used as a first line imaging technique
Class II	provides clinically relevant information and is frequently useful, but similar information may be provided by other imaging techniques
Class III	may provide clinically relevant information but is infrequently used because information from other imaging techniques is usually adequate
Class IV	does not provide clinically useful information
Inv	potentially useful, but still under investigation
N.B.	No Class I indication is provided for magnetic resonance imaging in patients with coronary artery disease

a.   Reproduced with permission from Sechtem et al., reference 10

implementation of very fast image acquisition methods ('pulse sequences') on commercially available hospital-based MR systems. Another step forward would be the application of MR contrast agents tailored to cardiac imaging. The advent of blood pool agents, and compounds specifically absorbed by ischemic myocardial tissue, for example, metabolism-incorporated contrast agents, is expected to improve further the results of cardiac MR techniques. A futuristic approach is the vizualisation of atherosclerotic plaques in the coronaries by MR imaging [49]. Recent studies have already shown the capability of intravascular MR imaging to accurately assess both plaque composition and size in aortic and femoral tissue [50,51]. When this will become a serious option in coronary arteries, it may offer important diagnostic and prognostic implications in patients with coronary artery disease.

Conclusions

With all the advances of the MR techniques in mind, the replacement of multiple diagnostic tests with one single MR test may have major effects on cardiovascular health care economics. To really prove this unique asset for MR imaging, time has come to institute adequate studies using comparative imaging modalities in order to have a better insight in cost/effectiveness of MR techniques. To this purpose, the Society of Cardiovascular Magnetic Resonance (SCMR) has launched a multicenter trial protocol entitled MARRVEL (Magnetic Resonance, Radionuclide Ventriculography and Echocardiography in Left ventricular function). This approach will hopefully lead to a significant contribution of cardiac MR techniques to the appropriate solution and better management of clinical problems in patients with manifestations of cardiac disease.

References

1. Underwood SR, Rees RSO, Savage PE *et al.* Assessment of regional left ventricular function by magnetic resonance. Br Heart J 1986;56:334-40.

2. Pattynama PMT, De Roos A, Van der Wall EE, Van Voorthuisen AE. Evaluation of cardiac function with magnetic resonance imaging. Am Heart J 1994;128:595-607.

3. Van Rossum AC, Visser FC, Sprenger M, Van Eenige MJ, Valk J, Roos JP. Evaluation of magnetic resonance imaging for determination of left ventricular ejection fraction and comparison with angiography. Am J Cardiol 1988;62:628-33.

4. Mohiaddin RH, Longmore DB. Functional aspects of cardiovascular nuclear magnetic resonance imaging. Techniques and application. Circulation 1993;88;264-81.

5. Van Rugge FP, Van der Wall EE, De Roos A, Bruschke AVG. Dobutamine stress magnetic resonance imaging for detection of coronary artery disease. J Am Coll Cardiol 1993;22;431-9.

6. Manning WJ, Atkinson DJ, Grossman W, Paulin S, Edelman RR. First-pass nuclear magnetic resonance imaging studies using gadolinium-DTPA in patients with coronary artery disease. J Am Coll Cardiol 1991;18:959-65.

7. Manning WJ, Li W, Edelman RR. A preliminary report comparing magnetic resonance coronary angiography with conventional angiography [published erratum appears in N Engl J Med 1990;330:152]. N Engl J Med 1993;328:828-32.

8. Mostbeck GH, Caputo GR, Higgins CB. MR measurement of blood flow in the cardiovascular system. AJR Am J Roentgenol 1992;159:453-61.

9. De Roos A, Van der Wall EE. Magnetic resonance imaging and spectroscopy of the heart. Curr Opin Cardiol 1991;6:946-52.

10. The clinical role of magnetic resonance in cardiovascular disease. Task Force of the European Society of Cardiology, in Collaboration with the Association of European Paediatric Cardiologists. Eur Heart J 1998;19:19-39.

11. Longmore DB, Klipstein RH, Underwood SR *et al.* Dimensional accuracy of magnetic resonance studies of the heart. Lancet 1985;1:1360-2.

12. Sechtem U, Pflugfelder PW, White RD *et al.* Cine MR imaging: potential for the evaluation of cardiovascular function. AJR Am J Roentgenol 1987;148:239-46.

13. Wetter DR, McKinnon GC, Debatin JF, Von Schulthess GK. Cardiac echo-planar MR imaging: comparison of single- and multiple shot techniques. Radiology 1995;194:765-70.

14. Rebergen SA, Van der Wall EE, Doornbos J, De Roos A. Magnetic resonance measurement of velocity and flow: technique, validation, and cardiovascular applications. Am Heart J 1993;126:1439-56.

15. Bottomley PA. MR spectroscopy of the human heart: the status and the challenges. Radiology 1994;191:593-612.

16. Beyerbacht HP, Vliegen HW, Lamb HJ *et al.* Phosphorus magnetic resonance spectroscopy of the human heart: current status and clinical implications. Eur Heart J 1996;17:1158-66.

17. Lamb HJ, Doornbos J, Den Hollander JA *et al.* Reproducibility of human cardiac 31P MR spectroscopy. NMR Biomed 1997;9:217-27.
18. Lamb HJ, Beyerbacht HP, Ouwerkerk R *et al.* Metabolic response of normal human myocardium to high-dose atropine-dobutamine stress studied by 31P-MRS. Circulation 1997;96:2969-77.
19. Pluim BM, Chin JC, De Roos A *et al.* Cardiac anatomy, function and metabolism in elite cyclists assessed by magnetic resonance imaging and spectroscopy. Eur Heart J 1996;17:1271-8.
20. Kersting-Sommerhoff BA, Diethelm L, Stanger P *et al.* Evaluation of complex congenital ventricular anomalies with magnetic resonance imaging. Am Heart J 1990;120:133-42.
21. Rebergen SA, Niezen RA, Helbing WA, Van der Wall EE, De Roos A. Cine gradient-echo MR imaging and MR velocity mapping in the evaluation of congenital heart disease. Radiographics 1996;16:467-81.
22. Kayser HWM, Schalij MJ, Van der Wall EE, Stoel BC, De Roos A. Biventricular function in patients with nonischemic right ventricle tachyarrhythmias assessed with MR imaging. AJR Am J Roentgenol 1997;169:995-9.
23. Rees RSO, Somerville J, Underwood SR *et al.* Magnetic resonance imaging of the pulmonary arteries and their systemic connections in pulmonary atresia: comparison with angiographic and surgical findings. Br Heart J 1987;58:621-6.
24. Rebergen SA, Ottenkamp J, Doornbos J, Van der Wall EE, Chin JGJ, De Roos A. Postoperative pulmonary flow dynamics after Fontan surgery: assessment with nuclear magnetic resonance velocity mapping. J Am Coll Cardiol 1993;21:123-31.
25. Rebergen SA, Chin JGJ, Ottenkamp J, Van der Wall EE, De Roos A. Pulmonary regurgitation in the late postoperative follow-up of tetralogy of Fallot. Volumetric quantitation by nuclear magnetic resonance velocity mapping. Circulation 1993;88:2257-66.
26. Niezen RA, Helbing WA, Van der Wall EE, Van der Geest RJ, Rebergen SA, De Roos A. Biventricular systolic function and mass studied with MR imaging in children with pulmonary regurgitation after repair for tetralogy of Fallot. Radiology 1996;201:135-40.
27. Rebergen SA, Helbing WA, Van der Wall EE, Maliepaard C, Chin JGJ, De Roos A. MR velocity mapping of tricuspid flow in healthy children and in patients who have undergone Mustard or Senning repair. Radiology 1995;194:505-12.
28. Groenink M, De Roos A, Mulder BJM, Van der Wall EE. The Marfan syndrome: effect of beta-blockers on entire aortic distensibility assessed with magmetic resonance imaging [abstract]. Circulation 1997;96(8 Suppl):I125.
29. Steffens JC, Bourne MW, Sakuma H, O'Sullivan M, Higgins CB. Quantification of collateral blood flow in coarctation of the aorta by velocity encoded cine magnetic resonance imaging. Circulation 1994;90:937-43.
30. Sechtem U, Theissen P, Heindel W *et al.* Diagnosis of left ventricular thrombi by magnetic resonance imaging and comparison with angiocardiography, computed tomography and echocardiography. Am J Cardiol 1989;64:1195-9.
31. Nienaber CA, Von Kodolitsch Y, Nicolas V *et al.* The diagnosis of thoracic aortic dissection by noninvasive imaging procedures. N Engl J Med 1993;328:1-9.
32. Van der Geest RJ, Buller VGM, Jansen E *et al.* Comparison between manual and semiautomated analysis of left ventricular volume parameters from short-axis MR images. J Comput Assist Tomogr 1997;21:756-65.
33. Buller VGM, Van der Geest RJ, Kool MD, Van der Wall EE, De Roos A, Reiber JHC. Assessment of regional left ventricular wall parameters from shortaxis magnetic resonance imaging using a three-dimensional extension to the improved centerline method. Invest Radiol 1997;32:529-39.
34. Van Rugge FP, Van der Wall EE, Spanjersberg SJ *et al.* Magnetic resonance imaging during dobutamine stress for detection and localization of coronary artery disease. Quantitative wall motion analysis using a modification of the centerline method. Circulation 1994;90:127-38.
35. Holman ER, Buller VGM, De Roos A *et al.* Detection and quantification of dysfunctional myocardium by magnetic resonance imaging. A new three-dimensional method for quantitative wall-thickening analysis. Circulation 1997;95:924-31.
36. Matheijssen NAA, Louwerenburg HW, Van Rugge FP *et al.* Comparison of ultrafast dipyridamole magnetic resonance imaging with dipyridamole SestaMIBI SPECT for detection of perfusion abnormalities in patients with one-vessel coronary artery disease: assessment by quantitative model fitting. Magn Reson Med 1996;35:221-8.
37. Vliegen HW, De Roos A, Bruschke AVG, Van der Wall EE. Magnetic resonance techniques for the assessment of myocardial viability: clinical experience. Am Heart J 1995;129:809-18.

38. Dendale P, Franken PR, Van der Wall EE, De Roos A. Wall thickening at rest and contractile reserve early after myocardial infarction: correlation with myocardial perfusion and metabolism. Coron Artery Dis 1997;8:259-64.

39. Baer FM, Voth E, Schneider CA, Theissen P, Schicha H, Sechtem U. Comparison of low-dose dobutamine-gradient-echo magnetic resonance imaging and positron emission tomography with [18F]fluorodeoxyglucose in patients with chronic coronary artery disease. A functional and morphological approach to the detection of residual myocardial viability. Circulation 1995;91:1006-15.

40. Lawson MA, Johnson LL, Coghlan L *et al.* Correlation of thallium uptake with left ventricular wall thickness by cine magnetic resonance imaging in patients with acute and healed myocardial infarcts. Am J Cardiol 1997;80:434-41.

41. Pennell DJ, Keegan J, Firmin DN, Gatehouse PD, Underwood SR, Longmore DB. Magnetic resonance imaging of the coronary arteries: technique and preliminary results. Br Heart J 1993;70:315-26.

42. Pennell DJ, Bogren HG, Keegan J, Firmin DN, Underwood SR. Assessment of coronary artery stenosis by magnetic resonance imaging. Heart 1996;75:127-33.

43. Post JC, Van Rossum AC, Hofman MBM, Valk J, Visser CA. Three-dimensional respiratory-gated MR angiography of coronary arteries: comparison with conventional coronary angiography. AJR Am J Roentgenol 1996;166:1399-404.

44. Wang Y, Rossman PJ, Grimm RC, Riederer SJ, Ehman RL. Navigator-echo-based real-time respiratory gating and triggering for reduction of respiration effects in three-dimensional coronary MR angiography. Radiology 1996;198:55-60.

45. Vliegen HW, Doornbos J, De Roos A, Jukema JW, Bekedam MA, Van der Wall EE. Value of fast gradient echo magnetic resonance angiography as an adjunct to coronary arteriography in detecting and confirming the course of clinically significant coronary artery anomalies. Am J Cardiol 1997;79:773-6.

46. Post JC, Van Rossum AC, Bronzwaer JGF *et al.* Magnetic resonance angiography of anomalous coronary arteries. A new gold standard for delineating the proximal course? Circulation 1995;92:3163-71.

47. Hoogendoorn LI, Pattynama PMT, Buis B, Van der Geest RJ, Van der Wall EE, De Roos A. Noninvasive evaluation of aortocoronary bypass grafts with magnetic resonance flow mapping. Am J Cardiol 1995;75:845-8.

48. Van der Wall EE, Vliegen HW, de Roos A, Bruschke AVG. Magnetic resonance imaging in coronary artery disease. Circulation 1995;92:2723-39.

49. Atalar E, Bottomley PA, Ocali O *et al.* High resolution intravascular MRI and MRS by using a catheter receiver coil. Magn Reson Med 1996;36:596-605.

50. Correia LCL, Atalar E, Kelemen MD *et al.* Intravascular magnetic resonance imaging of aortic atherosclerotic plaque composition. Arterioscler Thromb Vasc Biol 1997;17:3626-32.

51. Zimmermann GG, Erhart P, Schneider J, Von Schulthess GK, Schmidt M, Debatin JF. Intravascular MR imaging of atherosclerotic plaque: ex vivo analysis of human femoral arteries with histologic correlation. Radiology 1997;204:769-74.

16.   Real-Time Cardiovascular MR Imaging

Christopher J. Hardy

Summary

Cardiovascular MRI provides a flexible tool which should become increasingly important in the diagnosis and management of heart disease, combining a number of advantages in a single modality. It can generate thin sections from any angle, with no tissue interfaces to overcome. It offers a wide variety of contrast mechanisms to exploit, allowing enhanced visualization of moving blood, healthy and damaged myocardium, myocardial perfusion and strain, and cardiac anatomy. It is also noninvasive and, compared to x-ray angiography, relatively inexpensive. The speed of cardiac MRI pulse sequences has improved dramatically in recent years, offering the prospect of a rapid comprehensive cardiac MR exam which incorporates real-time interactive imaging as an integral component. Real-time MRI should be especially useful for rapid visualization of cardiac dynamics and blood flow, and for quickly locating oblique coronary scan planes prior to high-resolution coronary MR angiography.

Introduction

The rich variety of information available in MRI has enabled its use in assessing a wide range of parameters related to heart disease [1], including left-ventricular function [2-3], cardiac wall motion [4], myocardial perfusion [5-6] and strain [7-8], coronary anatomy [9 11] and flow [12], and even myocardial metabolism [13-14]. This raises the interesting possibility of the development of a comprehensive exam for coronary artery disease, which combines many or all of these assessments within a single exam. Until recently, the relatively slow speeds of most MRI scanners have .necessitated the use of ECG gating and respiratory compensation or breath holding to acquire cardiac images, often requiring tens of minutes per data set, making this possibility unlikely. However, advances in gradient and reconstruction hardware and in pulse sequence design have pushed maximum MR imaging rates into the range of 10 frames per second or better [15-16], making real-time interactive MRI now practical. High-speed MRI should play an important role in the context of an integrated cardiac MR exam, allowing for rapid, interactive progression from one stage of the exam to the next. It should prove particularly useful for real-time visualization of left ventricular function and wall motion abnormalities, for rapid location of oblique coronary scan planes, and for imaging under conditions of cardiac arrhythmia.

J.H.C. Reiber and E.E. van der Wall (eds.). What's New in Cardiovascular Imaging, 207–220.
©1998 Kluwer Academic Publishers.

High-speed MRI

The history of fast MRI is covered in a number of reviews [17-19]. A method for performing high-speed MRI was first proposed by Mansfield and Pykett [20], whose echo-planar imaging (EPI) sequence involved the traversal of all of k-space after a single NMR excitation. This soon evolved to a form which used blipped gradients [21-22], producing a rectilinear EPI k-space trajectory and corresponding pulse sequence diagram similar to that shown in Figures 1A and 1B, respectively. Resonant [23] and switched [24-26] gradient power tech-

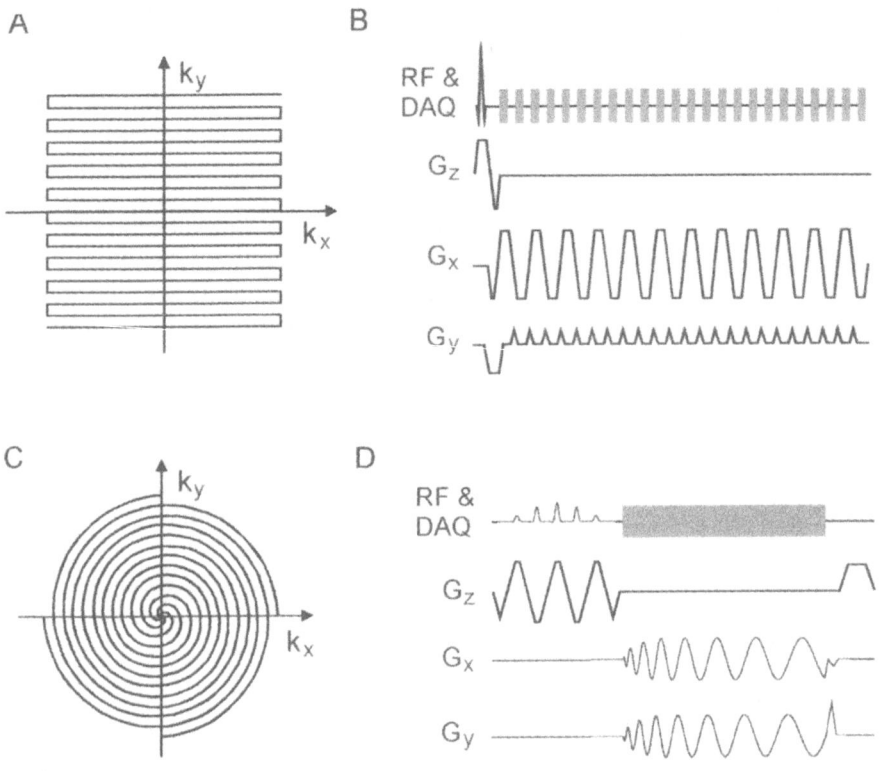

Figure 1. Rapid MRI imaging sequences. A) k-space trajectory for echo-planar sequence. B) Corresponding gradient, RF, and data-acquisition waveforms. C) k-space trajectory for interleaved spiral sequence. D) Corresponding waveforms for one of the interleaves.

nology and low-inductance, self-shielded coils [27-28] were developed to increase imaging speeds while minimizing artifacts, producing real-time [27,29] EPI movie loops and relatively high quality phase-contrast interleaved EPI images [30] of the heart. Alternatively, faster gradient speeds could be used to improve bandwidth and thus signal-to-noise ratio (SNR), while keeping imaging speed constant [31]. Rapid gradient-echo imaging techniques employing low-tip-angle RF excitation pulses [32-33] were also used to advantage in the heart, minimizing some artifacts associated with EPI, such as sensitivity to variations in magnetic field susceptibility, and chemical-shift artifacts.

Hybrid sequences such as RARE [34] and GRASE [35] use multiple gradient and RF refocusing pulses after an NMR excitation to produce T2-weighted snapshots with reduced sensitivity to chemical shift and field inhomogeneity compared to standard EPI sequences. However, the use of multiple RF refocusing pulses increases RF heating and MR-signal saturation effects, making these sequences less useful for continuous real-time imaging. Interleaved EPI pulse sequences [30,36] employ multiple excitation pulses with interleaved k-space trajectories to reduce the echo-train length, and minimize some of the artifacts associated with EPI pulse sequences, while maintaining some degree of imaging speed. Circular EPI trajectories [37] avoid the corners of k-space in order to improve speed, without yielding large sacrifices in spatial resolution. BURST imaging techniques [38] rely on a rapid sequence of RF pulses to generate multiple echoes during a constant readout gradient, removing the need for gradient switching, and producing ultrafast imaging rates, albeit with reduced resolution and SNR and with relatively high sensitivity to motion [39].

Another class of imaging sequence abandons rectilinear k-space trajectories altogether, in favor of curved paths which push the gradient slew rate more evenly over the entire sequence. The most successful of these has been the spiral trajectory [40-41] and its variant, the interleaved spiral, or pinwheel [10,37,41-42]. The spiral trajectory can be traversed at a nonuniform rate to produce constant gradient amplitudes or slew rates and thus maximize bandwidth [43]. A pinwheel trajectory and pulse sequence corresponding to one arm of the pinwheel are shown in Figures 1C and 1D, respectively. The NMR excitation pulse in this sequence is both spatially and spectrally selective [44], allowing the suppression of fat signals, which would otherwise cause blurring in a spiral acquisition. The advantages of reduced echo times gained by interleaving in EPI [30,36], also hold for interleaved spirals. Spirals have the further benefits of good flow characteristics [45] and relative insensitivity to motion [37], making them especially useful for cardiac imaging. Off-resonance and susceptibility effects can affect image quality, however, and measures such as automated field-map calculation and correction in the image reconstruction are generally necessary to prevent regional image blurring [46].

MR fluoroscopy

Rapid-imaging pulse sequences are most useful when employed in the context of a system capable of high-speed reconstruction and real-time image display. Such a system was first developed and demonstrated by Wright et al. [47], who used a workstation and array processor connected to a conventional MR scanner. Other experimental real-time whole-body MRI systems have since been developed [37,48-51], including those targeting cardiac [37,48] and interventional [50-51] applications. To improve imaging frame rates, a sliding reconstruction technique was introduced [52] which continually incorporates the most recently acquired lines of k-space to partially update the raw data set before reconstruction, with new reconstructions performed at a rate faster than the image acquisition rate. This allows the visualization of motion even when the basic repetition rate of the pulse sequence is not real time. The sliding reconstruction method has since been applied to interleaved-spiral imaging as well [37]. Spirals benefit from the fact that each interleaf samples the same range of spatial frequencies, including the center of k-space, providing a uniform response to motion. This is especially true when the interleaves are acquired in "bit-reversed" order rather than sequentially, since this causes any motion artifacts to be spread more diffusely [37].

M-mode MRI

In order to push MR imaging speeds into the range of 30 frames per second or higher, it is possible to trade away one spatial dimension to generate images analogous to M-mode ultrasound images. This is done by repeatedly exciting a column, or "pencil", of magnetization intersecting the heart, and reading out each time the MR signal along the length of the column (with use of a 1DFT reconstruction), to produce a display of heart motion which has time as one axis and position along the column as the other [53-54]. The pencil is excited by a single, low-tip-angle, two-dimensional selective-excitation pulse [55-57,43], which minimizes saturation of the MR signal. Figure 2A shows the basic M-mode pulse sequence. Here the initial pulse is the pencil-excitation pulse, which is immediately followed by a half-echo readout along the pencil axis. On scanners with maximal gradient slew rates of $120 \text{ T m}^{-1}\text{s}^{-1}$, and with a pencil diameter of 1 cm, the total time required to execute this sequence is on the order of 15 ms. The location of the pencil can be interactively set by drawing a line on a scout image while viewing a continuously scrolling M-mode display [48]. Figure 2B shows one such graphic prescription, with a corresponding M-mode trace displayed in Figure 2C. This type of image can be useful for rapidly assessing heart-wall motion and valve motion.

The above pulse sequence can be made velocity sensitive with the insertion of a bipolar gradient pulse between the excitation and readout, shown in Figure 2D. This pulse is inverted on alternate acquisitions and the signals subtracted to generate a phase-contrast M-mode image [54]. Figure 2E shows another pencil prescription, with the corresponding phase-contrast image displayed in Figure 2F. Here image intensity scales with velocity, and so static tissue is suppressed and a map of moving spins is generated, in this case from blood in the left ventricle and ascending aorta. One may alternatively calculate the phase of the signal before subtraction, to generate a phase-difference M-mode image, where the velocity direction can be displayed either using a gray-scale [48] or color [58] scheme. The velocity encoding of Figure 2D is in a direction along the pencil axis, but velocities can instead be encoded in other directions, for instance across the pencil, by moving the bipolar pulse to the y- or z-gradient axes. This method provides a good means of rapidly viewing anomalous blood-flow patterns in the heart and major vessels.

An alternative form of velocity encoding involves stepping the bipolar gradient through a range of values, as seen in Figure 2G, and performing a Fourier transform to produce velocity distribution profiles for different phases of the heart cycle [59], yielding a result analogous to Doppler M-mode ultrasound. Figure 2H shows the position of the pencil in the ascending aorta of a patient with Marfan syndrome and aortic insufficiency [60], and Figure 2I shows four of sixteen frames from the corresponding Fourier-encoded data set. Here the horizontal axis is position along the pencil and the vertical axis is velocity, with a range of ±80 cm/s. Positive blood velocities are evident in the ascending aorta in frame #5, and retrograde flow through the aortic valve is seen in frame #11 as negative velocities. This technique requires triggering the pulse sequence from the ECG, and acquiring signals over typically 16-32 cardiac cycles. However, if the bipolar pulse in Figure 2G is removed, and the constant readout gradient replaced with an oscillating triangular waveform, then Doppler-like

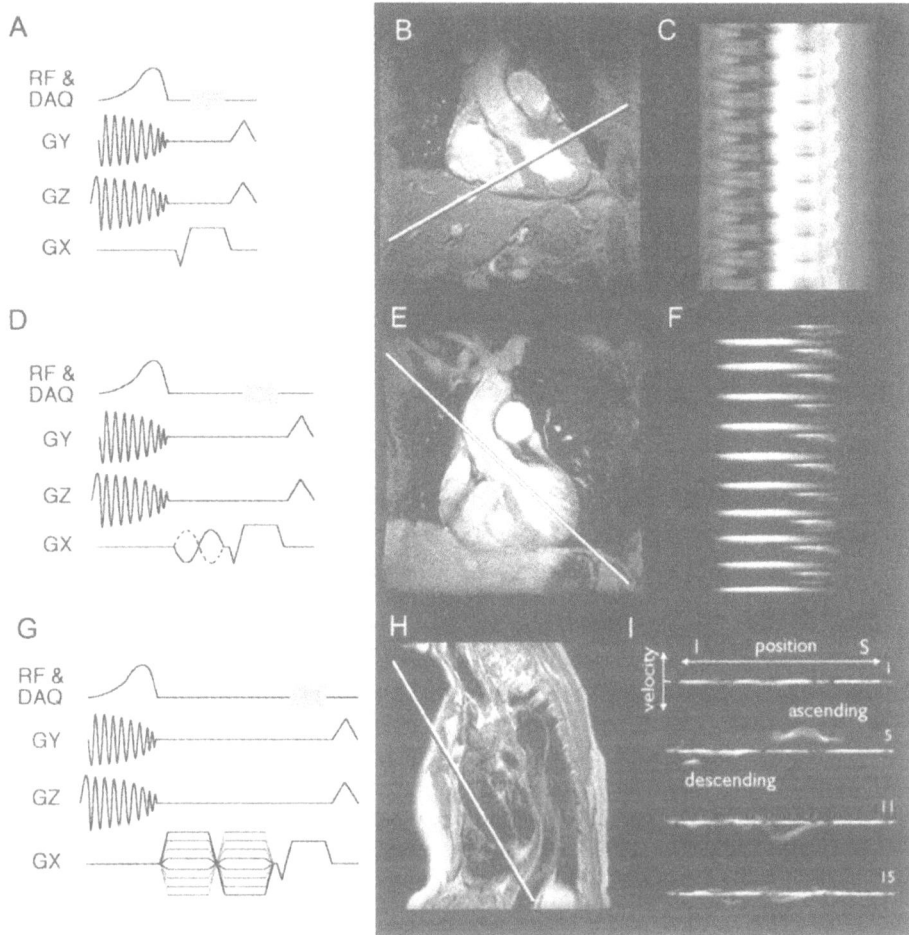

Figure 2. Pulse sequences (A,D,G), pencil prescription (shown as line) on scout images (B,E,H), and data (C,F,I) for M-mode (A,B,C), phase-contrast M-mode (D,E,F), and Fourier-velocity-encoded M-mode (G,H,I) sequences, showing heart motion and blood flow

velocity distributions can be captured in real time without the need for cardiac gating, at the cost of some spatial and velocity resolution [61].

M-mode MRI, while suffering from decreased time resolution relative to its ultrasound analog, also offers a number of advantages. The pencil in M-mode MRI can be oriented in an arbitrary manner, and does not need to be directed between the ribs. There is no divergence of the "beam" beyond a certain depth, and no scattering from interfaces between water, air, fat, and bone. Moreover, velocities can be encoded along any axis and can thus be measured in the same direction as the blood flow.

An interleaved version of the Fourier velocity-encoded M-mode sequence can be used to improve the effective time resolution of the technique, allowing rapid measurement of pulse-wave velocity in the aorta [60]. This in turn can be used to determine aortic distensibility, which is an important variable in the management of ventricular disease, and which may be useful for helping to determine the risk of sudden dissection or rupture of aortic aneurysms

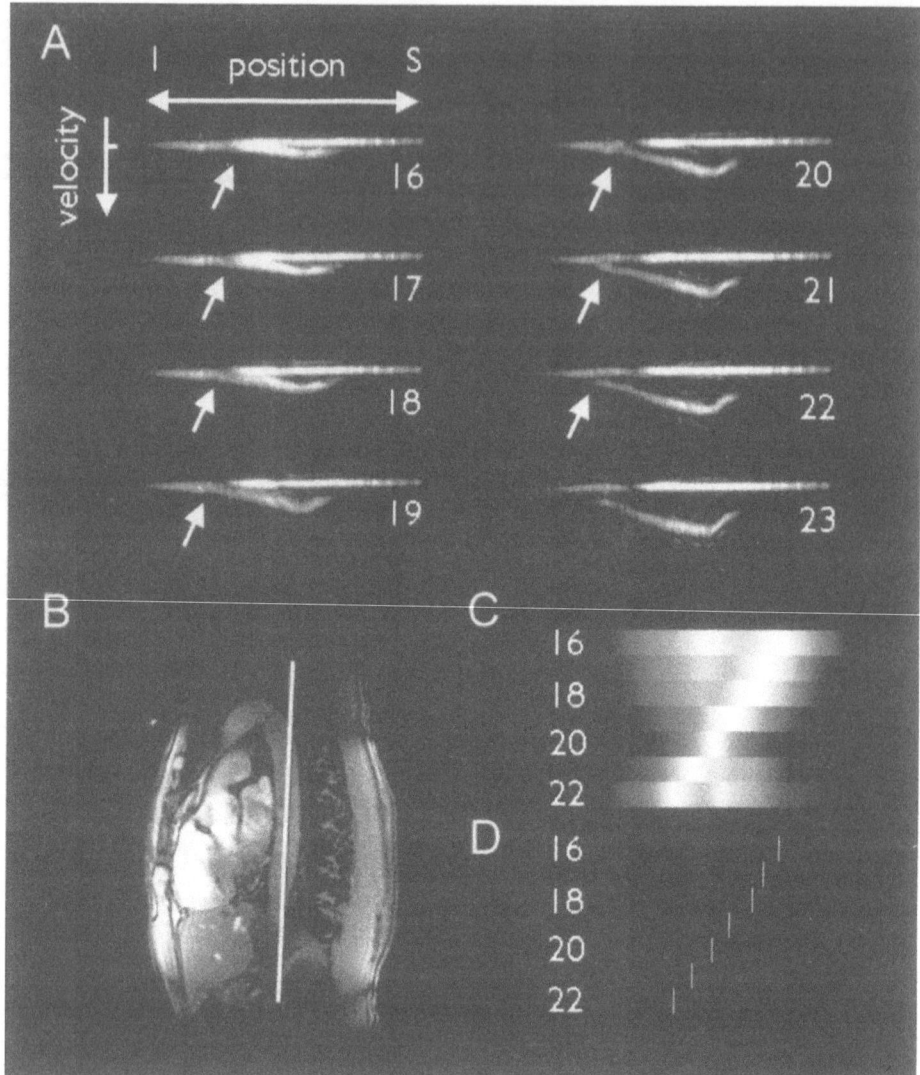

Figure 3. A) Eight frames (#16–#23) from a 128-frame interleaved Fourier-velocity-encoded M-mode data set, with pencil running along the descending aorta as shown by line in B). Arrows show propagation of velocity wave along the aorta. C) Cross-correlation of each frame with frame #20 yields functions whose peaks (D) show relative position of velocity wave.

[62]. Figure 3B shows the placement of the pencil excitation in a normal volunteer, and Figure 3A shows frames #16 through #23 from the subsequent 128-frame interleaved Fourier-encoded M-mode data set. Here the foot of the velocity wave can be seen propagating down the aorta (from right to left in the figure). This motion is especially striking when the data are played as a video loop. The relative position of the foot in each frame can be automatically quantified by cross-correlation of one frame with its neighboring frames. Figure 3C shows the result, for instance, when frame #20 is cross correlated with frames #16–#22. The peak of each correlation function, shown in Figure 3D, indicates the relative position of the

foot. A least-squares fit of the peaks yields a line whose slope is the average wave velocity in that portion of the vessel, giving a value of 364 ± 12 cm/s for this subject.

Real-time interactive cardiac MRI

High-speed MR pulse sequences with rapid image reconstruction and display provide fundamental new capabilities for cardiac MRI. To take full advantage of these, however, one must be able to interactively control the imaging plane and contrast parameters during real-time imaging. The first step toward such control was made by Holsinger et al., who interactively redirected a gradient-echo pulse sequence by entering new parameter values from the keyboard as the sequence was executing [63].

More recently, graphical tools [37,48,64-67] and interfaces to hardware devices [67-68] have been developed to provide highly intuitive methods for real-time scan-plane prescription, most in the context of cardiac MRI applications. A number of schemes have been demonstrated, all of which can be implemented during continuous imaging, permitting visualization of the beating heart during movement of the scan plane. Also, a colored 3D heart model [67,69] can be displayed near the MR imaging window, as shown in Figure 4. A semitransparent plane embedded in the model (Figure 4B) tracks in real time the location of the scan plane, displayed in Figure 4A, to enable the user to stay better oriented during interactive imaging. Alternatively, a cutaway view can be displayed, as seen in Figure 4C. One method for prescription within the real-time-imaging window is to "push" on various sectors of the current image with the mouse to tilt the scan plane about its center [64]. Alternatively, one of four colored icons (Figure 4D) can be dragged across the image, to reorient or offset the scan plane relative to its current location [67]. For instance, a curved arrow (shown in use in Figure 4A), can be dragged to spin the plane about its center. A scan-plane library (shown in Figure 4E) can be employed for rapid storage and retrieval of scan locations, with thumbnail images created to represent each location. Retrieval of a location is effected by selecting the appropriate thumbnail with the mouse. The advantage of these kinds of methods is that they are very intuitive, they allow the user to keep his eyes fixed on the imaging window during scan prescription, and they furnish essentially instantaneous visual feedback (via screen graphics) beyond that provided by the new images themselves.

Real-time interactive MRI should prove an excellent tool for assessing left ventricular function. An early study of this type was performed in a group of 30 patients with poor echocardiograms arising from inadequate acoustic windows [70]. Clear delineation of endocardium from blood for various wall segments in this population were obtained 36% of the time using echocardiography and 96% of the time with MRI. Moreover, inadequate visualization of all segments of any coronary distribution occurred 60% of the time with echocardiography and 0% with MRI for this group. The interactive MR exams were completed in less than 15 minutes in all 30 patients.

Real-time interactive MRI should also prove extremely useful for rapid localization of coronary scan planes prior to ECG-gated coronary MR angiography. The acquisition of complete 3D segmented gradient-echo data sets [11] to visualize the coronary arteries can be both time consuming and sensitive to motion, even with use of multiple breath holding or respiratory gating. Single-slice, transverse or oblique imaging [9] requires repetitive positioning of the scan plane at multiple locations along the coronary tree, with gated breath-held imaging at each location. In an alternate hybrid approach, real-time interactive imaging is

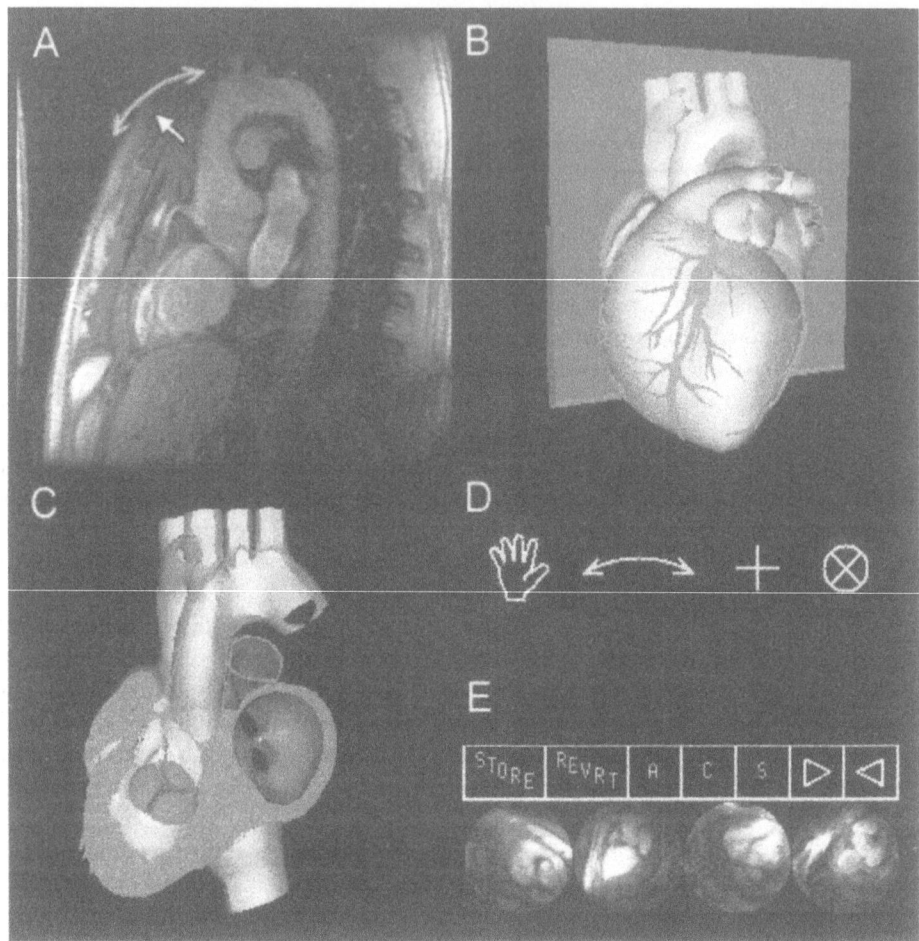

Figure 4. Graphical tools used for interactive cardiac MRI. Imaging window (A) shows current scan plane, whose position is continuously reflected in semitransparent embedded plane (B) or cutaway view (C) of colored 3D heart model. Colored icons (D) can be dragged across imaging window to rotate or offset scan plane, as shown in (A) for in-plane rotation. Scan-plane library (E) allows rapid storage and retrieval of scan locations (For color figure, see color section).

first used to locate an optimal oblique coronary scan plane. Then a limited number of contiguous slices are acquired around that plane within a breath hold with use of multi-slice spiral [71] or 2D segmented gradient-echo [67,72] imaging. Finally, if needed, a limited reformat of the data can be performed to produce images from relatively long sections of the coronaries. This approach yields relatively rapid visualization of portions of the coronary tree. Figure 5 shows a series of images captured from a real-time video segment, displaying the proximal right coronary artery. Visualization of the coronaries is good enough with this real-time spiral pulse sequence [37] to allow interactive prescription of optimal oblique planes in as little as 10 seconds [67]. Breath-held, ECG-gated images from two contiguous slices are shown in Figure 6. Here a dual-inversion-nulling pulse sequence was used to improve contrast with surrounding tissue [72].

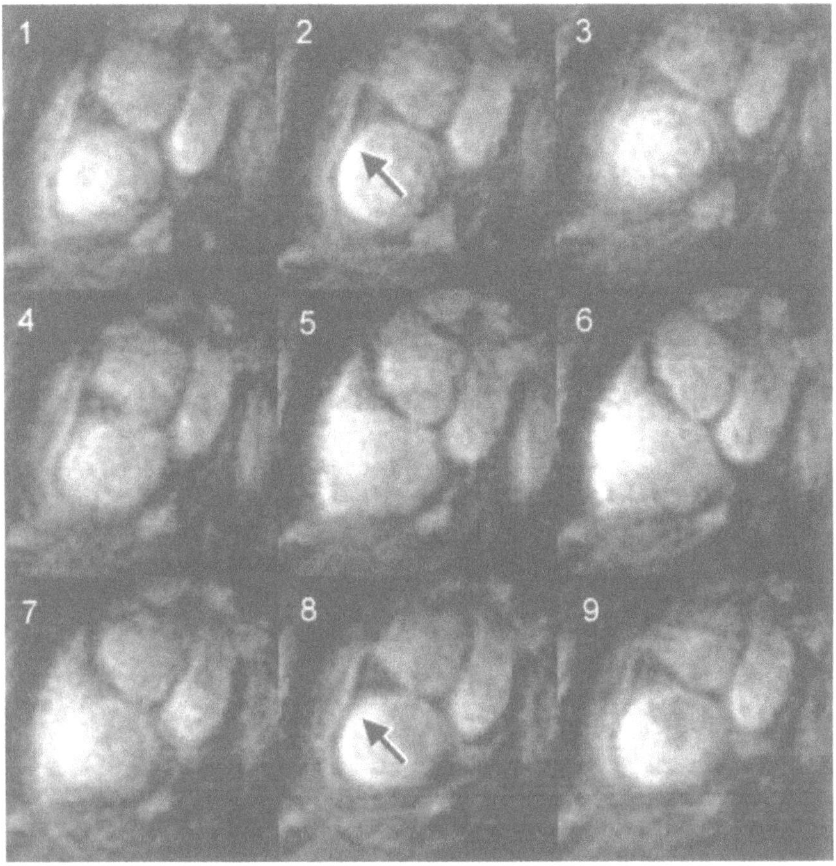

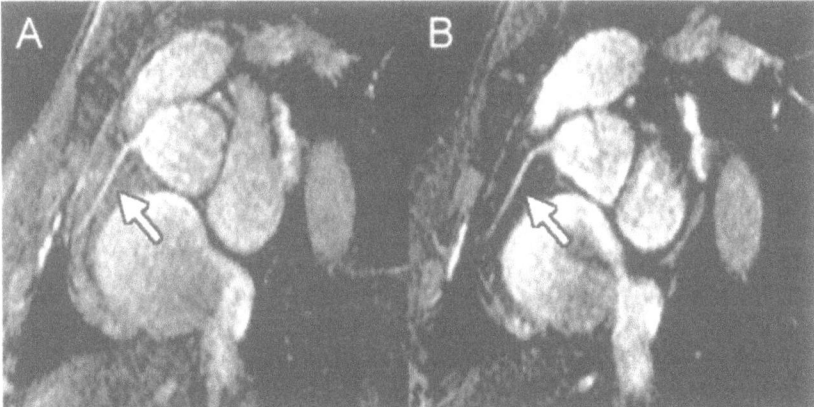

Figure 5. Continuous series of real-time spiral images, showing proximal right coronary artery (arrows) in selected frames.

Figure 6. Contiguous breath-held, ECG-gated MR images of proximal right coronary artery (arrows), acquired after real-time interactive localization of scan plane.

Conclusions

Recent improvements in gradient and reconstruction hardware, pulse sequence design, and user interface have made real-time interactive cardiac MRI now practical. This opens the possibilities for a flexible staged cardiac MRI exam which can be run in a variety of settings. A number of advances currently on the horizon promise to further increase the effectiveness of MRI in assessing coronary artery disease. More gains in reconstruction and display speed appear likely, as low-cost computer processing power continues to increase. Gradient speeds will probably show continued improvement as well, although we may soon enter a regime where peripheral nerve stimulation starts to become a consideration. Further refinement of MR pulse sequences is likely, with real-time capabilities being exploited to change the way clinically relevant parameters are measured.

The advent of intravascular MR contrast agents offers the promise of relatively high-contrast, high-resolution coronary MR angiography, providing greatly improved coronary visualization. Because these agents remain in the blood pool for relatively long periods, precise synchronization of the MR pulse sequence to the contrast injection is not necessary, and data can be collected over a longer interval of time. Early results have shown the potential benefits of MR stress testing for detecting and assessing the physiologic significance of coronary disease, with MRI pulse sequences employed to rapidly measure wall motion, perfusion, myocardial strain, or coronary flow before and during stress. MR-guided interventional procedures could one day become routine, with MRI used to direct the placement of catheters. Intravascular NMR receiver coils could potentially be used to image and characterize the composition of coronary plaques, for the purpose of determining the clinical risks associated with a particular lesion, and to predict its response to therapy. It is not yet clear which of these applications of cardiovascular MRI will demonstrate the most utility. However, whichever of these proves useful, real-time imaging seems likely to play an increasing role in the cardiovascular MRI exam of the future.

References

1. Van der Wall EE, Vliegen HW, De Roos A, Bruschke AVG. Magnetic resonance imaging in coronary artery disease. Circulation 1995;92:2723-39.
2. Van Rossum AC, Visser FC, Sprenger M, Van Eenige MJ, Valk J, Roos JP. Evaluation of magnetic resonance imaging for determination of left ventricular ejection fraction and comparison with angiography. Am J Cardiol 1988;62:628-33.
3. Underwood SR, Rees RSO, Savage PE *et al.* Assessment of regional left ventricular function by magnetic resonance. Br Heart J 1986;56:334-40.
4. White RD, Cassidy MM, Cheitlin MD *et al.* Segmental evaluation of left ventricular wall motion after myocardial infarction: magnetic resonance imaging versus echocardiography. Am Heart J 1988;115:166-75.
5. Atkinson DJ, Burstein D, Edelman RR. First-pass cardiac perfusion: evaluation with ultrafast MR imaging. Radiology 1990;174:757-62.
6. Wilke N, Simm C, Zhang J *et al.* Contrast-enhanced first pass myocardial perfusion imaging: correlation between myocardial blood flow in dogs at rest and during hyperemia. Magn Reson Med 1993;29:485-97.
7. Zerhouni EA, Parish DM, Rogers WJ, Yang A, Shapiro EP. Human heart: tagging with MR imaging - a method for noninvasive assessment of myocardial motion. Radiology 1988;169:59-63.
8. Axel L, Dougherty L. MR imaging of motion with spatial modulation of magnetization. Radiology 1989;171:841-5.
9. Edelman RR, Manning WJ, Burstein D, Paulin S. Coronary arteries: breath-hold MR angiography. Radiology 1991;181:641-3.

10. Meyer CH, Hu BS, Nishimura DG, Macovski A. Fast spiral coronary artery imaging. Magn Reson Med 1992;28:202-13.

11. Li D, Paschal CB, Haacke EM, Adler LP. Coronary arteries: three-dimensional MR imaging with fat saturation and magnetization transfer contrast. Radiology 1993;187:401-6.

12. Poncelet BP, Weisskoff RM, Wedeen VJ, Brady TJ, Kantor H. Time of flight quantification of coronary flow with echo-planar MRI. Magn Reson Med 1993;30:447-57.

13. Weiss RG, Bottomley PA, Hardy CJ, Gerstenblith G. Regional myocardial metabolism of high-energy phosphates during isometric exercise in patients with coronary artery disease. N Engl J Med 1990;323:1593-600.

14. Hardy CJ, Weiss RG, Bottomley PA, Gerstenblith G. Altered myocardial high- energy phosphate metabolites in patients with dilated cardiomyopathy. Am Heart J 1991;122:795-801.

15. Feinberg D. Fast MRI sequence design [abstract]. In: Syllabus of the ISMRM Fast MRI Workshop, Monterey, October 27-29, 1997. Berkeley: International Society for Magnetic Resonance in Medicine; 1997. p. 1-5.

16. Schmitt F. Gradient hardware considerations for fast MRI [abstract]. In: Syllabus of the ISMRM Fast MRI Workshop, Monterey, October 27-29, 1997. Berkeley: International Society for Magnetic Resonance in Medicine, 1997. p. 6-13.

17. Cohen MS, Weisskoff RM. Ultra-fast imaging. Magn Reson Imaging 1991;9:1-37.

18. Riederer SJ. Real-time imaging. In: Potchen EJ, Siebert JE, Haacke EM, Gottschalk A, editors. Magnetic resonance angiography: concepts & applications. St Louis: Mosby; 1993. p. 288-96.

19. Zientara GP. Fast imaging techniques. In: Jolesz FA, Young IR, editors. Interventional MR: techniques, methods and clinical experience. London: Martin Dunitz; 1998. p. 25-52.

20. Mansfield P, Pykett IL. Biological and medical imaging by NMR. J Magn Reson 1978;29:355-73.

21. Young IR, inventor. Nuclear magnetic resonance systems. US patent 4,355,282. 1979. August.

22. Edelstein WA, Hutchison JMS, Johnson G, Redpath TWT, Mallard JR, inventors. Methods of producing image information from objects. US patent 4,451,788. 1980. March.

23. Rzedzian RR, Pykett IL. Instant images of the human heart using a new, whole- body MR imaging system. AJR Am J Roentgenol 1987;149:245-50.

24. Hutchison JMS, Edelstein WA, Johnson G. A whole-body NMR imaging machine. J Phys E Sci Instrum 1980;13:947-55.

25. Mueller OM, Roemer PB, Park JN, Souza SP, Watkins RD. A 4-switch GTO speed-up inverter for fast-scan MRI [abstract]. Proc Soc Magn Reson Med 1992:589

26. Ideler KH, Nowak S, Borth G, Hagen U, Hausmann R, Schmitt F. A resonant multi purpose gradient power switch for high performance imaging [abstract]. Proc Soc Magn Reson Med 1992:4044.

27. Chapman B, Turner R, Ordidge RJ et al. Real-time movie imaging from a single cardiac cycle by NMR. Magn Reson Med 1987;5:246-54.

28. Roemer PB, Edelstein WA, Hickey JS. Selfshielded gradient coils [abstract]. Proc Soc Magn Reson Med 1986:1067-8.

29. Rzedzian RR. Real time MRI at 2.0 Tesla [abstract]. Proc Soc Magn Reson Med 1988:247.

30. McKinnon GC, Debatin JF, Wetter DR, Von Schulthess GK. Interleaved echo planar flow quantitation. Magn Reson Med 1994;32:263-7.

31. Reeder SB, McVeigh ER. The effect of high performance gradients on fast gradient echo imaging. Magn Reson Med 1994;32:612-21.

32. Henrich D, Haase A, Matthaei D. 3D-snapshot flash NMR imaging of the human heart. Magn Reson Imaging 1990;8:377-9.

33. Frahm J, Merboldt KD, Bruhn H, Gyngell ML, Hanicke W, Chien D. 0.3-Second FLASH MRI of the human heart. Magn Reson Med 1990;13:150-7.

34. Hennig J, Nauerth A, Friedburg H. RARE imaging: a fast imaging method for clinical MR. Magn Reson Med 1986;3:823-33.

35. Oshio K, Feinberg DA. GRASE (Gradient- and spin-echo) imaging: a novel fast MRI technique. Magn Reson Med 1991;20:344-9.

36. McKinnon GC. Ultrafast interleaved gradient-echo-planar imaging on a standard scanner. Magn Reson Med 1993;30:609-16.

37. Kerr AB, Pauly JM, Hu BS et al. Real-time interactive MRI on a conventional scanner. Magn Reson Med 1997;38:355-67.

38.   Hennig J, Mueri M. Fast imaging using Burst excitation pulses [abstract]. Proc Soc Magn Reson Med 1988:238.

39.   Jakob PM, Griswold M, Sodickson DK, Edelman RR. BURST imaging: New acquisition strategies [abstract]. In: Syllabus of the ISMRM Fast MRI Workshop, Monterey, October 27-29, 1997. Berkeley: International Society for Magnetic Resonance in Medicine; 1997. p. 162.

40.   Likes RS, inventor. Moving gradient zeugmatography. US patent 4,307,343. 1979. August.

41.   Meyer CH, Spielman D, Macovski A. Spiral fluoroscopy [abstract]. Proc Soc Magn Reson Med 1993:475.

42.   Hardy CJ, Bottomley PA. 31P spectroscopic localization using pinwheel NMR excitation pulses. Magn Reson Med 1991;17:315-27.

43.   Hardy CJ, Cline HE. Broadband nuclear magnetic resonance pulses with two- dimensional spatial selectivity. J Appl Phys 1989;66:1513-6.

44.   Meyer CH, Pauly JM, Macovski A, Nishimura DG. Simultaneous spatial and spectral selective excitation. Magn Reson Med 1990;15:287-304.

45.   Nishimura DG, Irarrazabal P, Meyer CH. A velocity k-space analysis of flow effects in echo-planar and spiral imaging. Magn Reson Med 1995;33:549-56.

46.   Irarrazabal P, Meyer CH, Nishimura DG, Macovski A. Inhomogeneity correction using an estimated linear field map. Magn Reson Med 1996;35:278-82.

47.   Wright RC, Riederer SJ, Farzaneh F, Rossman PJ, Liu Y. Real-time MR fluoroscopic data acquisition and image reconstruction. Magn Reson Med 1989;12:407-15.

48.   Hardy CJ, Darrow RD, Nieters EJ *et al.* Real-time acquisition, display, and interactive graphic control of NMR cardiac profiles and images. Magn Reson Med 1993;29:667-73.

49.   Crelier GR, Fischer SE, Arm E, Kunz P, Boesiger P. Realtime image reconstruction system for interactive magnetic resonance acquisition [abstract]. Proc Soc Magn Reson Med 1993:506.

50.   Schenck JF, Jolesz FA, Roemer PB *et al.* Superconducting open-configuration MR imaging system for image-guided therapy. Radiology 1995;195:805-14.

51.   Hardy CJ. High-speed interactive imaging for MRT [abstract]. Proc Soc Magn Reson 1995:489.

52.   Riederer SJ, Tasciyan T, Farzaneh F, Lee JN, Wright RC, Herfkens RJ. MR fluoroscopy: technical feasibility. Magn Reson Med 1988;8:1-15.

53.   Pearlman JD, Hardy CJ, Cline HE. Continual MR cardiography without gating: M-mode MR imaging. Radiology 1990;175:369-73.

54.   Hardy CJ, Pearlman JD, Moore JR, Roemer PB, Cline HE. Rapid NMR cardiography with a half-echo M-mode method. J Comput Assist Tomogr 1991;15:868-74.

55.   Pauly J, Nishimura D, Macovski A. A k-space analysis of small-tip-angle excitation. J Magn Reson 1989;81:43-56.

56.   Hardy CJ, Cline HE. Spatial localization in two dimensions using NMR designer pulses. J Magn Reson 1989;82:647-54.

57.   Hardy CJ, Cline HE, Bottomley PA. Correcting for nonuniform k-space sampling in two-dimensional NMR selective excitation. J Magn Reson 1990;87:639-45.

58.   Butts K, Hangiandreou NJ, Riederer SJ. Phase velocity mapping with a real time line scan technique. Magn Reson Med 1993;29:134-8.

59.   Dumoulin CL, Souza SP, Hardy CJ, Ash SA. Quantitative measurement of blood flow using cylindrically localized Fourier velocity encoding. Magn Reson Med 1991;21:242-50.

60.   Hardy CJ, Bolster BD Jr, McVeigh ER, Iben IET, Zerhouni EA. Pencil excitation with interleaved fourier velocity encoding: NMR measurement of aortic distensibility. Magn Reson Med 1996;35:814-9.

61.   Irarrazabal P, Hu BS, Pauly JM, Nishimura DG. Spatially resolved and localized real-time velocity distribution. Magn Reson Med 1993;30:207-12.

62.   Relvas MS, Bolster BD, Hardy CJ, Zerhouni EA. A non-invasive NMR method to measure aortic distensibility and diameter in patients at risk for dissection or rupture [abstract]. Proceedings of the SMR Workshop on Cardiovascular MRI: Present and Future, Santa Fe, Oct. 13-15, 1994. Berkeley: Society of Magnetic Resonance; 1994. p. 18.

63.   Holsinger AE, Wright RC, Riederer SJ, Farzaneh F, Grimm RC, Maier JK. Real- time interactive magnetic resonance imaging. Magn Reson Med 1990;14:547-53.

64.   Hardy CJ, Darrow RD. Interactive slice prescription schemes for rapid MR imaging of coronary arteries [abstract]. Proc Soc Magn Reson 1994:500.

65.   Hardy CJ, Darrow RD. Heartscape: an interactive cardiac scan-plane positioner [abstract]. Proc Int Soc Magn Res Med 1996:1496.

66. Debbins JP, Riederer SJ, Rossman PJ *et al.* Cardiac magnetic resonance fluoroscopy. Magn Reson Med 1996;36:588-95.

67. Hardy CJ, Darrow RD, Pauly JM *et al.* Interactive coronary MRI. Magn Reson Med. In press 1998.

68. Silverman SG, Collick BD, Figueira MR *et al.* Interactive MR-guided biopsy in an open-configuration MR imaging system. Radiology 1995;197:175-81.

69. Schroeder W, Martin K, Lorensen B. The visualization toolkit: an object-oriented approach to 3d graphics. Englewood Cliffs, NJ: Prentice-Hall; 1996.

70. Yang P, Kerr A, Liu A *et al.* Real-time interactive cardiac MRI for patients with suboptimal echocardiographic studies [abstract]. Proc Int Soc Magn Reson Med 1997:909.

71. Meyer CH, Hu BS, Kerr AB *et al.* High-resolution multi-slice spiral coronary angiography with real-time interactive localization [abstract]. Proc Int Soc Magn Reson Med 1997:439.

72. Hardy CJ, Dumoulin CL, Darrow RD. MR coronary angiography using a hybrid multi-slice technique with fat/muscle suppression and fluoroscopic localization [abstract]. Proc Int Soc Magn Reson Med 1997:440.

17. Left ventricular function under stress conditions by MRI

Markus B. Scheidegger, Marcus Spiegel & Peter Boesinger

Summary

Cardiac patients with ischemic heart disease often show normal cardiac function at rest. Abnormalities may be discovered by these functional examinations only during increased cardiac work. Therefore, cardiac function assessment under physiological or drug induced stress is a key part of a comprehensive cardiac examination. The value of MR cardiac imaging is limited without the ability to study the effects of stress on patients. A number of ways to stress patients in MR scanners has been considered or tested, however, most of them are either not practical or useful. Promising techniques are dynamic bicycle exercise and pharmacological stress testing by injection of either dipyridamole or dobutamine. In the majority of studies published in literature stress was applied pharmacologically. Commonly, short axis cine gradient echo images are acquired and regional wall motion abnormalities are studied. Generally, a good correlation between wall motion abnormalities and angiographic severity of coronary artery disease resulted. However, physical exercise would be a preferable form of stress. In this text, the feasibility of ergometer exercise in MR scanners is explored. The MR compatible equipment for supine bicycle exercise is described, and basic questions concerning patient safety are addressed. The MR sequences for imaging both for 5 seconds immediately after exercise, and for imaging during stress are described. They are based on gradient-echo echo-planar techniques (EPI). Imaging during stress can be done only with real time imaging using a new acquisition technique named turbo-field-echo-EPI, with an acquisition time of 75 ms per image. Short axis cine anatomical images suitable for qualitative wall motion assessment are presented, acquired within 5 seconds after exercise stop, as well as real time images acquired constantly during stress. Myocardial tagging is performed during exercise and within 5 seconds immediately after stress. The tagging data sets are suitable for a quantitative measurement of myocardial wall motion. Patient motion is the most severe problem to overcome. To this purpose, the acquisition needs to be extremely fast, in order to freeze motion. This is technically demanding, but with modern MR scanners it is possible to acquire cardiac images at a rate of approximately 10 images per second with a image resolution of approximately 2.5 mm.

From these preliminary experiments it is concluded that with some improvements in the imaging procedure and gradient performance of the MR system it is well feasible to perform left ventricular function assessment not only with pharmacological but also with physical stress using a bicycle ergometer.

J.H.C. Reiber and E.E. van der Wall (eds.). What's New in Cardiovascular Imaging, 221–232.
©1998 Kluwer Academic Publishers.

Introduction

In the last years, MRI has established its role in cardiovascular imaging, initially mainly for anatomical imaging. Recently, emphasis has been put more and more on cardiac function such as flow, myocardial motion, wall thickening, perfusion, coronary flow reserve, and even metabolism.

The ability to detect ischemic heart disease before myocardial infarction is very important, however, there are some potential pitfalls if using anatomical imaging only: myocardial ischemia can occur in the absence of disease of the epicardial coronary arteries, and, arterial disease can occur without causing myocardial ischemia. Therefore, the knowledge of coronary anatomy, although very important, is in principal inferior to functional tests. Cardiac patients with ischemic heart disease often show normal cardiac function at rest. Abnormalities may be discovered by these functional examinations only during increased cardiac work. Therefore, cardiac function assessment under physiological or drug induced stress is a key part of a comprehensive cardiac examination. The value of MR cardiac imaging is limited without the ability to study the effects of stress on patients.

Functional tests, beside the measurement of cardiac volumes and ejection fraction include:
- high resolution imaging during myocardial stress to evaluate regional wall motion,
- myocardial wall motion quantitation by tagging,
- spectroscopic imaging during stress to study metabolic evidence of ischemia,
- myocardial imaging in order to study regional deficits in perfusion during stress,
- and quantitation of coronary flow reserve.

Diagnostic tests under stress are very common in clinical cardiology; first of all the recording of the electrocardiogram (ECG) signal under bicycle exercise is to be mentioned. Also common are stress tests in nuclear medicine (Tl-201 and Tc-99m SestaMIBI myocardial perfusion imaging), both with either pharmacological or exercise induced stress [1-4]. Criteria are regional deficits in myocardial perfusion. However, the image resolution obtained is much less than even in low-resolution MR imaging of the heart.

Wall motion abnormalities are frequently assessed with echocardiographic stress tests, again either after injection of a stress inducing agent [5-7] or after treadmill exercise or during supine bicycle exercise [6,7].

Several different approaches may be considered for inducing stress in an MR environment:
1. Isometric exercise, as for instance with a hand dynamometer has been reported, however, muscle fatigue occurs quickly for isometric exercise, and the level of stress induced is limited [8-10]. For cardiac stress testing with largely increased cardiac stroke volume and heart rate, high levels of exercise are needed, which cannot be reached by handgrip type of exercise. The leg muscles, the largest muscle in the human body, must be involved in a dynamic exercise in order to reach a cardiac output close to maximum.
2. Cardiac pacing could also be considered [11], but pacing in any form (implanted pacemaker, invasive atrial pacing, or transesophageal cardiac pacing) is still strictly considered a contraindication for an MR examination, due to unresolved safety issues.
3. Cold-pressor stress [12], or mental stress are not further considered practical, due to either too small stress levels, high dependency on patient cooperation.
4. Pharmacological stress [13] (dipyridamole, dobutamine, or adenosine) seems to be a useful possibility, although an intravenous infusion is required, and side effects may occur.

Additionally, the time interval available for imaging under stress is restricted. The main advantage of pharmacological stress is the induction of stress without physical motion of the patient, i.e. no additional motion artifacts arise. MR examinations with pharmacologically induced stress have been reported [3,14-17].

5. Dynamic exercise: Schaefer et al. [18] presented a device for inducing stress by physical exercise within an MR magnet bore. However, dynamic exercise within an conventional MR magnet with a long magnet bore is difficult and considered unpleasant, and exercise during scanning poses considerable technical and methodological problems. Motion artifacts during exercise are often too high with conventional MRI sequences, due to a strongly amplified breathing motion, as well as some inevitable movements of the chest due to exercising. Therefore, reports on MRI using dynamic exercise have been rare in literature [19].

This text briefly summarizes results obtained with pharmacological stress application. However, the main emphasis is put on initial research experience with ergometer stress.

Stress examination in MRI: pharmacological stress application

The easiest way of stress application in an MR scanner is by means of pharmacological stress agents. A variety of agents can or have already been used in MR stress examinations.

Firstly, vasodilators have been used for induction of stress, mainly dipyridamole and adenosine. Dipyridamole is a potent coronary dilator, and thus has been used for assessment of perfusion deficits. It is often used in Tl-201 scintigraphy, and also in PET and SPECT [1,3,13,17].

The other agent category used [5-7,13-16,20,21] are Beta-agonists, among them dobutamine, dopamine, isoprenaline, and adrenaline. Dobutamine is a β-agonist which increases myocardial oxygen demand. This results in increased heart rate and blood pressure, less arrhythmias occur, and it provokes wall motion abnormalities. A number of studies has been published in literature [6,14-16] and others. Common is the assessment of regional wall motion abnormalities. To this purpose, mostly short axis cine gradient echo images are acquired, often at different levels of the heart. Generally, a significant correlation between detection of wall motion abnormality and the angiographic severity of coronary artery disease was found.

Physiologically induced stress during MR examinations

Beside the more widespread use and ease of application, there is a number of arguments in favor of dynamic physical exercise: Advantages of physical exercise stress testing over pharmacological stress include: the exercise load can be prescribed individually, both in load and in variation of the load pattern over time, and can be measured exactly. A controlled increase in cardiac output and myocardial oxygen demand can be provoked. We hypothesize, that dynamic exercise stress is the most preferable form of stress because it simulates most closely the stress experienced by the patient in daily life. In a comparison [22] of an echo stress test with exercise, dipyridamole and dobutamine in 100 patients with suspected or known coronary artery disease (CAD), physical exercise had the best sensitivity for diagnosis of CAD.

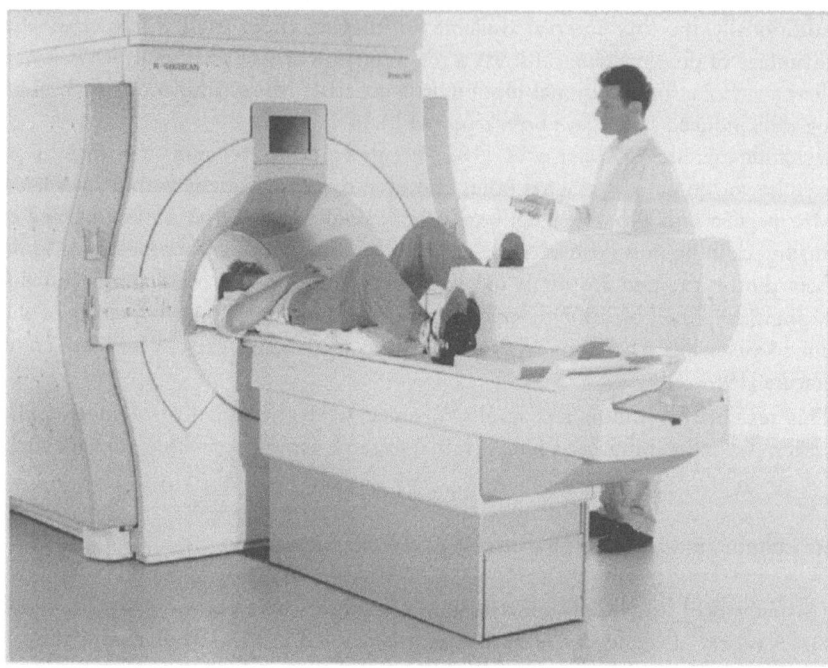

Figure 1. MR-compatible ergometer for supine leg exercise (Lode Medical Technology, Groningen, The Netherlands); volunteer with the exercise equipment for the MR scanner. A bicycle pedal drives electrical flywheel braking coils over a rubber chain transmission. The load is independent of the cycle speed and can be freely programmed over time within the range of 25 to 400 Watts. All protocols commonly used for cardiac stress examinations are available. The ergometer is built onto a standard patient bed of a Philips Gyroscan NT system (1.5 Tesla).

Wall motion abnormalities occurred always before any noticeable ST segment changes in the ECG when stress was physical.

In this text a number of fundamental questions is addressed concerning dynamic high level exercise in an MR magnet for cardiac imaging. A careful design of exercise apparatus, imaging and monitoring strategy have to be worked out, since motion artifacts are severe. Also, patient safety issues have to be addressed.

Equipment for physiological stress during MR examinations

Ergometer setup

In the following paragraph the setup of a MR compatible ergometer is described. In compact short bore MR magnets the legs of the patient are at least partly outside of the magnet bore while the heart is imaged. Patients are subjected to exercise in supine position using a programmable bicycle exercise equipment (Lode Medical Technology, Groningen, The Netherlands) altered to fit into an MR scanner environment. Figure 1 represents an image of a volunteer with the exercise equipment for the MR scanner. A bicycle pedal drives electrical flywheel braking coils over a rubber chain transmission. The load is independent of the cycle speed and can be freely programmed over time within the range of 25 to 400 Watts. All protocols commonly used for cardiac stress examinations are available. The ergometer is built onto a standard patient bed of a Philips Gyroscan NT system (1.5 Tesla).

Exercise protocol

The exercise protocol used in these preliminary studies consisted of a constant, cycling speed independent work load at various predefined levels from 33 Watts to 130 Watts, following an initial slow increase of 2 to 3 minutes to the defined work load. All volunteers were subjected to 4 different levels of stress: low level (33 Watt), intermediate-low (65 Watt), intermediate-high (99 Watt) and high-level (131 Watt), and the heart rate was monitored on a beat-to-beat basis at each level.

Monitoring and heart rate synchronization was obtained using peripheral pulse wave (PPU) and electrocardiographic (ECG) triggering. After the start of the imaging sequence all RR intervals of the electrocardiogram signal were recorded during the scan on an individual basis, in order to monitor heart rate recovery during the scan.

MR techniques for LV function assessment under physiological (ergometer) stress

Since it is extremely difficult to reach adequate image quality during heavy physical exercise with conventional MR imaging sequences, and since the electrocardiogram signal obtained from within an MR scanner during high level physical exercise is extremely distorted, most often too much to be used, the question comes up whether an exercise setup could be found with imaging immediately after repeated stops of exercise work. A *central* question is, whether scanning can be performed **during** exercise, or immediately **after** stopping it. The two different imaging strategies are hereafter referred to simply as *during*, and *after*, respectively. For the evaluation of advantages and disadvantages of these two different approaches the following questions need to be addressed: Does the time immediately after stopping exercise still represent the exercise state ? If yes, for how long periods is this true ? Therefore, a measure of exercise state is sought. We propose the heart beat rate as a valid measure for the stress state after exercise stop. The literature about heart rate recovery after stress [23-25] indicates, that only a very short time window in the order of less than 10 sec can be used immediately after stress, because the heart rate drops very quickly, at least in young trained subjects. However, the studies found in literature dealt with longer recovery periods, and no results were found in literature about the heart rate drop within the first 10 seconds.

Therefore, the heart rate drop was examined on a beat-to-beat basis after stopping bicycle exercise in the MR scanner at various levels of exercise, in order to acquire data about the heart rate recovery within the first 12 heart beats after exercise stop. The average heart rate dropped by only 4% within the first 10 heart beats immediately after stopping exercise. This change was smaller than changes measured during breath-holds of 10 heart beats duration at rest, therefore the influence of changing heart rate on the image quality is negligible, if MR images are acquired during the first 10 heart beats after exercise stop.

Imaging techniques have to be optimized for scanning both during and after stress to evaluate an ideal MR stress and imaging protocol. The imaging techniques included short axis anatomical imaging, and the assessment of myocardial wall motion by tagging [26].

Furthermore, in another study, quantitative flow measurements in the abdominal aorta were performed [27].

MR imaging protocols 'after'

The following type of MR scans were performed for LV functional evaluation:
• multi heart phase anatomical imaging for the qualitative assessment of contraction and wall motion abnormalities;
• quantitative wall motion analysis by CSPAMM [28] grid tagging

The protocols for imaging 'during' were also applied 'after', for comparison. A scan time interval of 10 heart beats was chosen for data acquisition immediately following an exercise-stop. MR imaging was synchronized to the ECG signal. Double oblique short and long axis anatomical images of the heart were acquired. Imaging protocol was based on a 2D multi heart phase gradient echo EPI technique with an EPI-factor of 9. Field-of-view was 200 mm x 186 mm, slice thickness 8 mm, the acquisition matrix was 128; thus the in-plane image resolution amounted to 2.34 x 2.96 mm per pixel. 12 heart phase images were acquired, the scans lasted 10 heart beats, i.e. usually 10 seconds at rest, and less than 5 seconds at the highest exercise levels. The volunteers were put in supine position and a linear surface coil (17 cm diameter) was put onto their chest. Scans were performed within a single inspiratory breath-hold of a maximum duration of 10 heart beats.

The CSPAMM tagging technique requires 4 acquisitions per phase encoding line to form a grid tagged image. Therefore, faster imaging sequences are required to keep the acquisition time within the requested 10 heart beats. The imaging protocol based on a 2D multiple heart phase TFEPI (CP3 cardiac SW patch, Philips Medical Systems) sequence. TFEPI (see Figure 2) is basically a multiple heart phase hybrid fast imaging sequence with k-space segmentation and EPI readout [29]. In each heart phase interval, 3 to 5 excitation pulses were applied, and each pulse was followed by an EPI readout train (9 to 13 EPI readouts). Prior to the acquisition of each heart phase a SPIR pulse was applied for fat suppression. Using the same geometrical scan parameters as above, but a reduced image resolution parallel to the stripes of only 30 %, imaging setups were found for CSPAMM imaging within 8 heart beats.

MR imaging protocols 'during'

Imaging during high levels of exercise essentially requires instant or real-time (RT) acquisition, thus data for one image have to be acquired during less than 70 to 100 ms. *During* exercise the following scans were performed: (1) multi heart phase anatomical imaging, and (2) quantitative wall motion analysis by SPAMM tagging [26]. The TFEPI sequence was used to obtain images of 2.3 mm x 3.9 mm resolution with a slice thickness of 8 mm within just 75 ms. Thus, a short axis slice is repeatedly imaged at a rate of 13 images per second.

Ergometric stress imaging in vivo

Exercise protocols could be performed for all volunteers. Undisturbed heart rate monitoring was obtained during all exercise levels using PPU. Using ECG it was only possible to moni-

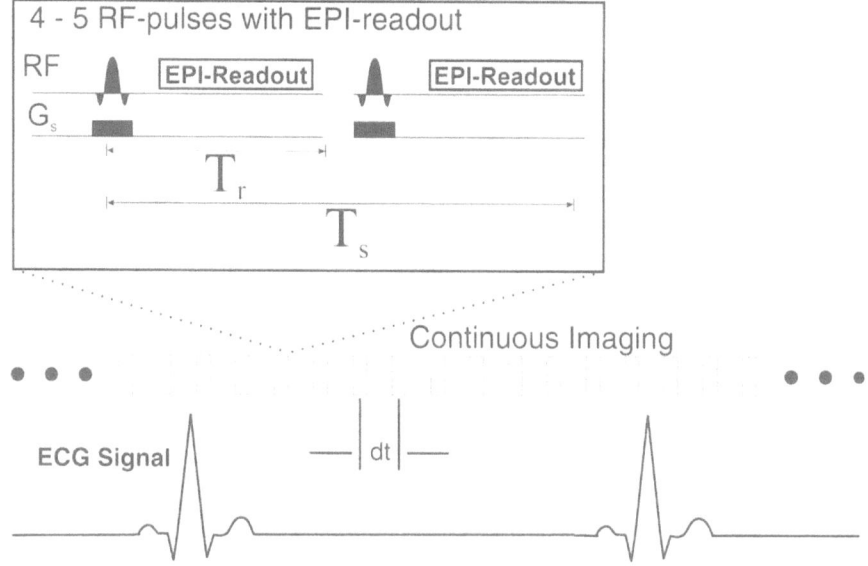

Figure 2. Ultrafast MR imaging sequence: TFEPI (= Turbo Field Echo Planar Imaging). It combines segmented k-space acquisition with echo planar (EPI) readout as in [29]. A slice selection (a) is immediately followed by a EPI-readout train (b). Slice selection and EPI readout are repeated multiple times (repetition time Tr) to split the k-space in multiple readouts. Total duration for one heart phase image is denoted as TS and the heart phase interval as dt. In a multiple-shot acquisition mode data from several (up to 10) heart beats are taken to form one image data set of 8 to 16 heart phase images. The sequence allows also for a real-time mode where each image is acquired during a time interval of approximately 75 ms.

tor heart rate up to exercise levels of approximately 65 watts corresponding to a heart rate in the range of 80-110 beats per minute. In all cases, the electrocardiogram, when disturbed to unreadability during exercise, recovered to a signal reliable for ECG triggering, immediately, i.e. within less than 2 heart beats. The scans started about 2 heart beats after exercise stop.

Imaging after exercise stop

Since the quality of the ECG signal immediately recovers after exercise stop, no triggering problems occur for the "after" protocol. RT imaging as well as imaging over 10 heart beats was successful in all cases in all volunteers. Due to very heavy breathing at the high levels of exercise, some sort of breath-holding or breathing reduction is absolutely necessary for the 10 heart beat protocol. Thus, the 10 heart beat protocol was performed with breath-holding after inspiration. Breath-holding at exhalation state was considered very strenuous, even for 5 seconds. For the tagging protocols immediately after exercising, a slice following CSPAMM tagging technique [28,30] was chosen. A complete CSPAMM experiment with grid tagging and a time resolution of 35 ms required also 8 heart beats. In Figure 3 a series of short axis anatomical images of a volunteer under ergometric stress acquired within 10 heart

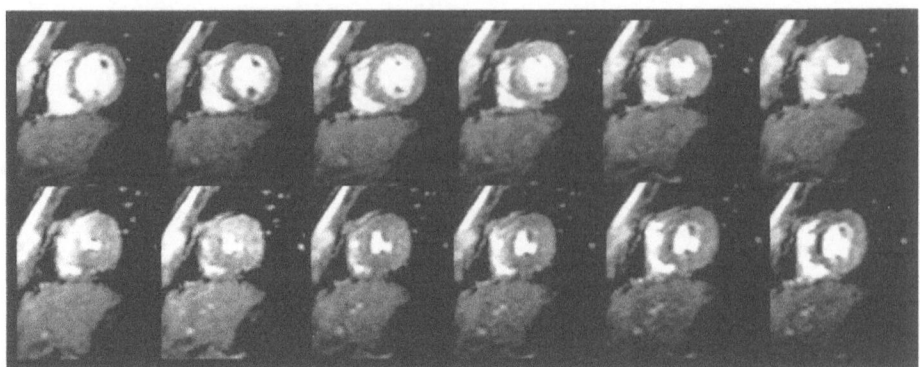

Figure 3. Short axis anatomical imaging for qualitative assessment of contraction and wall motion in a volunteer under ergometric stress. 12 heart phase images were acquired within 10 heart beats after pedaling stop at a heart rate of 130 beats per minute. Strong inflow of blood ensures a high contrast between myocardium and (very bright) blood.

beats after pedaling stop at a heart rate of 130 beats per minute is shown. Strong inflow of blood ensures a high contrast between myocardium and (very bright) blood.

Imaging during exercise

Using single heart beat (= real time (RT) = single shot) acquisition it was possible to acquire images also at the highest exercise levels explored in this protocol (130 Watt). The real time protocol was used in a "free run" mode, without ECG triggering. All data for one image were acquired within 75 ms or less, therefore triggering was not necessary, and differences in inspiration level from beat to beat did not influence the image quality. RT images during exercise were of similar, though at the average of a little bit lower quality, than the RT images acquired at rest. Since the resolution of the images parallel to the stripes can be much lower than perpendicular to the stripes, line tagging was performed, with a scan percentage of 35% of all ky-lines in phase encoding direction [26,30]. Thus, the time resolution for the real time tagging scans could be chosen to be 35 ms, half of that of the anatomical measurements. Only line tagging was performed for the RT protocol during exercise.

Figure 4 displays short axis anatomical images (left) and myocardial tagging images (right) at rest and *during* exercise with 120 Watts load. Images at rest are shown in the upper row, stress images in the lower row. The heart rate amounted to 62 beats per minute at rest, and to 132 beats per minute at the high level stress. All images were acquired in a real time mode, i.e. within a interval of 75 ms for the anatomical images, and within 30 ms for the line tagged images.

Safety considerations

Patient monitoring is a very critical issue, since ischemia is provoked with the stress testing [31]. Commercial equipment exists to monitor non-invasively blood pressure, oxygen saturation, and other vital parameters in MR scanners. The main and important difference com-

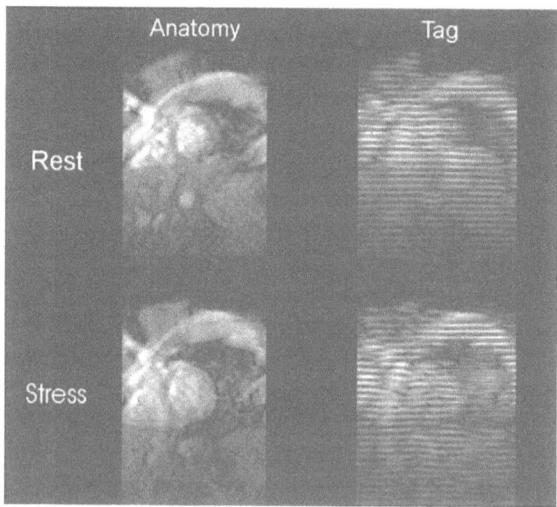

Figure 4. MR Imaging during high level ergometric exercise: Short axis anatomical images (left) and myocardial tagging images (right) at rest and during exercise with 120 Watts load. Images at rest are shown in the upper row, stress images in the lower row. The heart rate amounted to 62 beats per minute at rest, and to 132 beats per minute at the high level stress. All images were acquired in a real time mode, i.e. within a interval of 75 ms for the anatomical images, and within 30 ms for the line tagged images. Images were always acquired in a free run mode, covering 4-5 seconds, or 4-12 heart beats, respectively, and were normally viewed in a movie-mode.

pared to exercise testing outside of a magnetic field is the lack of a diagnostic ECG. This holds true also for MR studies at rest, and for pharmacologically induced stress.

Another difference in patient monitoring when compared to MR imaging at rest is the lack of a useable electrocardiogram signal at the high levels of physiologically induced exercise. However, the PPU heart rate monitoring was reliable throughout the exercise levels tested in this study. Therefore, heart rate can be monitored reliably. A carefully planned and trained emergency case scenario is mandatory. It is strongly recommended to use a trolley cart system, for emergency evacuations. In our test setup the whole ergometer together with the patient could be evaded out of the scanner and into another room using a trolley system in less than 20 seconds.

Together with the ability to take the patient out of the magnetic field in a very short time the basic patient safety concerns seems to be fulfilled, although other monitoring modalities might be wanted in addition. This statement, however, ignores the infrequent, but very dangerous cases of transmural ischemia, recognized in an ST-segment elevation; where some patients in such a situation do not feel strong discomfort. Therefore, it should be mentioned, and this is true for ergometric as well as for pharmacological stress evaluations, that the safety issues of MR stress testing are not yet fully solved. This is a reason we experimented with larger numbers of volunteers.

Problems and perspectives of MR examinations under ergometric stress

It seems possible to perform bicycle exercise in a standard whole body magnet independent of the posture of the person performing the exercise. All (young) volunteers could perform the protocols they were asked for, and useful images were acquired in all examinations.

Open problems

In some test cases, the diaphragm displacement caused by breathing was measured using a M-mode beam navigator placed perpendicularly through the dome of the right diaphragm. The diaphragm moved approximately 8 cm (!) in inferior-superior direction both during and immediately after exercise. Therefore, some sort of breathing motion control is an absolute necessity. Respiratory triggering or gating schemes prolong scan times too much, since imaging 'after' is restricted to a 10 heart beat interval. Inspiratory breath-holds were usually tolerated post exercise up to a duration of 5 sec. Breath-holding at an end-expiratory position was generally not tolerated. For registration of multiple slice images acquired over several heart beats, a proper fixation of the chest region is necessary. Nevertheless, registration of several sequentially acquired slice images is a problem, due to the heavy respiratory motion during exercise, or the deep inspirations taken for the breath-holds. MR-based control and correction schemes for this large breathing motion would be desirable, such as a navigator echo controlled image acquisition. However, due to the enhanced breathing, and due to the necessity to perform breath-holds at maximum inspiration, the reproduction of the inspiration level becomes a difficult issue. It is generally very difficult to repeat the same inspiration level at full inspiration. Therefore, slices acquired at rest and in inspiratory breath-holds 'after' often do not match with regard to their position in the heart. Additionally, a multiple slice data set of short axis images covering the ventricles to evaluate ejection fraction suffers from the same problem, and large errors can occur. In some cases a feedback of the breathing position as measured with a navigator beam across the diaphragm to the patient using a video-projection of a PC-screen was used. Generally feedback, resulted in an excellent reproduction of the breathing position. At rest, reproduction of the diaphragm within 1, maximally 2 mm was achieved.

Perspectives

It is possible to perform ECG triggered scans during exercise only at a low level exercise. PPU triggering is reliable at any level of exercise, but the high motion precludes scans extending over several heart beats. Thus, scanning during high level exercise (> 120 Watts, heart rate > 120 bpm) requires instant (=real time) scanning. The TFEPI sequence with a acquisition time of 65 to 80 ms per image fulfils this requirement. Anatomical images were of sufficient quality for evaluation of the chamber cross section and wall thickening [32]. Scanning immediately after stopping exercise resulted in generally better image quality, since breath-held scans were possible. Using fast imaging methods available on modern scanners it is possible to perform cardiac examinations both during and immediately post dynamic leg exercise.

When using a fast powerful gradient system images can be acquired in 40 to 50 ms with a increased resolution of approx. 2x2 mm, which should improve image quality. So far a simple surface coil was used. Sophisticated phased array coil will help improving the signal-to-noise ratio, or, if the coil sensitivity is used for phase encoding, the acquisition process can be speeded up considerably [33]. Using coil sensitivity encoding in our lab, at rest cardiac images have been acquired with a rate of 30 images/second, i.e. one anatomical MR image within 30 ms, freezing all cardiac motion.

With these technical improvements underway, it will be possible to perform cardiac exercise stress test in MR scanners, and access all the information cardiac MR is able to provide also under stress conditions.

References

1. Beer SG, Heo J, Iskandrian AS. Dipyridamole thallium imaging. Am J Cardiol 1991;67:18D-26D.
2. Freeman ML, Palac R, Mason J *et al.* A comparison of dobutamine and supine bicycle exercise for radionuclide cardiac stress testing. Clin Nucl Med 1984;9:251-5.
3. Pennell DJ, Underwood SR, Ell PJ, Swanton RH, Walker JM, Longmore DB. Dipyridamole magnetic resonance imaging: a comparison with thallium-201 emission tomography. Br Heart J 1990;64:362-9.
4. Kato Y, Kaneko K, Kondo T *et al.* Investigation of exercise stress whole-body thallium-201 scintigraphy: comparison between supine and sitting bicycle ergometer stress testing in patients with ischemic heart disease [Japanese]. Kaku Igaku 1988;25:39-48.
5. Izzat MB, Birdi I, Wilde P, Bryan AJ, Angelini GD. Comparison of hemodynamic performances of St. Jude Medical and CarboMedics 21 mm aortic prostheses by means of dobutamine stress echocardiography. J Thorac Cardiovasc Surg 1996;111:408-15.
6. McNeill AJ, Fioretti PM, el-Said SM, Salustri A, Forster T, Roelandt JR. Enhanced sensitivity for detection of coronary artery disease by addition of atropine to dobutamine stress echocardiography. Am J Cardiol 1992;70:41-6.
7. Rallidis L, Cokkinos P, Tousoulis D, Nihoyannopoulos P. Comparison of dobutamine and treadmill exercise echocardiography in inducing ischemia in patients with coronary artery disease. J Am Coll Cardiol 1997;30:1660-8.
8. Helfant RH, De Villa MA, Meister SG. Effect of sustained isometric exercise on left ventricular performance. Circulation 1971;44:982-93.
9. Kivowitz C, Parmley W, Donoso R, Marcus H, Ganz W, Swan HJC. Effects of isometric exercise on cardiac performance. The grip test. Circulation 1971;44:994-1002.
10. Kottmann W, Jette M, Schrader M, Claus J, Blumchen G. Fullungsdrucke (PCP, Einschwemmkatheter) unter kombinierter statischer (Handgriff) und dynamischer (Fahrradergometer) Belastung bei Postinfarktpatiente). Z Kardiol 1988;77:291-8.
11. Hofman MBM, De Cock CC, Van der Linden JC *et al.* Transesophageal cardiac pacing during magnetic resonance imaging: feasibility and safety considerations. Magn Reson Med 1996;35:413-22.
12. Greene MA, Boltax AJ, Lustig GA, Rogow E. Circulatory dynamics during the cold pressor test. Am J Cardiol 1965;16:54-60.
13. Fung AY, Gallagher KP, Buda AJ *et al.* The physiologic basis of dobutamine as compared with dipyridamole stress interventions in the assessment of critical coronary stenosis. Circulation 1987;76:943-51.
14. Pennell DJ, Underwood SR, Manzara CC *et al.* Magnetic resonance imaging during dobutamine stress in coronary artery disease. Am J Cardiol 1992;70:34-40.
15. Van Rugge FP, Van der Wall EE, De Roos A, Bruschke AVG. Dobutamine stress magnetic resonance imaging for detection of coronary artery disease. J Am Coll Cardiol 1993;22:431-9.
16. Van Rugge FP, Van der Wall EE, Spanjersberg SJ *et al.* Magnetic resonance imaging during dobutamine stress for detection and localization of coronary artery disease. Quantitative wall motion analysis using a modification of the centerline method. Circulation 1994;90:127-38.
17. Baer FM, Smolarz K, Jungehulsing M *et al.* Feasibility of high-dose dipyridamole-magnetic resonance imaging for detection of coronary artery disease and comparison with coronary angiography. Am J Cardiol 1992;69:51-6.
18. Schaefer S, Peshock RM, Raekey RW, Willerson JT. A new device for exercise MR imaging. AJR Am J Roentgenol 1986;147:1289-90.

19. Mohiaddin RH, Gatehouse PD, Firmin DN. Exercise-related changes in aortic flow measured with spiral echo-planar MR velocity mapping. J Magn Reson Imaging 1995;5:159-63.

20. Mannering D, Cripps T, Leech G *et al.* The dobutamine stress test as an alternative to exercise testing after acute myocardial infarction. Br Heart J 1988;59:521-6.

21. Rogers WJ, Power TP *et al.* 2D analysis of normal myocardial deformation during dobutamine stimulation using MRI tissue tagging. Proc Int Soc Magn Reson Med 1997:661.

22. Dagianti A, Penco M, Agati L *et al.* Stress echocardiography: comparison of exercise, dipyridamole and dobutamine in detecting and predicting the extent of coronary artery disease [published erratum appears in J Am Coll Cardiol 1995;26:114]. J Am Coll Cardiol 1995;26:18-25.

23. Darr KC, Basset DR, Morgan BJ, Thomas DP. Effects of age and training status on heart rate recovery after peak exercise. Am J Physiol. 1988;254:H340-3.

24. Cox RH. Exercise training and response to stress: insights from an animal model. Med Sci Sports Exerc 1991;23:853-9.

25. Shaw CE, McCully KK, Landsberg L, Posner J. The effect of a submaximal exercise orientation on cardiopulmonary cycle ergometer stress test results in older adults. J Cardiopulm Rehabil 1996;16:93-9.

26. Zerhouni EA, Parish DM, Rogers WJ, Yang A, Shapiro EP. Human heart: tagging with MR imaging-a method for noninvasive assessment of myocardial motion. Radiology 1988;169:59-63.

27. Pedersen EM, Kozerke S, Scheidegger MB *et al.* Fast flow measurements at different levels of ergometer exercise. Proc Int Soc Magn Reson Med 1997:115.

28. Fischer SE, McKinnon GC, Maier SE, Boesiger P. Improved myocardial tagging contrast. Magn Reson Med 1993;30:191-200.

29. McKinnon GC. Ultrafast interleaved gradient-echo-planar imaging on a standard scanner. Magn Reson Med 1993;30:609-16.

30. Fischer SE, McKinnon GC, Scheidegger MB, Prins W, Meier D, Boesiger P. True myocardial motion tracking. Magn Reson Med 1994;31:401-13.

31. Capezzuto A, Achilli A, Pontillo D, Sassara M, De Spirito S, Guerra R. Acute myocardial infarction shortly after a normal exercise stress test. Case reports. Angiology 1995;46:521-6.

32. Scheidegger MB, Spiegel M, Stuber M *et al.* Assessment of cqrdiac wall thickening and ejection fraction from real time mr images n patients with left ventricular dysfunction. Proc Int Soc Magn Reson Med 1998:554.

33. Pruessmann KP, Weiger M, Scheidegger MB *et al.* Coil sensitivity encoding for fast MRI. Proc Int Soc Magn Reson Med 1998:579.

18. Quantitation of global and regional left ventricular function by MRI

Rob J. van der Geest & Johan H.C. Reiber

Summary

Magnetic resonance imaging (MRI) provides several imaging strategies for assessing left ventricular function. As a three-dimensional imaging technique, all measurements can be performed without relying on geometrical assumptions. Global and regional function parameters can be derived from conventional or breath-hold cine MR imaging techniques. Velocity encoded cine MR imaging techniques can be applied during the same acquisition to provide quantitative information on flow velocity and volume in the heart and the greater arteries. Quantitative image analysis based on manual tracing of contours is a time consuming procedure and therefore not practical in routine clinical practice. This chapter describes the developments towards automated image analysis and contour detection techniques for cardiovascular MR imaging.

Introduction

The diagnosis of cardiovascular disease requires the precise assessment of both morphology and function. Nearly all aspects of cardiovascular function and flow can be quantified nowadays with fast magnetic resonance (MR) imaging techniques. Conventional and breath-hold cine MR imaging allows the precise and highly reproducible assessment of global and regional left ventricular function. Since MR imaging provides a three-dimensional data set for quantification of ventricular volumes and mass, it can be expected to have improved accuracy and inter-study reproducibility as compared to the results currently obtained from echocardiography [1,2]. Recently, segmented, fast cine MR imaging has been introduced to improve the time efficiency of functional evaluation of ventricular dimensions and function [3,4]. With this technological improvement, it has become possible to acquire multiple images at one particular anatomical level during a breath-hold period of about 16 seconds. It takes about 5 to 8 minutes to obtain a series of such images at the multiple levels encompassing the complete left ventricle, resulting in a complete three-dimensional data set.

Velocity encoded cine MR imaging (VEC-MRI), also called MR flow velocity mapping, is another MR imaging technique which plays an important role in the evaluation of ventricular performance [5]. VEC-MRI is a non-invasive method that provides accurate two-dimensional velocity maps anywhere in the cardiovascular system at high temporal resolution. VEC-MRI can be applied during the same MR examination in conjunction with other MR acquisitions, to provide measurements of stroke volume of both ventricles, quantifica-

J.H.C. Reiber and E.E. van der Wall (eds.). What's New in Cardiovascular Imaging, 233–246.
©1998 Kluwer Academic Publishers.

tion of valvular regurgitation, assessment of flow through the atrio-ventricular valves and coronary artery flow reserve [6-9].

Despite advances that have been made in the generation of new MR acquisition protocols and MR hardware, the analysis of the images often still relies on manual tracing of contours in many images. Reliable automated or semi-automated image analysis software would be very helpful to improve the clinical usefulness of cardiovascular MRI. Recent progress in MR imaging of the coronary arteries and myocardial perfusion imaging with contrast media, along with the further development of fast imaging sequences, suggest that MR imaging could evolve into a single technique ("one stop shop") for the evaluation of many aspects of heart disease. The reduction in MR acquisition times suggests that it may become feasible to carry out a comprehensive MR examination within an acceptable time period. As a result, even more images will be obtained during an MR examination and the need for automated or semi-automated image analysis software will only further increase.

In this chapter an overview will be given on some of the work that has been carried out towards the realization of computerized quantitative image analysis methods and (semi)automated contour detection software for cardiovascular MR imaging.

Assessment of global left ventricular function

By using multi-slice cine MR

Standard and breath-hold cine MR imaging provide accurate and highly reproducible measurements of left ventricular volumes, ejection fraction and myocardial muscle mass. Since multiple tomographic images are obtained, encompassing the entire heart, measurements of volumes and mass are not dependent upon the assumption of geometric models, as is required with X-ray angiography and echocardiography. In this regard, MR imaging has allowed the accurate quantification of left ventricular mass of abnormally shaped left ventricles due to myocardial infarction [10]. In extensive studies Maddahi and co-workers examined the effect of slice orientation and corrections for partial volume effect on the determination of myocardial mass, using Simpson's rule, in the dog model [11]. These studies have indicated that in vivo estimates of left ventricular myocardial mass are most accurate when the images are obtained in the short-axis plane of the heart. During such an examination multiple slices through the heart are acquired to encompass the complete ventricle in multiple phases within the cardiac cycle by using ECG-triggering. From the contours describing the endocardial and epicardial borders of the myocardium, ventricular volume and global function parameters can be derived including end-diastolic (ED) and end-systolic (ES) volumes, ejection fraction (EF), stroke volume (SV) and left ventricular mass. Since multiple phases are acquired within the cardiac cycle, also the dynamic changes in left ventricular volume may be studied. These dynamic processes can be described by the peak ejection rate (PER) and peak filling rate (PFR). Also the time offsets for these events, the time of PER (TPER) and PFR (TPFR) can be obtained.

By using VEC- MRI

VEC-MRI also plays an important role in the evaluation of global ventricular function. Application of this technique to the proximal portion of the ascending aorta allows the assessment of left ventricular systolic function by evaluating the flow over a complete cardiac cycle. Left ventricular stroke volume can be measured by integrating the flow over a complete cardiac cycle [6]. The clinical value of VEC-MRI has been proven in the evaluation of flow in the greater arteries [12,13]. Comparisons of cardiac output derived from chamber volume estimates and those measured by summation of aortic velocities in all frames show agreement to within 7% [14]. The results were also validated against Doppler echocardiography [15]. Since flow measurements are obtained at high temporal resolution over the complete cardiac cycle, VEC-MRI is especially useful in the evaluation of left and right ventricular diastolic function parameters by measuring flow over the atrio-ventricular valves. VEC-MRI has also been proven to be a valuable technique to quantitatively assess the severity of aortic or mitral valve insufficiency [7,16].

Assessment of regional ventricular function from short-axis multi-slice cine MR imaging

Two-dimensional approach

MRI acquisitions, in particular in the short-axis orientation, have proven their usefulness for the determination of left ventricular regional wall parameters [17-20]. In contrast to echocardiography and X-ray angiography which only provide good visualization of the endocardial borders of the myocardium, MRI also provides excellent depiction of the epicardial borders of the myocardium. This allows assessment of not only wall motion, but also wall thickening and thinning. It has been shown that wall thickening analysis is more sensitive in the detection of dysfunctional myocardium than wall motion analysis [21]. Local wall thickness can be derived from these acquisitions from manually or automatically defined endocardial and epicardial boundaries in each short-axis image. The assessment of true wall thickness requires measurements to be performed perpendicular to the myocardium; to this end, advanced two-dimensional (2D) algorithms such as the improved centerline method, were developed which performs accurate 2D wall thickness, irrespective of the chamber geometry [22,23]. It has been shown that the centerline method has some advantages over other wall motion models, which often rely on some definition of a reference point. Figure 1 illustrates the use of the 2D-centerline method for the assessment of regional myocardial wall thickness.

Three-dimensional approach

Since 2D-methods are confined to measurements within individual 2D images, the implicit assumption is made that the myocardial wall itself is always perpendicular to the acquisition plane. Because of the ellipsoidal cardiac geometry this assumption is rarely true, even when true short-axis images are obtained. In particular near the apex, the myocardium exhibits a through-plane curvature which causes the myocardium and imaging plane to intersect at an oblique angle. Also, the orientation of the myocardial wall with respect to the imaging planes may change from ED to ES, resulting in inaccurate wall thickening measurements.

Several groups have proposed methods for quantifying true three-dimensional wall thickness based on the three-dimensional data set of images [21,24-26]. These methods are based on volume element approaches and in some cases require additional tagged MR imaging acquisitions. A relatively uncomplicated algorithm, which is a straightforward extension to

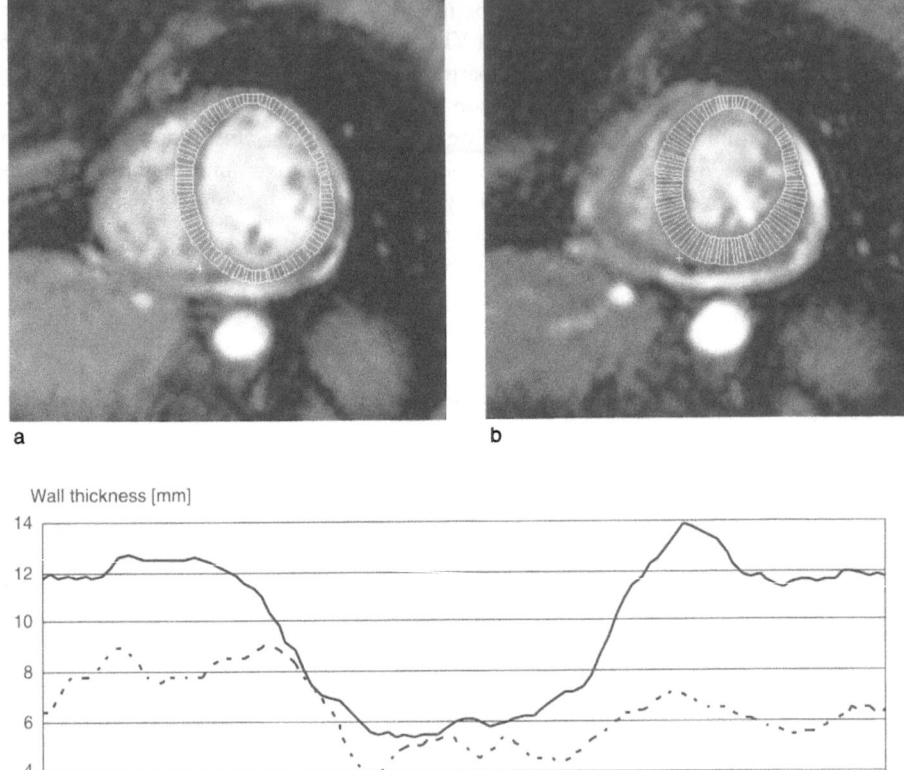

Figure 1. Wall thickness calculations performed by the 2D-centerline method in ED (a) and corresponding ES (b) image. The graph (c) shows the wall thickness as a function of the chord number starting at the indicated reference point (+) using clockwise numbering and demonstrates uniform increase in wall thickness from ED to ES for this normal volunteer.

the 2D-dimensional centerline method, was developed at our institution [27,28]. This 3D wall thickness calculation method performs the measurement of wall thickness perpendicular to the myocardium by correcting the overestimation present in the 2D-centerline method for each individual centerline chord. From the available endocardial and epicardial contours, the conventional 2D-centerline method is applied to compute in each imaging slice a centerline midway between the two contours and 2D-wall thickness measurements are obtained by constructing chords perpendicular to this centerline. Figure 2 illustrates that the angle of the myocardium with the imaging plane can be estimated by taking into account the centerpoint locations on the myocardium in the slices above and below the slice of interest. The

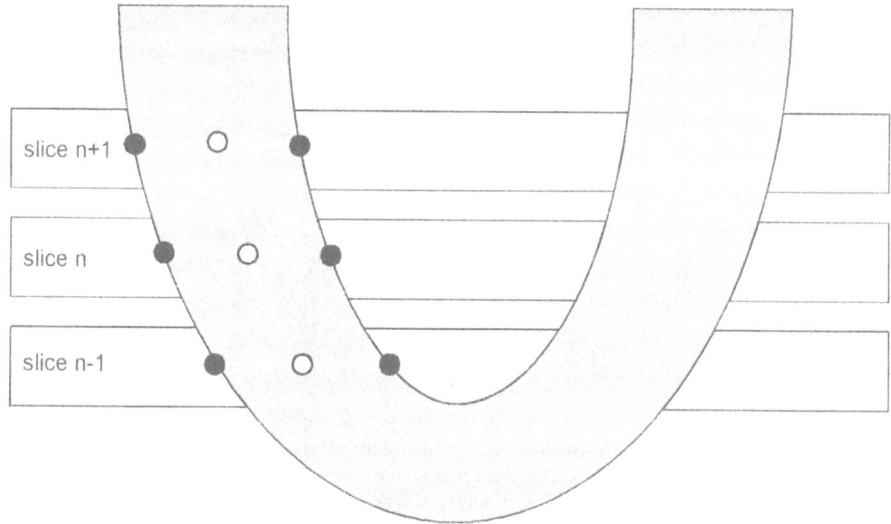

Figure 2. Centerline contour points (O) are computed midway between the endocardial and epicardial contour points (●). At each centerline point the local direction of the myocardium with the imaging plane is computed based on the centerline points in the slices above and below. The 3D-wall thickness (WT_{3D}) is computed from the 2D-wall thickness (WT_{2D}) according to $WT_{3D} = WT_{2D} \sin (\alpha)$.

overestimation in thickness measurement, WT_{2D}, obtained by the 2D- centerline method is a function of this angle according to:

$$WT_{3D} = WT_{2D} \sin (\alpha)$$

For each individual centerline chord this angle α can be computed and an estimation of the true 3D-wall thickness (WT_{3D}) is obtained.

To test the validity of this approach experiments were performed with phantom studies and imaging studies from healthy volunteers; the results will be described in the following paragraphs.

3D wall thickness in-vitro validation

To compare the accuracy and precision of the 3D wall thickness method with the conventional 2D method and the true wall thickness values, a software phantom with an overall true wall thickness of 10.0 mm was constructed. The phantom was given an approximate end-diastolic left ventricular shape and size to ensure a natural occurrence of systematic and random errors in the 2D measurements (Figure 3). The phantom was given a vertical, true short-axis orientation. Twelve similar phantoms were each created at a different, unique tilt angle from the short-axis orientation (from 5° to 60°, in 5° increments). All phantom study imaging parameters were chosen similar to the in-vivo normal acquisitions used in this study. The image resolution was 256x256 pixels at a field of view of 400x400 mm^2, resulting in an average wall thickness of 6.4 pixels. Slice thickness was 10.0 mm with no inter-slice

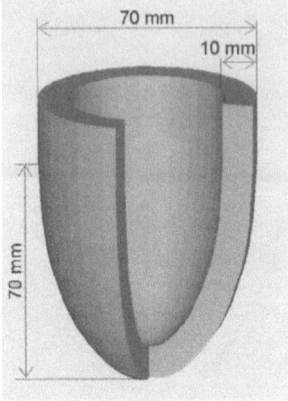

Figure 3. The software phantom which was constructed for validation of the new 3D- wall thickness calculation method. It consists of an ellipsoidal part with a diameter of 70 mm and a height of 70 mm extended at the base with a cylindrical part with a diameter of 70 mm. The phantom has an overall thickness of 10 mm.

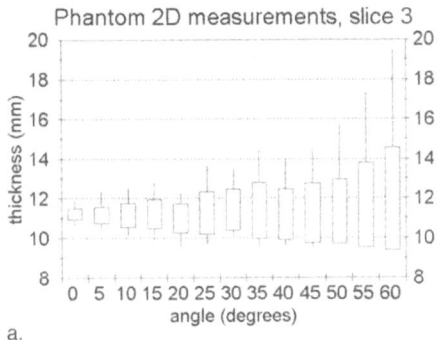

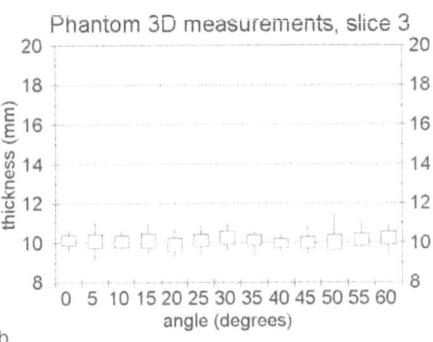

a.   b.

Figure 4. Bar graphs showing the estimated wall thickness of an apical slice of the phantom for different tilting degrees by using either the conventional 2D- (a) or new 3D-method (b). The slice is taken 30 mm above the apex.

distance. Figure 4 clearly demonstrates the improvement of the 3D-method as compared to the conventional 2D-approach. The 2D-method results in significant overestimations of wall thickness, even if the images are obtained in true short-axis orientation. In case the phantom is tilted, this overestimation becomes worse and also the variation in wall thickness estimation becomes larger. The results of the 3D-method shown in Figure 4b, demonstrates accurate wall thickness measurement even for large tilt angles.

3D wall thickness in-vivo validation

In the studies of normal volunteers, on the basis of theoretical considerations, the 3D-method was expected to demonstrate a decreased wall thickness in the apical slices, and an increased wall thickness homogeneity within individual images compared to the 2D-method. Table 1 lists the wall thickness measurements from 20 normal individuals by both the 2D and 3D methods, performed at each slice level (Apical / Low / Mid / Basal) in the two cardiac phases (ED/ES). The difference between both methods is also expressed as a percentage decrease in measured wall thickness implied by the 3D method's correction. All these differences including those at the highest slice level were statistically significant (p<0.05). Table 1 also lists the standard deviation (SD) of the 100 measurement chords within each single image, averaged over the 20 individuals. The 3D method also results in a smaller standard deviation compared to the 2D measurements, as is demonstrated by the percentage difference between the methods as listed in the same table.

Table 1: Wall thickness at four levels in 20 healthy volunteers[a]

	Apical	*Low*	*Mid*	*High*
ED-2D	6.52 mm (1.00)	6.92 mm (0.93)	7.09 mm (0.87)	7.62 mm (0.92)
ED-3D	5.79 mm (0.77)	6.32 mm (0.84)	6.90 mm (0.87)	7.56 mm (0.91)
ED-Diff.	11.24%* (22.90%)	8.67%* (10.13%)	2.57%* (0.31%)	0.73%* (0.90%)
ES-2D	11.43 mm (2.18)	12.90 mm (1.96)	13.30 mm (2.07)	12.84 mm (1.81)
ES-3D	10.63 mm (1.90)	12.22 mm (1.73)	12.97 mm (1.92)	12.73 mm (1.79)
ES-Diff.	6.96%* (12.89%)	5.28%* (11.64%)	2.51%* (7.44%)	0.92%* (1.47%)

a. Mean (in-slice SD) wall thickness in 20 healthy volunteers, and the percentual differences in mean values between the 2D and 3D methods. Both mean and SD were lower when calculated in 3D (*–p<0.05).

Three-dimensional visualization of regional function parameters

As described before, multi-slice, short-axis cine MR imaging allows high resolution and accurate assessment of regional left ventricular function. By using the centerline method for wall motion and wall thickening analysis, for each small segment of the myocardium the functional performance can be determined. By comparing the results of each individual segment with values derived from a database of normal values, an objective assessment of the total size of impaired myocardium can be derived [28]. In clinical practice, the spatial location and size of an abnormal portion of the myocardium is also of importance. Techniques to visualize the functional analysis results using dedicated three-dimensional (3D) displays, can be applied to fully benefit from the available 3D-information in the imaging data set. These three-dimensional displays are used to offer a good 3D-perception of the shape of the ventricle as seen from different viewing angles. Cine loops displaying the 3D-images of the ventricle in different phases within the cardiac cycle provide insight in patterns of myocardial contraction and relaxation. Functional data such as wall thickness or wall motion can be projected onto the 3D-displays using color-coding of the ventricular surface. By using standardized color coding schemes based on normal ranges computed from a large population of

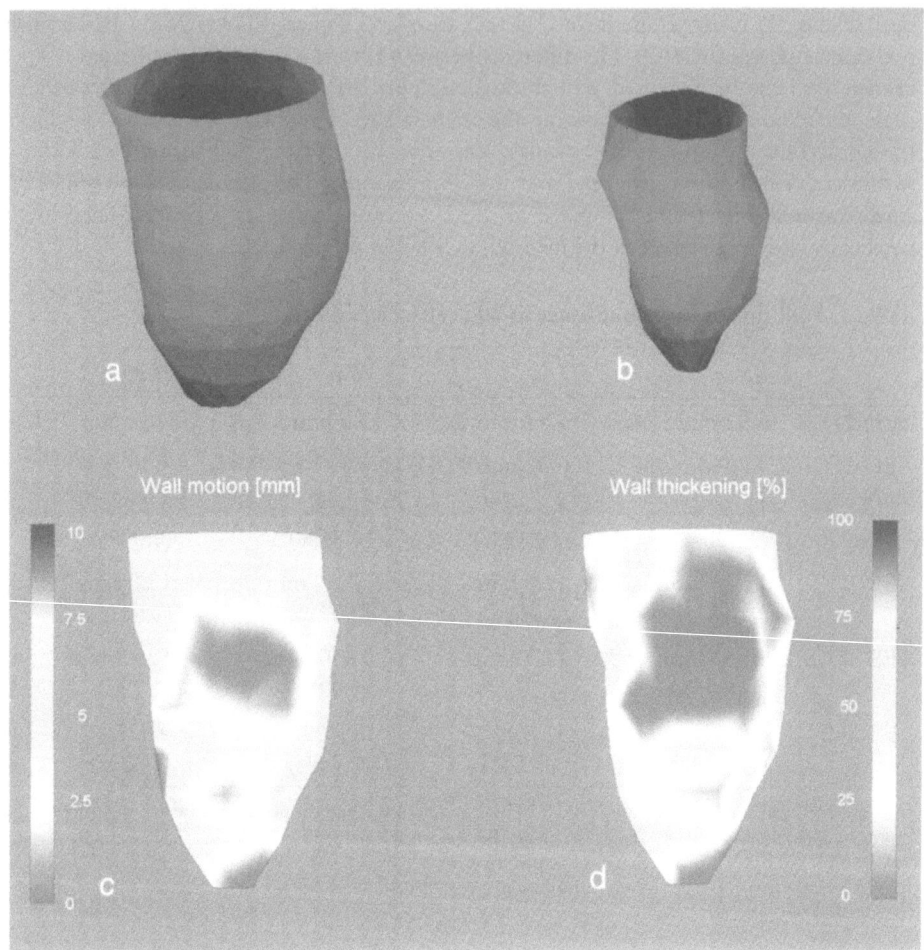

Figure 5. Surface rendered 3D-displays of the left ventricular endocardial surface of a normal volunteer in the ED (a) and ES (b) phases. The lower panel shows endocardial surfaces in the ES phase of an infarct patient. Functional information is projected on the surface by using a color coding scheme to display regional wall motion (c) and wall thickening (d) (For color figure, see color section).

healthy volunteers, the location, size and severity of myocardial abnormalities can easily be derived from such a display. Figures 5a and 5b show surface rendered displays of a left ventricle at end-diastole and end-systole. Depth cues such as shading and intensity cueing are used to provide better 3D perception. By enabling the interactive adjustment of the viewing angle or by showing the 3D displays in a cine mode, a further increase in the 3D perception of the displays can be obtained. The available functional data can be projected onto the surface of the myocardial shape to visualize the location and size of regions with abnormal ventricular performance (Figures 5c and 5d). The color coding scheme that is used for this purpose can be calibrated such that deviations from reference values are shown. Computation of a single display takes less than one second on a standard SUN Sparc 20 workstation. Pre-computed displays for a complete cardiac cycle can be displayed in real-time.

Automated contour detection in multi-slice cine MR short-axis images

It was mentioned earlier, that manual tracing of endocardial and epicardial contours in multi-slice cine MR images is a time-consuming and tedious procedure. On an average eight to ten imaging slices need to be studied in both the ED and ES phases. For clinical applications, this laborious analysis procedure is too time consuming and is subject to inter- and intra-observer variabilities [29]. Although the reported values for the variabilities are low, in a routine clinical setting one may expect to find more variations between more or less experienced observers. A considerable number of groups have contributed to the development of algorithms for the automated extraction of the endocardial and epicardial contours from short-axis cine MR imaging studies [30-32]. The automated contour detection algorithms developed at our laboratory follows a model-based approach and is directed at the definition of the endocardial and epicardial contours in all the phases and slices of an imaging study. The amount of user-interaction required to obtain reliable contours is limited, and is minimal in case the images are of good quality. The contour detection algorithm has been integrated in a software packages, MASS®, allowing semi-automated analysis of a multi-slice, multi-phase MR imaging study in less than 20 minutes. Manual tracing of the endocardial and epicardial contours in each of the images, would take three to four hours depending on the number of images and the image quality. A detailed description of the underlying contour detection algorithms has been described before [33].

The automated contour detection algorithm was validated on MR imaging studies from 10 infarct patients and 10 healthy volunteers. The two study groups were imaged on two different MR scanners with slightly different imaging protocols. In each of these studies the endocardial and epicardial contours were obtained by manual tracing and by using the automated contour detection algorithm. In this study, the user was allowed to correct clear failures of the automated contour detection, which was required for only two *epicardial* contours per study on an average. Manual editing of automatically detected *endocardial* contours was not allowed. In addition, also the contours in the most basal slice were obtained by manual tracing. Figure 6 shows a series of short-axis MR images with completely automatically detected contours. An evaluation of the level of agreement between the semi-automated contour detection and manual image analysis was performed for the assessment of global left ventricular volume parameters. In Table 2, the random and systematic differences are reported for a number of global left ventricular function parameters. Some underestimation of ventricular volumes can be observed in the group of normal volunteers. No statistically significant differences between the two analysis methods were found in the group of infarct patients. The random differences on the other hand are relatively small and in the same order of magnitude for both study populations. Since systematic errors are normally easier to overcome than random errors, it is suggested that the automated contour detection algorithm may need some further tuning for the type of scanner and acquisition protocol used for the normal volunteers. The automated contour detection algorithm results in a significant reduction in analysis time.

Automated quantification of aortic flow using flow velocity mapping

Application of velocity-encoded MRI (VEC-MRI) to the proximal portion of the ascending aorta allows the assessment of left ventricular systolic function by evaluating the flow over a

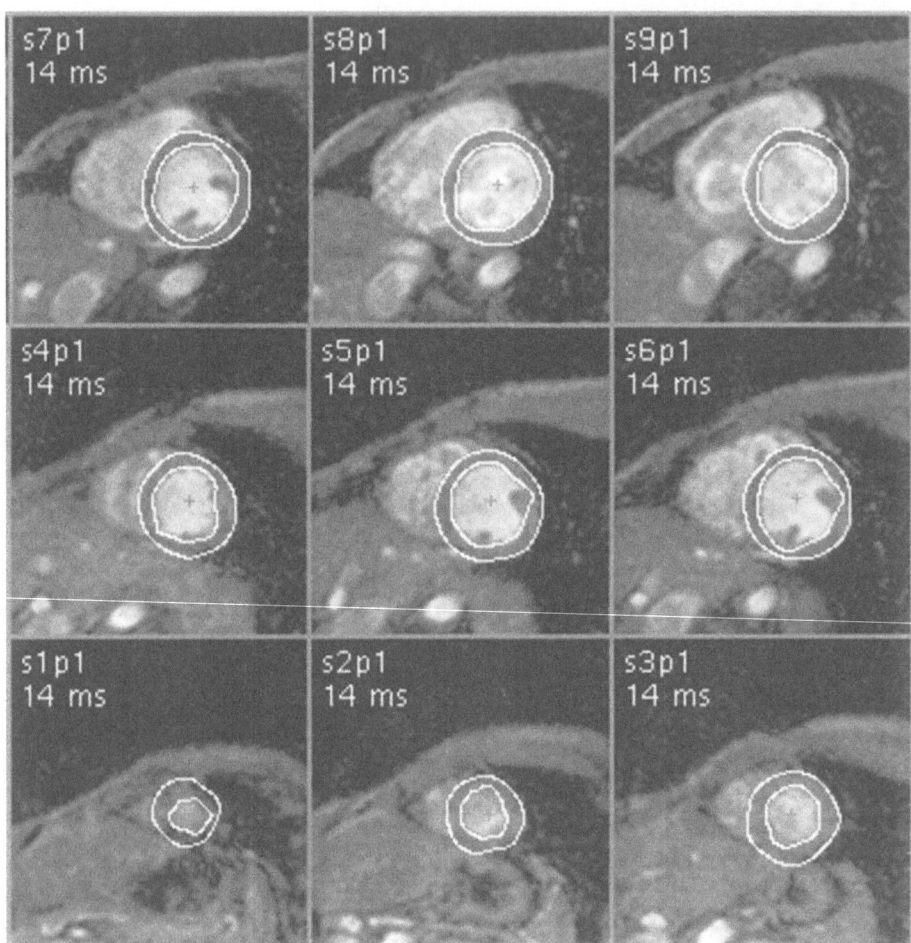

Figure 6. Series of images from apex to base of the left ventricle with completely automatically detected endocardial and epicardial contours.

complete cardiac cycle. Such a study requires a VEC-MRI acquisition in the transversal plane crossing the ascending aorta. The left ventricular stroke volume can be measured by integrating the flow over a complete cardiac cycle. For an accurate assessment of volume flow, contours describing the lumen of the vessels have to be obtained in the images. Manual contour tracing is still the most commonly used analysis method. Since in addition to the velocity encoded images also standard cine MR images are acquired during such an imaging study, the operator may choose in which image type contour tracing is performed. The in-plane motion of the greater vessels and changes in shape of the vessel cross section over the cardiac cycle requires the user to trace the luminal border of the vessel in each individual phase of the MR examination. An automated analysis method FLOW® was developed in our department to automatically detect the required contours in each of the cardiac phases [34]. This algorithm operates on the standard cine MR images which are obtained during a VEC-MRI acquisition.

Table 2: Systematic and random differences (auto-manual) in the assessment of left ventricular dimensions and functional parameters using either semi-automated or manual image analysis

Parameter	Normals (n=10)		Patients (n=10)		Overall (n=20)	
	Mean	SD	Mean	SD	Mean	SD
EDV [ml]	-13.4*	5.7	2.4	5.7	-5.5	9.7
ESV [ml]	-5.9*	4.9	-1.4	7.1	-3.6*	6.5
SV [ml]	-7.5*	4.4	3.8	7.6	-1.9*	8.4
EF [%]	1.4	3.0	2.1	4.9	1.7*	4.1
Mass [g]	22.8*	10.2	-8.2	16.2	7.3*	20.6

* indicates statistical significant difference between semi-automated and manually determined parameter ($p < 0.05$)

Contour detection software

The only user-interaction required, is the manual definition of an approximate center in one of the available images. In this first image radial scanlines are constructed at evenly spaced angular intervals starting at the center point. For each scan line the pixel with maximum edge strength is recorded. The search for edge pixels is limited to a distance of less than 20 mm from the indicated center point, representing a sufficiently large margin for most of the clinical cases. The mean gray value of these pixels is used as a threshold to obtain a rough estimation of the vessel area. The contour surrounding this segmented area is used as a model contour for the vessel boundary in this image. The position of the same vessel at another time frame can be estimated by shifting the model contour in a limited region around the initial location and examining the mean edge value measured in the modulus image along the contour points. At locations where high edge values are measured, a strong likelihood exists for being the desired contour location. If however, for each time frame, the contour would be detected at the location with maximum mean edge value, discontinuity of the contour position will be likely. Therefore, an algorithm was developed which finds the most likely contour position for each time frame, with the restriction that a contour is only allowed to displace 2 pixels (1.6 mm) from phase to phase. This particular part in the algorithm, which is based on dynamic programming, has proven to work very fast and reliable. After having found the correct contour location, a final optimized contour was detected by allowing small deformations of the model contour such that it would follow the edges in the modulus image. For this purpose a two-dimensional graph searching technique was used, known as minimum cost contour detection algorithm (MCA). The resulting contour was dilated by one pixel to be sure to encompass the complete region with flowing blood.

Evaluation

The automated analytical package FLOW® was validated on aortic flow velocity maps from a study population of 12 healthy volunteers (three men) with normal ECG and no history of cardiac malfunction. The images were obtained in the transversal orientation with a field of view of 200 x 140 mm, a scan matrix of 103 x 128 and a velocity sensitivity of 150 cm/s. Retrospective gating was applied to acquire images evenly spaced over a complete cardiac cycle resulting in twenty cardiac phases. Manual and automated image analyses were performed by two independent observers. The first observer repeated the automated and manual analyses after a two-week interval to avoid learning effects. The FLOW® quantification package ran on a commercially available SUN Sparc 20 workstation (Sun Microsystems, Mountain View, CA). The time required for manual analysis was 5-10 minutes. During automated analysis the user had to identify the approximate location of the center of the aorta in one of the available images. The total analysis time for automated analysis was less than 10 seconds.

Figure 7 shows an example of two flow curves obtained by manual and automated analysis. Stroke volume measurements were obtained by integrating the flow over the complete cardiac cycle. The mean left ventricular stroke volume (SV) obtained by VEC-MRI in the group of 12 volunteers was 86.4 ml (SD: 13.6 ml). No statistically significant differences were found between the results of manual and automated analyses. The mean difference between automated and manually assessed SV was 0.78 ml (SD: 1.99 ml). The intra-observer variability was 0.65 ml for manual analysis and 0.58 ml for automated analysis; the intra-observer variability was 0.99 ml for manual analysis and 0.90 ml for automated analysis. It can be concluded that the present automated contour detection algorithm performs equally well as the manual method in the determination of left ventricular stroke volume derived from VEC-MRI studies of the ascending aorta. The automated approach allows quantification of left ventricular stroke volume in less than 10 seconds.

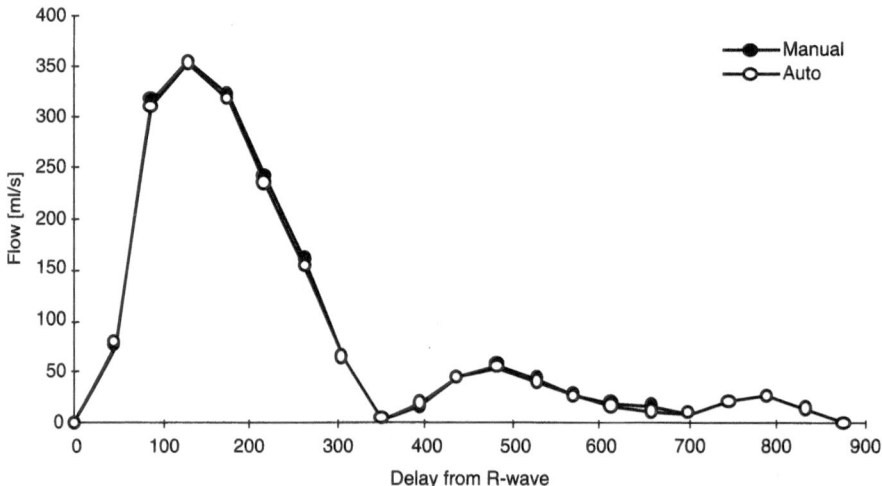

Figure 7. Example of flow curves obtained by manual tracing and automated contour detection.

Conclusion

Over the past few years the improvements in MRI hardware and software have resulted in a reduction of the imaging time required for a comprehensive cardiovascular MRI examination, thereby allowing the assessment of multiple aspects of cardiac function and anatomy. However, the clinical application of MRI for evaluation of cardiac function is still limited. Image analysis procedures which are based on manual contour tracing are too time consuming and require experienced observers. In order for MRI to become a valuable and routinely applicable imaging modality, the time required for quantitation of the many images should be reduced considerably. Automated analytical methods for left ventricular function and vascular flow measurements based on automated contour detection approaches have been developed. Validation studies of these new methods have confirmed their accuracy, precision, robustness and applicability for clinical research studies. These developments represent significant steps towards the routine use of cardiovascular MRI. However, more research and developmental work need to be carried out for other types of MR acquisitions.

References

1. Sakuma H, Fujia N, Foo TKF *et al.* Evaluation of left ventricular volume and mass with breath-hold cine MR imaging. Radiology 1993;188:377-80.
2. Young AA, Kramer CM, Ferrari VA, Axel L, Reichek N. Three-dimensional left ventricular deformation in hypertrophic cardiomyopathy. Circulation 1994;90:854-67.
3. Kramer CM, Lima JAC, Reichek N *et al.* Regional differences in function within noninfarcted myocardium during left ventricular remodeling. Circulation 1993;88:1279-88.
4. Lamb HJ, Doornbos J, Van der Velde EA, Kruit MC, Reiber JHC, De Roos A. Echo-planar MRI of the heart on a standard sytem: validation of measurements of left ventricular function and mass. J Comput Assist Tomogr 1996;20:942-9.
5. Szolar DH, Sakuma H, Higgins CB. Cardiovascular applications of magnetic resonance flow and velocity measurements. J Magn Res Imaging 1996;6:78-89.
6. Kondo C, Caputo GR, Semelka R, Foster E, Shimakawa A, Higgins CB. Right and left ventricular stroke volume measurements with velocity-encoded cine MR imaging: in vitro and in vivo validation. AJR Am J Roentgenol 1991;157:9-16.
7. Sondergaard L, Lindvig K, Hildebrandt P *et al.* Quantification of aortic regurgitation by magnetic resonance velocity mapping. Am Heart J 1993;125:1081-90.
8. Hundley WG, Li HF, Willard JE *et al.* Magnetic resonance imaging assessment of the severity of mitral regurgitation. Comparison with invasive techniques. Circulation 1995;92:1151-8.
9. Sakuma H, Blake LM, Amidon TM *et al.* Coronary flow reserve: noninvasive measurement in humans with breath-hold velocity-encoded cine MR imaging. Radiology 1996;198:745-50.
10. Shapiro EP, Rogers WJ, Beyar R *et al.* Determination of left ventricular mass by magnetic resonance imaging in hearts deformed by acute infarction. Circulation 1989;79:706-11.
11. Maddahi J, Crues J, Berman DS *et al.* Noninvasive quantitation of left ventricular myocardial mass by gated proton nuclear magnetic resonance imaging. J Am Coll Cardiol 1987;10:682-92.
12. Bogren HG, Klipstein RH, Firmin DN *et al.* Quantitation of antegrade and retrograde blood flow in the human aorta by magnetic resonance velocity mapping. Am Heart J 1989;117:1214-22.
13. Firmin DN, Nayler GL, Klipstein RH, Underwood SR, Rees RSO, Longmore DB. In vivo validation of MR velocity imaging. J Comput Assist Tomogr 1987;11:751-6.
14. Longmore DB, Klipstein RH, Underwood SR *et al.* Dimensional accuracy of magnetic resonance in studies of the heart. Lancet 1985;1:1360-2.
15. Karwatowski SP, Brecker SJD, Yang GZ, Firmin DN, Sutton MSJ, Underwood SR. Mitral valve flow measured with cine MR velocity mapping in patients with ischemic heart disease: comparison with Doppler echocardiography. J Magn Res Imaging 1995;5:89-92.

16.   Dulce MC, Mostbeck GH, O'Sullivan MM, Cheitlin V, Caputo GR, Higgins CB. Severity of aortic regurgitation: interstudy reproducibility of measurements with velocity-encoded cine MR imaging. Radiology 1992;185:235-40.

17.   Haag UJ, Hess OM, Maier SE *et al.* Left ventricular wall thickness measurements by magnetic resonance: a validation study. Int J Card Imaging 1991;7:31-41.

18.   Van Rugge FP, Van der Wall EE, Spanjersberg SJ *et al.* Magnetic resonance imaging during dobutamine stress for detection and localization of coronary artery disease. Quantitative wall motion analysis using a modification of the centerline method. Circulation 1994;90:127-38.

19.   Holman ER, Vliegen HW, Van der Geest RJ *et al.* Quantitative analysis of regional left ventricular function after myocardial infarction in the pig assessed with cine magnetic resonance imaging. Magn Reson Med 1995;34:161-9.

20.   Baer FM, Smolarz K, Theissen P, Voth E, Schicha H, Sechtem U. Regional 99mTc-methoxyisobutyl-isonitrile-uptake at rest in patients with myocardial infarcts: comparison with morphological and functional parameters obtained from gradient-echo magnetic resonance imaging. Eur Heart J 1994;15:97-107.

21.   Azhari H, Sideman S, Weiss JL *et al.* Three-dimensional mapping of acute ischemic regions using MRI: wall thickening versus motion analysis. Am J Physiol 1990;259:H1492-503.

22.   Sheehan FH, Bolson EL, Dodge HT, Mathey DG, Schofer J, Woo HK. Advantages and applications of the centerline method for characterizing regional ventricular function. Circulation 1986;74:293-305.

23.   Von Land CD, Rao SR, Reiber JHC. Development of an improved centerline wall motion model. Comput Cardiol 1990:687-90.

24.   Beyar R, Shapiro EP, Graves WL *et al.* Quantification and validation of left ventricular wall thickening by a three-dimensional volume element magnetic resonance imaging approach. Circulation 1990;81:297-307.

25.   Beyar R, Weiss JL, Shapiro EP, Graves WL, Rogers WJ, Weisfeldt ML. Small apex-to-base heterogeneity in radius-to-thickness ratio by three-dimensional magnetic resonance imaging. Am J Physiol 1993;264:H133-40.

26.   Dong SJ, MacGregor JH, Crawley AP *et al.* Left ventricular wall thickness and regional systolic function in patients with hypertrophic cardiomyopathy. A three-dimensional tagged magnetic resonance imaging study. Circulation 1994;90:1200-9.

27.   Buller VGM, Van der Geest RJ, Kool MD, Van der Wall EE, De Roos A, Reiber JHC. Assessment of regional left ventricular wall parameters from short axis magnetic resonance imaging using a three-dimensional extension to the improved centerline method. Invest Radiol 1997;32:529-39.

28.   Holman ER, Buller VGM, De Roos A *et al.* Detection and quantification of dysfunctional myocardium by magnetic resonance imaging. A new three-dimensional method for quantitative wall-thickening analysis. Circulation 1997;95:924-31.

29.   Pattynama PMT, Lamb HJ, Van der Velde EA, Van der Wall EE, De Roos A. Left ventricular measurements with cine and spin-echo MR imaging: a study of reproducibility with variance component analysis. Radiology 1993;187:261-8.

30.   Fleagle SR, Thedens DR, Stanford W, Pettigrew RI, Reichek N, Skorton DJ. Multicenter trial of automated border detection in cardiac MR imaging. J Magn Res Imaging 1993;3:409-15.

31.   Suh DY, Eisner RL, Mersereau RM, Pettigrew RI. Knowledge-based system for boundary detection of four-dimensional cardiac MR image sequences. IEEE Trans Med Imaging 1993;12:65-72.

32   Baldy C, Douek P, Croisille P, Magnin IE, Revel D, Amiel M. Automated myocardial edge detection from breath-hold cine-MR images: evaluation of left ventricular volumes and mass. Magn Reson Imaging 1994;12:589-98.

33.   Van der Geest RJ, Buller VGM, Jansen E *et al.* Comparison between manual and semi-automated analysis of left ventricular volume parameters from short axis MR images. J Comput Assist Tomogr 1997;21:756-65.

34.   Van der Geest RJ, Buller VGM, Reiber JHC. Automated quantification of flow velocity and volume in the ascending and descending aorta using MR flow velocity mapping. Comput Cardiol 1995:29-32.

19. Status of myocardial perfusion assessment by MRI

Stefan E. Fischer & Christine H. Lorenz

Summary

An integrated cardiac magnetic resonance exam has the potential to serve as a "one stop shop" imaging modality for the diagnosis of coronary artery disease. The combination of consistently attainable anatomic and functional information of an MR scan may replace a series of tests currently used in cardiology, such as stress echocardiography, cardiac catheterization with X-ray angiography and nuclear medicine tests. Such a cardiac MR examination may include imaging of at least the proximal part of the coronary arteries, the assessment of cardiac function under rest and stress conditions as well as the assessment of myocardial perfusion.

There exist a number of physical principles which generate image contrast dependent on the myocardial perfusion. However, the most promising method to assess myocardial perfusion with MRI is tracking of a contrast agent bolus and evaluating the uptake as well as the wash-out of the dye within the myocardium. Scientifically this concept has been proven to assess myocardial blood flow and even has been refined towards quantitative results, but only recent advances in MR instrumentation allow rapid imaging to cover the entire heart and therefore make these approaches potentially clinically useful.

Introduction

Integrated cardiac MR examination "one stop shop"

Currently the diagnosis of coronary artery disease requires a series of diagnostic imaging procedures such as nuclear medicine tests, echocardiographic stress tests, or cardiac catheterization including angiography. Some of these tests are invasive, and require X-ray or the injection of radionuclides. The combination of all these tests including hospitalization makes the diagnosis of patients with possible coronary artery disease consuming and expensive. Further, only in about half the patients undergoing the invasive procedure of X-ray angiography is an intervention such as PTCA or coronary artery bypass graft surgery necessary. On the other hand a short, one-hour integrated cardiac magnetic resonance imaging examination has the potential to be used to triage patients with suspected coronary artery disease towards either cardiac catheterization for PTCA or presurgical angiography or towards treatment with medicine only. The noninvasiveness of MR combined with excellent assessment of left and right ventricular cardiac function [1-7] including stress testing [8],

J.H.C. Reiber and E.E. van der Wall (eds.). What's New in Cardiovascular Imaging, 247–260.
©1998 Kluwer Academic Publishers.

and imaging of the proximal part of the coronary arterial tree [9,10] could provide the information necessary to make this triage decision accurate, fast and cost effective. An additional cornerstone of such an integrated cardiac exam is the possibility to assess myocardial perfusion with MRI.

The methods currently used clinically to measure myocardial blood flow involve the injection of a radioactive drug into the blood to make pictures of the heart with single positron emission computed tomography (SPECT) or positron emission tomography (PET). These types of studies have significant drawbacks. These include a limited ability to detect small areas of heart muscle with decreased blood flow, and limited ability to assess the pumping function of the heart. Because of these limitations, the results of these studies must typically be combined with those from other expensive imaging tests such as cardiac catheterization and echocardiography. There are two major reasons for pursuing myocardial blood flow measurement with MRI. First, MR perfusion assessment can easily be combined with imaging morphology and function of the heart and coronary arteries. Second, MRI has the potential to yield quantitative measurements of myocardial blood flow, that is, it could estimate the actual amount of blood going to each region of the heart muscle. No other imaging test except positron emission tomography (PET) has this ability, but PET is not widely available due to its expense.

MR perfusion assessment without contrast agents

Because of the high spatial resolution and ability of MRI to differentiate between different tissue characteristics, investigators have long sought to use MRI for characterization of ischemic heart disease. Two main classes of MRI techniques have been attempted for myocardial blood flow determination--those that use exogenous contrast agents, and those that do not. Perfusion assessment methods that don't require any contrast agent can be grouped according to their contrast mechanism: magnetization transfer [11,12], intra-voxel incoherent motion [13-16], oxygenation dependent susceptibility change [17,18] and arterial spin labeling [19,20].

Magnetization transfer (MT) imaging is a technique that takes advantage of a shift of magnetization between mobile protons and immobile protons. It is used clinically to suppress stationary tissue signal to improve contrast between flowing and stationary tissue (i.e. for MR angiograms). The signal changes due to MT weighting have been shown to be proportional to flow rate in an isolated heart preparation. However, the signal changes are extremely small, susceptible to motion artifacts, and cannot be quantitatively related to myocardial blood flow.

Diffusion imaging with MRI is a technique that is now in use primarily in evaluation of acute stroke. With this technique, large magnetic field gradients are used to dephase (or reduce) in tissue where random (Brownian) motion (diffusion) of protons is high. If one assumes that flow in capillaries can be modeled as 'pseudo-diffusion' due to the random orientation of the capillaries, then diffusion imaging can be used to assess the microcirculation. However, the technique is very susceptible to artifacts from bulk motion, making application in the heart extremely difficult, and the assumptions on the arrangement of the capillaries may not be accurate. Nonetheless, a few investigators have pursued this technique for myocardial blood flow assessment. Furthermore, the physiologic interpretation of the pseudo-diffusion coefficient is not clear at this point, rendering the technique only semi-quantitative at best.

Susceptibility-based imaging with MRI relies on changes in relative amounts of deoxyhemoglobin in blood which generate small changes in signal on gradient echo images due to local changes in magnetic susceptibility. This technique has been successfully employed in the brain for studying local cortical activation (fMRI). It has also been proposed as a method for measuring local oxygen saturation in myocardium. The information derived reflects oxygen level--a parameter not otherwise obtainable with imaging. The disadvantages of this technique include the requirement for high speed imaging, the fact that heart motion can result in dephasing that could mimic O2 deficits, and the current lack of a model to quantitative signal change. However, this technique appears very promising if the technical challenges can be overcome.

Arterial spin labeling is a technique that induces a contrast effect by altering the magnetization of protons in blood entering an organ. The tagged spins are then imaged as they pass through the organ of interest. Local perfusion can be estimated from a model describing the tagged spin behavior. This technique has been applied to isolated hearts and to the brain *in vivo*. Application to the brain *in vivo* has been possible because of the easy accessibility and relatively immobile nature of the carotid arteries. The advantage of the technique is that it is quantitative with perfusion proportional to apparent relaxation directly measurable by MR. The disadvantages for the heart are that it is difficult to tag the moving coronary arteries at their origin; knowledge of the tissue partition coefficient is needed; tissue T1 in absence of flow is required to obtain absolute perfusion; and the signal changes are quite small.

MRI contrast agent bolus tracking

While the non-contrast agent-based MR techniques are desirable, they have in common that myocardial blood flow-dependent signal changes are relatively small. Thus, contrast agents have been used to enhance the assessment of myocardial blood flow.

Basic principle and contrast behavior

In general, use of contrast agents and dynamic imaging with MRI follows similar principles as those used in radionuclide and indicator dilution methods. The approach can be described as follows: (1) inject a tracer and monitor the concentration of the tracer as a function of time in the blood and in the tissue of interest, and (2) describe the time-course of the concentration changes qualitatively [21-25] or by the use of mathematical models to extract quantitative values for myocardial blood flow [25-29]. A series of contrast agents is available for the use with MRI. The most commonly used agents are gadolinium-based complexes, such as Gd-DTPA [30], which leak from the blood pool into the extravascular space but do not pass through intact cell membranes. More recently developed contrast agents that stay in the vascular space, including iron oxides and Gd-DTPA-based molecules binding to blood protein albumin [31,32] are under investigation. Even though the pharmacodynamic properties of these agents are very different, they have basic contrast mechanisms in common. The paramagnetic particles of these contrast agents locally change the homogeneity of the magnetic field and therefore reduce spin-spin (T2 and T2*) as well spin-lattice relaxation times (T1). Whereas a shortening of T2 or T2* relaxation times accelerates the MR signal decay, a faster T1 relaxation yields in general an increased image intensity. The rate of decreasing T2* and T1 values as a function of contrast agent concentration varies from contrast agent to contrast agent. Basically the contrast in a MR image is always dependent on both T1 and T2 tissue relaxation times. However, by the application of contrast preparation schemes and by the proper choice of basic MR parameters, the image contrast can be adjusted to be more T1-weighted or T2-weighted, respectively. A T1-weighted sequence will show an increased intensity in a tissue with higher tracer concentration, and therefore can be used as a positive proof of perfusion. By using a sequence with a contrast behavior based on the T2-related signal change, non perfused tissue will keep the initial signal level, whereas the image intensity of normally perfused tissue decreases. Many variations on this general approach have been reported over the past few years. Figure 1 shows the contrast behavior of

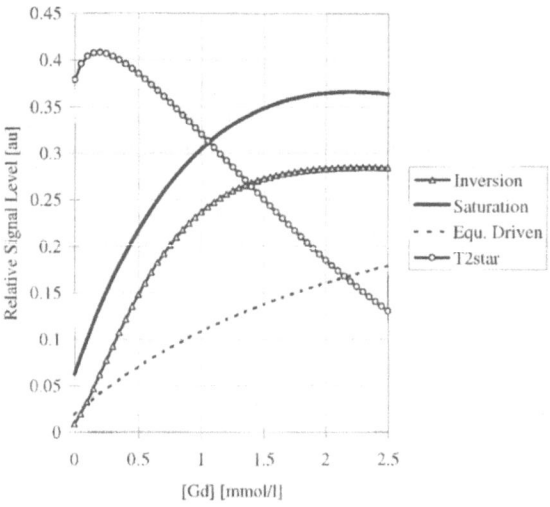

Figure 1. Contrast behavior of different MR imaging strategies. The simulated relative image intensity of selected imaging sequences is plotted as a function of the concentration of Gd-DTPA for an R-R interval of 800 ms. Solid line with triangles represents the contrast of an inversion recovery prepulses with a recovery time adjusted to null signal from myocardium without dye. The solid lines show the relative signal after a saturation prepulse 200 ms prior to the acquisition with TE = 5 ms and α = 30°. The dashed line gives the contrast assuming a constant repetitive excitation of the spins towards an steady state magnetization. Finally, the open circles represent a single shot EPI with TE = 25 ms, α = 35°, and no prepulse.

different imaging schemes including different contrast adjustment mechanisms. For these simulations a heart rate of 75 bpm was assumed, which means by obtaining an image in every heart beat the magnetization is never fully relaxed. Therefore the contrast range of the inversion prepulse is similar to that of the saturation prepulse. Whereas the inversion prepulse may null the signal from myocardium without contrast agent, the saturation pulse yields heart rate independent image signal intensity easier to convert into a T1 value or [Gd-DTPA]. Even for relatively short echo times, (TE of 1.2 ms for inversion recovery, and 4.5 ms for saturation recovery) a saturation of the relative signal level at a concentration of Gd-DTPA around 2 mmol/l can be observed. The equilibrium driven preparation schemes [33] rely on the [Gd], TR, and RF excitation angle-dependent steady state magnetization, and can be adjusted to be relatively linear over a wider range of contrast agent concentration.

However, the repetitive application of RF pulses, in this case every 5 ms with a flip angle of 20°, reduces the overall signal level. In contrast to the more T1 weighted sequences, a single shot sequence such as echo planar imaging (EPI) with a relatively long echo time of e.g. 25 ms yields an inverse contrast as a function of [Gd]. Variations include not only different image acquisition strategies but also the use of different contrast agents, such as intravascular agents or extracellular agents. Furthermore, different injection sites have been used such as left atrial injections and peripheral venous injection.

Status of MR instrumentation and image acquisition

The choice of the MR image acquisition sequence to assess myocardial perfusion is mainly driven by the pharmacokinetic properties of a particular contrast agent. Since the uptake in the myocardium of a contrast agent is within the range of a few seconds, and the slope of that uptake is an important parameter related to flow, the acquisition of an image in every heart beat interval is desirable. Until recently, inversion recovery TurboFLASH sequences were applied to track such a contrast agent bolus. The typical acquisition time of these TurboFLASH sequences, inversion recovery interval not included, was in the range of 500 ms per image. Thus, the acquisition was limited to a single slice assuming a normal cardiac frequency.

The dramatic progress in MR system performance over the past five years has changed the limitation of a MRI perfusion assessment completely. MR system performance is dependent on both strength and slew rate of the gradient system, on transition speed from radiofrequency excitation to signal reception and on the flexibility to apply a MR pulse sequence tailored to the specific imaging problem. However, reduction in scan time has always to be paid for with reduced signal-to-noise ratio or reduced image resolution. Therefore, advances in signal reception, such as better eddy current behavior of the system and phased array receiver coils are important system performance factors for perfusion imaging as well.

The increase in MR system performance yields a reduction of the scan time per image of a TurboFLASH approach on the order of 2.5 [28,34]. However, imaging strategies other than TurboFLASH have been proposed for the assessment of myocardial perfusion, which

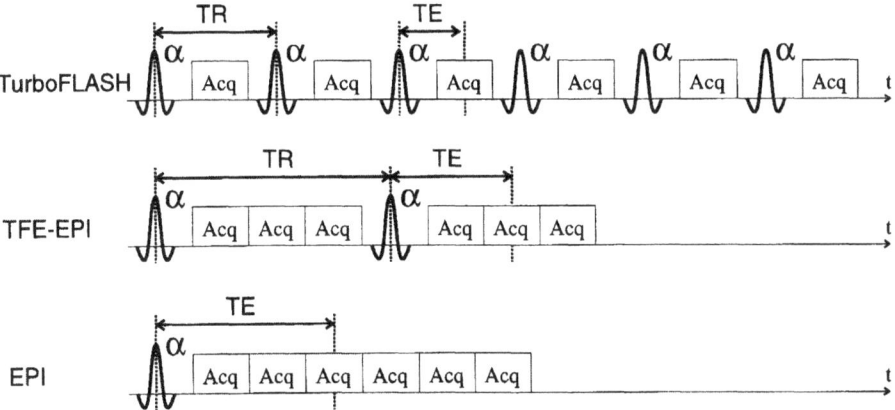

Figure 2. Timing of selected imaging sequences. Each sequence can be divided into an 'overhead' segment containing RF excitation and phase encoding and into an acquisition segment, comprised of the read-out gradients.

can further reduce scan time. Figure 2 compares the timing of a TurboFLASH sequence, an echo-planar imaging sequence (EPI) [35], and a hybrid sequence between TurboFLASH and EPI (TFE-EPI Turbo Field Echo Planar Imaging) [36-38]. In Table 1 typical image parameters and the basic contrast properties are summarized:

Table 1: Comparison of selected image acquisition sequences and contrast mechanisms

Sequence	Typical Parameters TE / TR /α (scan time per slice)	Dominant Contrast	Contrast Adjustment
TurboFLASH	1.2 ms / 2.4 ms / 18° (180 ms)	T1	Prepulses
TFE-EPI	4 ms / 10 ms / 30° (90 ms)	T1	Prepulses
EPI (single shot)	10-30 ms / RR / 45° (60 ms)	T2 or T2*	Echo Time

TurboFLASH. Recent developments of MR equipment have dramatically reduced echo time and therefore repetition time of a TurboFLASH sequence down to approximately 2 ms [34]. Such an approach now allows the assessment of multiple slices within a single heart beat. However, only about 50% of the acquisition time is effectively used for data sampling, and it is very unlikely that this ratio can be considerably improved due to limitations such as specific absorption rate (SAR) and time interval to switch from RF transmit to receive mode. The large number of RF excitations is only possible by a reduction of the RF excitation flip angle.

EPI. The most effective pulse sequences in terms of read-out/overhead time ratio are EPI sequences. Echo planar imaging sequences combined with state of the art gradient systems can be used to reduce imaging time dramatically and allow the acquisition of multiple slices per heart beat as well. However, single shot EPI for the estimation of Gd concentration suffers from the superposition of signal enhancement due to T1 reduction and susceptibility related signal decay. The relatively long echo time of a single shot methods, however, can be used to get an inverse contrast behavior as compared to a T1 weighted sequence as shown for the "T2*" curve in Figure 1.

TFE-EPI. The greater flexibility in pulse sequences of state-of-the-art clinical scanners allows the generation of a hybrid sequence between TurboFLASH and EPI. The advantage of such a segmented EPI sequence is the increased acquisition speed as compared to TurboFLASH since only a few RF excitations are required. Compared to single shot EPI the image contrast with respect to the Gd concentration can be adjusted by the short echo time in case of half k-space acquisition, using a saturation prepulse to be sensitive to T1 changes over a range up to 2 mmol/l.

Image evaluation and quantification

Different perfusion rates of the tissue are characterized by the magnitude and the speed of the contrast agent uptake. In the case of Gd-DTPA as compared to a purely intravascular contrast agent, the properties of the contrast agent wash-out phase contain additional information. To track the transit of the contrast agent through the myocardium images have to be obtained at least every 1-2 seconds over approximately 30 seconds to cover the first-pass of the contrast agent through the myocardium or over several minutes to cover both wash-in and wash-out. Rather than just looking at single images of the image time series, time-intensity curves of different segments of the myocardium are compared for a more objective measure. The processing steps can be summarized as followed:

Segmentation of different regions of interest in the myocardium and calculation of mean signal intensity values.

- Calibration of the time signal intensity curves to time [Gd] concentration curves. The contrast agent concentration can be determined from the assessment of the longitudinal relaxation, T1. By additional scans, i.e. prior to the injection, T1 values of blood and myocardium can be determined [39,40] and used to calibrate the subsequent T1 weighted scans.
- Extraction of qualitative measures from the time-intensity curves, such as slope of uptake, mean transit time, peak contrast agent concentration, time to peak.

For a quantitative assessment of perfusion rates the [Gd] time curve in the aorta or the left ventricle has to be determined to serve as the input function for the pharmacokinetic modeling of the contrast agent transit [41,42]. However many of these models have to make assumptions of extraction and distribution volume [43,44]. In the case of Gd-DTPA the leakage of the contrast agent into the extracellular space has to be modeled as well [45,46]. Recently, a few studies have validated their results with microsphere measurement of myocardial blood flow.

Complete heart coverage

Figure 3 shows a schematic of an interleaved multiple slice acquisition and contrast adjustment strategies for the different type of sequences. The relatively long acquisition time of TurboFLASH requires a prepulse prior to the acquisition of each slice. To pack imaging of

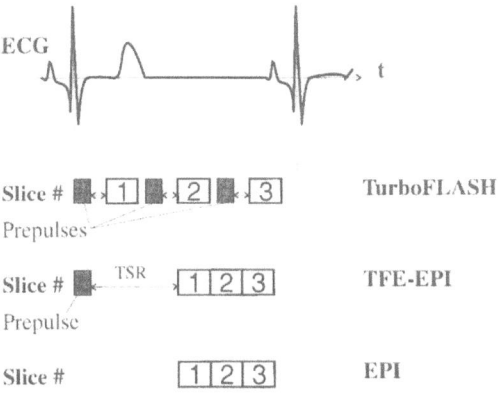

Figure 3. Examples of multiple slice acquisition schemes including prepulses to adjust the contrast properties.

multiple slices into a single heart beat the saturation recovery time is relatively short and therefore suboptimal for detecting small Gd-DTPA concentration changes in the myocardium. For the TFE-EPI sequence the acquisition of four slices can be completed in as little as 400 ms. Therefore a single prepulse affecting all slices can generate a sufficient contrast in all the slices. Since each slice is obtained at a different saturation recovery time, each slice has to be calibrated separately. The T2* weighted single shot EPI sequence does not require any prepulse and therefore is the most efficient sequence. However, single shot EPI sequences are very sensitive to flow and off resonance effects yielding still relatively poor image quality.

Figure 4 shows one out of 6 slices acquired every other heart beat by the use of a TFE-EPI

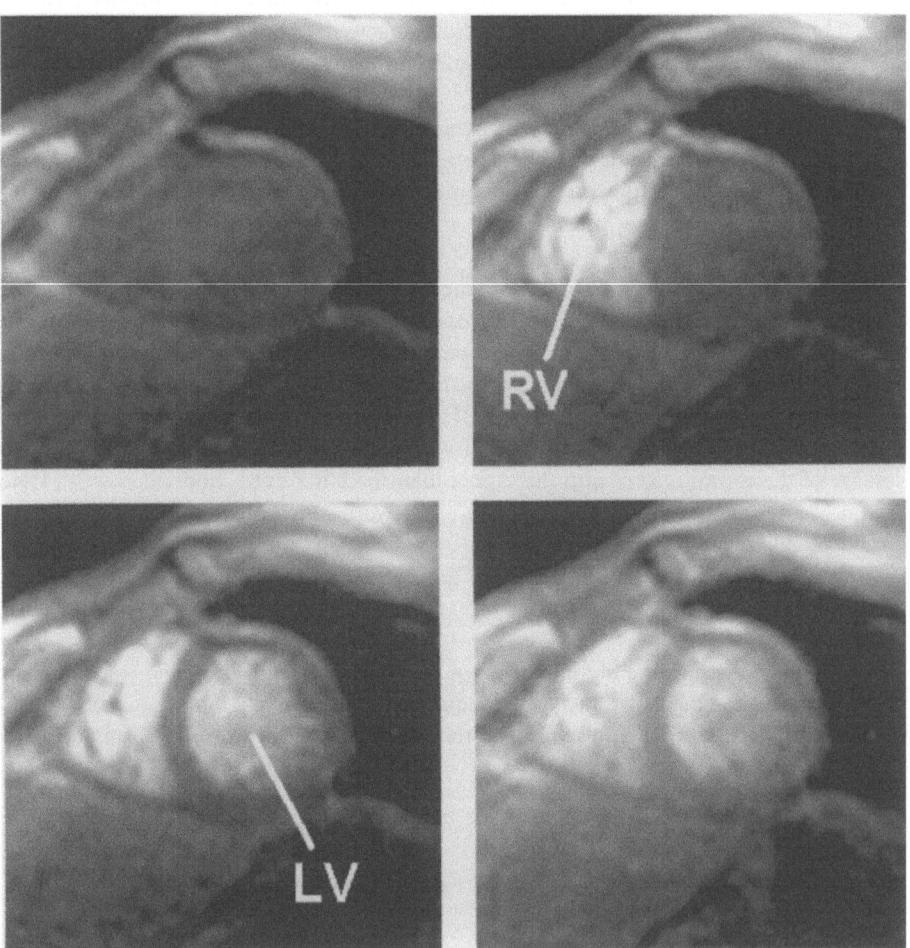

Figure 4. One of 3 slices acquired in one heart beat interval by a TFE-EPI sequence prior to the injection of Gd-DTPA (upper-left), during the first right ventricular passage (upper right), left ventricular passage (bottom left) and during the wash-in into the myocardium (bottom right).

sequence acquired with a 1.5 T whole body scanner (Gyroscan ACS-NT, Philips Medical Systems, Best, The Netherlands) equipped with a 105 T/m/s fast gradient systems. The imaging parameters were as followed.

- 90° prepulse 400 ms prior to acquisition of center slice
- Acquisition of 6 slices, 3 per heart beat
- Rectangular field-of-view: 280 mm x 210 mm
- Scan matrix: 128 x 96
- Half scan or asymmetrical k-space coverage: half scan is essential to reduce the echo time and to reduce scan time per slice.
- 9 RF excitations per image
- RF flip angle sequencing, in order to keep the excited magnetization constant.
- Time between RF excitations 11 ms.
- 128 x 128 to 128 x 96 scan matrix
- 6 k-space lines per RF excitation, second echo is closest to center k-space.
- Echo time: 5 ms, by the use of echo shifting.
- Scan time per image: 100 ms

The same slice obtained during late diastole is shown prior to peripheral intravenous injection of a 0.05 mmol/kg bolus of Gd-DTPA as well as during right ventricular passage and left ventricular passage and during the wash-in into the myocardium.

Perfusion reserve

MR perfusion assessment methods can be used to compare perfusion rates at rest and with vasodilation analogous to nuclear medicine stress tests [47]. Figure 5 gives an example of the

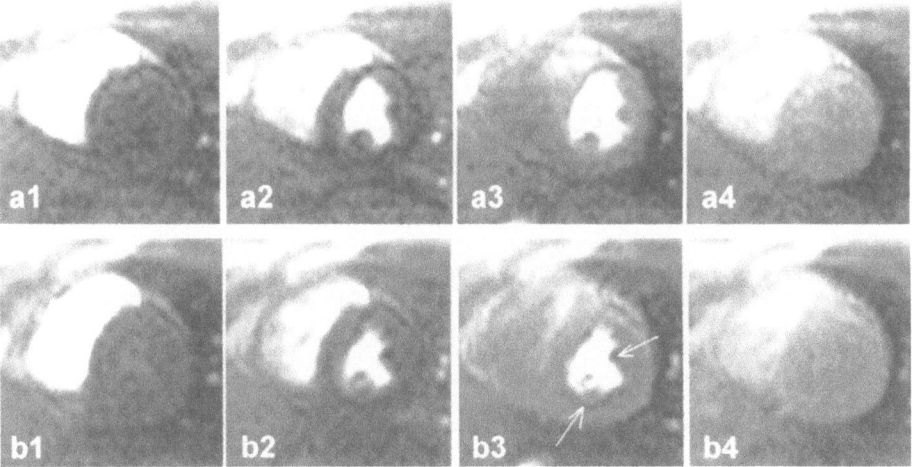

Figure 5. One of 3 slices of a patient with symptoms of angina at different time points of the contrast agent's transit through right and left ventricle and myocardium. The images a1-a4 were obtained at rest, whereas b1-b4 are part of a time series obtained during vasodilation by infusion of adenosine. (Courtesy of Dr. M. Jerosch-Herold, University of Minnesota Medical School).

assessment of perfusion reserve. A short axis slice from a patient is shown at rest (heart rate 73 bpm) during the passage of 0.025 mmol/kg Gd-DTPA bolus applied with a venous catheter through the right ventricle (t = 0 s), the left ventricle (t = 3.3 s), the first pass through the myocardium (t = 7.4 s) and at t = 14 s. In the same slice during vasodilation (heart rate of 104 bpm) during the infusion of 0.14 mg/kg/min adenosine, (t = 0 s, 2.9 s, 4.6 s, 10 s) dark areas during the first pass can be observed. In this example a TurboFLASH sequence on a 1.5 T Vision (Siemens Medical Systems, Erlangen, Germany) with TR / TE / flip angle of 2.2/1.5/18° was used. In the same study of 9 patients with symptoms of angina, a positive exercise stress test of angina with normal epicardial coronary artery flow reserve (CFR) measured with intravascular 12 MHz Doppler wire showed an excellent correlation with the noninvasively assessed myocardial perfusion reserve (r=0.84, MR perfusion reserve = 0.004 + 0.98 CFR).

Transmural perfusion differences

Compared to PET and SPECT, high resolution of MR perfusion scans in the range of 2 mm x 2 mm with a slice thickness of 5-8 mm enables the detection of myocardial blood flow differences between endocardium and epicardium. Figure 6 shows two time intensity curves in endocardial (circles) and epicardial (triangle) regions of a patient with "syndrome-X" and a coronary flow reserve in the left anterior descending coronary artery of 1 to 2.2. The fitting of a two compartment model (solid and dashed line) using the time-intensity curve in the cavity of the left ventricle as a input function yielded a ratio of 1.8 to 1 between epicardial and endocardial perfusion rates.

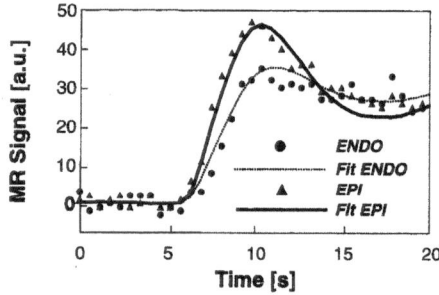

Figure 6. Comparison of time-intensity curves during vasodilation in a patient with syndrome-X. The fitting of the time-intensity curves with a two compartment model yielded a epi/endocardial perfusion ratio of 1.8. (Courtesy of Dr. M. Jerosch-Herold, University of Minnesota Medical School).

Discussion and outlook

The feasibility of MRI to detect perfusion defects by tracking the transit of an MR contrast through the myocardium has been demonstrated in various studies. By the deconvolution of the myocardial time-intensity curves with the arterial input function even absolute perfusion rates can be calculated. The second hurdle of MR perfusion methods towards a clinical application has been overcome by the advances in MR instrumentation and pulse sequences. The short scan times allow coverage of the entire heart with better spatial resolution than nuclear medicine methods and sufficient temporal resolution to detect small differences in the uptake of the contrast agent.

Before these methods can be evaluated with large multi-center clinical studies, image evaluation has to be improved. The large number of images (dynamic scans of multiple slices) and the fact that the perfusion information can only be derived from the time-intensity diagram over the whole series rather than from a single image requires computer-assisted image evaluation and data postprocessing. The first steps towards a perfusion map of the heart include segmentation of heart wall as well as blood pool for the determination of the input function. Automatic segmentation of the myocardium in this case is not trivial. On one hand the image contrast changes dramatically during the transit of the contrast agent causing problems in the determination of thresholds for image intensity or gradients used for segmentation. On the other hand the duration of the dynamic scans is longer than most patients can hold their breath. Thus, even though the images are triggered with respect to the heart's motion, respiratory motion causes translation in the range of several times the slice thickness of an MR scan. Thus, not always the same tissue is imaged in the same slice for each of the dynamic scans. Therefore the evaluation of time-intensity curves becomes more difficult as does the segmentation of the myocardium, since the shape of the heart section varies with the respiratory motion. After a time-intensity curve in each volume of interest is extracted from the image set, relevant parameters for a qualitative perfusion assessment, such as slope of the contrast agent uptake or mean transit time have to be derived from these curves. For a more quantitative perfusion rate evaluation, pharmacokinetic model fitting of the time-intensity curve of each segment of the myocardium has to be performed. However, the modeling of the Gd-DTPA uptake is an additional hurdle for the clinical use of MR perfusion quantification, since assumptions of extraction efficiency and water exchange rates between vascular and extracellular space are part of the models. However, it is very likely that intravascular contrast agents, will be available for human use in the near future which will simplify the modeling. Finally, display methods for the resulting three-dimensional regional myocardial blood flow need to be developed.

Further advances in MR perfusion assessment will include use of intravascular contrast agents and the real-time correction of the slice position to compensate for respiratory motion.

However, the most important advantage of MR myocardial blood flow assessment is the ability to combine perfusion assessment with the evaluation of global and regional heart wall motion, and possibly with the imaging of the proximal part of the coronary arterial tree all in the same scanning session.

Conclusions

Assessment of myocardial perfusion and flow reserve is a critical component in the evaluation of patients with ischemic heart disease. The concept of tracking the transit of an MR contrast agent through the myocardium in order the assess perfusion defects has been proven at least in a single slice. State of the art MR hardware and pulse sequences are feasible to generate images with a contrast agent concentration dependent contrast covering the entire heart with sufficient temporal resolution. The better spatial resolution of MR images as compared to SPECT or PET enables the assessment of transmural perfusion differences. Used in conjunction with MR methods to image the proximal part of the coronary arteries and cardiac function, MR perfusion assessment can complete the one-stop-shop cardiac examination for the diagnosis of ischemic heart disease.

Acknowledgments

The authors like to thank Dr. Michael Jerosch-Herold, Dr. Norbert Wilke, Dr. Robert F. Wilson and Dr. Arthur E. Stillman from the University of Minnesota Medical School, Minneapolis, MN, USA for their contribution on myocardial perfusion reserve quantification. Further, we would like to acknowledge help from Dr. Samuel A Wickline and Lars O. M. Johanson, Cardiology, Barnes-Jewish Hospital St. Louis, MO, USA.

Reference

1. Goldman MR, Pohost GM, Ingwall JS, Fossel ET. Nuclear magnetic resonance imaging: potential cardiac applications. Am J Cardiol 1980;46:1278-83.
2. Waterton JC, Jenkins JP, Zhu XP, Love HG, Isherwood I, Rowlands DJ. Magnetic resonance (MR) cine imaging of the human heart. Br J Radiol 1985;58:711-6.
3. Schiebler M, Axel L, Reichek N *et al.* Correlation of cine MR imaging with two- dimensional pulsed Doppler echocardiography in valvular insufficiency. J Comput Assist Tomogr 1987;11:627-32.
4. Lorenz CH, Walker ES, Graham TP Jr, Powers TA. Right ventricular performance and mass by use of cine MRI late after atrial repair of transposition of the great arteries. Circulation 1995;92(9 Suppl):II233-9.
5. Shapiro EP, Rogers WJ, Beyar R *et al.* Determination of left ventricular mass by magnetic resonance imaging in hearts deformed by acute infarction. Circulation 1989;79:706-11.
6. Matheijssen NA, Baur LH, Reiber JH *et al.* Assessment of left ventricular volume and mass by cine magnetic resonance imaging in patients with anterior myocardial infarction intra-observer and inter-observer variability on contour detection. Int J Card Imaging 1996;12:11-9.
7. Zerhouni EA, Parish DM, Rogers WJ, Yang A, Shapiro EP. Human heart: tagging with MR imaging- a method for noninvasive assessment of myocardial motion. Radiology 1988;169:59-63.
8. Pennell DJ, Underwood SR, Manzara CC *et al.* Magnetic resonance imaging during dobutamine stress in coronary artery disease. Am J Cardiol 1992;70:34-40.
9. Manning WJ, Edelman RR. Magnetic resonance coronary angiography. Magn Reson Q 1993;9:131-51.
10. Hofman MB, Paschal CB, Li D, Haacke EM, van Rossum AC, Sprenger M. MRI of coronary arteries: 2D breath-hold vs 3D respiratory-gated acquisition. J Comput Assist Tomogr 1995;19:56-62.
11. Balaban RS, Chesnick S, Hedges K, Samaha F, Heineman FW. Magnetization transfer contrast in MR imaging of the heart. Radiology 1991;180:671-5.
12. Prasad PV, Burstein D, Edelman RR. MRI evaluation of myocardial perfusion without a contrast agent using magnetization transfer. Magn Reson Med 1993;30:267-70.
13. Le Bihan D, Turner R, Moonen CT, Pekar J. Imaging of diffusion and microcirculation with gradient sensitization: design, strategy, and significance. J Magn Reson Imaging 1991;1:7-28.
14. Le Bihan D. Theoretical principles of perfusion imaging. Application to magnetic resonance imaging. Invest Radiol 1992;27(Suppl 2):S6-11.
15. Moseley ME, Sevick R, Wendland MF *et al.* Ultrafast magnetic resonance imaging: diffusion and perfusion. Can Assoc Radiol J 1991;42:31-8.
16. Turner R, Le Bihan D, Maier J, Vavrek R, Hedges LK, Pekar J. Echo-planar imaging of intravoxel incoherent motion. Radiology 1990;77:407-14.
17. Atalay MK, Reeder SB, Zerhouni EA, Forder JR. Blood oxygenation dependence of T1 and T2 in the isolated, perfused rabbit heart at 4.7T. Magn Reson Med 1995;34:623-7.
18. Dardzinski BJ, Sotak CH. Rapid tissue oxygen tension mapping using 19F inversion-recovery echo-planar imaging of perfluoro-15-crown-5-ether. Magn Reson Med 1994;32:88-97.
19. Detre JA, Zhang W, Roberts DA *et al.* Tissue specific perfusion imaging using arterial spin labeling. NMR Biomed 1994;7:75-82.
20. Williams DS, Grandis DJ, Zhang W, Koretsky AP. Magnetic resonance imaging of perfusion in the isolated rat heart using spin inversion of arterial water. Magn Reson Med 1993;30:361-5.
21. Atkinson DJ, Burstein D, Edelman RR. First-pass cardiac perfusion: evaluation with ultrafast MR imaging. Radiology 1990;174:757-62.

22. Manning WJ, Atkinson DJ, Grossman W, Paulin S, Edelman RR. First-pass nuclear magnetic resonance imaging studies using gadolinium-DTPA in patients with coronary artery disease. J Am Coll Cardiol 1991;18:959-65.

23. Wilke N, Jerosch-Herold M, Stillman AE *et al.* Concepts of myocardial perfusion imaging in magnetic resonance imaging. Magn Reson Q 1994;10:249-86.

24. Eichenberger AC, Schuiki E, Kochli VD, Amann FW, McKinnon GC, von Schulthess GK. Ischemic heart disease: assessment with gadolinium-enhanced ultrafast MR imaging and dipyridamole stress. J Magn Reson Imaging 1994;4:425-31.

25. Burstein D, Taratuta E, Manning WJ. Factors in myocardial "perfusion" imaging with ultrafast MRI and Gd-DTPA administration. Magn Reson Med 1991;20:299-305.

26. Keijer JT, van Rossum AC, van Eenige MJ *et al.* Semiquantitation of regional myocardial blood flow in normal human subjects by first-pass magnetic resonance imaging. Am Heart J 1995;130:893-901.

27. Fritz-Hansen T, Rostrup E, Larsson HBW, Søndergaard L, Ring P, Henriksen O. Measurement of the arterial concentration of Gd-DTPA using MRI: a step toward quantitative perfusion imaging. Magn Reson Med 1996;36:225-31.

28. Wendland MF, Saeed M, Yu KK *et al.* Inversion recovery EPI of bolus transit in rat myocardium using intravascular and extravascular gadolinium-based MR contrast media: dose effects on peak signal enhancement. Magn Reson Med 1994;32:319-29.

29. Kraitchman DL, Wilke N, Hexeberg E *et al.* Myocardial perfusion and function in dogs with moderate coronary stenosis. Magn Reson Med 1996;35:771-80.

30. Johnston DL, Liu P, Lauffer RB *et al.* Use of gadolinium-DTPA as a myocardial perfusion agent: potential applications and limitations for magnetic resonance imaging. J Nucl Med 1987;28:871-7.

31. Dolan RP, Prasad PV, Wielopolski PA *et al.* First-pass myocardial imaging with MS-325, an intravascular MRI contrast agent. Proc Int Soc Magn Reson Med 1996;686.

32. Lauffer RB, Parmelee DJ, Ouellet HS *et al.* MS-325: a small-molecule vascular imaging agent for magnetic resonance imaging. Acad Radiol 1996;3(Suppl 2):S356-58.

33. Judd RM, Reeder SB, Atalar E, McVeigh ER, Zerhouni EA. A magnetization- driven gradient echo pulse sequence for the study of myocardial perfusion. Magn Reson Med 1995;34:276-82.

34. Laub G, Somonetti O. Assessment of myocardial perfusion with saturation- recovery TurboFLASH sequences. Proc Int Soc Magn Reson Med 1996;179.

35. Saeed M, Wendland MF, Yu KK *et al.* Identification of myocardial reperfusion with echo planar magnetic resonance imaging. Discrimination between occlusive and reperfused infarctions. Circulation 1994;90:1492-501.

36. McKinnon GC. Ultrafast interleaved gradient-echo-planar imaging on a standard scanner. Magn Reson Med 1993;30:609-16.

37. Fischer SE, Wickline SA, Lorenz CH. Multiple Slice hybrid imaging sequence for myocardial perfusion measurement. Proc Int Soc Magn Reson Med 1996;682.

38. Schwitter J, Debatin JF, Von Schulthess GK, McKinnon GC. Normal myocardial perfusion assessed with multishot echo-planar imaging. Magn Reson Med 1997;37:140.-7

39. Look DC, Locker DR. Time saving in measurement of NMR and EPR relaxation times. Rev Sci Instrum 1970;41:250.

40. Gowland P, Mansfield P. Accurate measurement of T1 in vivo in less than 3 seconds using echo planar imaging. Magn Reson Med 1993;30:351-4.

41. Akbudak E, Conturo TE. Arterial input function from MR phase imaging. Magn Reson Med 1996;36:809-15.

42. Donahue KM, Weisskoff RM, Parmelee DJ *et al.* Dynamic Gd-DTPA enhanced MRI measurement of tissue cell volume fraction. Magn Reson Med 1995;34:423-32.

43. Tong CY, Prato FS, Wisenberg G *et al.* Techniques for the measurement of the local myocardial extraction efficiency for inert diffusible contrast agents such as gadopentate dimeglumine. Magn Reson Med 1993;30:332-6.

44. Tong CY, Prato FS, Wisenberg G *et al.* Measurement of the extraction efficiency and distribution volume for Gd-DTPA in normal and diseased canine myocardium. Magn Reson Med 1993;30:337-46

45. Donahue KM, Burstein D, Manning WJ, Gray ML. Studies of Gd-DTPA relaxivity and proton exchange rates in tissue. Magn Reson Med 1994;32:66-76.

46. Judd RM, Atalay MK, Rottman GA, Zerhouni EA. Effects of myocardial water exchange on T1 enhancement during bolus administration of MR contrast agents. Magn Reson Med 1995;33:215-23.

47. Pennell DJ, Mavrogeni SI, Forbat SM, Karwatowski SP, Underwood SR. Adenosine combined with dynamic exercise for myocardial perfusion imaging. J Am Coll Cardiol 1995;25:1300-9.

20.

Nuclear cardiology: which clinical questions can be answered now and in the future?

Jamshid Maddahi

Summary

Nuclear cardiology has now become an established method for diagnosis and evaluation of coronary artery disease (CAD). Since its introduction about two and a half decades ago, myocardial perfusion scintigraphy has become the most commonly performed method in the field of nuclear cardiology and has advanced significantly. Clinical applications have expanded from diagnosis to risk stratification of CAD and assessment of a variety of clinical conditions such as myocardial infarction, left ventricular dysfunction, and revascularization. More recently, cost-effectiveness of these procedures has been demonstrated in a variety of clinical settings. This chapter provides an overview of the clinical questions that can be answered, by myocardial perfusion imaging, now and in the future.

Detection of coronary artery disease

Diagnostic accuracy of various methods

Table 1 summarizes sensitivities, specificities, and normalcy rates for various myocardial perfusion imaging methods for detection of CAD [1]. The combined reported sensitivity and specificity of thallium-201 (Tl-201) imaging by planar acquisition and qualitative analysis, in a total of 4678 patients, are 82% and 88% respectively. In order to overcome subjectivity of interpretation inherent in qualitative visual analysis of myocardial perfusion images, several methods for semi-quantitative analysis of images have been developed [1]. These methods have proven to be clinically useful by reducing inter-observer variability of image interpretation and providing an objective measure of the size of perfusion defects. These methods, however, do not replace physician interpretation of images and are regarded as an expert "second opinion". The method of imaging has evolved from the conventional planar method to single photon emission computed tomography (SPECT). From the technical point of view, SPECT reduces overlap of various myocardial regions and improves image contrast. The literature results for the SPECT method, as compared to the planar imaging method, showed a slightly higher sensitivity, due to improved image contrast. More detailed studies subsequently showed that the sensitivity of SPECT was superior to the planar imaging method, particularly in patients with single-vessel disease, mild to moderate coronary

J.H.C. Reiber and E.E. van der Wall (eds.). What's New in Cardiovascular Imaging, 261–278.
©1998 Kluwer Academic Publishers.

stenosis, and those without prior myocardial infarction. The specificity of SPECT imaging, however, was lower than the planar imaging method. This was in part due to more sources of artifact during SPECT image acquisition and processing. It was also noted that the specificity of SPECT further decreased from 91% to 43% from 1984 to 1990 [2]. This decline of specificity with time is likely to be due, in part, to an increase in referral bias in the more recent studies. Although the true, unbiased specificity of the SPECT technique has not been determined, it may be implied from the normalcy rate of 89% which was observed in patients with a low likelihood of CAD prior to SPECT imaging. The sensitivity of myocardial perfusion imaging for detecting CAD, not only is influenced by the method of imaging, but also by the clinical characteristics of the patient who is being studied. It has been shown that the sensitivity of Tl-201 SPECT imaging is higher in patients with prior myocardial infarction (MI) than those without MI (99% vs. 85%, respectively) and is higher in patients with triple-vessel CAD than those with double and single-vessel CAD (95%, 93%, and 83%, respectively). The sensitivity of SPECT Tl-201 imaging for detecting moderate coronary stenoses (50%-70% narrowing) is 63% and for those with severe coronary narrowing (70%-100%) is 88% [2].

Table 1: Sensitivities, specificities, and normalcy rates for various myocardial perfusion imaging methods for detection of coronary artery disease (CAD)[a]

Imaging method	# of patients	Sensitivity	Specificity	Normalcy rate
Planar Tl-201, Qualitative	4678	82%	88%	—
Planar Tl-201, Quantitative	800	89%	68%	88%
SPECT Tl-201, Qualitative	818	90%	77%	—
SPECT Tl-201, Quantitative	1578	91%	70%	89%
SPECT Tc-99m sestamibi, Quantitative	161	89%	36%	81%
Dipyridamole Tl-201	1272	87%	81%	—
PET, Qualitative and Quantitative	507	94%	83%	96%

a. Tl-201=Thallium-201 scintigraphy, SPECT= single photon computed tomography, PET= positron emission tomography.

In recent years, technetium-99m (Tc-99m) labeled myocardial perfusion tracers (Tc-99m sestamibi and Tc-99m tetrofosmin), have become clinically available. These agents offer several advantages over Tl-201. They are better suited for standard gamma cameras which perform best at the 140 keV photon peak of technetium-99m. As a result of a higher photon peak, soft tissue attenuation is less prominent than Tl-201. Furthermore, due to the short half life (six hours) of Tc-99m and the prompt hepatobiliary and renal excretion, up to 30 mCi can be administered as a single dose while keeping the radiation to the target organ (small intestine) at less than five rads. The higher administration dose of Tc-99m labeled agents, compared to Tl-201, results in a far greater count rate and high count density images. The higher photon flux also allows electrocardiographic gating of planar or tomographic images and the performance of first pass studies [1]. Since Tc-99m sestamibi and Tc-99m tetrofosmin do not redistribute significantly separate injections of the agent are necessary, one during exercise and the second at rest, to assess reversibility of myocardial perfusion defects.

A significant development in stress myocardial perfusion imaging was availability of Pharmacologic stress testing, as a substitute for treadmill exercise, in patients who are unable to exercise because of peripheral vascular, musculoskeletal, or neurologic diseases or they cannot achieve an adequate exercise heart rate due to lack of motivation, poor physical condition, or taking beta/calcium channel-blocking medications. Of the three available pharmacological stress testing agents, two (dipyridamole and adenosine) are coronary vasodilators that increase myocardial blood flow 3 to 5 times the resting level in myocardial regions that are supplied by normal coronary arteries. In myocardial regions that are supplied by diseased coronary arteries, the hyperemic response to these agents is attenuated or blood flow actually decrease below the resting level. In patients with coronary artery disease, therefore, infusion of dipyridamole or adenosine induces disparity in regional myocardial perfusion similar to that achieved with exercise testing. Adenosine is a direct coronary vasodilator and activates the adenosine A2 receptors in the coronary arterial wall. This leads to increase in adenosine cyclase and c-AMP levels, decreased transmembrane calcium uptake, and ultimately, to coronary vasodilation [1]. Dipyridamole exerts its effect by raising endogenous adenosine blood levels through blocking the cell membrane transport and reuptake of endogenous adenosine [1]. The third pharmacological stress agent, dobutamine, is predominantly a beta-1 agonist that increases heart rate, myocardial contractility, and systolic blood pressure [1]. Thus, the coronary vasodilatory effect of dobutamine is similar to that of physiologic exercise. Dobutamine is reserved for patients who cannot undergo stress testing with dipyridamole or adenosine because of history of asthma or advanced heart block. It is generally felt that the risk of serious events is similar to that seen with exercise. Combined major adverse events among 73.806 patients who were evaluated with dipyridamole TI-201 testing [3] included cardiac death (0.95 per 10.000), nonfatal myocardial infarction (1.76 per 10.000), nonfatal sustained ventricular arrhythmias (0.81 per 10.000), transient cerebral ischemic attacks (1.22 per 10.000), and severe bronchospasm (1.22 per 10.000). Such risks may be diminished by careful screening of patients who are referred for dipyridamole stress testing and proper attention to the aforementioned contraindications of dipyridamole testing. The safety of adenosine pharmacological stress was recently updated in 9.256 patients [4] and are considered similar to dipyridamole, with the added side effect of different degrees of temporary AV block that resolve after termination of infusion. The pooled literature results (table 1) as well as studies in patients who underwent both maximal exercise and pharmacologic stress testing have shown that the two modes of stress testing have similar sensitivities and specificities for detection of CAD.

PET is increasingly being used for the noninvasive evaluation of CAD [4]. The pooled literature results suggest that the specificity and normalcy rate of PET is higher than the SPECT method (table 1) [4]. This is most likely related to lower false positive rate of PET which is attained by routine application of attenuation correction. This difference between PET and SPECT, however, is likely to diminish with increasing application of gating and attenuation correction to SPECT studies that are expected to improve identification of attenuation artifacts.

Cost-effectiveness of nuclear cardiology in detecting CAD

In patients suspected of having coronary artery disease (CAD), noninvasive testing has been playing an increasing role in selecting patients who would require coronary angiography for either the "definitive" diagnosis of CAD or as a prelude to planning myocardial revascularization by percutaneous transluminal coronary angioplasty (PTCA) or coronary artery bypass grafting (CABG). Exercise electrocardiography and stress myocardial perfusion imaging using planar, SPECT, or PET methods are commonly used for these purposes. The accuracies and costs of these tests are different from one another and their utilization is highly variable and subjective. A challenging task facing cardiology today is to objectively assess the cost relative to effectiveness of these testing modalities for diagnosis and management of CAD. We used a mathematic to define cost-effective utility of nuclear cardiology testing for diagnosis of CAD and selection of appropriate candidates for coronary angiography, according to quantitative methods of decision analysis [5,6,7]. Clinical utility or effectiveness was defined in terms of percent correct diagnosis of CAD. Cost was defined as dollars of medical expenditure. Six competing strategies were compared in subsets of patients with different pretest likelihoods of CAD, based on age, sex, and symptoms. Nuclear cardiology testing was the most cost-effective initial modality of choice in patients with an intermediate pretest likelihood of CAD. In patients with a low likelihood of CAD, nuclear cardiology testing was cost-effective in the subgroup of patients who had abnormal exercise treadmill electrocardiograms. In patients with a high pretest likelihood of CAD, direct referral to coronary angiography was the most cost-effective strategy for diagnosis of CAD. Several studies in the literature support the conclusions that are drawn from our modeling approach to cost-effective diagnosis of CAD [7].

Detection of disease in individual coronary arteries

The coronary arteries and their branches supply different regions of the left ventricular (LV) myocardium. Based on the known anatomic relationship between coronary arteries and various myocardial regions and actual study of patients with single and multivessel CAD and with myocardial perfusion studies, general guidelines have been developed for assignment of various myocardial regions to specific coronary arteries. Table 2 summarizes the pooled literature sensitivities and specificities of the different myocardial perfusion imaging methods for detection of disease in the left anterior descending (LAD), left circumflex (LCX), and right coronary (RCA) arteries [1]. As shown, improvement of sensitivity for detection of disease in individual coronary arteries has been reported using the SPECT technique, particularly for detection of disease in the LCX coronary artery. This improved sensitivity may be related to improved defect contrast and decreased overlap between myocardial regions that result from SPECT imaging. The ability to detect disease in individual coronary arteries makes the SPECT technique suitable for detection and localization of ischemia, as a guide to selection of patients for percutaneous coronary angioplasty. Furthermore, multivessel, and potentially high risk, CAD may be identified. The pooled literature results [1] demonstrate that 69% (291/423) of patients with three-vessel coronary artery disease are correctly identified as such by the SPECT imaging method.

Table 1: Sensitivities and specificities for various myocardial perfusion imaging methods for detection of coronary artery disease (CAD) in different coronary arteries[a]

Imaging method	*LAD*		*LCX*		*RCA*	
	Sens	*Spec*	*Sens*	*Spec*	*Sens*	*Spec*
Planar Tl-201, Qualitative	69%	94%	37%	95%	65%	85%
Planar Tl-201, Quantitative	77%	74%	50%	85%	91%	59%
SPECT Tl-201, Qualitative	74%	86%	57%	94%	88%	83%
SPECT Tl-201, Quantitative	80%	83%	72%	85%	83%	85%
SPECT Tc-99m sestamibi, Quantitative	69%	76%	70%	80%	77%	85%

a. Tl-201 = Thallium-201 scintigraphy, SPECT = single photon computed tomography, LAD = left anterior descending, LCX = left circumflex, RCA = right coronary artery, Sens = sensitivity, Spec = specificity

Risk stratification in patients with known or suspected CAD

During the last decade and a half, clinical application of myocardial perfusion imaging has evolved from diagnosis to risk stratification of CAD. The prognostic application of myocardial perfusion imaging plays an important role in patient management; the decision between myocardial revascularization and medical therapy depends on the risk of coronary events on medical therapy versus the risk of myocardial revascularization procedure.

Identification of patients at low risk for coronary events

In 1983, Brown et al. [8] demonstrated that among 61 patients with suspected coronary artery disease who had a negative exercise myocardial perfusion study, none died during an average of 46 months of follow up and 3 developed myocardial infarction during this period (0.85% event rate per year). These initial results were subsequently confirmed by several studies [1]. In a total of 2.825 patients without myocardial infarction and with a normal Tl-201 exercise myocardial perfusion planar study, reported in 13 separate publications, the weighted average incidence of cardiac death per year is 0.24%, ranging from 0 to 0.7%. Furthermore, the average incidence of developing myocardial infarction is 0.53% per year ranging from 0 to 1.4%. These results suggest that a normal exercise myocardial perfusion study in patients without prior myocardial infarction is associated with a very low likelihood of coronary events during the subsequent year. The observed coronary event rates in this population, is very similar to patients with normal coronary arteries. This suggests that further cardiac catheterization or intervention is not justified in these patients. Association between a normal stress myocardial perfusion study and low coronary event rate has also been reported, in rather small groups of patients, using Tl-201 SPECT, Tc-99m sestamibi SPECT, atrial pacing planar Tl-201 stress testing and dipyridamole stress planar Tl-201 imaging [9] and PET [10]. An implication of excellent prognosis in patients with normal stress myocardial perfusion study is that the subgroup with coronary disease and normal perfusion studies also have good prognosis. The question whether normal thallium-201 studies would have the same benign predictive value in patients with angiographic significant CAD, has been addressed in a recent study by Brown and Rowen [11]. These investigators demonstrated that of 75 patients with significant coronary artery disease who had normal exercise planar Tl-201 myocardial perfusion studies, 1 patient developed non-fatal myocardial infarction 28 months after the Tl-201 study, yielding an annual event rate of 7% per year. In comparison, 2 of the 101 patients with normal exercise planar Tl-201 studies who had either normal coronary arteries (14 patients) or a low likelihood of CAD, developed hard events (non-fatal MI at 28 months and cardiac death at 23 months), yielding an annual event rate of 1% per year. These results imply that a normal exercise Tl-201 myocardial perfusion study, even in the presence of significant coronary artery disease, carries a very benign prognosis with a very low rate of hard cardiac events.

Identification of patients with high risk CAD

Extensive literature has documented the powerful prognostic role of an abnormal myocardial perfusion study. In this regard, the following scintigraphic parameters have emerged as significant prognostic indicators: 1) the size (extent) and severity of perfusion defects, 2) increased lung uptake of Tl-201, implying increased pulmonary capillary wedge pressure, and 3) transient postexercise ischemic dilation of the left ventricle. The extent of myocardial ischemia may not be always inferred by the number of diseased coronary arteries. This is due to the fact that the size of myocardial ischemia is influenced by the size of the supplying coronary artery; the location, severity and the number of coronary narrowings; and the status of collateral blood flow. On stress myocardial perfusion studies, the extent of myocardial hypoperfusion may be expressed by the number of myocardial segments with a defect or the actual percent of total LV myocardium with perfusion defects. The severity of hypoperfusion (reflecting the severity of underlying coronary artery disease) may be measured by the degree of reduction of activity in the defect zone. These defects could be further categorized to reflect infarcted myocardium (if they are nonreversible) or viable but jeopardized myocardium (if they are reversible). Several investigators have evaluated the relation between the size of myocardial hypoperfusion and subsequent coronary events. Brown et al. [8] showed, by stepwise logistic regression analysis, that in 100 patients without prior myocardial infarction, potential predictors of cardiac death or myocardial infarction were the number of transient Tl-201 defects, total number of Tl-201 defects and the number of diseased vessels by angiography. Importantly, after the number of transient Tl-201 defects (which had the highest significant chi-squared value) was included in the logistic regression model, no other predictor was found to be significant. In the study of Ladenheim et al. [12], involving 1.689 patients without prior myocardial infarction, stepwise logistic regression identified only 3 independent predictors of annual coronary events; the number of myocardial regions with reversible hyperperfusion, the magnitude of hypoperfusion, and achieved heart rate. Increased pulmonary uptake of Tl-201 may be quantified by several approaches and abnormal values have been observed in patients with extensive coronary disease. Furthermore, several studies have shown that increased pulmonary uptake of Tl-201 is a significant predictor of future cardiac events in univariate and multivariate statistical analyses. Transient post exercise dilation of the left ventricle is a specific marker of multivessel critical stenoses [1] and is a marker of poor prognosis. Transient dilation of the left ventricle with Tc-99m sestamibi imaging and following pharmacologic stress testing, is less common but its significance is similar to exercise testing.

Incremental prognostic power of myocardial perfusion imaging

The incremental prognostic power of stress Tl-201 myocardial perfusion imaging in comparison with other parameters such as clinical variables, exercise treadmill results and coronary angiography, has been extensively evaluated. Four of the reported studies have addressed the incremental value of exercise Tl-201 imaging over and above clinical, exercise ECG, and angiographic variables. Brown et al. [8] showed that the number of transient Tl-201 defect was a better predictor of future cardiac events as compared with clinical, ECG and angiographic data. Kaul and associates [13] showed the number of diseased vessels was an important independent predictor of cardiac events, but it did not add significantly to the overall ability of the exercise Tl-201 test to predict events. Furthermore, information obtained from Tl-201 imaging alone was marginally superior to that obtained from cardiac catheterization alone and significantly superior to that obtained from exercise testing alone in determining the occurrence of events. In addition, unlike the exercise Tl-201 test, which could predict the occurrence of all categories of events, catheterization data were not able to predict the occurrence of non-fatal myocardial infarction. These data suggested that exercise Tl-201 imaging is superior to data from both exercise testing alone and cardiac catheterization alone for predicting future events in patients with chronic CAD who have undergone both exercise Tl-201 imaging and catheterization for the evaluation of chest pain. In another study, Kaul et al. [14] showed that the number of diseased vessel was the single most important predictor of future events followed by the number of segments demonstrating redistribution on delayed Tl-201 images, except in the case of non-fatal myocardial infarction, for which redistribution was the most important predictor of future events. When CAD was defined as 70% or greater luminal diameter narrowing, the number of diseased vessels significantly lost its power to predict events. In this study, when exercise Tl-201 stress test results were considered as a whole (in conjunction with change in heart rate from rest to exercise, ST segment depression on the ECG, and ventricular premature beats on exercise), they were as powerful as cardiac catheterization data. Of note, combination of both catheterization and exercise Tl-201 data was superior to either alone for determining future events. In a subsequent study by Pollack and associates [15] showed that Tl-201 imaging provided significant additional prognostic information compared with clinical and exercise stress test data. In a subgroup of patients in whom lung/heart Tl-201 ratio had been analyzed, coronary angiography did not provide additional prognostic information. In this subgroup of patients, the combination of clinical and exercise Tl-201 variables provided greater prognostic information than the combination of clinical and angiographic data. In the remaining subgroup of patients in whom the lung/heart ratio had not been analyzed, coronary angiography provided incremental prognostic information compared with clinical and exercise Tl-201 data alone.

In a recent study by Berman et al [16], a similar approach was used to assess the incremental prognostic power of exercise Tc-99m sestamibi SPECT in 1702 patients with known or suspected ischemic heart disease, who were followed up for a mean of 20 Å 5 months. Of these patients, 1.282 had normal and 420 had an abnormal rest ECG findings. The subgroup with normal rest ECG findings were divided into two subsets; 548 with a low (<15%) pretest likelihood of CAD and 734 with an intermediate or high (>15%) pretest likelihood of CAD. In the 548 patients with a low pretest likelihood of CAD, coronary event rate was 0.5%. Although myocardial perfusion imaging in these patients appeared to provide some risk stratification, the impact was not statistically significant and nuclear testing in this sub group was not cost-effective. In the 734 patients with an intermediate to high likelihood of CAD, a low post ECG likelihood of CAD was associated with a low hard event rate of 1.7%. In these patients, a normal scan was associated with a significantly lower hard event rate (0%) than an abnormal scan (6.2%) but, the prognostic use of nuclear exercise testing, could not be justified on the basis of cost. On the other hand, in patients with a post exercise ECG likelihood of >15%, scan results stratified patients into high and low risk groups (7.9% vs 0.7%) and the use of exercise nuclear testing was an economically superior clinical strategy. In the 420 patients with uninterpretable exercise ECG responses, nuclear exercise testing had incremental prognostic value in all patients regardless of their pretest likelihood of CAD. Cost analysis, however, demonstrated that nuclear exercise testing was cost-effective only in those with an intermediate to high likelihood of coronary disease.

Cost-effectiveness of nuclear cardiology for prognosis of CAD

Referral to coronary angiography is often influenced by the prognostic, as well as the diagnostic implications of the pre angiographic test results. In other words, patients who are identified to be at high risk on medical therapy are more appropriate candidates for coronary angiography as a prelude to possible myocardial revascularization. Because these invasive procedures are indicated only in patients who are at high risk with medical therapy, nuclear cardiology procedures, by virtue of incremental prognostic information, identify appropriate candidates for more invasive procedures, aimed at improving survival. Based on the published reports [16,17], strategies for cost effective prognostication of CAD depend on not only the patient's pretest likelihood of CAD but also the status of the rest electrocardiogram [7]. In patients with a normal rest electrocardiogram, a low pretest likelihood of CAD indicates a low risk for cardiac events with medical therapy. Therefore coronary angiography is not indicated in these patients. Patients with an intermediate likelihood of CAD should first undergo exercise electrocardiographic testing; a negative would indicate a low risk for cardiac events and a positive response would indicate the need for nuclear cardiology testing for further cost-effective risk stratification. In patients with a high pretest likelihood of CAD, the combined exercise electrocardiographic and nuclear cardiac testing is the most cost-effective strategy; a negative or a positive nuclear test result would imply low or high risk, respectively. The latter patients would then be candidates for coronary angiography. In all patients with an abnormal rest electrocardiogram, the most cost-effective strategy is uniform referral to nuclear cardiac testing (which is performed in conjunction with exercise electrocardiography), regardless of the pretest likelihood of CAD; a negative or a positive nuclear test result would indicate low or high risk for coronary events, respectively. The latter group would be proper candidates for referral to coronary angiography.

Impact of nuclear cardiology procedures on patient management and outcome

The impact of exercise myocardial perfusion imaging on the subsequent need for coronary angiography and revascularization as well as patient outcome has been studied by several investigators [18,19]. In the study of Bateman and colleagues [19], the impact of myocardial perfusion scintigraphy on subsequent coronary angiographic rates was determined in 4.162

patients in a cardiology practice. In this study, the vast majority of patients had known CAD (more than one third had prior infarction and more than two thirds had prior PTCA or CABG) and 60% of the scans had reversible perfusion defects. Of patients with reversible defects, 32% were followed up by angiography versus 3.5 % without reversible defects. Among studies with reversible defects, subsequent angiography rate was 60% for those showing high risk reversibility, compared with 9% for all other studies demonstrating reversibility. Multivariate logistic regression identified high risk and any reversibility as the strongest predictors of angiography. Their findings suggested that the referring cardiologists, even in this highly biased environment of selfreferral, placed more emphasis on the scintigraphic findings than on any other characteristic in deciding on whether subsequent angiography should be performed; patients who had no perfusion defects rarely were referred for angiography, whereas the majority of those with high risk scintigraphic findings were studies angiographically. In this study, emphasis on reversibility rather than any scintigraphic abnormality suggested the logical desire to assess invasively and if possible revascularize those with sizeable regions of jeopardized myocardium.

Risk stratification following myocardial infarction

In survivors of myocardial infarction, many high risk clinical and laboratory variables have been identified. These variables include recurrent angina, left ventricular failure, shock, conduction abnormalities, malignant arrhythmias, and decreased left ventricular ejection fraction. In subset of patients with uncomplicated myocardial infarction (asymptomatic and without evidence of severe left ventricular dysfunction) one year mortality ranges from 2 to 7.5% [20]. The aim of noninvasive testing prior to discharge of uncomplicated MI patient, therefore, is the identification of patients who are at relatively lower or higher risk for subsequent death or recurrent infarction on the basis of residual ischemic myocardium, either adjacent to or remote from the infarction. In 1983, Gibson et al. [21] compared the predictive value of predischarge of maximal exercise Tl-201 imaging with clinical, exercise treadmill, and coronary angiographic data. They demonstrated that presence of reversible Tl-201 defects involving multiple vascular territories and increased lung uptake of Tl-201 were significant prognostic indicators than these patients. The combination of these Tl-201 variables had significantly greater sensitivity for predicting future cardiac events as compared with exercise treadmill and coronary angiographic data. With wide application of thrombolytic therapy in acute phase of myocardial infarction, the role of myocardial perfusion imaging for risk stratification of patients following myocardial infarction has changed [22]. In patients treated with thrombolytic therapy, Tl-201 redistribution is still more prevalent than ST segment depression (48% versus 14%) but the prevalence of inducible ischemia is less than that observed in the pre-thrombolytic era (59% for Tl-201 redistribution and 32% for ST segment depression) [22]. Therefore, although fewer ischemic responses are observed in patients who undergo reperfusion therapy, detection of ischemia is better achieved with exercise perfusion imaging than exercise ECG alone. In the four published studies, the positive and negative predictive accuracy of myocardial perfusion imaging for prediction of future cardiac events has been 40% and 93%, respectively [1,9]. Availability of pharmacologic coronary vasodilation with dipyridamole and adenosine has provided a unique opportunity for early post-myocardial infarction (MI) risk stratification using myocardial perfusion imaging. With pharmacologic vasodilation, maximum hyperemia may be achieved without the undesired effects of maximal exercise testing such as increase of myocardial oxygen consumption (due to significant increase in heart rhythm blood pressure) and increase in intraventricular pressure and possible adverse effects on ventricular remodeling due to increase of systolic and mean blood pressure during exercise. In 4 studies that have employed dipyridamole pharmacologic coronary vasodilation and thallium-201 imaging early following uncomplicated myocardial infarction, the positive and negative predictive accuracies have been 30% and 94%, respectively [1,9]. Of note, in a recent study by Mahmarian et al. [23], adenosine coronary vasodilation and Tl-201 imaging were utilized to predict cardiac death, myocardial infarction, unstable angina and congestive heart failure in a total of 92 patients during 15 month follow up after uncomplicated myocardial infarction. Presence of reversible defect involving 5% of the left ventricle was 50% sensitive and 97% specific for predicting subsequent coronary events.

Assessment of myocardial viability in ischemic cardiomyopathy

Coronary artery disease is the most common cause of heart failure in the United States. According to the National Heart, Lung, and Blood Institute, there are 400.000 new cases of heart failure and over 200.000 deaths from heart failure each year. Currently, over 2 million Americans have heart failure. In addition, ischemic cardiomyopathy comprises a major overlapping group with patients in congestive heart failure; it constitutes about 40-50% of patients referred for heart transplantation in the United States. Hence, the management of these patients has become an important focus of the health care industry. The reported mortality of patients with ischemic cardiomyopathy is high but variable, ranging from 15% to 60% per year [24]. In the clinical management of patients with CAD and poor LV function, the available therapeutic choices are medical therapy, revascularization (coronary artery bypass surgery or percutaneous transluminal coronary angioplasty), or cardiac transplantation. One year survival after cardiac transplantation is currently favorable at approximately 90%. Cardiac transplantation, however, cannot be performed in the majority of candidates due to shortage of donor hearts, resulting in a large number of patients on the waiting list with an annual mortality rate of about 30% [24]. Moreover, cardiac transplantation is an expensive procedure. It is well recognized that poor ventricular function and heart failure may improve after coronary revascularization in some patients. In the CASS study [25], coronary artery bypass surgery was beneficial in patients with severe left ventricular dysfunction, not only in promoting their survival but also in improving their function status. However, myocardial revascularization in patients with poor LV function is associated with 5%-37% mortality [24], therefore, revascularization should be recommended in the subgroup of patients with poor LV function in whom is intervention is very likely to reverse regional and global LV dysfunction and result in improvement of symptoms and enhanced survival. Prior to the development of cardiac imaging techniques, the decision as to which patients with ischemic cardiomyopathy might benefit from revascularization was a difficult one. While diagnostic techniques conventionally used in the preoperative assessment of these patients allow one to assess coronary artery anatomy and disease as well as wall motion and ejection fraction, they fall short in giving us useful information concerning the reversibility of dysfunctional myocardial segments. Nuclear cardiology techniques (various Tl-201 imaging protocols, PET assessment of myocardial metabolism, and more recently Tc-99m sestamibi imaging) have been extensively evaluated for their ability to predict reversibility of dysfunctional LV myocardium.

Prediction of post revascularization recovery of regional LV dysfunction

Table 3 summarizes the results from reported literature on the value of Tl-201 myocardial scintigraphy and myocardial perfusion-fluoro deoxyglucose (FDG) PET imaging for predicting post revascularization improvement of regional LV contractile dysfunction. The pooled literature positive and negative predictive values of PET imaging are both 83% [24]. The predictive value of Tl-201 myocardial scintigraphy depends on the imaging protocol and the interpretive criterion. With both rest-redistribution and stress-redistribution-reinjection protocols, defect reversibility criterion has a high positive predictive value and a relatively lower negative predictive value for post revascularization improvement of regional LV dysfunction. Use of the alternative interpretation criterion of Tl-201 uptake on the redistribution image, is associated with a lower positive predictive value and a higher negative predictive value [26].

Table 2: Positive and negative predictive values of various Thallium-201 (Tl-201) myocardial scintigraphy protocols and myocardial perfusion-Fluoro-deoxyglucose (FDG) positron emission tomography (PET) imaging for predicting post revascularization improvement of regional left ventricular (LV) contractile dysfunction

Imaging method	Positive predictive value	Negative predictive value
Perfusion-FDG PET imaging	83%	83%
Rest-redistribution Tl-201 imaging		
Defect reversibility	80%	63%
Uptake on the redistribution image	67%	81%
Stress-redistribution-reinjection Tl-201 imaging		
Defect reversibility	79%	72%
Uptake on the redistribution image	47%	94%

Prediction of post revascularization recovery of global LV dysfunction

The average positive and negative predictive values of rest-redistribution Tl-201 scintigraphy, in three published studies, are 70% and 77%, respectively [26]. Literature reports on the value of PET for predicting improvement in LV ejection fraction (EF) are predominantly presented as comparison between pre and post revascularization LVEF's in patients with and those without significant PET viability. The average LVEF significantly increased from pre to post revascularization in patients who had the PET pattern of perfusion-metabolism mismatch [24]. In three of five studies in which LVEF was also determined in patients who did not have the PET pattern of perfusion-metabolism mismatch, LVEF remained unchanged or decreased following revascularization [24].

Prediction of post revascularization improvement in heart failure symptoms

Since most patients with poor LV function suffer from heart failure symptoms, an important goal in assessing myocardial viability is to predict recovery of heart failure symptoms following myocardial revascularization. This question has been addressed by two groups of investigators, using myocardial perfusion-FDG metabolism PET imaging. Eitzman and colleagues [27] used PET to assess myocardial viability in 82 patients with poor LV function (average LVEF=34%). Improvement in heart failure, by at least one class, was related to the PET pattern (presence or absence of mismatch) and type of treatment (revascularization or medical therapy). More patients in the subgroup with mismatch who underwent revascularization than the other subgroups had improvement in heart failure class [27]. Di Carli et al. [28] performed perfusion-DG metabolism PET studies in 93 patients with LV dysfunction (average LVEF=25%) who were followed up for an average of 13.6 months and of whom 66 had severe heart failure symptoms. In the medically treated patients as a group, the severity of heart failure symptoms did not change significantly during the follow-up period. In contrast, a significant improvement in heart failure symptoms was observed only in the subgroup of patients with mismatch who underwent revascularization. Stated differently, in the 34 patients with heart failure who underwent revascularization, 71% of the subgroup with PET mismatch pattern prior to surgery had improvement in heart failure symptoms while only 31% of patients without PET mismatch pattern had improvement in heart failure symptoms. In a more recent study by Di Carli et al. [29], the total extent of a PET mismatch correlated linearly and significantly with a percent improvement in functional state after coronary artery bypass grafting. A blood flow metabolism mismatch of >18% was associated with a sensitivity of 76% and age specificity of 78% for predicting a change in functional state after revascularization. Patients with large mismatches (>18%) achieved a significantly higher functional state compared to those with minimal or no PET mismatch (<5%). These data suggest that the PET pattern of myocardial viability not only predicts recovery of regional and global LV dysfunction after myocardial revascularization, but it also identifies the subgroup of patients with poor LV function and heart failure who are most likely to show relief of heart failure symptoms as a result of revascularization. Furthermore, in patients with ischemic cardiomyopathy, the magnitude of improvement in heart failure symptoms after coronary bypass surgery is related to the preoperative extent and magnitude of myocardial viability as assessed by PET imaging. Patients with large perfusion metabolism mismatches exhibit the greatest clinical benefit after revascularization.

Prediction of the potential for improvement in survival following revascularization

A major goal of noninvasive diagnostic procedures in the assessment of CAD is to evaluate prognosis and to assess the potential of survival benefit from a treatment plan. In the study of Di Carli et al. [28],univariate analysis indicated that the extent of mismatch was the only predictor of survival. Heart failure class, current constructive pulmonary disease, sex, age, prior myocardial infarction, presence of Q waves on the resting electrocardiogram, diabetes, hypertension, presence of angina, LVEF, extent of PET matched and revascularization were not predictors of survival in the univariate analysis. A stepwise Cox model analysis was performed to determine the prognostic contribution of mismatch when covariates with borderline significance in the univariate analysis were included in the model. The extent of mismatch and revascularization were the only predictors of survival. The relative risk (haz-

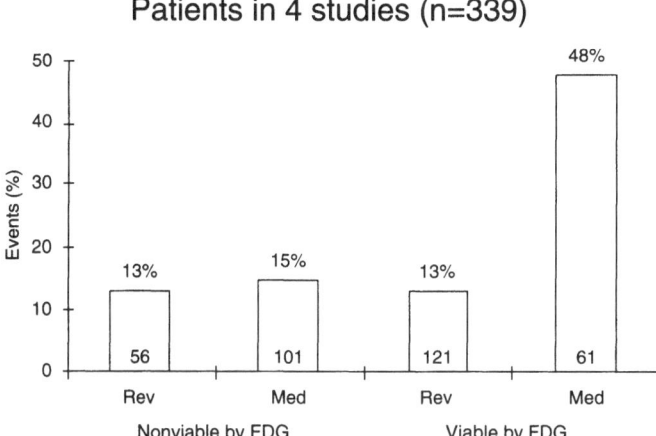

Figure 1. Results of four published studies (27,28,30,31), relating patients' annual mortality (events %) to the positron emission tomographic pattern of myocardial viability by perfusion-Fluoro-deoxyglucose (FDG) imaging and the methods of treatment. Rev= revascularization, Med= medical therapy.

ard) of cardiac death associated with mismatch increased by 3.5% with each unit of increment in the percent extent of mismatch, i.e., the more extensive the mismatch, the higher the risk of dying during the follow-up period. In contrast, revascularization was associated with a positive effect on survival, decreasing the risk of cardiac death by 28%. These data were further analyzed to assess the value of mismatch for risk stratification of patients on medical therapy and myocardial revascularization using a life-table analysis. The estimated annual survival of patients with mismatch was lower than that of patients without mismatch. Furthermore, the annual survival probability of patients without mismatch was similar between the revascularized and medical therapy subgroups. Figure 1 summarizes the results of four published studies [27,28,30,31], relating patients' prognosis to the PET pattern of viability and the method of treatment (revascularization vs medical therapy). The average annual mortality of patients with the PET pattern of mismatch was significantly higher in patients who were treated medically as compared to those who underwent revascularization (48% vs 13%, respectively). In patients who did not have the PET mismatch pattern, annual mortality was similar in the medically treated and revascularized patients (15% and 13%, respectively).

Cost effectiveness of PET in management of candidates for heart transplantation

Cardiac transplant has been the ultimate therapy for end-stage heart failure; however, because of the limited number of available donor hearts, the waiting period for heart transplant by eligible recipients has been prolonged, ranging from eight months to two years. By detecting the presence of sufficient amount of viable (hibernating) myocardium, potential candidates for myocardial revascularization may be identified. Such approach, not only lowers the number of patients who are waiting for transplant, but it reduces the overall cost of patient care by offering coronary artery bypass surgery to patients who would otherwise undergo cardiac transplantation which is more costly. Duong et al. [32], showed that among

112 candidates for cardiac transplantation with ischemic cardiomyopathy (LVEF 35%), Thirty were found to have evidence of PET mismatch in 2 regions of the myocardium and also had suitable coronary targets. All these 30 patients were subsequently taken off the transplant list and underwent coronary artery bypass graft surgery. The operative mortality was 10% and 2 more patients died later in the follow-up period, with an overall mortality of 16.7%. Of the remaining 82 patients who had either minimal or no evidence of PET mismatch, 33 patients underwent cardiac transplantation and 49 were left on medical therapy. The perioperative mortality for cardiac transplantation was 6.1% and 4 additional patients died during the follow up period, yielding an overall mortality of 18.2% for patients undergoing cardiac transplantation. Therefore, in this study, PET assessment of myocardial viability in cardiac transplant candidates allowed identification of adequate hibernating tissue in 27% of patients who were subsequently referred for coronary artery bypass graft surgery with similar perioperative and long term survival rates as compared to those patients who were referred to cardiac transplantation. In these 112 patients, use of a PET-based algorithm for management of ischemic cardiomyopathy resulted in $3.8 million of savings in the overall patient care, primarily by identifying candidates in whom coronary artery bypass surgery could be offered as an alternative to the more costly cardiac transplantation procedure.

Future directions

Improved diagnostic accuracy of SPECT imaging

This is primarily being accomplished by compensating for attenuation and scatter. The current trends in scatter correction takes advantage of the multi-energy sampling capabilities of the new digital detectors which acquire data from different regions of energy simultaneously. Multiple techniques differ from each of other primarily by the location and width of the energy windows used, sampling regions to integrate the scatter data and the algorithms to predict and correct the data. Image reconstruction is done using iterative algorithms which work by modeling the SPECT acquisition using mathematical representation of the image formation process and initial estimate of the tracer distribution and the attenuation map. Iterative algorithms yield successful more accurate approximation of the two tracer distribution by including additional information affecting the image process such as attention and scatter. Such algorithms can be categorized as statistical or analytical. In the future, it may be important to add also depth resolution compensation to allow for differences in resolution as a function of the distance between the heart and the detector. Attenuation/scatter programs for myocardial SPECT imaging are now commercially available and initial results from multicenter trials are promising. They provide a significant achievement towards true quantitative SPECT imaging and improved diagnostic accuracy.

Absolute quantitation of myocardial perfusion

At the present, absolute quantitation of myocardial blood flow and quantitation of myocardial blood flow reserve is only feasible by the PET technique [33]. Overall, many factors affect resting myocardial blood flow, hyperemic myocardial blood flow, and thus myocardial blood flow reserve in normal individuals. This normally observed variability limits application of absolute measurement of myocardial blood flow and quantitation of myocardial flow reserve in detecting true abnormalities in patients suspected of having CAD. It should be noted, however, that these measurements are useful within the same individual before and after a given intervention and thus could be used to monitor effect of therapeutic interventions such as cardiovascular conditioning, cessation of smoking, reduction of mental stress, and lowering of plasma lipids [33]. Quantitative PET has also been used to study myocardial blood flow syndrome-X, hypertrophic cardiomyopathy and cardiac transplant vasculopathy. In these conditions, myocardial blood flow is effected uniformly; no significant regional differences in myocardial blood flow are present. Therefore, absolute quantitation of myocardial blood flow and flow reserve offer a theoretical advantage over relative quantitation of myocardial blood flow in evaluating these conditions [33].

Imaging myocardial sympathetic innervation

I-123 MIBG (metaiodobenzylguanidine) is available in Japan and Europe but has not undergone multicenter clinical trials in the United States. It is a norepinephrine analog that is stored in the vesicles in the sympathetic nerve terminals [34]. The myocardial uptake, washout and mediastinal-to-myocardial ratio reflect sympathetic activity and tone which have been shown to be important prognostic markers in patients with heart failure. A rapid myocardial washout and a high mediastinal-to-myocardial ratio identifies patients at high risk. This tracer appears to be well suited for the study of patients with heart failure and also in the study of patients with serious ventricular arrhythmias [34].

Imaging myocardial fatty acid metabolism

I-123 labeled fatty acids have undergone many modifications since the initial report in 1965. Radiolabeled iodophenylpentadecanoic acid (IPPA) undergoes rapid beta oxidation in the mitochondria and the presence of the phenyl group prevents nonspecific deiodination and the rapid release of free iodine. The additional of a methyl group to this long chain fatty acid (BMIPP) slows the oxidation and results in prolonged myocardial retention. I-123 IPPA has completed phase III clinical trials in the United States and is awaiting approval by the FDA for detecting myocardial viability in patients with ischemic cardiomyopathy. In Japan and Europe, I-123 BMIPP is often combined with perfusion tracers such as thallium-201 to detect myocardial viability. Extensive literature indicates that a mismatch pattern (larger BMIPP defect than thallium defect) is a marker of high risk patients and a marker of recovery of LV function in patients with acute coronary syndromes. BMIPP appears to have a unique memory feature that is attributed to metabolic stunning such that an episode of myocardial ischemia can be detected by BMIPP imaging even hours after the ischemic episode has subsided and perfusion pattern and wall motion abnormality have normalized. This feature may make it ideal for emergency room imaging in patients presenting with chest pain syndromes [34].

Imaging myocardial hypoxia

Radiopharmaceuticals that incorporate nitroimidazole moieties have been developed to detect regional tissue oxygen tension. In 1981, it was suggested that this class of compounds could be used for the direct visualization of tissue hypoxemia. Assessment of tissue oxygen tension maybe the best indicator of the balance between myocardial blood flow and oxygen consumption. Several such compounds have been evaluated: The positron emitting radiotracer F-18 misonidazole and Tc-99 labeled nitroimidazole BMS-181321. The nitroimidazole are believed to passively diffuse across the cell membrane and once in the cytoplasm, nitro-reduction occurs independent of oxygen tension. In the presence of normal oxygen tension, the radical anion $(R-NO_2)$ interacts with oxygen yielding superoxide and noncharged misonidazole; the noncharged misonidazole then diffuses out of the cell. In the presence of low tissue oxygen tension, the misonidazole anion is reduced further yielding nitro so compounds and hydroxylamines which have a lower permeability and are retained within the cells. Another compound BMS-194796 is a more hydrophilic nitroimidazole than BMS-181321 and has higher myocardial retention following transient ischemia and less retention in the liver. Thus the class of nitroimidazole compounds offer promise for positive imaging of ischemic myocardium [34].

Thrombus and atherosclerotic plaque imaging

Several blood components can be labeled for thrombus imaging. These include red blood cells, some of the clotting factors, fibrinogen, fibrin and platelets. The composition of arterial thrombus differs from venous thrombus; the arterial thrombus is being platelet rich while the venous thrombus is fibrin rich. Thus the selection of which imaging agent to use is determined to a great extent on the type of thrombus that is clinically suspected. Other factors that are important for thrombus imaging include: the delivery rate of the radiolabeled agent to the thrombus site; the specificity of the binding site for active thrombosis; number of binding sites; affinity of radiolabeled compounds for binding sites; detachment rate; clearance of background activity and the size of the agents. The ultimate goal is to be able to image the atherosclerotic plaque especially the unstable plaque responsible for unstable angina pectoris, acute myocardial infarction or sudden death. This field is rapidly advancing, for example it is known that smooth muscle hyperplasia plays an important role in the formation of the atherosclerotic plaque. It is likely that in the process of plaque formation there is also transformation of these muscle cells from the contractile phenotype to the synthetic phenotype. This is associated with up regulation of the purine P_2 receptors. Technetium 99m AP4A has been used to image these receptors in an animal model with atherosclerosis [34].

References

1.   Maddahi J. Myocardial perfusion imaging for the detection and evaluation of coronary artery disease. In: Skorton DJ, editor. Marcus Cardiac imaging. 2nd ed. Philadelphia: Saunders; 1996. p. 971-96.
2.   Maddahi J, Rodrigues E, Berman DS, Kiat H. State-of-the-art myocardial perfusion imaging. Cardiol Clin 1994;12:199-222.
3.   Lette J, Tatum JL, Fraser S *et al.* Safety of dipyridamole testing in 73.806 patients: the multicenter dipyridamole safety study. J Nucl Cardiol 1995;2:3-17.
4.   Cerqueira MD, Verani MS, Schwaiger M, Heo J, Iskandrian AS. Safety profile of adenosine stress perfusion imaging: results from the Adenoscan Multicenter Trial Registry. J Am Coll Cardiol 1994;23:384-9.
5.   Maddahi J, Czernin J. Absolute quantitation of myocaridal blood flow: the technical and clinical prospects for single-photon emission computed tomography. J Nucl Cardiol 1996;3(6 pt 2):S60-5.
6.   Gambhir SS, Hoh CK, Phelps ME, Madar I, Maddahi J. Decision tree sensitivity analysis for cost-effectiveness of FDG-PET in the staging and management of non-small-cell lung carcinoma. J Nucl Med 1996;37:1428-36.

7. Maddahi J, Gambhir SS. Cost-effective selection of patients for coronary angiography. J Nuc Cardiol 1997;4(2 pt 2):S141-51.

8. Brown KA, Boucher CA, Okada RO *et al.* Prognostic value of exercise thallium-201 imaging in patients presenting for evaluation of chest pain. J Am Coll Cardiol 1983;1:994-1001.

9. Heller GV, Brown KA. Prognosis of acute and chronic coronary artery disease by myocardial perfusion imaging. Cardiol Clin 1994;12:271-89.

10. Maddahi J, Ashouri S, Rokhsar S, Flamm H, Schelbert H, Phelps M. Prognostic value of a normal rest-stress myocardial perfusion positron emission tomography (PET): a long term follow up study [abstract]. J Am Coll Cardiol 1998;31(2 Suppl A):479A.

11. Brown K, Rowen M. Prognostic value of a normal exercise myocardial perfusion imaging study in patients with angiographyically significant coronary artery disease. Am J Cardiol 1993;71:865-7.

12. Ladenheim ML, Pollock BH, Rozanski A, *et al.* Extent and severity of myocardial hypoperfusion as predictors of prognosis in patients with suspected coronary artery disease. J Am Coll Cardiol 1986;7:464-71.

13. Kaul S, Finkelstein DM, Homma S, Leavitt M, Okada RD, Boucher CA. Superiority of quantitative exercise thallium-201 variables in determining long-term prognosis in ambulatory patients with chest pain: a comparison with cardiac catheterization. J Am Coll Cardiol 1988; 12:25-34.

14. Kaul S, Lilly D, Gascho J *et al.* Prognostic utility of the exercise thallium- 201 test in ambulatory patients with chest pain: comparison with cardiac catheterization. Circulation 1988;77:745-58.

15. Pollock SG, Abbott RD, Boucher CA, Beller GA, Kaul S. Independent and incremental prognostic value of tests performed in hierarchial order to evaluate patients with suspcted coronary artery disease. Validation of models basedon these tests. Circulation 1992;85:237-48.

16. Berman DS, Hachamovitch R, Kiat H *et al.* Incremental value of prognostic testing in patients with known or suspected ischemic heart disease: a basis for optimal utilization of exercise technetium-99m sestamibi myocardial perfusion single-photon emission computed tomography. J Am Coll Cardiol 1995;26:639-47.

17. Ladenheim ML, Kotler TS, Pollock BH, Berman DS, Diamond GA. Incremental prognostic power of clinical history, exercise electrocardiography and myocardial perfusion scintigraphy in suspected coronary artery disease. Am J Cardiol 1987;59:270-7.

18. Nallamothu N, Pancholy SB, Lee KR, Heo J, Iskandiran AS. Impact on exercise single-photon emission computed tomographic thallium imaging on patient management and outcome. J Nucl Cardiol 1995;2:334-8.

19. Bateman TM, O'Keefe JH, Dong VM, Barnhart C, Ligon RW. Coronary angiographic rates after stress single-photon emission computed tomographic scintigraphy. J Nucl Cardiol 1995;2:217-23.

20. Epstein SE, Palmeri ST, Patterson RE. Current conepts: evaluation of patients after acute myocardial infarction: indications for cardiac catheterization and surgical intervention. N Engl J Med 1982;307:1487-92.

21. Gibson RS, Watson DD, Craddock G, *et al.* Prediction of cardiac events after uncomplicated myocardial infarction: a prospective study comparing predischarge exercise thallium-201 scintigraphy and coronary angiography. Circulation 1983;68:321-36.

22. Gimple LW, Beller GA. Assessing prognosis after acute myocardial infarction in the thrombolytic era. J Nucl Cardiol 1994;1:198-209.

23. Mahmarian JJ, Pratt CM, Nishimura S, Abren A, Verani MS. Quantitative adenosine 201-Tl single-photon emission computed tomography for the early assessment of patients surviving acute myocardial infarction. Circulation 1993;87:1197-210.

24. Maddahi J, Blitz A, Phelps M, Laks H. The use of positron emission tomography in the management of patients with ischemic cardiomyopathy. Adv Card Surg 1996;7:163-88.

25. Alderman EL, Fisher LD, Litwin P *et al.* Results of coronary artery surgery in patients with poor left ventricular function (CASS). Circulation 1983;68:785-95.

26. Maddahi J, Schelbert H, Brunken R, Di Carli M. Role of thallium-201 and PET imaging in evaluation of myocardial viability and management of patients with coronary artery disease and left ventricular dysfunction. J Nucl Med 1994;35:707-15.

27. Eitzman D, Al-Aouar Z Kanter HL *et al.* Clinical outcome of patients with advanced coronary artery disease after viability studies with positron emission tomography. J Am Coll Cardiol 1992;20:559-65.

28. Di Carli MF, Davidson M, Little R *et al.* Value of metabolic imaging with positron emission tomography for evaluating prognosis in patients with coronary artery disease and left ventricular dysfunction. Am J Cardiol 1994;73:527-33.

29. Di Carli MF, Asgarzadie F, Schelber HR *et al.* Quantitative relation between myocardial viability and improvement in heart failure symptoms after revascularization in patients with ischemic cardiomyopathy. Circulation 1995;92:3436-44.

30. Tamaki N, Kawamoto M, Takahashi N *et al.* Prognostic value of an increase in fluorine-18 deoxyglucose uptake in patients with myocardial infarction: comparison with stress thallium imaging. J Am Coll Cardiol 1993;22:1621-7.

31. Lee KS, Marwick TH, Cook SA *et al.* Prognosis of patients with left ventricular dysfunction, with and without viable myocardium after myocardial infarction. Relative efficacy of medical therapy and reascularization. Circulation 1994;90:2687-94.

32. Duong TH, Hendi P, Fonarow G *et al.* Role of positron emission tomographic assesment of myocardial viability in the management of patients who are referred for cardiac transplantation [abstract]. Circulation 1995;92(8 Suppl):I123.

33. Maddahi J, Czernin J. Absolute quantitation of myocardial blood flow: the technical and clinical prospects for single-photon emission computed tomography. J Nucl Cardiol 1996;3(6 pt 2):S60-5.

34. Iskandiran AE, Maddahi J. Nuclear cardiology: new developments and future directions. J Nucl Cardiol 1997;4(2 pt 2):S189-92.

21.

State-of-the-art in myocardial perfusion SPECT imaging

Ernest V. Garcia, Tracy L. Faber,
C. David Cooke & Russell D. Folks

Summary

State-of-the-art instrumentation and computer methods in myocardial perfusion SPECT imaging are now either available or soon to be available to clinicians worldwide. Advancements in instrumentation such as multiple detector systems and attenuation correction techniques have resulted in myocardial perfusion images with higher spatial and contrast resolution, more counts, and less degradation due to radiation absorption and scatter. Advancements in computer methods have evolved in key areas such as: multiple gated SPECT acquisition, automation, measurement of functional parameters, three-dimensional displays, image fusion and the use of artificial intelligence in decision support systems. These advancements in computers methods applied to higher quality images from the instrumentation advancements have resulted in tools which allow the clinicians to make a more comprehensive and accurate assessment of their patients' myocardial status. These advancements continue to strengthen the already strong role of myocardial perfusion SPECT imaging in the diagnosis and prognosis of patients with coronary artery disease.

Introduction

Major technical advancements in instrumentation and computer methods are finding their way from the research laboratories to routine clinical use. Advancements in instrumentation include the use of multiple detector systems to increase imaging performance and attenuation correction methods to compensate for physical factors that degrade image quality and quantitative accuracy.

The most dramatic advancements have been realized in new computer methods. The availability of affordable computers with ever increasing speed, memory and application software have allowed the development and implementation of state-of-the-art clinical tools to facilitate the acquisition, processing, analysis, display and interpretation of myocardial perfusion SPECT studies. These advancements include: a) the acquisition of multiple gated projections to allow simultaneous assessment of myocardial perfusion and function, b) total automation of the reconstruction and slice reorientation process, c) total automation of identifying and isolating the left ventricular (LV) myocardium for quantification of myocardial perfusion and function, d) total automation of LV endocardial and epicardial border definition for assessment of regional and global functional parameters, e) three-dimensional

J.H.C. Reiber and E.E. van der Wall (eds.). What's New in Cardiovascular Imaging, 279–292.
©1998 Kluwer Academic Publishers.

(3D) display of myocardial distributions for improved visualization of myocardial perfusion and function, f) image fusion techniques to register 3D coronary vasculature reconstructed from coronary arteriography onto 3D myocardial perfusion distributions for the comprehensive assessment of myocardial physiology and anatomy, and g) expert systems and artificial neural nets to assist the physician in interpreting these results. The rest of this chapter discusses these advancements in detail.

Advances in instrumentation

Multiple detector systems

SPECT acquisitions with single-head detectors usually take from 20 to 40 minutes due to the relatively low number of photons per unit time that are counted and since a considerable number of counts per pixel are required to generate diagnostic images. The use of multiple detectors immediately increases the throughput of a laboratory by decreasing the total time required to acquire the same number of counts. For 180° orbit SPECT acquisition of the heart, the optimal detector configuration is two heads separated 90° apart, since the full orbit may be acquired in half the time with only a 90° motion. For optimal 360° acquisition the triple-headed systems are preferred with each head separated by 120° [1]. This decrease in acquisition time also reduces patient discomfort and patient movement. The increase in sensitivity may also be traded for an increase in resolution resulting in studies with higher spatial and contrast resolution that are easier to interpret.

Attenuation correction

There are physical phenomena that degrade the degree with which the myocardial counts represent tracer activity and thus diagnostic accuracy. These are: a) the variable attenuation [absorption and scatter] by the thorax of the photons emitted from the myocardium, b) the incorrect counting of photons scattered into the detector's crystal, and c) the limited and variable nature of the spatial resolution across the myocardial tracer distribution. Variable attenuation correction methods are presently being commercialized to compensate for (a) above. This correction requires a transmission source mounted on the SPECT system that allows the acquisition of a transmission study. Emission and transmission studies should be acquired simultaneously to prevent increased acquisition time and misregistration. This simultaneous acquisition requires an additional correction (d) for the additional scatter generated from the patient into the transmission source's photopeak. These studies are used by an iterative reconstruction algorithm running on state-of-the-art workstations to generate attenuation corrected images. These attenuation corrected images, although usually of higher diagnostic quality that uncorrected images, are not generally corrected for (b), (c) and sometimes (d) above. This can result in images with "unfamiliar" artifacts. Another limitation is that most commercialized attenuation correction procedures do not allow for simultaneous R-wave synchronized multiple gated acquisition.

Because there is so much variability in the implementation of these correction methodologies it is wise to delay the use of a specific implementation until extensive clinical results are documented characterizing the accuracy of each approach. Ficaro et al. reported on a clinical trial of his correction technique applied to patients from his institution which yielded increased sensitivity and particularly increased specificity for detecting coronary artery disease (CAD) [2]. Hendel et al. has reported on a multicenter clinical trial that used the ExSPECT algorithm developed at Emory to correct for attenuation, scatter and depth dependent resolution [3]. This evaluation showed a highly statistically significant increase in normalcy rate with no loss in sensitivity. Normalcy rate is the rate of detecting patients with low likelihood of CAD as being normal. In light of these and other findings, experts recommend that attenuation corrected studies should only be interpreted side by side with the non-corrected studies in order to optimize diagnostic accuracy.

Advances in computer methods

Most commercial nuclear medicine computer systems now have the capability of acquiring and reconstructing multiple-gated tomographic studies. This feature has promoted the use of SPECT for assessing cardiac global and regional function, including the assessment of left ventricular ejection fraction, LV end-diastolic and systolic volumes, and LV myocardial wall motion and thickening. These assessments are being primarily investigated using gated SPECT imaging of the Tc-99m myocardial perfusion tracers and more recently with thallium-201.

Oblique reorientation and reslicing

Most cardiac images are viewed in a standard format, consisting of short axis, horizontal long axis, and vertical long axis slices. Short axis slices are also necessary for some automatic perfusion quantification algorithms. Generation of these standard sections from the original transaxial images has been performed interactively, requiring the user to mark the location of the left ventricular axis. In the past few years, some automatic techniques for performing this task have become commercially available [4,5].

These two approaches start by identifying the left ventricular region in the transaxial images, using a threshold-based approach that includes knowledge about expected position, size, and shape of the LV. Once isolated, the approach described by Germano et al. [4] uses the original data to refine the estimate of the myocardial surface. Normals to an ellipsoid fit to the LV region are used to resample the myocardium; a gaussian function is fit to the profiles obtained at each sample. The best fit gaussian is used to estimate the myocardial center for each profile, and after further refinement based on image intensities and myocardial smoothness, the resulting mid-myocardial points are fit to an ellipsoid whose long axis is used as the final LV long axis. The method was tested on 400 patient images, and the result compared to interactively denoted long axes. Failure of the method was described as either not localizing the LV, presence of significant hepatic or intestinal activity in the 'LV' region of the image, or greater than 45° difference between automatically and interactively determined axes. With these criteria, the method was successful in 394 of the 400 cases.

Mullick et al. [5] use a more complex heuristic technique to determine the optimal LV threshold and isolate it from other structures. After this is accomplished, they use the segmented data directly to determine the long axis. The binary image is tessellated into triangular plates, and the normal of each plate on the endocardial surface is used to 'Point to' the LV long axis. The intersection of these normals (or near-intersections) are collected and fit to a 3-d straight line, which is then returned as the LV long axis. This method was tested on 124 patient datasets, and the automated long axis orientation was compared to interactively determined angles. Failure was described as a failure to isolate the left ventricle, and this method succeeded in 116 of 124 cases.

Automated perfusion quantification

Data-based methods for identifying a patient's myocardial perfusion abnormalities from Tl-201 SPECT studies have been previously developed and commercialized by investigators at Cedars-Sinai Medical Center [6] and Emory University [7] and reported as early as 1985. These methods utilized a statistically defined database of normal patients to be used as a pattern to compare prospective CAD patients. Although these methods have been extensively validated and proven to be clinically valuable in standardizing and objectifying myocardial perfusion scans, they have been limited by several deficiencies.

Five major limitations have been identified with these early approaches. One limitation has been the extensive operator interaction. This results in a reduced objectivity and reproducibility of the program. By automating the process this limitation has been overcome, as was partially addressed in the previous section. A second limitation has been the failure to sample the count distribution perpendicular to the myocardial wall, particularly at the apex. This usually results in artifactually increasing the counts from the apical region. A third limitation has been the lack of databases for perfusion tracers other than Tl-201. Comparison of patients acquired with different tracers and/or different protocols to the Tl-201 database often leads to incorrect identification of abnormalities. A fourth limitation has been the inability of these data-based approaches to compensate for attenuation in a patient whose attenuating tissue (such as breast and diaphragm) is significantly more than those of the normal patients selected for the normal database. This almost always leads to artifactually defining these photopenic regions as hypoperfused myocardium. The fifth limitation has been the inability of the polar map display to represent accurately the true extent and location of an abnormality. This is due to the warping created by transforming a three-dimensional distribution into a two dimensional polar map. This limitation results in underestimating the extent of hypoperfused apical regions and overestimating the extent of hypoperfused basal regions.

More recently, investigators working at Emory University and Cedars-Sinai Medical Center have developed [8] and extensively validated [9] a new data-based quantitative package known as CEqual® (Cedars-Emory Quantitative Analysis) designed to overcome the above-mentioned limitations. The attributes of this approach are described below.

Methods. This quantitative method uses several image identification techniques (e.g. image clustering, filtered thresholding, and specified threshold constraints) for isolation of the left myocardium from the remainder of the image. Once the left myocardium is identified, the apical and basal image slices, the (x, y) coordinates of the central axis of the ventricular chamber, and a limiting radius for the maximum count circumferential profile search are determined automatically. In the majority of cases, operator interaction is required only for verification of automatically determined parameters. If at any time the program fails to locate any of the features, it will branch to an interactive mode and require the operator to select the parameters manually.

The CEqual technique has been developed to generate count profiles from a hybrid, two-part, three-dimensional sampling scheme of stacked short-axis slices. In this approach the apical region of the myocardium is sampled using spherical coordinates, and the rest of the myocardium is sampled using cylindrical coordinates. This approach promotes a radial sampling which is mostly perpendicular to the myocardial wall for all points and thus results in a more accurate representation of the perfusion distribution with minimal sampling artifacts. Following operator verification of the automatically derived features, the three-dimensional maximum count myocardial distribution is extracted from all stacked short axis tomograms [8]. Maximum count circumferential profiles, each comprised of 40 points, are automatically generated from the short-axis slices using this 2-part sampling scheme. These profiles are generated for the stress and rest myocardial perfusion distributions. A normalized percent change between stress and rest is also calculated as a reversibility circumferential profile. The most normal region of the stress distribution is used for normalizing the rest to the stress distribution.

New databases. Using the CEqual approach, normal limits were defined from a group of patients with less than 5% probability of coronary artery disease. Gender matched normal databases have been defined and validated for the following SPECT protocols: 1. Low dose rest, high dose stress, one-day Tc-99m sestamibi (Cardiolite) protocol; 2. High dose stress and rest two-day Tc-99m sestamibi protocol; 3. Stress-redistribution Tl-201 protocol; 4. Rest Tl-201/ stress Tc-99m sestamibi dual isotope protocol; and 5. Low dose stress, high dose rest Tc-99m Tetrofosmin (Myoview) one day protocol. All protocols used treadmill exercise to stress the patients.

Display

Once perfusion has been quantified, the quantitative data must be displayed. SPECT perfusion data requires complex methods of display in order to present the larger amount of information clearly and logically. Polar maps were developed as a way to display the quantified perfusion data of the entire left ventricle in a single picture. More recently, three-dimensional displays have been adopted by many researchers, hospitals, and manufacturers as a more natural way to present the information.

Polar maps. Polar maps, or bull's-eye displays, are the standard for viewing circumferential profiles. They allow a quick and comprehensive overview of the circumferential samples from all slices by combining these into a color-coded image. The points of each circumferential profile are assigned a color based on normalized count values, and the colored profiles are shaped into concentric rings. The most apical slice processed with circumferential profiles forms the center of the polar map, and each successive profile from each successive short axis slice is displayed as a new ring surrounding the previous. The most basal slice of the left ventricle makes up the outermost ring of the polar map.

The use of color can help identify abnormal areas at a glance, as well. Abnormal regions from the stress study can be assigned a black color, thus creating a blackout map. Blacked-out areas that normalize at rest are color-coded white, thus creating a whiteout reversibility map. Additional maps, e.g., a standard deviation map that shows the number of standard deviations below normal of each point in each circumferential profile, can aid in evaluation of the study by indicating the severity of any abnormality.

Polar maps, while offering a comprehensive view of the quantitation results, distort the size and shape of the myocardium and any defects. There have been numerous improvements in the basic polar map display to help overcome some of these problems. For instance, 'distance-weighed' maps are created so that each ring is the same thickness. These maps have been shown to be useful for accurate localization of abnormalities. 'Volume-weighed' maps are constructed such that the area of each ring is proportional to the volume of the corresponding slice. This type of map has been shown to be best for estimating defect size. However, more realistic displays have been introduced which do not suffer from the distortions of polar maps.

3-Dimensional displays. Three-dimensional graphics techniques can be used to overlay results of perfusion quantification onto a representation of a specific patient's left ventricle. This representation is generated using endocardial or epicardial surface points extracted from the perfusion data. For example, the method used at Emory for detecting the surface of the myocardium starts with the coordinates of the maximal myocardial count samples created during perfusion quantification. The coordinates of each sampled point are filtered to remove noise. By assuming that the myocardium is 1cm thick at end diastole, an estimate of the endocardial surface can be generated by subtracting a distance of 5mm from the myocardial center point. Adding 5mm estimates the epicardial surface. Other investigators have also used the surface model for displaying myocardial perfusion.

Once extracted, boundary points can be connected into triangles or quadrilaterals, which are in turn connected into a polygonal surface representing the endocardial and/or epicardial surface. Once a surface is generated, perfusion is displayed by assigning to each triangle or quadrilateral a color corresponding to the counts extracted from the myocardium at that sample during a quantification process. Colors can be interpolated between triangles to produce a continuum of colors across the myocardium, or the triangles can be left as patches of distinct color.

Surface models can generally be displayed using standard computer graphics packages, allowing rotations and translations of the model, positioning of one or more light sources, and adjustment of the model's opacity (the amount of light shining through the model) or reflectance (the amount of light reflecting off of the model). Figure 1 shows the 3-dimensional representation of a patient's processed myocardial perfusion study.

Integration of multimodality cardiac imagery

Often, more than one type of imaging procedure is used to evaluate patients for cardiac disease. Coronary angiography is the gold standard for diagnosis of coronary artery stenosis; magnetic resonance imaging is performed to determine gross anatomy, and SPECT is used to evaluate myocardial perfusion. There are major advantages in automatically reorienting and rescaling multimodality images so that they are in the same position and orientation as each other, and in displaying their information in a unified manner. This process is termed multimodality registration, fusion, or unification. While physicians frequently perform this image integration mentally, automating the processes may improve their ability to assimilate the large amount of data and to draw meaningful conclusions from it. Following automatic unification, comparisons between information contained in the studies are straightforward, since cardiac structures can be viewed in the same orientation or sliced in the same manner. Cause and effect relationships may be more apparent, and anatomy and physiology may be

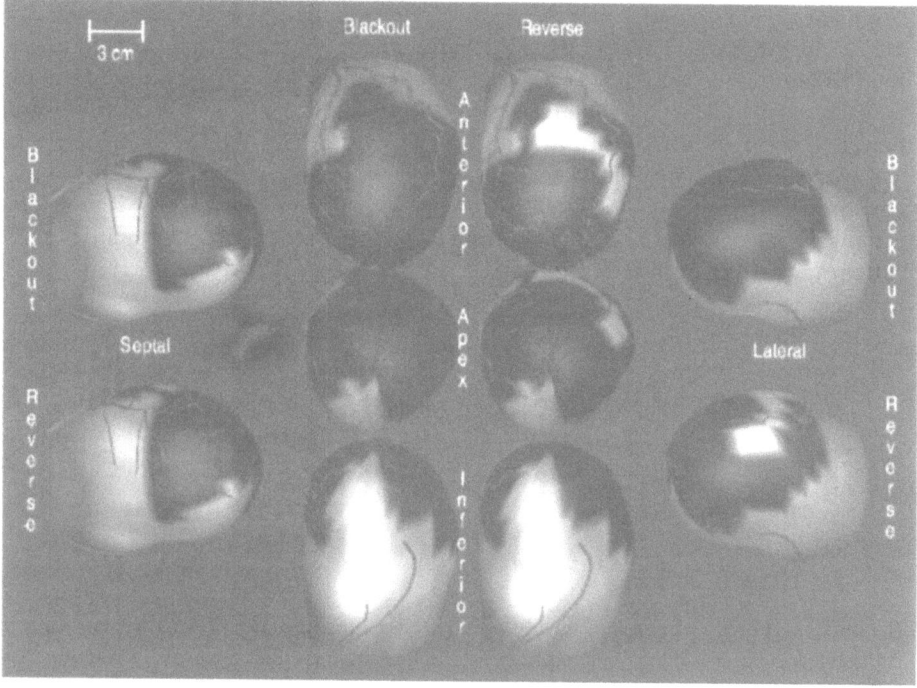

Figure 1. Three-dimensional display of the myocardial perfusion distribution. This is a 3-D display of a patient's myocardial perfusion distribution depicted from different orientations after the distribution has been compared to a dual isotope normal data base (Tc-99m sestamibi stress/ TI-201 rest). The colors are indicative of the amount of tracer uptake which is related to myocardial perfusion with the lighter colors representing higher myocardial flow. The "Blackout" results highlights in black the regions of the stress study which were statistically abnormal. The "Reverse" results highlights in white the regions of the rest study that statistically improved at rest and were found at stress to be abnormal. Superimposed is a generic set of coronaries to be used as a road map to assign a region of the myocardium to a vascular territory. This patient exhibits extensive anterolateral and anteroseptal stress perfusion defects with partial reversibility at rest (For color figure, see color section).

more easily compared. In the following sections, four approaches to automatic integration of cardiac nuclear medicine images with other modality data are described.

Registration of myocardial perfusion and magnetic resonance images. Registration of SPECT perfusion images with magnetic resonance (MR) images of the same patient was first demonstrated by Faber et al. [10]. This method requires that endocardial surfaces be detected in both sets of images. The end-diastolic and end-systolic frames are then determined using the chamber volumes computed from those surfaces. A cost function consisting of the distance of the MR end-diastolic surface from the SPECT end-diastolic surface plus the distance of the MR end-systolic surface from the SPECT end-systolic surface is minimized over translation and rotation in three dimensions. The resulting transform is then applied to the SPECT image itself, along with an interpolation between frames, so that the images match in both time and space. Therefore, myocardial thickening observed in MR images can be directly compared to perfusion information evaluated from the SPECT images in the same areas of the heart.

Registration of SPECT and coronary angiographic data. Ideally, accurate assessment of the extent and severity of coronary artery disease requires the integration of physiologic information derived from SPECT perfusion images and anatomic information derived from coronary angiography. This integration has been performed by registering a 3-d left ventricular model representing myocardial perfusion with the patient's own 3-d coronary artery tree, and presenting both in a single unified display. The patient-specific coronary arterial tree is obtained from a 3-d geometric reconstruction performed on simultaneously acquired, digital, biplane angiographic projections, or from two single plane projections acquired at different angles [11]. The 3-d reconstructed arterial tree is approximated by successive conical segments, and scaled and rotated to fit onto the myocardial surface. The left and/or right coronary arteries are registered with the myocardial perfusion surface model by automatically minimizing a cost function that describes the relationships of the coronary artery tree with the interventricular and atrioventricular groove and the surface of the myocardium. Figure 1 illustrates this unified display. Recent reports have described preliminary validations of this technique in animal studies [12]; human study validations are currently being performed. Similar work has been reported by Krause et al. [13].

Gated SPECT acquisition and reconstruction

Acquisition consists of performing multiple gated acquisition at each of the planar projections for the same total time per projection. These acquisitions are usually obtained over 180% at one minute or less per projection so as to maintain the total study time to within 30 minutes to an hour. Because of both the short acquisition time per projection and the consideration of reconstruction times, the number of frames per cardiac cycle are kept to a minimum, i.e., between 8 and 16. It has been shown that although 16 frames result in slightly better accuracy for determining regional function, 8 frames are adequate and take less space and processing time [14]. Although several imaging protocols are used, the most popular one is to gate the stress Tc-99m perfusion study in order to simultaneously obtain a stress perfusion distribution but a resting functional distribution. This offers promise for screening patients who have not had a previous myocardial infarction with a single acquisition [15].

The reconstruction process is the same as that of non-gated SPECT except that each of the frames per cardiac cycle have to be shuffled so that individual projection sets are created for each frame of the cardiac cycle. Once reconstructed into transaxial slices, each set is reconstructed along the same oblique angles in order to generate vertical, horizontal and short axis slices that have the same orientation from frame to frame. The program then reshuffles back each of the slices from each of the 8 individual tomographic sets into sets of 8 frames, multiple-gated tomographic slices which may be displayed in a closed-loop cine format for assessment of cardiac function.

Visual assessment of myocardial thickening

Assessment of myocardial thickening uses the fact [16] that objects such as myocardial walls smaller than two spatial resolution distances in thickness (~26 mm) exhibit a maximal count which is proportional to the thickness of the object. This is sometimes referred as the partial-volume effect. Thus visual assessment consists of determining if each region of the myocardium brightens as the myocardium thickens at end-systole. If a region brightens (or changes in color) then is must be thickening. If it thickens then it must be viable, although a sub-endocardial MI cannot be ruled out since it is a combination of necrotic and viable tissue.

Increased specificity. It has been shown that cine display of the beating myocardial perfusion distribution throughout the cardiac cycle has been useful in identifying imaging artifacts, particularly attenuation artifacts. DePuey et al. have shown that visual assessment of myocardial thickening may differentiate MI from artifacts since fixed defects with decreased function probably represent MI, whereas attenuation artifacts either have normal function or at least do not demonstrate markedly reduced function [17]. In a study of 551 consecutive patients referred for evaluation of CAD of 78 patients with fixed defects and no clinical MI 60 had normal defect function. Because most of the fixed defects with normal systolic function occurred in women with anterior fixed defects or men with inferior fixed defects, these were most likely attenuation artifacts. With this assessment patients with unexplained fixed defects decreased from 14% to 3%.

Quantification of global and regional function

Quantification of global and regional parameters requires knowledge of the endocardial and (depending on the parameter being determined) the epicardial surface throughout the cardiac cycle. These surface points may be manually assigned or automatically detected. Manual methods are subjective and time consuming. The automated methods use either boundary (edge) detection or geometric modeling.

St. Luke's-Roosevelt approach. In this approach reported by DePuey et al. [17] using a manual method and Nichols et al. [18] using an automated method endocardial borders are defined from mid-ventricular vertical and horizontal long-axis slices. The manual method used operator definition of the borders corresponding to a 34% count level of the maximum count. The automated method automatically determined the LV center. Endocardial borders at end-diastole (ED) and end-systole were generated by searching inward from the location of the maximal counts along the myocardium to the previously pre-determined threshold. Once the endocardial borders are defined at ED and ES, LVEF is then computed by the Simpson's rule method, corrected for the average resolution (point spread function) of the SPECT camera.

Validation of the manual method using EFs from 30 patients who had undergone planar gated blood pool imaging yielded correlation coefficients ranging from .79 to .88 depending on the operator with inter- and intra-observer reproducibility of r = 0.75. The automated method was also validated using 75 patients who had undergone equilibrium gated blood pool imaging yielding a correlation of r = .87 and in 65 patients who had undergone gated first pass also yielding a correlation of r = .87. Inter- and intra-observer agreement was also assessed (r = .92 and .94, respectively) resulting in a significant improvement over the manual methods.

Cedars-Sinai approach. In the approach reported by Germano et al. [4,19] automatic border definition is done using thresholds of a Gaussian function pre-calibrated to a phantom. Although it has been shown that the spatial resolution of SPECT is too low to actually measure the edges of the endocardial surface, the pre-calibration to a phantom and the high tolerance of the EF calculation to these borders results in clinically useful results. This approach has become popular because it was the first to offer commercially totally automatic processing from beginning to end [4] for both Tc-99m sestamibi and Tl-201. The initial publication reported successful complete automatic oblique axis reorientation in 93.6% of 700 processed studies; more recent reports using prospective patients report an 83% total success rate [19]. The approach also automated segmentation and contouring of the LV's endocardial and epicardial surfaces claiming a 100% success rate in 65 patients [19] and a correlation with first pass data of r = .909, SEE = 6.87%.

Emory approach. In the approach developed at Emory [14,20] geometric modeling is used. The model uses the maximal count circumferential profile points obtained from the perfusion quantification of the LV as the center of the myocardium. The program assumes that the myocardial thickness at end-diastole (ED) is 1 cm throughout and calculates myocardial thickening throughout the cardiac cycle by using Fourier analysis. This analysis assumes that the change in count is proportional to the change in thickness, a by-product of the partial-volume effect described above. By determining the center and absolute thickness of the LV myocardium at ED, the center of the myocardium throughout the cardiac cycle, and the percent thickening from frame-to-frame 3D geometric models of the endocardial and epicardial surfaces are created for each time interval in the cardiac cycle. Once the orientation of the LV is determined, either manually or using commercially available automatic reorientation algorithms, the program generation of the endocardial and epicardial surfaces is totally automatic. These surfaces are then used for all the necessary measurements of global and regional function such as ED and ES volumes, LV myocardial mass and LV ejection fraction.

Faber et al. [21] have used this methodology to validate these functional parameters. Using a cohort of 80 patients who had undergone first-pass ventricular angiography at two institutions (Emory and St.Luke's-Roosevelt) to compare against the determination of LVEF as 100* (EDV-ESV)/EDV resulted in the following correlation: y=.94x +5.4%, r = .82, SEE = 8.5%. Faber et al. [22] have also performed a sensitivity analysis which shows that these calculations are quite insensitive of the assumptions used. This analysis showed that even if the true ED myocardial thickness was 1.5 cm over the entire ventricle rather than the 1.0 assumed by this approach the EF error would only be 6%.

Faber et al. [21] have also used this methodology in patients who have undergone gated MR to validate ED and ES volumes, LV myocardial mass [23] and LV ejection fraction as well as the actual shapes of the surfaces [24]. These validations yielded excellent results.

Cooke et al. [14] have also reported that using a Fourier analysis methodology clinically useful determinations of myocardial thickening can be obtained even when using the 8 gated frame methodology and even when the counts in a hypoperfused wall fall to 5% of the normal count level. This Fourier analysis determines the phase and amplitude of the counts changes throughout the cardiac cycle for each 3D myocardial sample. Figures 2 and 3 show the functional results of the patient example illustrated in Figure 1.

Artificial intelligence techniques applied to SPECT

Interpretation of medical images by decision-support systems has made significant progress in recent years, mostly due to the implementation of artificial intelligence (AI) techniques. Expert systems and neural networks are two AI techniques that are currently being applied in myocardial perfusion SPECT imaging.

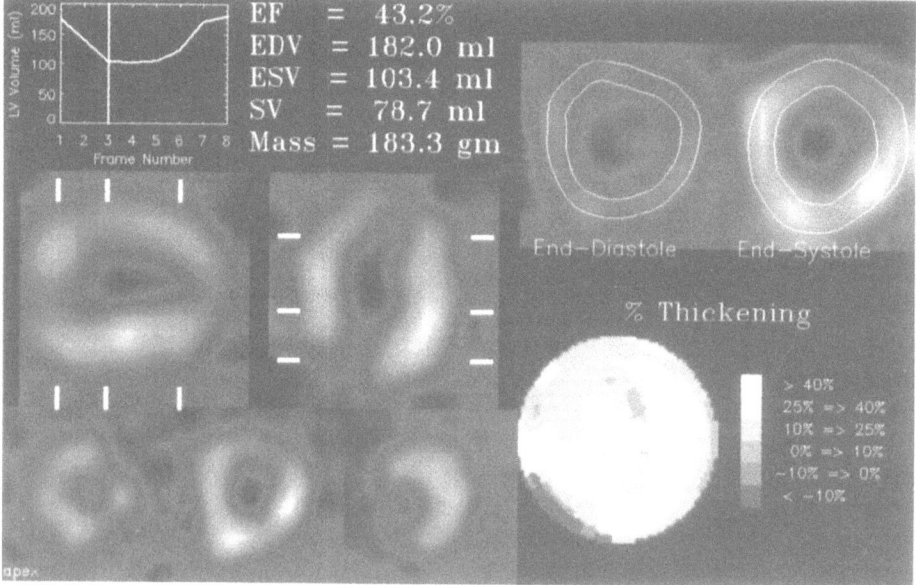

Figure 2. Display of myocardial function parameters for the patient shown in Figure 1. This comprehensive report includes the patient's LV volume-time curve, ejection fraction (EF), end-diastolic volume (EDV), end-systolic volume (ESV), stroke volume (SV) and total LV mass as calculated using the Emory CEqual-EGS approach. The report also includes in the lower right panel a polar map of myocardial thickening as measured using amplitude and phase analysis. The map is color coded to correspond to the % thickening color bar on its right. The lower left panel may be used for a cinematic display of the LV to visually assess wall motion and wall thickening (For color figure, see color section).

An example of the power of expert systems is found in PERFEX® (PERfusion EXpert), a preliminary system which has been developed and validated to assist in diagnosing coronary artery disease from 3-D myocardial perfusion distributions [25]. This type of approach has the potential for standardizing the image interpretation process. The use of neural networks has also been used by different groups in nuclear cardiology to identify which coronaries are expected to have stenotic lesions for a specific hypoperfused distribution [26].

Conclusion

Perfusion quantification methods will continue to evolve with and adapt to nuclear cardiology and the changing needs of physicians in specific, and to nuclear medicine technology and the health care system in general. The high level of automation already achieved in myocardial perfusion imaging is unmatched by any other cardiac imaging modality, and continues to be its major strength. In addition, strong statistical evaluations of the accuracy and validity of the various techniques have been made possible simply because of the large amount of objectivity and standardization in the automated processes. These strengths should be built upon and enhanced to demonstrate the value of nuclear cardiology in patient management, and most importantly, to maintain the highest quality clinical care.

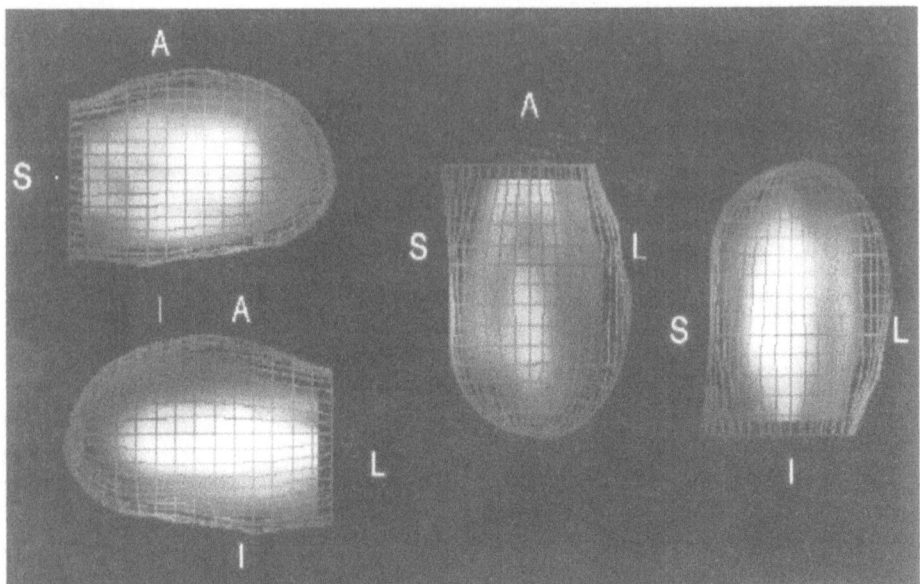

Figure 3. Three-dimensional display of myocardial function. This is a 3-D display of a patient's myocardial endocardial surface at end-diastole (mesh) and at end-systole (solid surface) depicted from different orientations. This display may be viewed in a dynamic fashion to visually assess wall motion as the excursion of the wall and wall thickening as the change in color. The color is a function of both myocardial perfusion and myocardial thickness. A myocardial segment that increases in color brightness indicates thickening and thus viable myocardium. This patient exhibits extensive anterolateral and anteroseptal resting wall motion and wall thickening abnormalities. (Abbreviations: A = anterior, S = septal, L = lateral and I = inferior) (For color figure, see color section).

Several methods are now commercially available that provide an accurate determination of left ventricular ejection fraction and other parameters of global and regional function from gated SPECT myocardial perfusion studies of Tc-99m perfusion agents and Tl-201. The methods vary in their degree of automation, approach for endocardial and epicardial surface definition, accuracy of determining absolute volume, accuracy of determining regional function and methods of display. It is highly recommended that all perfusion studies be complemented by the quantitative measurement of LVEF from gated SPECT perfusion studies.

These advancements coupled with the advancements in instrumentation such as the use multiple detectors and correction methodologies continue to strengthen the already strong clinical role of myocardial perfusion SPECT imaging.

References

1.   Garcia EV. Quantitative myocardial perfusion single-photon emission computed tomographic imaging: Quo vadis? (Where do we go from here?). J Nucl Cardiol 1994;1:83-93.
2.   Ficaro EP, Fessler JA, Ackerman RJ, Rogers WL, Corbett JR, Schwaiger M. Simultaneous transmission/emission myocardial perfusion tomography. Diagnostic accuracy of attenuation corrected 99mTc-sestamibi single-photon emission computed tomography. Circulation 1993;3:463-73

3.   Hendel RC, Berman DS, Cullom SJ, Follansbee WP, Braymer WK, Heller GH. Diagnostic value of SPECT myocardial perfusion imaging utilizing attenuation and scatter correction with resolution compensation: results of a multicenter trial. Circulation 1997;8:I-308.

4.   Germano G, Kavanagh PB, Su HT *et al.* Automatic reorientation of 3-dimensional transaxial myocardial perfusion SPECT images. J Nucl Med 1995;36:1107-14.

5.   Mullick R, Ezquerra NF. Automatic determination of left ventricular orientation from SPECT data. IEEE Trans Med Imag 1995;14:88-99.

6.   Garcia EV, Van Train K, Maddahi J *et al.* Quantification of rotational thallium- 201 myocardial tomography. J Nucl Med 1985;26:17-26.

7.   DePasquale E, Nody A, DePuey G *et al.* Quantitative rotational thallium-201 tomography for identifying and localizing coronary artery disease. Circulation 1988;77:316-27.

8.   Garcia EV, Cooke CD, Van Train KF *et al.* Technical aspects of myocardial perfusion SPECT imaging with Tc-99m sestamibi. Am J Cardiol 1990;66:23-31E.

9.   Van Train KF, Garcia EV, Maddahi J *et al.* Multicenter trial validation for quantitative analysis of same-day rest-stress technetium-99m-sestamibi myocardial tomograms. J Nucl Med 1994;35:609-168.

10. Faber TL, McColl RW, Opperman R, Corbett JR, Peshock RM. Spatial and temporal registration of cardiac SPECT and MR images: Methods and evaluation. Radiology 1991;179:857-64.

11. Peifer JW, Ezquerra NF, Cooke CD *et al.* Visualization of multimodality cardiac imagery. IEEE Trans on Biomed Engineering 1990;37:744-56.

12. Faber TL, Klein JL, Folks RD *et al.* Automatic unification of 3-d cardiac perfusion with 3-d coronary artery anatomy, In Computers in Cardiology, IEEE Computer Society, Los Alamitos, California 1996, in press.

13. Krause T, Fischer R, Solzback U. 3-d fusion of myocardial perfusion scintigraphy and coronary angiography [abstract]. J Nucl Med 1996;37:218P.

14. Cooke CD, Garcia EV, Cullom SJ, Faber TL, Pettigrew RI. Determining the accuracy of calculating systolic wall thickening using a fast fourier transform approximation: a simulation study based on canine and patient data. J Nucl Med 1994;35:1185-92.

15. Chua CT, Germano G, Maurer G, Van Train K, Friedman J, Berman D. Gated technetium-99m sestamibi for simultaneous assessment of stress myocardial perfusion, postecercise regional ventricular function and myocardial viability. Correlation with echocardiography and rest thallium-201 scintigraphy. J Am Coll Cardiol 1994;23:1107-14.

16. Galt JR, Garcia EV, Robbins W. effects of myocardial wall thickness on SPECT Quantification. IEEE Trans Med Imaging 1990;9:144-50.

17. DePuey EG, Rozanski A. Using gated technetium-99m-sestamibi SPECT to characterize fixed myocardial defects as infarct or artifact. J Nucl Med 1995;36:952-5.

18. Nichols K, DePuey EG, Rozanski A. Automation of gated tomographic left ventricular ejection fraction. J Nucl Med 1996;3:475-82.

19. Germano G, Kiat H, Kavanagh PB *et al.* Automatic quantification of ejection fraction from gated myocardial perfusion SPECT. J Nucl Med 1995;36:2138-47.

20. Vansant JP, Faber TL, Folks RD, Rao JM, Garcia EV. Resting left ventricular volumes and ejection fraction from gated SPECT: correlation to first pass [abstract]. Circulation, 1995;92:I11.

21. Faber TL, Cooke CD, Folks RD, Vansant JP, Klein JL, Garcia EV. An integrated processing program for analysis of left ventricular function and perfusion. Computers in Cardiology 1997;24:697-700.

22. Faber TL, Cooke CD, Vansant JP, Garcia EV. Sensitivity of an Automated ejection fraction calculation from gated perfusion tomograms to modeling assumptions [abstract]. J Nuc Med 1996;37:213P.

23. Faber TL, Folks RD, Cooke CD, Vansant JP, Pettigrew RI, Garcia EV. Left ventricular mass from ungated perfusion images: Comparison to MRI. J Nucl Med 1997;38:20P.

24. Faber TL, Cooke CD, Peifer JW *et al.* Three-dimensional displays of left ventricular epicardial surface from standard cardiac SPECT perfusion quantification techniques. J Nucl Med 1995;36:697-703.

25. Garcia EV, Cooke CD, Krawczynska E *et al.* Expert system interpretation of technetium-99m sestamibi myocardial perfusion tomograms: enhacements and validation. Circulation 1995;92:I-10.

26. Hamilton D, Riley PJ, Miola UJ, Amro AA. A feed forward neural network for classification of bull's-eye myocardial perfusion images, Eur J Nucl Med 1995;22:108-15.

22. State of the art in the assessment of ventricular function by gated SPECT

Berthe L.F. van Eck-Smit

Summary

The developments of 99m-technetium (^{99m}Tc) labeled perfusion agents, multi-headed gamma cameras and computer software programs have made tomographic techniques suitable for clinical use. Tomography has the advantage of superior diagnostic capabilities that result from increased image contrast and three-dimensional data representation. Nowadays, there are two major nuclear tomographic modalities for the assessment of left ventricular function i.e. gated blood pool SPECT and gated myocardial perfusion SPECT. The diagnostic efficacy of gated blood pool SPECT has been validated by compating it with planar blood pool imaging, contrast ventriculography, echocardiography, and MRI. The more recently developed gated myocardial perfusion SPECT has mainly been compated with planar blood pool measurements and contrast ventriculography. Both gated SPECT modalities demonstrated to be an accurate method for the assessment of left ventricular function in patients with and without coronary artery disease.

Introduction

In the last decades cardiovascular radionuclide tomography has become one of the corner stones of the noninvasive assessment of myocardial perfusion and function. The development of ^{99m}Tc labeled perfusion agents, multi-headed gamma cameras and computer software programs made tomographic techniques suitable for clinical use. Tomography has the advantage of superior diagnostic capabilities that result from increased image contrast and three-dimensional data representation. Nowadays, there are two major nuclear tomographic modalities for the assessment of left ventricular function: Gated blood pool single photon emission computed tomography (SPECT) and gated myocardial perfusion SPECT.

Gated blood pool SPECT

Left ventricular ejection fraction (LVEF) has proven to be one of the most powerful predictors of survival in patients with coronary artery disease [1-8]. Planar gated blood pool radionuclide angiography (RNA) is an established modality widely used for the noninvasive assessment of global and regional ventricular function. The method was first described by Strauss et al. in 1971 [9]. Since then the quantitative measurement of LVEF and qualitative

J.H.C. Reiber and E.E. van der Wall (eds.). What's New in Cardiovascular Imaging, 293–298.
©1998 Kluwer Academic Publishers.

assessment of regional wall motion by RNA has proven to be an accurate and reproducible way of assessing LV function. The mean inter- and intra-observer variability is < 2% and the inter-study variability is < 5% [10,11]. However, planar imaging suffers from the same problems as all imaging modalities using projectional images. With two-dimensional compression of three-dimensional data, important structures in such images may be hidden or masked by objects in front or behind these. To overcome some of the major limitations of planar imaging, SPECT may be used. An advantage of gated SPECT over planar studies is the analysis of the cardiac blood pool in three dimensions. Moreover, the tomographic technique allows reconstruction of images in any plane, resulting in complete separation of the cardiac chambers and yielding slices of the heart without overlapping counts from background tissue. This results in an increase in contrast resolution and the ability to discern differences in tracer concentration in neighboring structures [12]. Although the SPECT technique has been available for more than fifteen years, its development and widespread clinical utilization have been hampered by four closely related factors: prolonged acquisition time, large data sets, excessive processing time and limited system sensitivity of single detector tomographic systems. The development of multi-detector gamma cameras and advances in computer hardware and software have made gated blood pool SPECT practical.

Gated SPECT imaging of the left ventricular blood pool

Gated SPECT RNA is generally performed after in vivo labeling of autologous red blood cells with 740 MBq (20 mCi) of ^{99m}Tc pertechnetate 20 minutes after administration of stannous pyrophosphate. Acquisition of SPECT data is usually performed with 8 to 24 frames per cardiac cycle. Sixteen time intervals are considered adequate for an accurate assessment of systolic function [13].

Ideally gated SPECT studies are acquired at 3° increments over a range of 360°, with acquisition matrices of 128 x 128 pixels. These strategies will minimize the occurrence of artifacts.

Analysis of images: left ventricular ejection fraction and volumes

Global left ventricular volumes and left ventricular ejection fraction can be calculated using a surface-rendering method to define the ventricular volume of interest. The voxels within this volume are summed at each time frame throughout the cardiac cycle. When the total number of left ventricular voxels are multiplied by the calibrated volume per voxel, the left ventricular volume can be determined without geometric assumption. To determine the borders of the left ventricle either an iso-count contour can be employed or the second-derivate (gradient) can be searched for within the individual slices [14-21].

Wall motion is often assessed visually or semi-quantitatively [17], although quantitative analysis has been described with increasing frequency. The methods employed include endocardial surface tracking from iso-count contours or gradient- determined endocardial searches [15,19-21], and phase analysis [22,23].

Clinical applications and comparison with other imaging modalities

The primary clinical implication of gated blood pool SPECT is the evaluation of patients with coronary heart disease. Many studies have demonstrated the diagnostic efficacy of gated

SPECT in comparison with planar blood pool imaging and contrast ventriculography [15,17,24,25]. Studies comparing gated blood pool SPECT with contrast ventriculography or echocardiography have found that SPECT blood pool studies identified wall motion abnormalities as well or better than the modalities compared [15,17,24,26]. Gated SPECT studies appear to be of greatest value in the identification of wall motion abnormalities involving the inferior, posterior, and mid- to-basal septal segments. As the analysis of contrast ventriculography and echocardiography is performed on single or biplane projections, these methods have geometric limitations which will result in sampling bias, especially in case of myocardial infarction.

Despite the limitations of contrast ventriculography and echocardiography, Murano et al. reported an excellent linear correlation between left ventricular end-diastolic volume assessed by gated SPECT and echocardiography (r=0.98, P<0.01) and between gated SPECT and contrast ventriculography (r=0.89, P<0.01)in a population of 20 patients, including 13 patients with ischemic heart disease, 3 patients with hypertrophic cardiomyopathy and 2 patients with dilated cardiomyopathy [27].

In a direct comparison of gated blood pool tomography with [11]CO positron emission tomography (PET) and gated myocardial perfusion imaging using ^{99m}Tc-Sestamibi, Cross et al. reported a positive correlation (r=0.89, P<0.001) between PET and SPECT in normal controls and in patients with proven left ventricular dysfunction [28].

Assessment of left ventricular function and wall motion with gated blood pool SPECT was compared with magnetic resonance imaging (MRI) and ^{99m}Tc-Sestamibi gated myocardial perfusion imaging by Faber et al. [21]. Automatic motion measurements in the apical and mid ventricular regions of both SPECT modalities agreed well with MR images of the same patients; the average error in these areas was 0.32 mm. The largest error was found in the septal region, whereby the largest differences and standard deviations were found in the basal regions.

In a recent study by Chin et al., right and left ventricular ejection fractions determined by gated blood pool SPECT was compared with MRI and conventional first pass planar scintigraphy in 18 patients [29]. Absolute ventricular volumes showed excellent correlation with MRI for both right ventricular volumes (r=0.91, slope= 0.90, SEE = 15.7) and left ventricular volumes (r=0.96, slope= 0.88, SEE = 18.2). For left ventricular ejection fraction there was also an excellent correlation between gated blood pool SPECT and MRI.

Gated myocardial perfusion imaging

Myocardial perfusion imaging using ^{99m}Tc-labeled agents has become a commonly used procedure for the evaluation of ischemic heart disease. The ability for the combined assessment of perfusion and left ventricular function from gated SPECT perfusion images has only recently been demonstrated [30-40].

Gated myocardial perfusion SPECT is generally performed 1 hour after i.v. administration of 500-750 MBq (15-20 mCi) of ^{99m}Tc-Sestamibi or [99m]Tc- Tetrofosmin. Acquisition of SPECT data is performed with 8 or 16 frames per cardiac cycle. Most gated myocardial SPECT studies are acquired at 3°-6° increments over a range of 360°, with acquisition matrices of 64 x 64 pixels.

Analysis of images

In summary, the measurement of left ventricular ejection fraction is based on changes in endocardial surface position [30-36] or based on changes in count density during the cardiac cycle [37-40]. Most of the reported software programs are commercially available and easily installed on modern gamma camera computer systems. The majority of these programs automatically select, analyze, quantitate, and display the key image data in myocardial perfusion studies. In contrast to most other imaging techniques, the procedure is virtually operator independent.

Clinical applications and comparison with other imaging modalities

Measurements of ejection fraction and assessment of wall motion have been tested in patients and have been compared with other imaging modalities. In most studies left ventricular ejection fraction measurements correlated excellently with planar radionuclide angiography [32,34,35] and contrast ventriculography [31] showing correlation coefficients ranging from 0.70-0.93.

Conclusion

Tomographic imaging is a natural extension of the technologies of planar gated blood pool imaging and myocardial perfusion imaging. The most important additional value of tomography to gated blood pool imaging seems to be the improved assessment of wall motion abnormalities and optional measurement of right ventricular function. Gated SPECT has expanded the applications of myocardial perfusion imaging to include the evaluation of left ventricular size and regional wall motion. The accuracy of both new modalities for the assessment of left ventricular function and the detection of wall motion abnormalities correlate well with other imaging modalities such as contrast ventriculography, echocardiography and MRI.

References

1.   Shaw LJ, Peterson ED, Kesler K, Hasselblad V, Califf RM. A meta-analysis of predischarge risk stratification after acute myocardial infarction with stress electrocardiographic, myocardial perfusion, and ventricular function imaging. Am J Cardiol 1996;78:1327-37.
2.   Borges-Neto S, Shaw LJ, Kesler K *et al.* Usefulness of serial radionuclide angiography in predicting cardiac death after coronary artery bypass grafting and comparison with clinical and cardiac catheterization data. Am J Cardiol 1997;79:851-5.
3.   Nicrd P, Corbett JR, Firth BG *et al.* Prognostic value of resting and submaximal exercise radionuclide ventriculography after acute myocardial infarction in high-risk patients with single and multivessel disease. Am J Cardiol 1983;52:30-6.
4.   Corbett JR, Dehmer GJ, Lewis SE *et al.* The prognostic value of submaximal exercise testing with radionuclide ventriculography before hospital discharge in patients with recent myocardial infarction. Circulation 1981;64:535-44.
5.   Iskandrian AS, Hakki AH, Goel IP, Mundth ED, Kane-Marsch SH, Schenk CL. The use of rest and exercise radionuclide ventriculography in risk stratification in patients with suspected coronary artery disease. Am Heart J 1985;110:864-72.

6.   Iqbal A, Gibbons RJ, Zinsmeister AR, Mock MB, Ballard DJ. Prognostic value of exercise radionuclide angiography in a population-based cohort of patients with known or suspected coronary artery disease. Am J Cardiol 1994;74:119-24.

7.   Johnson SH, Bigelow C, Lee KL, Pryor DB, Jones RH. Prediction of death and myocardial infarction by radionuclide angiocardiography in patients with suspected coronary artery disease. Am J Cardiol 1991;67:919-26.

8.   Shaw LJ, Heinle SK, Borges-Neto S, Kesler K, Coleman RE, Jones RH. Prognosis by measurements of left ventricular function during exercise. J Nucl Med 1998;39:140-6.

9.   Strauss HW, Zaret BL, Hurley PJ, Natarajan TK, Pitt B. A scintiphotographic method for measuring left ventricular ejection fraction in man without cardiac catheterization. Am J Cardiol 1971;28:575-80.

10.   Wackers FJ, Berger HJ, Johnstone DE *et al.* Multiple gated cardiac blood pool imaging for left ventricular ejection fraction: validation of the technique and assessment of variability. Am J Cardiol 1979;43:1159-66.

11.   Hecht HS, Josephson MA, Hopkins JM, Singh BN. Reproducibility of equilibrium radionuclide ventriculography in patients with coronary artery disease: response of left ventricular ejection fraction and regional wall motion to supine bicycle exercise. Am Heart J 1982;104:567-74.

12.   Fischman AJ, Moore RH, Gill JB, Strauss HW. Gated blood pool tomography: a technology whose time has come. Semin Nucl Med 1989;19:13-21.

13.   Bacharach SL, Green MV, Borer JS. Instrumentation and data processing in cardiovascular nuclear medicine: evaluation of ventricular function. Semin Nucl Med 1979;9:257-74.

14.   Tauxe WN, Soussaline A, Todd-Pokropek A *et al.* Determination of organ volume by single-photon emission tomography. J Nucl Med 1982;23:984-7.

15.   Gill JB, Moore RH, Tamaki N *et al.* Multigated blood-pool tomography: new method for the assessment of left ventricular function. J Nucl Med 1986;27:1916-24.

16.   Underwood SR, Walton S, Laming PJ *et al.* Left ventricular volume and ejection fraction determined by gated blood pool emission tomography. Br Heart J 1985;53: 216-22.

17.   Corbett JR, Jansen DE, Lewis SE *et al.* Tomographic gated blood pool radionuclide ventriculography: analysis of wall motion and left ventricular volumes in patients with coronary artery disease. J Am Coll Cardiol 1985;6:349-58.

18.   Myers RW, Bails RP, Reed VR *et al.* Angiocardiography with the seven-pinhole collimator: evaluation of methodology and accuracy in assessing global and regional left ventricular function. Clin Nucl Med 1982;7:151-6.

19.   Faber TL, Stokely EM, Peshock RM, Corbett JR. A model-based four dimensional left ventricular surface detector. IEEE Trans Med Imaging 1991;10:321-9.

20.   Ekman M, Lomsky M, Stromblad SO, Carlsson S. Closed-line integral optimization edge detection algorithm and its application in equilibrium radionuclide angiocardiography. J Nucl Med 1995;36:1014-8.

21.   Faber TL, Akers MS, Peshock RM, Corbett JR. Three-dimensional motion and perfusion quantification in gated single-photon emission computed tomograms. J Nucl Med 1991;32:2311-7.

22.   Yamashita K, Tanaka M, Asada N *et al.* A new method of three dimensional analysis of left ventricular wall motion. Eur J Nucl Med 1988;14:113-9.

23.   Graf G, Mester J, Clausen M *et al.* Reconstruction of Fourier coefficients: a fast method to get polar amplitude and phase images of gated SPECT. J Nucl Med 1990;31:1856-61.

24.   Underwood SR, Walton S, Ell PJ, Jarritt PH, Emanuel RW, Swanton Rh. Gated blood pool emission tomography: a new technique for the investigation of cardiac structure and function. Eur J Nucl Med 1985;10:332-7.

25.   Bartlett ML, Srinivasan G, Barker WC, Kitsiou AN, Dilsizian V, Bacharach SL. Left ventricular ejection fraction: comparison of results from planar and SPECT gated blood-pool studies. J Nucl Med 1996;37:1795-9.

26.   Cerqueira MD, Harp GD, Ritchie JL. Quantitative gated blood pool tomographic assessment of regional ejection fraction: definition of normal limits. J Am Coll Cardiol 1992;20:934-41.

27.   Murano K, Narita M, Kurihara T. Left ventricular function assessed by multigated blood pool single photon emission tomography with 99m Tc [Japanese]. J Cardiol 1992;22:245-53.

28.   Cross SJ, Lee HS, Metcalfe MJ, Norton MY, Evans NT, Walton S. Assessment of left ventricular regional wall motion with blood pool tomography: comparison of 11CO PET with 99Tcm SPECT. Nucl Med Commun 1994;15:283-8.

29.   Chin BB, Bloomgarden DC, Xia W et al. Right and left ventricular volume and ejection fraction by tomographic gated blood-pool scintigraphy. J Nucl Med 1997;38:942-8.

30.   Germano G, Kiat H, Kavanagh PB *et al.* Automatic quantification of ejection fraction from gated myocardial perfusion SPECT. J Nucl Med 1995;36:2138-47.

31.   Williams KA, Taillon LA. Left ventricular function in patients with coronary artery disease assessed by gated tomographic myocardial perfusion images. Comparison with assessment by contrast ventriculography and first-pass radionuclide angiography. J Am Coll Cardiol 1996;27:173-81.

32.   De Puey EG, Nichols K, Dobrinsky C. Left ventricular ejection fraction assessed from gated technetium-99m-sestamibi SPECT. J Nucl Med 1993;34:1871-6.

33.   Najm YC, Timmis AD, Maisey MN *et al.* The evaluation of ventricular function using gated myocardial imaging with Tc-99m MIBI. Eur Heart J 1989;10:142-8.

34.   Yang KTA, Chen HD. A semi-automated method for edge detection in the evaluation of left ventricular function using ECG-gated single photon emission tomography. Eur J Nucl Med 1994;21:1206-11.

35.   Boonyaprapa S, Ekmahachai M, Thanachaikun N, Jaiprasert W, Sukthomya V, Poramatikul N. Measurement of left ventricular ejection fraction from gated technetium-99m sestamibi myocardial images. Eur J Nucl Med 1995;22:528-31.

36.   Everaert H, Franken PR, Flamen P, Goris M, Momen A, Bossuyt A. Left ventricular ejection fraction from gated SPECT myocardial perfusion studies: a method based on the radial distribution of count rate density across the myocardial wall. Eur J Nucl Med 1996;23:1628-33.

37.   Marcassa C, Marzullo P, Parodi O, Sambuceti G, L'Abbate A. A new method for noninvasive quantitation of segmental myocardial wall thickening using technetium-99m 2-methoxy-isobutyl-isonitrile scintigraphy: results in normal subjects. J Nucl Med 1990;31:173-7.

38.   Mochizuki T, Murase K, Fujiwara Y, Tanada S, Hamamoto K, Tauxe WN. Assessment of systoloc thickening with thallium-201 ECG-gated single-photon emission computed tomography: a parameter for local left ventricular function. J Nucl Med 1991;32:1496-500.

39.   Calnon DA, Kastner RJ, Smith WH, Segalla D, Beller GA, Watson DD. Validation of a new count-based gated single photon emission computed tomography method for quantifying left ventricular systolic function: comparison with equilibrium radionuclide angiography. J Nucl Cardiol 1997;4:464-71.

40.   Smith WH, Kastner RJ, Calnon DA, Segalla D, Beller GA, Watson DD. Quantitative gated single photon emission computed tomography imaging: a counts-based method for display and measurement of regional and global ventricular systolic function. J Nucl Cardiol 1997;4:451-63.

23.   Assessment of myocardial viability by FDG imaging with SPECT

Jeroen J. Bax, Frans C. Visser, Jan-Hein Cornel, Paolo M. Fioretti, Arthur van Lingen, Ernst E. van der Wall & Cees A. Visser

Summary

The use of F18-fluorodeoxyglucose (FDG) imaging with single photon emission computed tomography (SPECT) to assess myocardial viability has been introduced recently. Several centers have now gained experience with cardiac FDG SPECT imaging; this report provides a summary of the currently available data on FDG SPECT. A good agreement between FDG PET and FDG SPECT has been shown in various studies. Studies in patients undergoing revascularization show that FDG SPECT can predict improvement of regional and global left ventricular (LV) function after revascularization. Improvement of global LV function requires the presence of a substantial amount of viable tissue. Initial results in patients with ischemic cardiomyopathy undergoing revascularization suggest that FDG SPECT can also predict improvement of heart failure symptoms. Thus, FDG SPECT appears useful in the pre-operative evaluation of patients with depressed LV function (secondary to chronic coronary artery disease) undergoing revascularization.

FDG imaging can also provide prognostic information. Positron emission tomographic studies with FDG have demonstrated that the presence of viable tissue is associated with a high mortality when these patients are treated medically. Currently, no prognostic FDG SPECT studies are available. Additional studies are needed to determine whether FDG SPECT can also provide this prognostic information.

Introduction

In patients with reduced left ventricular (LV) function due to chronic coronary artery disease, reversal of LV dysfunction is possible after adequate revascularization. To explain this improvement of LV function following revascularization, the concepts of hibernation and repetitive stunning have been proposed [1]. Hibernation is defined as a condition of chronically reduced perfusion accompanied by a reduction of contractile function, which can be reversed after coronary revascularization [1]. Recent studies however have shown that many regions with "hibernating" myocardium had near-normal perfusion [2-4]. Accordingly, Vanoverschelde has proposed the term "repetitive stunning", assuming that recurrent attacks of ischemia may result in a chronic depression of contractile function [1].

Independent of the underlying mechanism of the chronic dysfunction, assessment of viability is nowadays becoming implemented in the decision-making process concerning the

J.H.C. Reiber and E.E. van der Wall (eds.). What's New in Cardiovascular Imaging, 299–310.
©1998 Kluwer Academic Publishers.

optimal therapeutic approach in individual patients with ischemic cardiomyopathy. It is well-known that medical treatment of this subset of patients carries a poor prognosis [5]. Excellent long-term survival has been reported following heart-transplantation; this approach however is unable to meet the increasing demand for donor hearts [5]. In addition, revascularization may offer an alternative therapeutic strategy in patients with LV dysfunction due to chronic coronary artery disease. Although survival benefit following revascularization as compared to conventional medical therapy was demonstrated [6], revascularization of these patients is associated with a relatively high (peri-)operative morbidity and mortality [7]. Therefore, the clinical challenge is to identify the patients with jeopardized but viable myocardium and predict adequately improvement of LV function after revascularization.

A large variety of techniques has been introduced to assess viable myocardium, including scintigraphic techniques [8], low-dose dobutamine echocardiography [9] and magnetic resonance techniques [10]. Metabolic imaging with F18-fluorodeoxyglucose (FDG) and positron emission tomography (PET) is considered a very accurate technique to assess viability [11]. Many studies have indeed demonstrated that FDG PET can adequately predict functional recovery after revascularization [12]. Currently, the availability of PET facilities is limited and much effort has been invested to develop single photon emission computed tomographic (SPECT) imaging with FDG using 511 keV collimators [13-16]. In this review the current status of FDG SPECT imaging is discussed.

FDG SPECT study protocol and viability criteria

Optimal identification of jeopardized but viable myocardium requires integration of information on contractile function, perfusion and metabolic status of the myocardium. In our previous studies the following protocol was used. First, wall motion was evaluated by resting two-dimensional echocardiography to identify regions with contractile dysfunction. Next, resting perfusion was assessed by early thallium-201 SPECT [17] and metabolic activity was evaluated by FDG SPECT. The FDG studies were performed during hyperinsulinemic glucose clamping [18]; this approach has been demonstrated to yield the best image quality in FDG PET studies [18] and to minimize heterogeneity in myocardial FDG uptake [19]. Different FDG-perfusion patterns were observed (Table 1). Viability on FDG SPECT in seg-

Table 1: FDG-perfusion patterns

Tissue characterization	contraction	perfusion	FDG uptake
transmural scar	↓	severe ↓	severe ↓
nontransmural scar	↓	mild ↓	mild ↓
stunning	↓	N	N / ↑
hibernation	↓	↓	N / ↑

ments with contractile dysfunction was defined when perfusion was normal (consistent with repetitive stunning) or when increased FDG uptake was present in perfusion defects (FDG-perfusion mismatch, consistent with hibernation). Scar tissue was characterized by a concordant reduction in perfusion and FDG uptake (FDG-perfusion match). An example of a patient with a FDG-perfusion mismatch is demonstrated in Figure 1. In these studies we have applied sequential perfusion-FDG imaging; more recently the use of dual-isotope dual-acquisition has been validated [14,20,21]. This approach is less time-consuming and avoids misalignment between the FDG and perfusion study.

TL/FDG SPECT

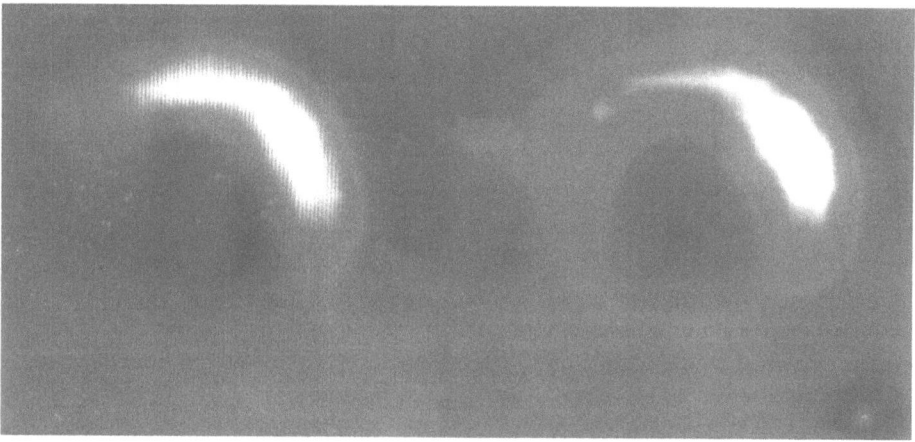

Figure 1. Corresponding short-axis slices of a patient with a perfusion defect on the early thallium-201 image (representing perfusion, left) in the infero-septal region and relatively increased FDG uptake (representing glucose utilization) in the septum. The area of FDG-perfusion mismatch represents viable myocardium (from reference 11, with permission) (For color figure, see color section).

Developments in patient preparation prior to FDG imaging

Myocardial FDG uptake depends mainly on the plasma levels of FFA and insulin [22]. High insulin levels promote cardiac FDG uptake, whereas high FFA levels inhibit FDG uptake. As stated in the previous paragraph, the hyperinsulinemic euglycemic clamp was used to optimize FDG image quality. With the infusion of insulin, cardiac FDG uptake is stimulated directly and indirectly (by depression of peripheral lipolysis thereby lowering plasma FFA levels). For clinical routine however, the use of the hyperinsulinemic euglycemic clamp may be too time-consuming and laborious. Recently, Knuuti et al. [23] have demonstrated that oral administration of a nicotinic acid derivative (Acipimox, Byk, The Netherlands) may be an alternative to clamping. Acipimox inhibits peripheral lipolysis, thus reducing plasma FFA levels. Knuuti and colleagues [23] have performed a direct comparison between hyperinsulinemic euglycemic clamping and Acipimox in 12 patients with coronary artery disease. During both protocols plasma levels of the various substrates were measured. As expected, insulin levels were high during clamping and low after Acipimox administration. Importantly, plasma levels of FFA were comparably low after Acipimox and during clamping. The myocardial FDG uptake patterns were compared visually, showing no differences.

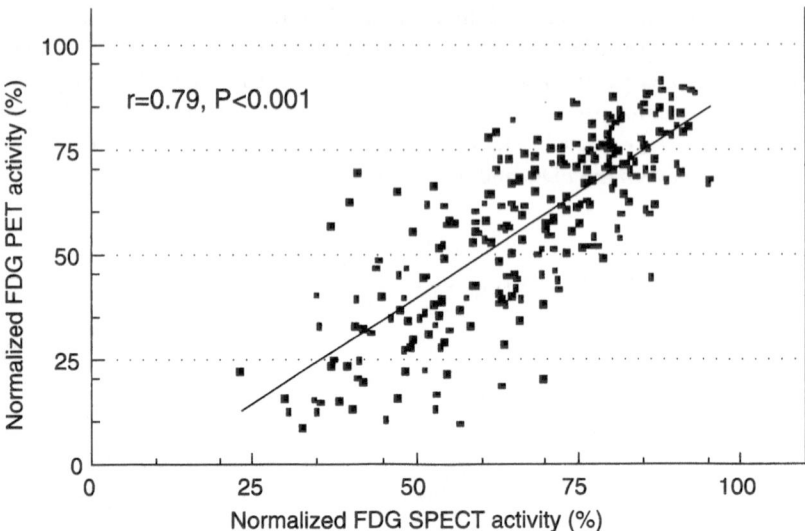

Figure 2. Scatter plot showing the relation between the normalized FDG PET and FDG SPECT activities (from reference 14, with permission).

Radioactivity levels (blood and myocardium) were computed from the images, revealing higher FDG activities in the myocardium and blood after Acipimox as compared to the clamping protocol. The myocardium-to-blood ratio (frequently used as a measure of image quality) was comparable after both approaches. Importantly, no side-effects of Acipimox (besides flushing) were observed. Similar results were obtained with the FDG SPECT approach [24]. Hence, the use of Acipimox may further facilitate routine FDG imaging.

Comparison between FDG SPECT and FDG PET

Several studies have compared FDG PET with FDG SPECT [15,25-27], showing a good agreement between PET and SPECT in the assessment of viable myocardium. Martin et al. [26] evaluated myocardial viability in 9 patients with FDG PET and FDG SPECT. Eight of 9 patients had perfusion-FDG matches, indicating necrotic tissue and 4 patients had additional regions of perfusion-FDG mismatch, suggesting viable myocardium. The number, size and location of the matches and mismatches were not different between PET and SPECT. Similar findings were reported by 2 other studies [25,27]. A similar study was performed at the Free University Hospital Amsterdam in combination with the PET Center Groningen, except that the PET data were analyzed quantitatively and the SPECT data semi-quantitatively [14]. In Figure 2, the relation between the normalized FDG PET and FDG SPECT activities is shown. Moreover, all segments with normalized FDG uptake <40% on SPECT were nonviable by PET, whereas in the segments with FDG uptake >90% only 3% of the segments were nonviable by PET. Consequently, the frequency of viable segments by PET increased from 0% in the segments with FDG uptake <40% on SPECT, to 97% in the segments with FDG uptake >90% on SPECT (Figure 3). The main shortcoming of these comparative studies is the lack of outcome after revascularization.

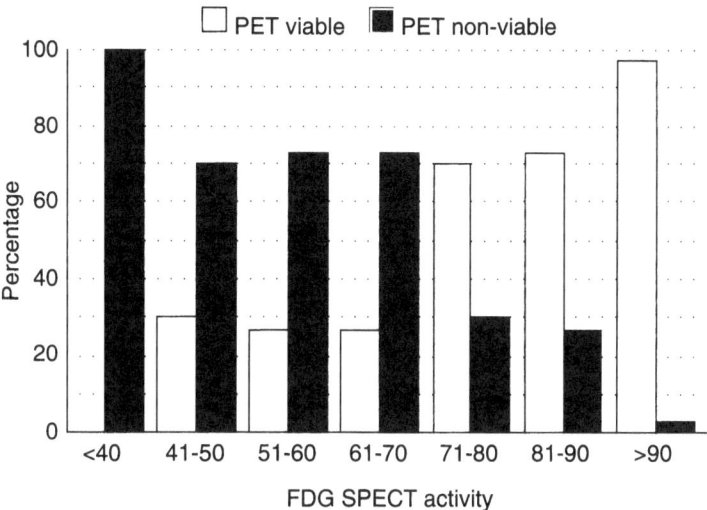

Figure 3. Bar graph demonstrating the relation between the normalized FDG SPECT activity and viability on FDG PET (from reference 11, reproduced with permission).

FDG SPECT to predict functional outcome after revascularization

Other studies have focused on the prediction of functional outcome after revascularization [28,29]. In a recent study, we have evaluated the use of FDG SPECT in the prediction of improvement of regional wall motion after revascularization [29]. We prospectively studied 20 patients who were already scheduled for revascularization (12 CABG and 8 PTCA). Recovery of function, as assessed by echocardiography 3 months after the revascularization, served as the gold standard for viable myocardium. Of the 17 segments classified viable by FDG SPECT, 14 (82%) improved in regional wall motion after revascularization. In contrast, only 3 of 28 (11%) segments classified nonviable on FDG SPECT improved in function after revascularization. In the viable segments the mean wall motion score improved from 1.5 ± 0.7 to 0.7 ± 0.7 (P<0.01, see Figure 4); in the nonviable segments the mean wall motion score remained unchanged (1.7 ± 0.6 versus 1.7 ± 0.5, ns). These data indicate that FDG SPECT can predict improvement of regional function after revascularization.

Clinically more important is the prediction of improvement of global LV function. In another study, we have evaluated prediction of improvement of LV ejection fraction (EF) after revascularization by FDG SPECT in 22 patients with depressed LV function (LVEF <30%) [28]. The patients were arbitrarily divided into 2 groups: 14 patients had ≥3 viable, dysfunctional segments on FDG SPECT and 8 patients had 2 or less viable, dysfunctional segments. The LVEF increased significantly in the first group, from 25 ± 6% to 32 ± 6% (P<0.01) after revascularization (Figure 5). In the second group, the LVEF remained unchanged after the revascularization (24 ± 6% vs 25 ± 6%, ns).

Finally, preliminary data are available on the prediction of improvement of heart failure symptoms after revascularization. Thirty-two patients with ischemic cardiomyopathy (mean LVEF 28 ± 6%) undergoing revascularization were studied. Heart failure symptoms (func-

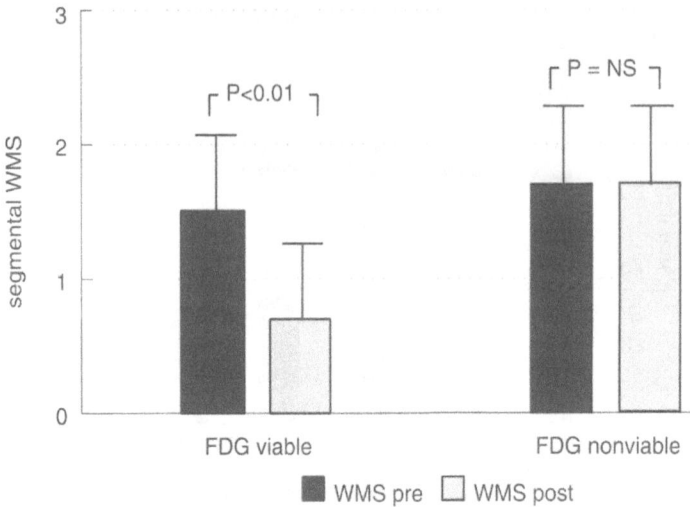

Figure 4. Bar graph showing the mean wall motion score (WMS) in segments with and without viability on FDG SPECT. In the viable segments the mean WMS decreased significantly after revascularization, whereas the mean WMS remained unchanged in the nonviable segments (data based on reference 28).

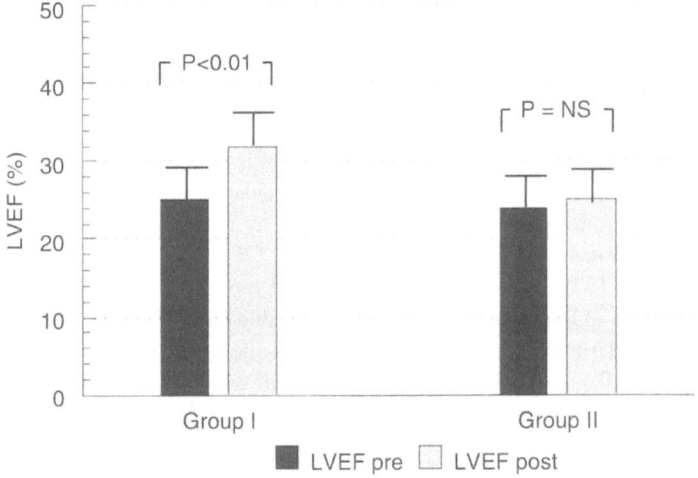

Figure 5. Bar graph showing the improvement in left ventricular ejection fraction (LVEF) after revascularization in patients with substantial viability on FDG SPECT (≥3 viable dysfunctional segments, group I). In the patients without substantial viability (2 or less dysfunctional viable segments, group II) the LVEF remained unchanged (from reference 29 with permission).

tional status) were graded according to the New York Heart Association (NYHA) criteria, before and 3 months after revascularization. In patients (n=18) with ≥3 viable segments, LVEF improved from 27 ± 8% to 34 ± 9% (P<0.05) and the NYHA functional status decreased from 2.9 ± 0.3 to 1.5 ± 0.7 (P<0.01). Conversely, in patients (n=14) with 2 or less

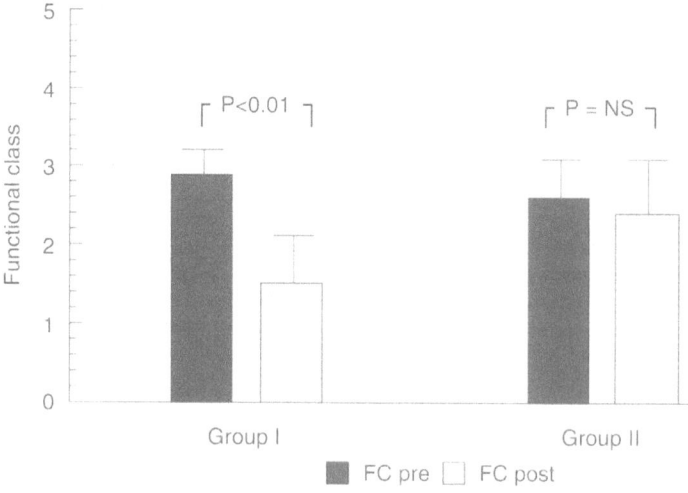

Figure 6.
Bar graph demonstrating the change in heart failure symptoms after revascularization. Group I: patients with ≥3 viable dysfunctional segments on FDG SPECT; group II: patients with 2 or less dysfunctional viable segments (data based on reference 30). FC: Functional Class according to the NYHA criteria.

viable segments the LVEF (31 ± 8% versus 31 ± 8%, ns) and the functional status (2.6 ± 0.5 vs 2.4 ± 0.7, ns) remained unchanged (Figure 6) [30].

Comparison between FDG SPECT and stress echocardiography

Echocardiography during the infusion of incremental doses of dobutamine has also been used to identify viable myocardium and predict improvement of LV function after revascularization [9]. While FDG imaging detects preserved metabolic activity in dysfunctional myocardium, the hallmark of viability during dobutamine echocardiography is the presence of contractile reserve in dysfunctional tissue. When improvement of contractile function occurs during dobutamine infusion, improvement of function is likely to occur after coronary revascularization. A recent meta-analysis concerning the different "viability-techniques and their accuracy to predict improvement of function revealed that dobutamine echocardiography has a higher specificity but a lower sensitivity as compared to FDG imaging [12]. Hence, some segments may not demonstrate contractile reserve, but may still exhibit residual glucose metabolism. We recently compared both techniques in 40 patients with a depressed LV function (LVEF 31 ± 16%). Resting echocardiography showed akinesia in 165 segments. Viability was detected by FDG SPECT in 55 segments, with 38 demonstrating contractile reserve. On the other hand, only 7 of the 113 segments classified nonviable by FDG SPECT showed a contractile reserve during dobutamine echocardiography (Figure 7). Comparable results have been reported in studies comparing FDG PET with dobutamine echocardiography [31-33]. Segments with contractile reserve and metabolic activity are likely to recover function after revascularization, but further studies are needed to assess the

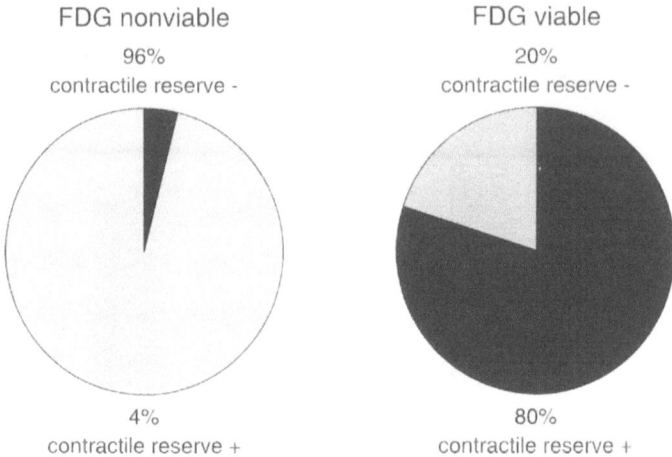

Figure 7. Pie chart showing the relation between contractile reserve and preserved metabolic activity in chronic dysfunctional myocardium. Segments without metabolic activity seldomly exhibit contractile reserve (left). In addition, a substantial percentage of segments with metabolic activity fails to demonstrate contactile reserve (right).

functional fate after revascularization of the segments with preserved metabolic activity without contractile reserve.

Future directions

Various FDG PET studies have recently demonstrated that this technique may also provide prognostic information on morbidity and mortality. Several retrospective studies [34-37] have recently shown that the presence of a mismatch pattern in patients who are treated medically is associated with a higher morbidity and mortality. Di Carli et al. [36] performed a retrospective analysis of 93 patients with severely depressed LV function who previously underwent FDG PET imaging; the mean follow-up period was 14 months. Forty-three patients were revascularized and 50 patients were treated medically. The patients were subsequently divided into 4 groups depending on the treatment (medical versus revascularization) and on the presence or absence of a mismatch pattern. The highest mortality (42%) was observed in the group of patients with a mismatch pattern who were treated medically (Figure 8). The authors also demonstrated that angina and symptoms of congestive heart failure improved significantly in the group of patients with a mismatch who underwent revascularization, in contrast to the other groups [36].

Currently, no prognostic FDG SPECT data are available and future studies are necessary to determine whether FDG SPECT yields similar prognostic information as compared to FDG PET.

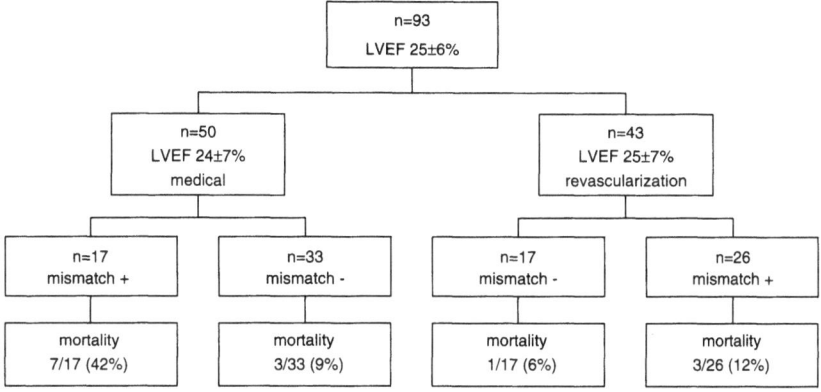

Figure 8. Flow chart showing the relation between therapy, viability (according to the FDG PET study) and mortality. The highest mortality was observed in the patients who were treated medically and who had a mismatch pattern on FDG PET (data based on reference 36).

Conclusions

The currently available data have clearly demonstrated the feasibility of FDG SPECT. Several studies have shown a good agreement between FDG PET and FDG SPECT. Results in patients undergoing revascularization illustrated that FDG SPECT can predict improvement of regional and global LV function after revascularization. Also, substantial viability on FDG SPECT was predictive for improvement of heart failure symptoms after revascularization, indicating improvement of quality of life in these patients.

A good agreement between FDG imaging and dobutamine echocardiography can be obtained, although future studies are needed to compare their predictive accuracy; these studies also need to focus on the outcome of the discordant segments, in particular the segments without contractile reserve but with metabolic activity.

Finally, several studies have shown that FDG PET provides prognostic information; future studies need to establish the prognostic value of FDG SPECT.

References

1. Vanoverschelde JLJ, Wijns W, Borgers M *et al.* Chronic myocardial hibernation in humans. From bedside to bench. Circulation 1997;95:1961-71.
2. Vanoverschelde JLJ, Wijns W, Depre C *et al.* Mechanisms of chronic regional postischemic dysfunction in humans. New insights from the study of noninfarcted collateral-dependent myocardium. Circulation 1993;87:1513-23.
3. Marinho NVS, Keogh BE, Costa DC, Lammerstma AA, Ell PJ, Camici PG. Pathophysiology of chronic left ventricular dysfunction. New insights from the measurement of absolute myocardial blood flow and glucose utilization. Circulation 1996;93:737-44.
4. Mäki M, Luotolahti M, Nuutila P *et al.* Glucose uptake in the chronically dysfunc tional but viable myocardium. Circulation 1996;93:1658-66.
5. Louie HW, Laks H, Milgalter E *et al.* Ischemic cardiomyopathy. Criteria for coronary revascularization and cardiac transplantation. Circulation 1991;84(5 Suppl):III290-5.

6. Pigott JD, Kouchoukos NT, Oberman A, Cutter GR. Late results of surgical and medical therapy for patients with coronary artery disease and depressed left ventricular function. J Am Coll Cardiol 1985;5:1036-45.

7. Mickleborough LL, Maruyama H, Takagi Y, Mohamed S, Sun Z, Ebisuzaki L. Results of revascularization in patients with severe left ventricular dysfunction. Circulation 1995;92(9 Suppl]:II73-9.

8. Dilsizian V, Bonow RO. Current diagnostic techniques of assessing myocardial viability in patients with hibernating and stunned myocardium [published erratum appears in Circulation 1993;87:2070]. Circulation 1993;87:1-20.

9. Cornel JH, Bax JJ, Fioretti PM. Assessment of myocardial viability by dobutamine stress echocardiography. Curr Opin Cardiol 1996;11:621-6.

10. Van der Wall EE, Vliegen HW, De Roos A, Bruschke AVG. Magnetic resonance imaging in coronary artery disease. Circulation 1995;92:2723-39.

11. Bax JJ, Visser FC, Van Lingen A, Cornel JH, Fioretti PM, Van der Wall EE. Metabolic imaging using F18-fluorodeoxyglucose to assess myocardial viability. Int J Card Imaging 1997;13:145-55; discussion 157-60.

12. Bax JJ, Wijns W, Cornel JH, Visser FC, Fioretti PM, Boersma E. Accuracy of currently available techniques for prediction of functional recovery after revascularization in patients with left ventricular dysfunction due to chronic coronary artery disease: comparison of pooled data. J Am Coll Cardiol 1997;30:1451-60.

13. Bax JJ, Visser FC, van Lingen A et al. Feasibility of assessing regional myocardial uptake of ^{18}F-fluorodeoxyglucose using single photon emission computed tomography. Eur Heart J 1993;14:1675-82.

14. Bax JJ, Visser FC, Blanksma PK et al. Comparison of myocardial uptake of fluorine-18-fluorodeoxyglucose imaged with PET and SPECT in dyssynergic myocardium. J Nucl Med 1996;37:1631-6.

15. Sandler MP, Videlefsky S, Delbeke D et al. Evaluation of myocardial ischemia using a rest metabolism/stress perfusion protocol with fluorine-18 deoxyglucose/technetium-99m MIBI and dual-isotope simultaneous-acquisition single-photon emission computed tomography. J Am Coll Cardiol 1995;26:870-8.

16. Bax JJ, Cornel JH, Visser FC et al. Prediction of recovery of myocardial dysfunction after revascularization. Comparison of fluorine-18-fluorodeoxyglucose/thallium-201 SPECT, thallium-201 stress-reinjection SPECT and dobutamine echocardiography. J Am Coll Cardiol 1996;28:558-64.

17. Melin JA, Becker LC. Quantitative relationship between global left ventricular thallium uptake and blood flow: effects of propranolol, ouabain, dipyridamole, and coronary artery occlusion. J Nucl Med 1986;7:641-52.

18. Knuuti MJ, Nuutila P, Ruotsalainen U et al. Euglycemic hyperinsulinemic clamp and oral glucose load in stimulating myocardial glucose utilization during positron emission tomography. J Nucl Med 1992;33:1255-62.

19. Gropler RJ, Siegel BA, Lee KJ et al. Nonuniformity in myocardial accumulation of fluorine-18-fluorodeoxyglucose in normal fasted humans. J Nucl Med 1990;31:1749-56.

20. Bax JJ, Valkema R, Visser FC et al. FDG SPECT in the assessment of myocardial viability. Comparison with dobutamine echo. Eur Heart J 1997;18(Suppl D):D124-9.

21. Rambaldi R, Poldermans D, Bax JJ, Fioretti PM, Krenning EP, Valkema R. Assessment of myocardial viability by dobutamine stress echo and simultaneous Tc99m-tetrofosmin/18-Fluorodeoxyglucose SPECT [abstract]. J Nucl Cardiol 1997;4:S110.

22. Camici P, Ferrannini E, Opie LH. Myocardial metabolism in ischemic heart disease: basic principles and application to imaging by positron emission tomography. Prog Cardiovasc Dis 1989;32:217-38.

23. Knuuti MJ, Yki-Järvinen H, Voipio-Pulkki LM et al. Enhancement of myocardial [fluorine-18]fluorodeoxyglucose uptake by a nicotinic acid derivative. J Nucl Med 1994;35:989-98.

24. Bax JJ, Veening MA, Visser FC et al. Optimal metabolic conditions during fluorine-18 fluorodeoxyglucose imaging; a comparative study using different protocols. Eur J Nucl Med 1997;24:35-41.

25. Burt RW, Perkins OW, Oppenheim BE et al. Direct comparison of fluorine-18- FDG SPECT, fluorine-18-FDG PET and rest thallium-201 SPECT for the detection of myocardial viability. J Nucl Med 1995;36:176-9.

26. Martin WH, Delbeke D, Patton JA et al. FDG-SPECT: correlation with FDG- PET. J Nucl Med 1995;36:988-95.

27. Chen EQ, MacIntyre J, Go RT et al. Myocardial viability studies using fluorine- 18-FDG SPECT: a comparison with fluorine-18-FDG PET. J Nucl Med 1997;38:582-6.

28. Bax JJ, Cornel JH, Visser FC *et al.* The role of fluorine-18-deoxyglucose single photon emission computed tomography in predicting reversibility of regional wall motion abnormalities after revascularization. In: Van der Wall EE, Blanksma PK, Niemeyer MH, Paans AM, editors. Cardiac positron emission tomography. Viability, perfusion, receptors and cardiomyopathy. Dordrecht: Kluwer Academic Press; 1995. p. 75-85.

29. Bax JJ, Cornel JH, Visser FC *et al.* Prediction of improvement of contractile function in patients with ischemic ventricular dysfunction after revascularization by fluorine-18-fluorodeoxyglucose single photon emission computed tomography. J Am Coll Cardiol 1997;30:377-83.

30. Bax JJ, Visser FC, Cornel JH *et al.* Prediction of improvement of LVEF and heart failure symptoms by FDG SPECT [abstract]. J Am Coll Cardiol. In press 1998.

31. Sawada S, Elsner G, Segar DS *et al.* Evaluation of perfusion and metabolism in dobutamine-responsive myocardium. J Am Coll Cardiol 1997;29:55-61.

32. Melon PG, De Landsheere CM, Degueldre C, Peters JL, Kulbertus HE, Pierard LA. Relation between contractile reserve and positron emission tomographic patterns of perfusion and glucose utilization in chronic ischemic left ventricular dysfunction: implications for identification of myocardial viability. J Am Coll Cardiol 1997;30:1651-9.

33. Sun KT, Czernin J, Krivokapich J *et al.* Effects of dobutamine stimulation on myocardial blood flow, glucose metabolism, and wall motion in normal and dysfunctional myocardium. Circulation 1996;94:3146-54.

34. Lee KS, Marwick TH, Cook SA *et al.* Prognosis of patients with left ventricular dysfunction, with and without viable myocardium after myocardial infarction. Relative efficacy of medical therapy and revascularization. Circulation 1994;90:2687-94.

35. Eitzman D, Al-Aouar Z, Kanter HL *et al.* Clinical outcome of patients with advanced coronary artery disease after viability studies with positron emission tomography. J Am Coll Cardiol 1992;20:559-65.

36. Di Carli MF, Davidson M, Little R *et al.* Value of metabolic imaging with positron emission tomography for evaluating prognosis in patients with coronary artery disease and left ventricular dysfunction. Am J Cardiol 1994;73:527-33.

37. Vom Dahl J, Altehoefer C, Sheehan FH *et al.* Effect of myocardial viability assessed by technetium-99m-sestamibi SPECT and fluorine-18-FDG PET on clinical outcome in coronary artery disease. J Nucl Med 1997;38:742-8.

24.　What are the niches for SPECT versus PET versus MRI?

Jens C. Stollfuss, Frank M. Bengel & Markus Schwaiger.

Summary

Nuclear medicine techniques are the most widely validated diagnostic procedures for noninvasive assessment of myocardial perfusion and metabolism. Large patient populations have been evaluated to assess diagnostic accuracy and define prognostic values. SPECT performed under resting and stress conditions using Tc-99m labeled flow tracers has a high diagnostic, cost-effective performance for detection and location of coronary artery disease. Positron emission tomography using FDG for assessment of residual viability in patients with severely impaired left ventricular function remains the gold standard for other methods evolving in the field of metabolic CV imaging. Currently, PET is the only method that has the potential to offer non-invasive true quantitative measurements of myocardial blood flow and flow reserve.

MRI probably has the greatest potential for future developments in cardiac imaging due to its technical diversity. In clinical routine, it offers great potential for detailed anatomical imaging of the heart and great vessels in adults and children with complex myocardial disease, flow evaluation in patients with valvular disease as well as information on global and regional myocardial function. Functional MR imaging directed towards assessment of ischemic heart disease and metabolic activity is beginning to evolve. Current research and development with high field spectroscopic MRI, interventional MRI, metabolic contrast agents and high resolution vessel wall characterization may eventually find clinical application in CV MRI.

Introduction

Diseases of the cardiovascular (CV) system are cumulatively representing the number one cause of death in industrialized countries. Thus, there is need for a better understanding of the fundamental anatomic, histologic and physiologic manifestations of the disease processes affecting the heart and the vasculature. Prevention of CV disease, the improved accuracy of their diagnosis, optimal therapeutic planning and cost-effective, minimal risk monitoring are objectives to be addressed. Several established imaging procedures are currently available for effective CV imaging. Nuclear medicine techniques have limited anatomic resolution, but are well established and validated for the functional assessment of CV diseases, thereby providing noninvasive information about myocardial perfusion and metabolism. Positron emission tomography (PET) offers potential to provide true quantitative measurements of

J.H.C. Reiber and E.E. van der Wall (eds.). What's New in Cardiovascular Imaging, 311–322.
©1998 Kluwer Academic Publishers.

physiologic processes like myocardial blood flow and oxygen consumption. However, there is a trend away from the application of radionuclides toward other techniques without radiation burden and with higher spatial resolution. The technologic diversity of magnetic resonance imaging (MRI) allows 3-dimensional imaging of the CV system based on definition of high resolution anatomy, intracardiac and intravascular blood flow, cardiac chamber contraction and regional myocardial mechanics. Additional functional applications for cardiovascular MRI, like myocardial perfusion imaging and tissue characterization are beginning to evolve and must compete with established methods in the field of functional CV imaging. In the following, an overview on the classical state-of-the-art applications in SPECT, PET and MRI is given with a focus on competitive and complementary aspects of these applications in clinical routine and research.

Technical background and recent developments

Single photon emission tomography (SPECT)

SPECT is routinely applied for myocardial perfusion imaging, resulting in an accurate characterization of localization and severity of perfusion abnormalities [1]. Multi-headed cameras have been developed to increase count statistics and reduce acquisition time. A methodological problem of myocardial SPECT comes from the inhomogeneous attenuation of photons in the thorax. Photon attenuation reduces specificity of image analysis, especially for obese patients and women with large breasts [2]. With the development of multi-headed cameras, methods to overcome this problem have been introduced. In addition to emission data, transmission images are acquired simultaneously using external radioactive sources [3]. Recently, Ficaro et al. compared the diagnostic accuracy of attenuation corrected and non-corrected SPECT images for the detection of coronary artery disease, demonstrating improved accuracy of myocardial perfusion imaging using SPECT in conjunction with attenuation-correction [4]. Further methodological improvement can be expected from additional correction for scatter due to high liver uptake and activity from tissue surrounding the myocardium [5].

Another promising approach is the development of electrocardiographic gating for both positron emission tomography (PET) and SPECT systems. Historically, electrocardiographic gating was performed in conjunction with planar radionuclide angiography (RNA), representing a reproducible and largely observer independent tool to assess global and regional left ventricular function [6]. With the advanced multi-headed camera systems, gating can also be applied to myocardial perfusion studies. By performing gated SPECT, it is possible to augment perfusion data with additional information on regional and global left ventricular function without increasing imaging time. Resting left ventricular ejection fraction, the most important measure of cardiac performance and prognosis in patients with coronary artery disease (CAD), can be derived from gated perfusion studies and have been validated against conventional radionuclide imaging [7]. Regional wall motion and wall thickening may also be addressed by gated perfusion SPECT and may provide incremental information, especially in areas with reduced perfusion [8]. In the future, quantitative approaches toward regional wall motion and wall thickening may also be established (Figure 1).

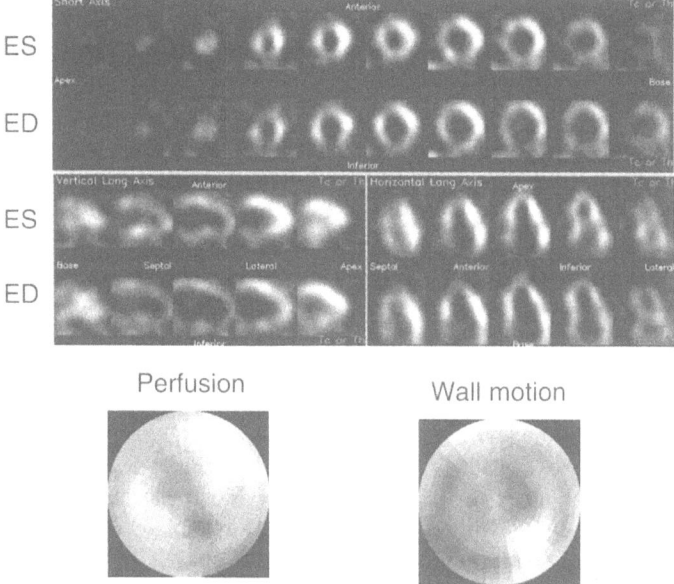

Figure 1. Gated myocardial perfusion SPECT. Corresponding end-systolic (ES) and end-diastolic (ED) slices are displayed as a report page. Additionally, software tools are applied to calculate polar maps of regional perfusion and wall motion (endocardial shortening), which may add to visual image analysis. As expected in this case of a patient with three vessel CAD; there is inhomogeneous perfusion as well as wall motion.

Various photon emitting tracers are in routine use for SPECT imaging. Thallium-201 (Tl-201) was introduced in the mid-seventies as an agent with superior physiological properties and is still in wide clinical use [9]. As a monovalent cation, it behaves similarly to potassium and is actively taken up by the myocardium via the sodium/potassium-ATP-ase [10]. Because cell membrane integrity is a prerequisite for Tl-201 uptake, preserved activity also reflects myocardial viability. Imaging protocols have been introduced that aim at the enhanced detection of myocardial viability by reinjection Tl-201 at rest after the routine stress-redistribution imaging procedure [11].

Technetium-99m (Tc-99m) is widely and readily available and several Tc-99m labeled perfusion tracers have been recently introduced. Among those, Tc-99m sestamibi is the most established. This cationic complex passively crosses the cell membrane and is then bound to mitochondria. Due to intracellular retention, a relevant redistribution is not observed, leading to the necessity of separate stress and rest injections. While Tc-99m sestamibi uptake is proportional to blood flow at lower flow ranges, the retention underestimates blood flow at higher flow ranges. This effect seems to be even more pronounced in new flow tracers such as Tc-99m tetrofosmin and Tc-99m Q12, indicating a potential limitation of these tracers [12]. Apart from the usefulness as a perfusion tracer, there is also evidence that Tc-99m sestamibi and Tc-99m tetrofosmin uptake may reflect myocardial viability [13,14].

Positron emission tomography

The basic principle of PET is the detection of photon-coincidences derived from positron/ electron annihilation using a detector ring system. Compared to SPECT, PET provides higher spatial resolution. Photon attenuation along the coincidence lines is precisely and easily corrected by the use of individual transmission scans with external radioactive sources. In addition, dynamic scanning can be performed due to high temporal resolution. Dynamic data can then be fitted to compartment models. Using this technique, absolute quantitative values of physiological and biochemical processes can be obtained, e.g. quantitative blood measurements and quantification of glucose and oxygen consumption.

Recently, efforts have been made to visualize positron emitting tracers with conventional gamma camera systems using high energy collimators resulting in myocardial 511 keV SPECT. Sensitivity and specificity of SPECT and PET for detection of myocardial viability was investigated using a single injection of (18F)-fluorodeoxyglucose (FDG) [15]. Furthermore, rotating multi-purpose dual-headed cameras have been developed to provide the opportunity for SPECT imaging of conventional tracers as well as coincidence imaging of positron emitting tracers [16]. Although both approaches, 511 keV SPECT and coincidence imaging are at the expense of absolute quantification, they may be promising for a wider clinical application. However, the uncollimated use of SPECT devices for coincidence imaging leads to a 3D imaging of the chest with a relatively high scatter fraction. The implementation of attenuation correction to these systems is mandatory for imaging of the heart in order to achieve acceptable image quality (Figure 2).

MCD Imaging with Attenuation Correction
Cardiac Viability Study

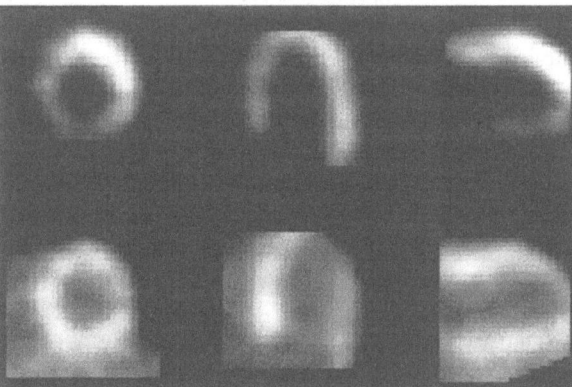

FDG no corr.
MCD

FDG att. corr.
MCD

Figure 2. This figure shows a multi-coincidence study (SPECT device) using FDG with (lower row) and without (upper row) attenuation correction of the same patient. Note that the activity in the inferior wall would be severely underestimated without application of attenuation correction.

For assessment of regional myocardial blood flow, several positron emitting tracers have been used. Noninvasive quantitative blood flow measurements have contributed significantly to an improved understanding of the effect of risk factors and therapeutic approaches on coronary microcirculation [17,18]. The introduction of (18F)-fluorodeoxyglucose

(FDG) has been a breakthrough in noninvasive diagnosis of myocardial viability [19]. Preserved FDG-uptake reflects intact glucose utilization and therefore, myocardial viability. Ischemia results in enhanced FDG uptake, probably due to increased sacrolemmal translocation of glucose transporter proteins [20]. A FDG PET study is usually performed after oral glucose loading or under hyperinsulemic euglycemic clamping to ensure maximal stimulation of myocardial glucose uptake by insulin. Further positron emitting tracers are available for noninvasive assessment of myocardial metabolism and the cardiac sympathetic nervous system. Theoretically, PET radiochemistry allows for the production of an almost unlimited variety of biomolecules to trace the physiology of the heart.

SPECT as well as PET systems have been in clinical use for imaging of the cardiovascular system for more than a decade. Robust and stable hard and software systems have been developed for assessment of cardiovascular perfusion and function. However, at the current clinical state both PET and magnetic resonance imaging (MRI) systems dedicated to professional cardiovascular imaging are not widely available. MRI systems have disadvantages coming from the lack of commercially available software, problems with ECG-gating and monitoring of the patient due to the magnetic field. In addition to practical advantages, SPECT and PET techniques allow sensitive imaging of physiological CV processes in vivo, thereby needing only very small amounts of tracer substances in the range of micrograms.

Clinical applications

Assessment of ischemic heart disease

Myocardial perfusion imaging using SPECT is a well established tool for the primary detection of coronary artery disease. Stress tests are applied to increase coronary blood flow. The development of ischemia or regional flow heterogeneity is then used to deduce the presence of stenoses. In addition to physical exercise protocols (treadmill or bicycle), various pharmacological agents such as dipyridamole, adenosine and dobutamine are available for stress testing [21]. Recent research efforts focused on the establishment of cost-effective strategies for detection of coronary artery disease. Based on Bayes theorem, cost-effectiveness can be calculated by decision tree models [22]. The effectiveness of nuclear medicine techniques is highly dependent on the pre-test likelihood of CAD, which can be estimated by risk factors, age, sex and symptoms [23]. Traditionally, exercise electrocardiography is performed first. Positive responders subsequently undergo radionuclide imaging for preselection for coronary angiography. However, it has been shown that the most effective strategy in patients with intermediate likelihood includes myocardial perfusion imaging by SPECT in combination with exercise testing as the primary diagnostic procedure [22]. Patients with high likelihood for CAD (>70%) should be directly referred to coronary angiography [24].

Apart from the primary diagnosis of CAD, perfusion scintigraphy plays an important role in patients with known CAD. The hemodynamic relevance of known stenosis can be assessed by the presence, extent and severity of a stress-induced perfusion defect. Culprit lesions in patients with symptomatic multivessel disease are identified by the localization of perfusion defects. Subsequently, perfusion scintigraphy can be repeated after intervention to assess the short-term efficacy. In patients with multivessel disease, Breisblatt et al. demonstrated that approximately half of the patients showed scintigraphic evidence of ischemia in a second vascular territory after angioplasty of a culprit vessel. In the case of a normal scintigram after angioplasty, on the other hand, a second intervention was necessary in only 13% during a follow-up period of one year [25]. These data suggest the importance of a complete revascularization to eliminate stress-induced ischemia. Myocardial perfusion scintigraphy also provides high accuracy for the noninvasive, long-term follow-up after interventional procedures by assessing patency of coronary bypass grafts as well as the long-term effect of percutaneous transluminal coronary angioplasty. Most probably due to higher spatial resolution and the use of individual correction for photon attenuation, PET resulted in higher diagnostic accuracy for detection of CAD compared to SPECT [26,27]. The possibility to perform quantitative blood flow and flow reserve measurements using dynamic PET may also provide earlier diagnosis of CAD compared to SPECT, which relies on qualitative evaluation of regional perfusion abnormalities [28].

However, there is increasing evidence that the greatest value of nuclear imaging is found in the risk assessment rather than pure diagnosis of CAD [29]. The amount of infarcted myocardium and the extent of jeopardized myocardium are prognostic factors which are reflected by the extent and severity of perfusion defects. In a recent study, Haas et al. investigated viability assessment by (13N)-ammonia and FDG PET with respect to postoperative recovery and early outcome [30]. They found that selection of patients for coronary artery bypass grafting on the basis of PET data in conjunction with clinical status and angiography led to postoperative recovery with fewer complications and a significant decrease of early mortality compared to decision making on the basis of clinical data and angiographic results alone.

Global left ventricular function can be assessed additionally by gated SPECT. Myocardial perfusion imaging provides information for risk stratification that cannot be derived from clinical history, risk factors, resting or exercise ECG of coronary angioplasty. In a very large patient group without known CAD (n=2200), Hachomovitch and colleagues compared different models for risk factor stratification including clinical data only, clinical and exercise data, and nuclear medicine data [31]. They found a significantly larger receiver operator characteristics area for the model including nuclear data compared to those without nuclear data, demonstrating the incremental value of myocardial perfusion SPECT for risk stratification. In some studies, it has been shown that patients without known CAD and a normal perfusion scan have excellent prognosis. The mean cardiac rate (infarction or death) among 3573 patients with proven CAD and normal scintigram was only 0.9% [32]. Such prognostic testing may guide further therapeutic decision making in patients with low risk for subsequent myocardial infarction or death. This testing also identifies the patient population who can be initially treated by anti-ischemic medication and risk factor modification. In patients at higher risk, ischemia targeted or complete revascularization may be added to medical therapy depending on the degree of perfusion abnormalities [33]. Such testing-driven, risk-sensitive therapeutic strategies are likely to improve quality and overall cost-effectiveness of CAD treatment. Nuclear cardiology may be a key factor in this regard.

Only few data are available concerning MRI for detection of coronary artery disease. Myocardial ischemia, in general, is associated with increased myocardial signal as a result of prolonged relaxation times on T1 images [34]. However, in a clinical setting the detection of myocardial intensity changes from induced reversible ischemia, moreover ischemia at rest, has not been reliable. In contrast to irreversible injured myocardium, reversibly ischemic myocardium does not necessarily alter myocardial relaxation times or intensity in the early phase. It also failed to distinguish between reversible and irreversible damages to the myocardium, as determined by nuclear imaging [35]. Using ultrafast sequences, a direct relation has been shown experimentally between myocardial blood flow and signal intensity after administration of gadolinium-chelates [36]. In patients with and without the use of pharmacological stress agents, several different patterns in intensity versus time curves have been observed after a bolus administration of gadolinium-chelates [37]. Some investigators observed, qualitatively, an abnormal delay in signal increase in hypoperfused myocardium. These areas correlated well with abnormal areas on nuclear perfusion imaging [38]. Others showed decreased peak signal intensity in hypoperfused areas [37]. A current limitation using ultrafast GE sequences is that the left ventricle can only be partially sampled (usually 1-3 anatomical levels), whereas experimental EPI methods would theoretically allow to generate a multi-slice tomography to generate a 3D perspective. Although the current results concerning perfusion imaging using MRI are promising, more work is needed to define its importance in relation to established nuclear medicine methods [39]. At the current stage of development, myocardial perfusion imaging is the primary domain of nuclear imaging. However, direct visualization of coronary arteries is also possible using MRI techniques and will be the ultimate challenge in the field of research [40].

Assessment of myocardial viability

In patients with chronic CAD and left ventricular dysfunction, it is well known that impaired function is not always an irreversible process related to prior myocardial infarction. There are different mechanisms thought to explain the underlying pathophysiology of dysfunctional but viable myocardium. "Hibernating myocardium" is defined as dysfunctional due to chronic hypoperfusion, while "repetitive stunned myocardium" is continuously dysfunctional due to repetitive ischemia. Clinically, both processes may co-exist and be difficult to distinguish. However, a major characteristic of both hibernating as well as repetitive stunned myocardium is an improvement in function after restoration of blood flow. Thus, functional recovery after revascularization can be predicted by the assessment of extent and localization of viable myocardium.

Several nuclear medicine imaging protocols have been employed for the detection of myocardial viability. The combined use of a flow tracer (e.g. (13N)-ammonia) and FDG as a metabolic tracer for PET imaging is well accepted as the gold standard for viability assessment [19]. Ischemically compromised but still viable myocardium is defined by a "mismatch" between severely reduced blood flow and preserved or even enhanced FDG uptake in the myocardium. Currently, polar map techniques can be used to quantitate the extent of scar and mismatch as percent of the whole ventricle (Figure 3). The amount of viable myocardium is not only predictive for functional improvement after revascularization, but is also prognostic for reduced perioperative risk and improved long term outcome [41], as well as improved heart failure symptoms [42]. If scar is the predominant cause of reduced left ventricular function, the patient will not benefit from revascularization and should be treated medically or should even undergo heart transplantation. On the other hand, if reasonable amounts of viable myocardium are detected in patients scheduled for heart transplantation, the strategy may be changed towards bypass surgery. As a guide to adequate therapy, the use of nuclear techniques for viability assessment not only improves outcome, but also reduces overall costs for the management of patients with ischemic cardiomyopathy [43].

Extensive experience for determination of viability has also been made with the single photon emitter Tl-201, which reflects both perfusion and cell membrane integrity. It has been shown that chronically hypoperfused, but still viable myocardium, presents as a defect

REPORT PAGE

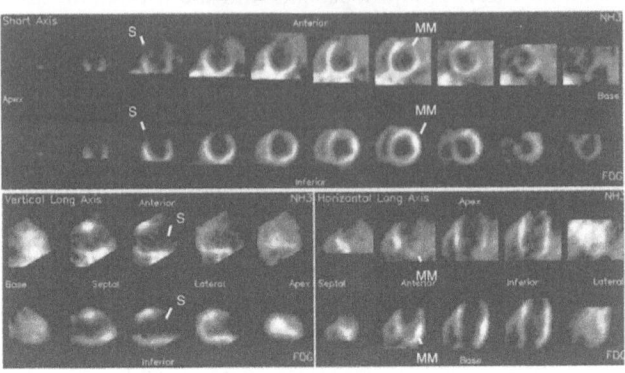

POLAR MAP ANALYSIS

Ammonia   FDG   Viability-Map

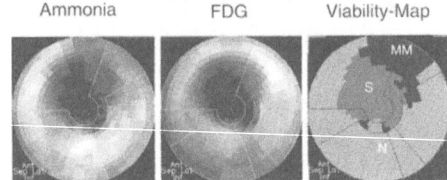

Figure 3. PET viability study of a patient with ischemic cardiomyopathy using (13N)- ammonia (NH3) as flow tracer, and (18F)-fluorodeoxyglucose (FDG) as metabolic tracer. Corresponding slices along the short and long axes of the ventricle are displayed on the top. In the basal area of the anterolateral wall , a markedly reduced flow (upper row) but preserved FDG uptake (lower row) was observed. This flow/metabolism mismatch (MM) indicates the presence of ischemically compromised but viable myocardium. In the apex and the distal anterior wall, a scar (S) with reduction of both flow and FDG uptake was observed. The polar-map analysis can be used to quantitate the size of abnormalities. In this case, the mismatch area (MM) includes 15% of the left ventricle, while 31% are scar (S) and 54% are normal (N).

in stress and early redistribution images, but shows a late fill-in phenomenon after reinjection of thallium at rest [11]. In comparison to FDG PET, Tl-201 reinjection imaging has comparable diagnostic accuracy [44]. However, disadvantages of PET and SPECT techniques include the limited spatial resolution compared to MRI. Myocardial scarring after infarction may involve the whole myocardial wall or only subendocardial layers depending on the severity and duration of ischemia. However, differentiated viability assessment of endocardial and epicardial myocardial layers is not possible by nuclear techniques due to limited anatomical resolution. In addition, scar size can be overestimated due to partial volume effects. Techniques with higher resolution are, therefore, desirable.

MRI procedures for detection of myocardial viability are beginning to evolve. Several studies performed in various animal models have been promising in characterizing reversible and irreversible injuries to myocardium due to myocardial infarction based on signal intensity changes after administration of gadolinium-chelates [45,46].

However, studies in patients with occlusive and reperfused myocardial infarction have not consistently shown that contrast enhanced MRI is effective for differentiating these two types of myocardial infarction. [47]. The capabilities of more basic forms of MRI, such as cine, to provide functional information about myocardium in combination with assessment of diastolic wall thickness and systolic wall thickening makes it suitable for detection of myocardial viability [48]. A comparison of cine low dose dobutamine stress with positron emission tomography in patients with chronic MI showed that the use of these parameters was very accurate in assessing myocardial viability. Wall thickening was found to be a better predictor of residual metabolic activity than was end-diastolic wall thickness [49]. However, more work is needed to define the role of functional MRI for detection of viability in a clinical setting. At the current stage of development, PET using FDG remains the gold standard for detection of residual myocardial viability after myocardial infarction.

Summary

In general, nuclear medicine techniques are the most widely validated techniques for noninvasive assessment of myocardial perfusion and metabolism. Large patient populations have been evaluated to assess diagnostic accuracy and define prognostic values. SPECT performed under resting and stress conditions using Tc-99m labeled flow tracers has a high diagnostic, cost-effective performance for detection and location of coronary artery disease especially in patients with intermediate likelihood for having coronary artery disease CAD. Technical advances in SPECT acquisition, such as patient individual attenuation and scatter correction, give hope for an improvement in overall accuracy. A clinical progress represents the simultaneous assessment of perfusion and global and regional left ventricular function by gated SPECT.

Positron emission tomography using FDG for assessment of residual viability in patients with severely impaired left ventricular function remains the gold standard for other methods evolving in the field of metabolic cardiovascular imaging. Currently, PET is the only method that has the potential to offer noninvasive true quantitative measurements of myocardial blood flow and flow reserve, thereby offering a clinical potential for investigation of patients with normal coronary angiogram presenting with angina pectoris. From a scientific point of view, PET also can be used to monitor the effect of risk factor modification on endothelial function.

MRI probably has the greatest potential for future developments in cardiac imaging due to its technical diversity. In clinical routine, it offers great potential for detailed anatomical imaging of the heart and great vessels in adults and children with complex myocardial disease as well as flow evaluation in patients with valvular disease. It offers unique technically superior information on left ventricular ejection fraction and regional myocardial functional parameters. Functional MRI directed towards assessment of ischemic heart disease and metabolic activity is beginning to evolve. However, it is difficult to predict which relatively expensive technological advances currently under investigation have a future role in cardiovascular imaging. In the field of anatomical imaging of the heart and vasculature, MRI must compete with well accepted and less expensive procedures like e.g. echocardiography. Current research and development with high field spectroscopic MRI, interventional MRI, metabolic contrast agents and high resolution vessel wall characterization may, however, eventually find clinical application to future work in cardiovascular MRI.

References

1. DePasquale EE, Nody AC, DePuey EG *et al.* Quantitative rotational thallium-201 tomography for identifying and localizing coronary artery disease. Circulation 1988;77:316-27.

2. DePuey EG Garcia EV. Optimal specificity of thallium-201 SPECT through recognition of imaging artifacts. J Nucl Med 1989;30:441-9.

3. Ficaro EP, Fessler JA, Ackermann RJ, Rogers WL, Corbett JR, Schwaiger M. Simultaneous transmission-emission thallium-201 cardiac SPECT: effect of attenuation correction on myocardial tracer distribution. J Nucl Med 1995;36:921-31.

4. Ficaro EP, Fessler JA, Shreve PD, Kritzman JN, Rose PA, Corbett JR. Simultaneous transmission/emission myocardial perfusion tomography. Diagnostic accuracy of attenuation-corrected 99mTc-sestamibi single-photon emission computed tomography. Circulation 1996;93:463-73.

5. Galt JR, Cullom SJ, Garcia EV. SPECT quantification: a simplified method of attenuation and scatter correction for cardiac imaging. J Nucl Med 1992;33:2232-7.

6. Schelbert HR, Verba JW, Johnson AD *et al.* Nontraumatic determination of left ventricular ejection fraction by radionuclide angiocardiography. Circulation 1975;51:902-9.

7. Germano G, Kiat H, Kavanagh PB *et al.* Automatic quantification of ejection fraction from gated myocardial perfusion SPECT. J Nucl Med 1995;36:2138-47.

8. Berman DS, Germano G. Evaluation of ventricular ejection fraction, wall motion, wall thickening, and other parameters with gated myocardial perfusion single-photon emission computed tomography. J Nucl Cardiol 1997;4(2 pt 2):S169-71.

9. Strauss HW, Harrison K, Langan JK, Lebowitz E Pitt B. Thallium-201 for myocardial imaging. Relation of thallium-201 to regional myocardial perfusion. Circulation 1975;51:641-5.

10. Nielsen AP, Morris KG, Murdock R, Bruno FP, Cobb FR. Linear relationship between the distribution of thalium-201 and blood flow in ischemic and nonischemic myocardium during exercise. Circulation 1980;61:797-801.

11. Dilsizian V, Rocco TP, Freedman NM, Leon MB, Bonow RD. Enhanced detection of ischemic but viable myocardium by the reinjection of thallium after stress-redistribution imaging. N Engl J Med 1990;323:141-6.

12. Matsunari I, Haas F, Nguyen NT *et al.* Comparison of sestamibi, tetrofosmin and Q12 retention during vasodilation in porcine myocardium [abstract]. Circulation 1997;96(8 Suppl):I687.

13. Udelson JE, Coleman PS, Metherall J *et al.* Predicting recovery of severe regional ventricular dysfunction. Comparison of resting scintigraphy with 201Tl and 99mTc-sestamibi. Circulation 1994;89:2552-61.

14. Matsunari I, Fujino S, Taki J *et al.* Myocardial viability assessment with technetium-99m-tetrofosmin and thallium-201 reinjection in coronary artery disease. J Nucl Med 1995;36:1961-7.

15. Bax JJ, Visser FC, Blanksma PK *et al.* Comparison of myocardial uptake of flourine-18-fluorodeoxyglucose imaged with PET and SPECT in dyssynergic myocardium. J Nucl Med 1996;37:1631-6.

16. Ziegler SI, Enterrottacher A, Boning G *et al.* Performance characteristics of a dual head coincidence camera for the detection of small lesions [abstract]. J Nucl Med 1997;38(5 Suppl):206P.

17. Czernin J, Barnard RJ, Sun KT *et al.* Effect of short-term cardiovascular conditioning and low-fat diet on myocardial blood flow and flow reserve. Circulation 1995;92:197-204.

18. Dayanikli F, Grambow D, Muzik O, Mosca L, Rubinfire M Schwaiger M. Early detection of abnormal coronary flow reserve in asymptomatic men at high risk for coronary artery disease using positron emission tomography. Circulation 1994;90:808-17.

19. Tillisch J, Brunken R, Marshall R *et al.* Reversibility of cardiac wall-motion abnormalities predicted by positron tomography. N Engl J Med 1986;1986:884-8.

20. Young L, Renfu Y, Russell R *et al.* Low-flow ischemia leads to translocation of canine heart GLUT-4 and GLUT-1 glucose transporters to the sacrolemma in vivo. Circulation 1997;95:415-22.

21. Orlandi C. Pharmacology of coronary vasodilation: a brief review. J Nucl Cardiol 1996;3(6 pt 2):S27-30.

22. Maddahi J Gambhir SS. Cost-effective selection of patients for coronary angiography. J Nucl Cardiol 1997;4(2 pt 2):S141-51.

23. Diamond GA, Forrester JS. Analysis of probability as an aid in the clinical diagnosis of coronary-artery disease. N Engl J Med 1979;300:1350-8.

24. Patterson RE, Eisner RL, Horowitz SF. Comparison of cost-effectiveness and utility of exercise ECG, single photon emission computed tomography, positron emission tomography, and coronary angiography for diagnosis of coronary artery disease. Circulation 1995;91:54-65.

25. Breisblatt WM, Barnes JV, Weiland F Spaccavento LJ. Incomplete revascularization in multivessel percutaneous transluminal coronary angioplasty: the role for stress thallium-201 imaging. J Am Coll Cardiol 1988;11:1183-90.

26. Schelbert HR, Wisenberg G, Phelps ME *et al.* Noninvasive assessment of coronary stenoses by myocardial imaging during pharmacologic coronary vasodilation. VI. Detection of coronary artery disease in human beings with intravenous N-13 ammonia and positron computed tomography. Am J Cardiol 1982;49:1197-207.

27. Tamaki N, Yonekura Y, Senda M *et al.* Value and limitation of stress thallium- 201 single photon emission computed tomography: comparison with nitrogen-13 ammonia positron tomography. J Nucl Med 1988;29:1181-8.

28. Dayanikli F, Grambow D, Muzik O, Mosca L, Rubinfire M, Schwaiger M. Early detection of abnormal coronary flow reserve in asymptomatic men at high risk for coronary artery disease using positron emission tomography. Circulation 1994;90:808-17.

29. Berman DS Hachamovitch R. Risk assessment in patients with stable coronary artery disease: incremental value of nuclear imaging. J Nucl Cardiol 1996;3(6 pt 2):S41-9.

30. Haas F, Haehnel CJ, Picker W *et al.* Preoperative positron emission tomographic viability assessment and perioperative and postoperative risk in patients with advanced ischemic heart disease. J Am Coll Cardiol 1997;30:1693-700.

31. Hachamovitch R, Berman DS, Kiat H *et al.* Exercise myocardial perfusion SPECT in patients without known coronary artery disease: incremental prognostic value and use in risk stratification. Circulation 1996;93:905-14.

32. Brown KA. Prognostic value of thallium-201 myocardial perfusion imaging in patients with unstable angina who respond to medical treatment. J Am Coll Cardiol 1991;17:1053-7.

33. Miller DD, Gersh BJ. Risk-sensitive therapeutic strategies for coronary artery disease: toward testing-driven therapy in stable angina patients with low-to intermediate risk cardiac imaging results. J Nucl Cardiol 1997;4:409-17.

34. Scholz TD, Martins JB Skorton DJ. NMR relaxation times in acute myocardial infarction relative influence of changes in tissue water and fat content. Magn Reson Med 1992;23:89-95.

35. Ahmad M, Johnson RF Jr, Fawett HD, Schreiber MH. Magnetic resonance imaging in patients with unstable angina: comparison with acute myocardial infarction and normals. Magn Reson Imaging 1988;6:527-34.

36. Miller DD, Holmvang G, Gill JB *et al.* MRI detection of myocardial perfusion changes by gadolinium-DTPA infusion during dipyridamole hyperemia. Magn Reson Med 1989;10:246-55.

37. Manning WJ, Atkinson DJ, Grossmann W, Paulin S, Edelman RR. First-pass nuclear magnetic resonance imaging studies using gadolinium-DTPA in patients with coronary artery disease. J Am Coll Cardiol 1991;18:959-65.

38. Wilke N, Jerosch-Herold M, Stillman AE *et al.* Concepts of myocardial perfusion imaging in magnetic resonance imaging. Magn Reson Q 1994;10:249-86.

39. Steffans JC, Sakuma H, Bourne MW, Higgins CB. Magnetic resonance imaging in ischemic heart disease. Am Heart J 1996;132:156-73.

40. Van der Wall EE, De Roos A, Van Voorthuisen AE, Bruschke AVG. Magnetic resonance imaging: a new approach for evaluating coronary artery disease? Am Heart J 1991;121:1203-20.

41. Haas F, Hahnel C, Sebening F, Meisner H, Schwaiger M. Effect of preoperative PET viability on peri- and postoperative risk [abstract]. J Am Coll Cardiol 1996;27(Suppl A):300A.

42. DiCarli MF, Asgarzadie F, Schelbert HR *et al.* Quantitative relation between myocardial viability and improvement in heart failure symptoms after revascularization in patients with ischemic cardiomyopathy. Circulation 1995;92:3436-44.

43. Beller GA. Selecting patients with ischemic cardiomyopathy for medical treatment, revascularization, or heart transplantation. J Nucl Cardiol 1997;4(2 pt 2):S152-7.

44. Bonow RO. Identification of viable myocardium. Circulation 1996;94:2674-80.

45. Schaefer S, Malloy CR Katz J *et al.* Gadolinium-DTPA enhanced nuclear magnetic resonance imaging of reperfused myocardium: identification of the myocardial bed at risk. J Am Coll Cardiol 1988;12:1064-72.

46. Masui T, Saeed M, Wendland MF, Higgins CB. Occlusive and reperfused myocardial infarcts: MR imaging differentiation with nonionic-Gd-DTPA-BMA. Radiology 1991;181:77-83.

47. De Roos A, Van Rossum AC, Van der Wall E *et al.* Reperfused and nonreperfused myocardial infarction: diagnostic potential of Gd-DTPA-enhanced MR imaging. Radiology 1989;172:717-20.

48.   Baer FM, Smolarz K, Jungehulsing M *et al.* Chronic myocardial infarction: assessment of morphology, func-
       tion, and perfusion by gradient echo magnetic resonance imaging and 99mTc-methoxyisobutyl-isonitrile
       SPECT. Am Heart J 1992;123:636-45.
49.   Baer FM, Voth E, Schneider CA, Theissen P, Schicha H Sechtem U. Comparison of low-dose dobutamine-
       gradient-echo magnetic resonance imaging and positron emission tomography with [18F]fluorodeoxyglu-
       cose in patients with chronic coronary artery disease. A functional and morphological approach to the
       detection of residual myocardial viability. Circulation 1995;91:1006-15.

25.

Echocardiography: where are we now and where are we heading?

Michael H. Picard

Summary

Two-dimensional echocardiography plays a critical role in the care of patients with both acute and chronic cardiac diseases. Tremendous advances in this noninvasive imaging technology have occurred of the last 35 years and current and future innovations are progressing at a rapid pace. Advances in instrumentations, such as harmonic imaging, new applications of echocardiography in the operating room, and new developments in myocardial contrast echocardiography are just a few examples of new developments that are currently available to enhance care. In addition, advances in computer processing speed and storage capability means that the vision of the "digital echo lab" is close to reality. This new application, with its potential to speed the acquisition, interpretation, transmission and storage of echocardiograms, should enable this image modality to maintain its position of importance as we look to the future of medicine.

Introduction

In the 35 years since Edler first applied ultrasound for diagnosis of heart disease [1], tremendous strides have been made. Ultrasonic imaging and Doppler techniques are now used on a daily basis to enhance patient care in a cost effective manner [2,3] and improve our understanding of cardiac physiology [4]. Despite the tremendous advances which have occurred over the last 35 years, current and future innovations in this imaging technique are more exciting for clinical cardiologists than the advances to date (Table 1). These include advances in instrumentation (harmonic imaging), new applications of echocardiography (intraoperative and three-dimensional echocardiography), new adjunctive agents for use in assessing myocardial perfusion, and the introduction of digital image acquisition and storage.

Advances in instrumentation

Modifications in image processing and transducer production have brought about tremendous changes in image quality. Digital imaging platforms utilizing broad band transducers now can send and receive a range of frequencies. The manner in which these signals are pro-

J.H.C. Reiber and E.E. van der Wall (eds.). What's New in Cardiovascular Imaging, 323–332.
©1998 Kluwer Academic Publishers.

Table 1: Example of recent advances in echocardiography

---

1. Instrumentation

    harmonic imaging

2. New techniques and applications

    intraoperative echocardiography

    three-dimensional echocardiography

    contrast echocardiography

        left ventricular opacification / endocardial border enhancement

        Doppler signal enhancement

        myocardial perfusion

   use in clinical trials with echocardiographic endpoints

        LV volume and function

        LV mass

  small animal echocardiography

    transgenic models

3. Digital echocardiography

    tele-echocardiography

---

cessed results in wide capabilities and flexibility for the echocardiographer. The advances described below have resulted in improvements in transthoracic echocardiograms to such a degree that the transthoracic echocardiogram can be utilized with more confidence even in clinical situations previously reserved for transesophageal echocardiography.

For example, while transthoracic images on adult patients were typically best obtained using ultrasound frequencies between 2 and 3.5 MHz, now the same patients can be imaged at higher frequencies. This results in improvements in spatial resolution particularly for assessment of valve morphology, small structures such as the left atrial appendage and even myocardial fiber orientation [5].

While in the past, a major limitation to two-dimensional echocardiographic imaging was relatively low frame rates (approximately 30 Hz), the newest instruments can perform with frame rates greater than 150 Hz. This results in improvements in temporal resolution particularly for subtle cardiac motion.

Although initially introduced to enhance signal detection from echocardiographic contrast agents, harmonic imaging has now been applied to the "non contrast" image resulting in dramatic improvements in delineation of cardiac structures, particularly endocardial border definition [6,7]. Using this approach, specific frequencies are transmitted and then specific multiples of the frequency are received and used for construction of the image. For example, 2.5 MHz can be transmitted and then while a whole range of frequencies are received only the 5 MHz or "second harmonic" signals are used. Although it was initially thought that only contrast microbubbles produced harmonic frequencies because of their specific resonant properties, it is now known that tissue alters the transmitted ultrasound pulse to produce harmonic signals. Specifically clutter signal and artifactual signals are reduced using this technique (Figure 1).

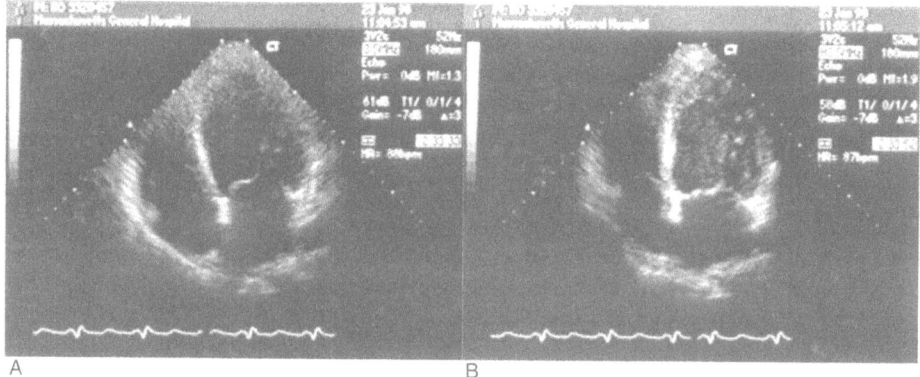

Figure 1. An example of improvement in left ventricular endocardial border delineation with harmonic imaging during transthoracic echocardiography. A. Apical four chamber view with 3.5 MHz transducer. B. Same view using harmonic imaging. Note the improvement in identification of all borders particularly the apical and lateral endocadium.

New clinical applications of echocardiography

In addition to improvements in instrumentation, there continue to be new ways in which we apply echocardiography both in clinical practice and in research. In clinical settings this includes: 1) the use of transesophageal echocardiography in the operating room in conjunction with cardiac surgery, 2) evolving protocols utilizing exercise and pharmacologic stress to diagnose the spectrum of coronary artery disease, 3) new methods for quantitation of valvular regurgitation and intracardiac hemodynamics using Doppler, and 4) use of contrast agents to assess myocardial perfusion.

In parallel with new innovations in cardiac surgical techniques, intraoperative transesophageal echocardiography now has become an integral part of many procedures (Table 2). The goal is that the information provided to the surgeon can assist in the design of the appropriate operation, reduce the duration of the procedure and improve outcome.

Current uses for intraoperative echocardiography include: 1) assessing valve morphology in order to determine best approach to repair [8,9], 2) post-operative assessment of adequacy of valve repair [10], 3) determining etiology for difficulty encountered upon weaning from cardiopulmonary bypass, 4) imaging of the aorta to identify "high risk" aortic atheroma prior to identifying best sites for cannulation and cross clamping of the aorta [11], 5) identification of air in the heart, 6) early detection of myocardial ischemia/regional wall motion abnormalities, 7) assessing extent of aortic dissection, 8) identification of left atrial and appendage thrombi, 9) assessing prosthetic valve function and paravalvular leaks, and 10) guidance of minimally invasive procedures - by imaging cardiac structures which previously would have been directly visualized and by confirming the position of intravascular catheters/vents/drains and endo-aortic occlusion devices.

Design modifications in the future will allow surgeons to use miniaturized transducers for epicardial and epi-aortic imaging in addition to the continued use of transesophageal imag-

Table 2: Echocardiography during cardiac surgery

1. Assessment of valve morphology prior to repair
2. Post-operative assessment of adequacy of valve repair
3. Determination of etiology for difficulty encountered upon weaning from cardiopulmonary bypass
4. Imaging of the aorta to identify "high risk" aortic atheroma

   • identification of best sites for cannulation / cross clamping of the aorta

5. Identification of air in the heart
6. Early detection of myocardial ischemia (regional wall motion abnormalities)
7. Assessment of extent of aortic dissection
8. Identification of left atrial and appendage thrombi
9. Assessment of prosthetic valve function / paravalvular leaks
10. Guidance of minimally invasive procedures

   • confirming the position of percutaneously placed intravascular catheters and endo-aortic occlusion devices required for cardiopulmonary bypass
   • imaging cardiac structures previously directly visualized

ing. Three-dimensional echocardiography with its unique display capabilities should have a future role in surgical planning. However, development of interactive display/workstations which will allow the surgeon correcting congenital heart lesions to pre-operatively plan complex procedures by segmenting or dissecting a three-dimensional echocardiographic image on such a workstation in a manner mimicking the operation is still required.

Recent improvements in gas filled microbubbles combined with enhancements in instrumentation (intermittent and harmonic imaging) have the potential to revolutionize the field of noninvasive imaging. When properly constructed, the microbubbles reflect sound and thus their appearance in cardiac chambers and myocardium can be easily identified by an increased signal during transthoracic two-dimensional echocardiography. At present, the intravenous administration of these contrast agents, which pass through the right heart and pulmonary circuit, results in left ventricular cavity opacification and thus enhanced detection of endocardial borders. This has the potential to improve the quality of echocardiograms in patients who provide technical challenges to imaging and also to improve the ability to assess both Doppler signals [12], and regional and global left ventricular function [13].

To date, the most successful studies of myocardial contrast echocardiography for assessing perfusion beds has been with direct injections into the left heart. Such studies have demonstrated the ability to accurately predict infarct size from risk area [14], delineate the presence of collateral vessels often not appreciated by angiography [15] and, quantitate the presence of "no reflow" after successful recanalization of an occluded coronary artery [16].

Although not yet ready for widespread clinical applications, the greatest excitement of this contrast technique is that it should allow assessment of myocardial perfusion at the bedside without need for radiation exposure. Specifically this includes identification of the success of reperfusion therapy in acute myocardial infarction, the outpatient diagnosis of significant coronary artery disease, assessment of the physiologic significance of coronary collateral vessels, assessment of myocardial perfusion before and after interventions, and as an adjunct to stress echocardiography to relate coronary anatomy and physiology to ventricular structure and function. Once algorithms can successfully quantitate coronary flow [17], contrast agents and echocardiography can be combined with coronary vasodilators to assess coronary flow reserve, thus allowing discrimination between degrees of coronary artery disease.

New applications of echocardiography in research

Echocardiography now plays an expanding role in both clinical and experimental research settings to answer important fundamental questions. Increasingly echocardiography is being used as a primary endpoint in clinical trials. For example, echocardiography has been instrumental in studies of: 1) left ventricular mass regression after treatment of hypertension [18], 2) treatment of cardiogenic shock [19], 3) new strategies for treating heart failure [20], 4) treatment of myocarditis [21] and 5) catheter based coronary interventions [22].

The development of genetically altered small animals has enhanced our understanding of the role of specific genes in disease states and the basic mechanisms underlying cardiac physiology [23]. Under- or over-expression of specific gene products in mice have produced models with decreased or increased cardiac function [24,25], cardiac hypertrophy [26-28], congenital heart defects [29] and accelerated atherosclerosis [30,31]. The challenge in this setting has been to develop methods to assess these phenotypic changes. The first methods were histologic and required sacrifice of the animal models. Thus long term follow-up of an individual animal was not possible to assess natural history. Next, invasive methods for measuring ventricular pressures and performing angiography were perfected [32]. Again the preparation required for these invasive approaches often preclude serial studies and the tenuous hemodynamic states of many of these preparations are altered by the required deep anesthesia and thoracotomy [33]. Challenges to high quality echocardiographic imaging in mice include the small size of the heart (10 x 5 mm) and the rapid resting heart rate (600-700 bpm). Advances in parallel processing and broad band transducers have resulted in the ability to obtain images of the murine heart with high frequency transthoracic echocardiographic transducers operating at high frame rates, thus providing optimal representation of both cardiac structure and motion throughout the cardiac cycle (Figure 2). Furthermore, additional modifications in technique and instruments have enabled visualization and quantitation of murine right ventricular function [34,35] and neonatal mice [36]. Contrast echocardiographic techniques have now been applied to these models to assist in understanding alterations in the myocardial circulation (Figure 2C) [37].

Digital echocardiography

In the past, one of the weaknesses of echocardiography in comparison to most other imaging techniques was that, although the data were initially acquired in a digital format, it was converted to analog format for presentation and archiving on videotape. Thus, later processing of the image and other tasks such as quantitation or border detection were difficult. In addition, the tedious process of searching through long segments of videotape record made comparison of multiple studies on the same patient time consuming. In the past, if the digital data were to be used for image representation, extensive compression of the files was necessary for standard computers to handle or store the data especially when color Doppler or

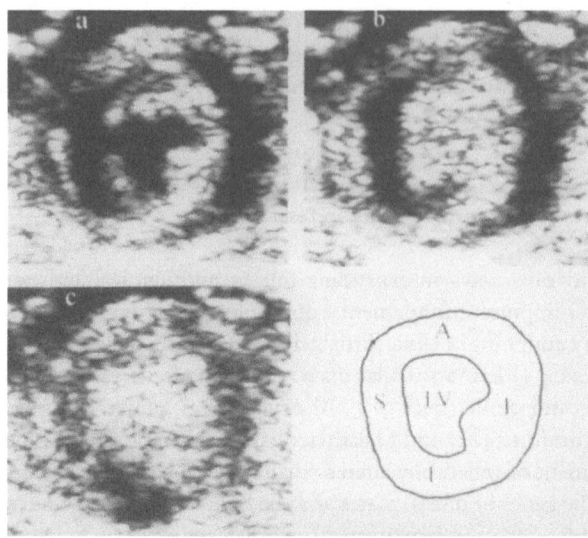

Figure 2. Examples of murine transthoracic echocadiography. A) Short axis view at mid ventricular level performed with 13 MHz linear array probe. B) Same view after jugular venous injection of contrast microbubbles. Opacification of the left ventricular cavity is homogeneous. C) Five beats after appearance of the contrast in the left ventricular cavity, passage of contrast is noted in the myocardial segments as an increase in the videointensity of the segments (compared to A). The lack of signal in the inferior wall is due to attenuation of signal by the contrast in the left ventricular cavity. D) Schematic of the left ventricle delineating segments. LV - left ventricular cavity; A - anterior wall; S - septum; L - lateral; I - inferior.

multiple cardiac cycles were included. This made transmission of echocardiographic studies for off-site review a challenge.

However now that both echocardiographic instruments and computers have matured, this modality can be maintained in digital format. The next stage of development of echo labs will be facilities where the digitally acquired images are transferred throughout the hospital from the echo machine over networks to high capacity storage media. The studies then will be able to be interpreted on computer workstations. The advantages of the digital echocardiographic laboratory are multiple and include ease of interpretation, storage, comparison, quantitation, processing and transfer. The prospects for telemedicine with this approach are expansive. When combined with high speed transmission strategies or use of the world wide web, clinical applications include the potential for real-time expert review of emergency procedures from a distance thus reducing delays in patient care [38]. With improvements in border detection, automated endocardial border detection is possible leading to rapid assessment of left ventricular volumes and ejection fractions [39]. When combined with opacification of the blood pool with intravenous contrast agents, this task can be even more simplified. Thus, it is possible that in the future, transthoracic echocardiograms specifically performed for left ventricular function assessment can be rapidly acquired, consisting of a brief series of views performed during the continuous infusion of contrast microbubbles in a concentration high enough to constantly opacify the left ventricle and that an ejection fraction will be automatically quantitated after the application of algorithms which detect the contrast silhouette.

The ability to acquire, manipulate and store echocardiographic images in digital format has led to advances in three-dimensional imaging and other novel strategies. For example, dynamic holographic echocardiographic images of the heart can not only be constructed but also printed by holographic laser printers, thus allowing the representation of cardiac motion on printable two-dimensional media [40]. By tilting the images in relation to a light source, these hand-held prints provide visualization of cardiac structures with the same resolution and accuracy of a standard two-dimensional echocardiogram and provide visualization of motion. A major advantage of this technology is that all of the information is provided on one page, thus making storage and incorporation into the medical record quite easy.

Conclusion

In summary, tremendous accomplishments have resulted in the development of echocardiography over the last 35 years. Its versatility has resulted in its position as an important tool in the care of patients with heart disease. Enhancements currently under development are even more exciting and will ensure both the long term practicality and viability of this ultrasound technique in the medical imaging field.

References

1. Edler I, Herz CH. The use of ultrasonic relfectoscope for the continuous recording of movements of heart walls. Kungl Fysiogr Sallsk I Lund Forhandl 1954;24:5.
2. Picard MH. Transesophageal echocardiography: Advantages and indications in the era of health care reform. Int J Cardiac Imaging 1995;11(Suppl 1):1-4.
3. Krumholz HM Douglas PS Goldman L Waksmonski C. Clinical utility of transthoracic two-dimensional and Doppler echocardiography. J Am Coll Cardiol 1994;24:125-31.
4. Picard MH, Wilkins GT, Ray PA, Weyman AE. Natural history of left ventricular size and function after acute myocardial infarction. Assessment and prediction by echocardiographic endocardial surface mapping. Circulation 1990;82:484-94.
5. Hunziker PR, Liel-Cohen N, Scherrer-Crosbie M, Buck T, Levine RA, Picard MH. Determination of myocardial fiber architecture in man by high-resolution echocardiography. J Am Coll Cardiol 1998;31(Suppl A):478A.
6. Bednarz J, Spencer KT, Mor-Avi V, Korcarz CE, Rafter P, Lang RM. Can harmonic imaging without contrast enhancement aid in the echocardiographic evaluation of left ventricular function?]abstract]. Circulation 1997;96(8 Suppl):I584.
7. Pyles JM, Sawada SG, Feigenbaum H, Segar DS. Enhanced endocardial visualization using harmonic imaging without contrast [abstract]. Circulation 1997;96(8 Suppl):I585.
8. David TE, Armstrong S, Sun Z, Daniel L. Late results of mitral valve repair for mitral regurgitation due to degenerative disease. Ann Thorac Surg 1993;56:7-14.
9. Foster GP, Isselbacher EM, Rose GA, Torchiana DF, Akins CW, Picard MH. Accurate localization of mitral regurgitant defects using multiplane transesophageal echocardiography. Ann Thorac Surg. In press 1998.
10. Marwick TH, Stewart WJ, Currie PJ, Cosgrove DM. Mechanisms of failure of mitral valve repair: an echocardiographic study. Am Heart J 1991;122:149-56.
11. Wareing TH, Davila-Roman VG, Daily BB *et al.* Strategy for the reduction of stroke incidence in cardiac surgical patients. Ann Thorac Surg 1993;55:1400-8.
12. Willliams MJA, McClements BM, Picard MH. Improvement of transthoracic pulmonary venous flow Doppler signal with intravenous injection of sonicated albumin. J Am Coll Cardiol 1995:26;1741-6.
13. Hundley WG, Kizilbash A, Afridi I, Franco F, Peshock, Grayburn PA. Intravenous dodecafluoropentane improves determination of left ventricular function during transthoracic echocardiography [abstract]. J Am Coll Cardiol 1997;29(Suppl A):520A.

14. Kaul S, Pandian NG, Okada RD, Pohost GM, Weyman AE. Contrast echocardiography in acute myocardial ischemia: I. In vivo determination of total left ventricular "area at risk". J Am Coll Cardiol 1984;4:1272-82.

15. Ragosta M, Camarano G, Kaul S, Powers ER, Sarembock IJ, Gimple LW. Microvascular integrity indicates myocellular viability in patients with recent myocardial infarction. New insights using myocardial contrast echocardiography. Circulation 1994;89:2562-9.

16. Ito H, Tomooka T, Sakai N et al. Lack of myocardial perfusion immediately after successful thrombolysis. A predictor of poor recovery of left ventricular function in anterior myocardial infarction. Circulation 1992;85:1699-705.

17. Wei K, Jayaweera AR, Firoozan S, Linka A, Skyba DM, Kaul S. Quantification of myocardial blood flow with ultrasound-induced destruction of microbubbles administered as a contrast venous infusion. Circulation 1998;97:473-83.

18. Papademetriou V, Gottdiener JS, Narayan P et al. Hydrochlorothiazide is superior to isradipine for reduction of left ventricular mass: results of a multicenter trial. The Isradipine Study Group. J Am Coll Cardiol 1997;30:1802-8.

19. Hochman JS, Menon V, Connery C et al. Outcome of patients undergoing cardiac surgery during hospitalization for cardiogenic shock (CS) complicating acute MI [abstract]. Circulation 1997;96(8 Suppl):I435.

20. Scherrer-Crosbie M, Cocca-Spofford D, DiSalvo TG, Semigran MJ, Dec GW, Picard MH. Effect of vesnarinone on cardiac function in patients with severe congestive heart failure. Am Heart J. In press 1998.

21. Mendes LA, Picard MH, Dec GW, Davidoff R. Early development of sphericity in active myocarditis: association with left ventricular volume and function. Myocarditis Treatment Trial (MTT) Investigators. J Am Soc Echocardiogr 1994;7:S39.

22. Williams MJA, Dow CJ, Newell JB, Palacios IF, Picard MH. Prevalence and timing of regional myocardial dysfunction after rotational coronary atherectomy. J Am Coll Cardiol 1996;28:861-9.

23. Steudel W, Scherrer-Crosbie M, Bloch KD et al. Sustained pulmonary hypertension and right ventricular hypertrophy after chronic hypoxia in mice with congenital deficiency of nitric oxide synthase 3. J Clin Invest. In press 1998.

24. Milano CA, Allen LF, Rockman HA et al. Enhanced myocardial function in transgenic mice overexpressing the beta 2-adrenergic receptor. Science 1994;264:582-6.

25. D'Angelo DD, Sakata Y, Lorenz JN et al. Transgenic Galphaq overexpression induces cardiac contractile failure in mice. Proc Natl Acad Sci U S A 1997;94:8121-6.

26. Gottshall KR, Becker KD, Hunter JJ, Chien KR. A genetic model of cardiac hypertrophy in MLC-ras mice. J Card Fail 1996;2(4 Suppl):S28-34.

27. Hirota H, Yoshida K, Kishimoto T, Taga T. Continuous activation of gp130, a signal-transducing receptor component for interleukin 6-related cytokines, causes myocardial hypertrohy in mice. Proc Natl Acad Sci U S A 1995;92:4862-6.

28. Geisterfer-Lowrance AA, Christe M, Conner DA et al. A mouse model of familial hypertrophic cardiomyopathy. Science 1996;272:731-4.

29. Ewart JL, Cohen MF, Meyer RA et al. Heart and neural tube defects in transgenic mice overexpressing the Cx43 gap junction gene. Development 1997;124:1281-92.

30. Plump AS, Smith JD, Hayek T et al. Severe hypercholesterolemia and atherosclerosis in apolipoprotein E-deficient mice created by homologous recombination in ES cells. Cell 1992;71:343-53.

31. Ishibashi S, Brown MS, Goldstein JL, Gerard RD, Hammer RE, Herz J. Hypercholesterolemia in low density lipoprotein receptor knockout mice and its reversal by adenovirus-mediated gene delivery. J Clin Invest 1993;92:883-93.

32. Rockman HA, Ono S, Ross RS et al. Molecular and physiological alterations in murine ventricular dysfunction. Proc Natl Acad Sci U S A 1994;91:2694-8.

33. Hoit BD, Ball N, Walsh RA. Invasive hemodynamics and force-frequency relationships in open- versus closed-chest mice. Am J Physiol 1997;273:H2528-2533.

34. Scherrer-Crosbie M, Steudel W, Hunziker PR, Foster GP, Zapol WM, Picard MH. Validation of three dimensional transesophageal echocardiography for right ventricular volumes and function in mice [abstract]. Circulation 1997;96(8 Suppl):I698.

35. Scherrer-Crosbie M, Steudel W, Hunziker PR, Foster GP, Zapol WM, Picard MH. Validation of transesophageal echocardiography for the assessment of right ventricular hypertrophy in the mouse [abstract]. Circulation 1997;96(8 Suppl):I699.

36. Fatkin D, Aristizabal O, Srinivasan S *et al.* Noninvasive in vivo assessment of cardiac function in the neonatal murine heart using high frequency (50 Mhz) ultrasound backscatter microscopy [abstract]. Circulation 1997;96(8 Suppl):I738.

37. Scherer-Crosbie M, Steudel W, Hunziker PR, Liel-Cohen N, Zapol WM, Picard MH. Noninvasive assessment of myocardial perfusion in mice: a contrast echocardiography study [abstract]. J Am Coll Cardiol 1998;31(Suppl A):438A.

38. Trippi JA, Lee KS, Kopp G, Nelson DR, Yee KG, Cordell WH. Dobutamine stress tele-echocardiography for evaluation of emergency department patients with chest pain. J Am Coll Cardiol 1997;30:627-32.

39. Picard MH, Bosch HG, Morrissey RL, Reiber JHC. Automated echocardiographic ventricular volume quantitation: validation of a new border detection method [abstract]. Circulation 1994;90(4 Suppl):I608.

40. Hunziker PR, Klug MA, Scherrer-Crosbie M *et al.* Dynamic holographic imaging of the beating human heart. Circulation 1997;96(8 Suppl):I698.

26.

Intravenous echocontrast for assessment of left ventricular function and perfusion

Thomas H. Marwick

Summary

New echocardiographic contrast agents are being approved by regulatory authorities. These microbubbles have greater reflectivity and persistence than the previously available compounds. This review summarizes the important technical considerations surrounding these compounds and the processes required to image them. Echocardiographic contrast will be used for opacification of the left ventricle (particularly during stress echocardiography), Doppler enhancement, and assessment of myocardial perfusion. Of these indications, the prospect of assessment of myocardial perfusion is the most attractive, but also most difficult. This chapter discusses some of the pitfalls of qualitative evaluation, and the development of post processing techniques to solve these limitations.

Introduction

Echocardiographic contrast agents promise a new dimension to echocardiography. The impact of these agents on the clinical application of echocardiography is likely to be great, and at least as marked as the changes provoked by the introduction of color Doppler or transesophageal echocardiography in the last 10 years. The major indications for contrast echocardiography will be delineation of the ventricular cavity and identification of myocardial perfusion. While these aims seem simple, the acquisition of reliable data for both purposes is quite complex, and before discussing the clinical applications of contrast echo, this chapter will review some basic concepts regarding contrast agents, imaging and analysis.

Technical considerations for contrast echocardiography

Contrast agents

Echo contrast enhancement is based upon strong reflection of ultrasound from gas liquid interfaces. Such interfaces magnify the backscatter of ultrasound by up to 10^{12}, compared with only two-fold increases in backscatter from solid-liquid interfaces. Thus, the presence of microbubbles within the ventricular cavity clearly separates blood from endocardium, and

J.H.C. Reiber and E.E. van der Wall (eds.). What's New in Cardiovascular Imaging, 333–350.
©1998 Kluwer Academic Publishers.

this distinction is several orders of magnitude greater than the usual signal which delineates the tissue blood interface. The size of microbubbles is greater than the wavelength of ultrasound, so the agents scatter rather than reflect incident ultrasound. The strength of the backscatter signal is proportionate to the 6th power of the radius of the bubbles [1], although bubble size is constrained by the need to pass through the circulation. Backscatter is also proportionate to the amount of contrast present, so administration of greater concentrations increases left sided opacification [2]. The use of bolus injections in the presence of heart failure and other conditions which increase pulmonary transit time, is associated with reduction of LV opacification due to dilution of the bolus.

Echocardiographic contrast agents have been used for over 30 years [3], predominantly for the recognition of right heart pathology, enhancement of right sided Doppler signals at rest and exercise [4] and identification of cardiac shunts. The most widely used agent for right heart evaluation is agitated normal saline, and the best opacification is obtained by mixing a small amount of blood prior to agitation. Application of the technique to left sided and intra-coronary injections required reduction of bubble size, which was accomplished by sonication [5]. This was also found to denature albumen and contribute to a stable bubble shell. Microbubbles formed by this technique have a uniform bubble size <10 microns in diameter (average 5 microns). This technique permitted the production of air-filled bubbles of contrast agent (Renografin) or albumin, which have been used for studies of the coronary circulation via catheter injection [6-8].

For intravenous use, microbubbles need to be small and persistent. For both safety and efficacy, bubbles need to be small enough to traverse the capillaries; embolization in the lungs would reduce the delivery of contrast to the heart, and embolization of the coronary circulation may produce untoward events. After intravenous injection, contrast agents may be filtered by the lungs, destroyed by mechanical pressure [9,10], or dissolve within the circulation. Persistence of the contrast effect is required for several minutes if complete imaging is to be feasible. The persistence of microbubbles (T) is expressed by the equation:

$$T = r^2 \cdot \rho / 2D \cdot Cs$$

Thus, persistence is proportionate to the square of the radius and the density of the gas, and inversely proportionate to diffusivity and the saturation constant. As the size of the bubbles is limited by the need to traverse the microcirculation, persistence can best be increased by increasing the density of the gas, and selecting gases of low diffusivity and solubility.

Intravenous contrast agents which are currently available or under development are listed in Table 1 [11]. The first generation agents, Albunex [12,13] and Levovist are air-filled bubbles which produce modest frequency and degrees of LV opacification, but rarely myocardial opacification. The only air-filled second generation agent is Quantison Depot, in which the high diffusivity of air is controlled by the bubble membrane. Generally, the second generation agents have been based upon the use of perfluorocarbons to increase density and reduce diffusivity of the bubble contents [14]. The main distinction between these agents is between those that are free flowing, compared with agents which have prolonged persistence in the coronary circulation related to local deposition. At present, the clinical experience with the 2nd generation agents is limited; initial impressions do not suggest that there is a substantial difference between them in terms of safety or efficacy.

Table 1: Commercially produced echocardiographic contrast agents for MCE from venous injections. Modified from Kaul [11]

Name	Manufacturer	Distributor (USA)	Size (μm)	Conc.[a]	Shell composition	Gases	Indication (eventual[b])
Free-following tracers							
Albunex	Molecular Biosystems	Mallinckrodt Medical	4.3	0.5	Denatured albumin	Air	LVO, MCE[c]
Optison	Molecular Biosystems	Mallinckrodt Medical	3.9	0.8	Denatured albumin	Air/perfluoropropane	LVO, MCE
Aerosomes	ImaRx Pharmaceutical	Dupont-Merck	-	-	Lipids and surfactants	Air/perfluoropropane	LVO, MCE
Imagent	Alliance	Not determined	5.0	0.5	No shell; surfactant stabilized	Air/perfluoropropane	LVO, MCE
BR1	Bracco	Bracco	2.5	0.2	Lipids and surfactants	Air/H_2SF_6	LVO, MCE
Levovist	Schering	Berlex	2-4	-	No shell; surfactant stabilized	Air	LVO
Sonovist	Schering	Berlex	1-2	-	Cyanoacrylate	Air	LVO, MCE
N100100	Nycomed	Nycomed	4-6	-	No information released	Air	LVO, MCE
Deposit tracers							
Quantison depot	Andaris	Not determined	10.0	0.015	Denatured albumin (very thick shell)	Air	MCE[c]
Echogen	Sonos	Abbott	3-5	1000	No shell; surfactant stabilized	Dodecafluoropentane	LVO, MCE

a.   Concentration 10^{-9} (in vitro measurements)
b.   Indications for most pending FDA approval
c.   For left heart (LV, aortic root, or direct coronary injections) only

Ultrasound technology and myocardial contrast

The current generation of ultrasound equipment is not optimized for contrast echocardiography. Thresholding (Figure 1) prevents the recognition of low levels of activity (insufficient to be differentiated from baseline noise). At the other end of the spectrum of signal amplitude, excessive backscatter may saturate the system. Nonetheless, development of new echo contrast agents has enabled LV opacification and Doppler enhancement with standard ultrasound equipment.

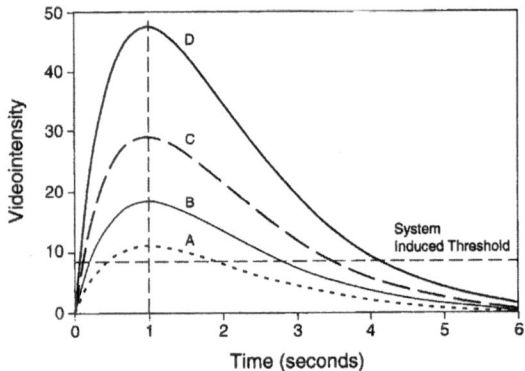

Figure 1. Effect of contrast dose on duration of detectable myocardial contrast effect. Greater doses (e.g. C or D) attain threshold most rapidly and last longer, giving the longest effect.

The presence of contrast within the LV may reduce the distinction between cavity and endocardium, particularly if the gains are too high. Moreover, great challenges surround the identification of coronary flow with contrast echo techniques. The major problem is that intra-myocardial blood volume accounts for <10% of total myocardial volume, so that the contribution of contrast, and particularly increments of contrast volume have limited impact on the backscatter from the wall. Indeed, the increment in brightness may be no greater than that due to the inherent noise of the image. Increasing the delivery of contrast increases the backscatter from the myocardium, but is limited by the production of attenuation from overlying segments, as well as increases of LV cavity intensity. Several techniques have been developed which enhance the ability to identify contrast within the myocardial blood volume.

1. Harmonic imaging. The use of the harmonic imaging increases the distinction between contrast and myocardium. The physical basis of this phenomenon is illustrated in Figure 2. Oscillation of the bubbles in response to ultrasound leads to reflection of waves at twice, or multiples of the frequency of the incident ultrasound [15]. The harmonic response is dependent on shell stiffness (rigid shells are more difficult to oscillate) and bubble size (small bubbles require higher transmitted frequencies). Fortuitously, bubbles of appropriate size to pass through the lungs are also highly resonant, using the typical frequency for diagnostic ultrasound. Using a broad-band transducer, the ultrasound device therefore transmits at one frequency and selectively receives at twice this frequency. This technique has improved contrast enhancement and improved delineation of the endocardial border, by permitting reduction

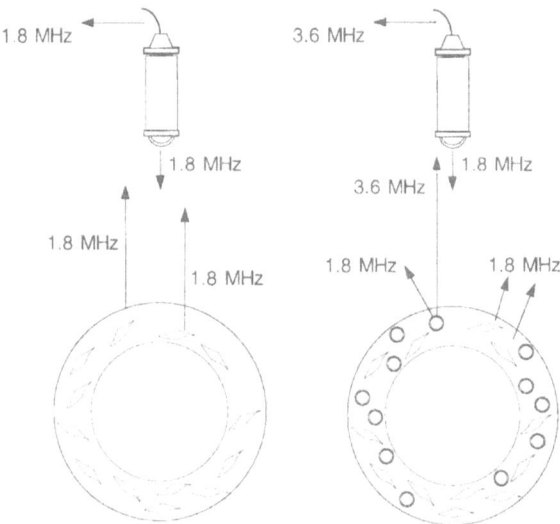

Figure 2. Physical basis of harmonic imaging. Ultrasound is reflected at harmonics of the insonating frequency. The reception of these removes clutter from non-contrast images and dramatically improves delineation of LV cavity and myocardium.

of the overall gain settings, and therefore reducing the signal from myocardium. The LV opacification may be seen with this technique in situations where it was previously not, and the duration of opacification is also prolonged.

2. Doppler imaging. Movement of the myocardium produces signals of low frequency and high amplitude, which are normally filtered in the course of acquiring Doppler images of blood flow. Alteration of gain and filter settings permits myocardial Doppler data to be derived for velocity, acceleration, or power. If the blood component is enhanced by contrast effect, power or energy Doppler imaging of myocardial blood flow may be differentiated from adjacent tissue by combination with harmonic imaging [16].

3. Triggered imaging. Exposure of microbubbles to ultrasound contributes to their destruction [17]. Indeed, the apical segments of the ventricle are usually less well opacified than the remainder of the ventricle, based upon the intensity of the scan lines close to the transducer. Exposure of the bubbles to ultrasound at only one point in every cardiac cycle, or even every few cardiac cycles, reduces bubble destruction, and therefore increases both persistence and intensity of myocardial opacification [18]. There is no consensus as to the optimal timing of triggering. We have favored diastolic triggering, because the heart is in a more uniform and reproducible position during diastole, and on theoretical grounds, coronary perfusion is maximal. However, systolic triggering is favored if quantitative approaches are used (see below), because larger regions of interest may be drawn, without including signals from the LV cavity and bright endocardial and epicardial targets.

Image acquisition

1. Equipment settings. In respect of equipment, it seems likely that harmonic imaging will be the technique of choice, with no apparent down-side, for both delineation of the LV cavity and assessment of myocardial perfusion. Lower frequency imaging increases bubble destruction, so the highest possible imaging frequency is desirable [19]. A more difficult decision is the selection of continuous vs. intermittent imaging. For wall motion assessment, continuous imaging is preferable. Triggered imaging is more desirable if the purpose of the study is mainly examination of myocardial perfusion, and this is particularly the case if visual interpretation is planned - certainly, triggered and continuous imaging are likely to be combined in future protocols. The selection of end-diastolic or end-systolic triggering remains an unresolved issue, with advantages for each. Similarly, optimal triggering intervals need to be defined, and although myocardial opacification is better with greater intervals between the triggers, this has the disadvantage of making the examination more difficult, particularly in respect of maintaining the same image orientation.

Power (measured as mechanical index) is correlated closely with detection of adequate contrast effect, but is also an important determinant of bubble destruction. We usually start the study with the lowest power which gives good opacification (usually MI 0.7 to 0.8), and use higher power settings when triggered imaging is performed (MI 1.0). A wide dynamic range should be selected, to maximize the gray scale. Overall gain is unrelated to power, and should be increased as necessary to optimize the image, as it has no effect on bubble destruction. Lateral gain control may sometimes be useful for enhancing the baseline delineation of the anterior and lateral walls, and of producing homogeneous levels of gain at baseline. The image focus is usually placed at the junction of the upper two-thirds and lower third of the image. A linear post processing curve is preferable.

2. Imaging technique. The technique of contrast echocardiography will likely require a slightly different approach from standard 2D echocardiography. The parasternal views may be limited by attenuation of the posterior wall due to overlying contrast within the left ventricular cavity, although the use of low dose infusions has minimized this effect. Apical views also pose limitations, related to bubble destruction in the apex, reduction of visualization in the lateral and anterior walls (related to anisotropy and overlying lung - Figure 3) and inabil-

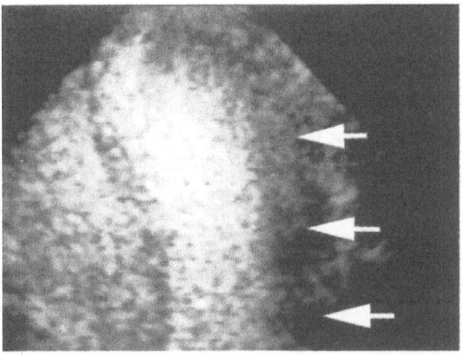

Figure 3. Artifact giving the appearance of a perfusion defect in the lateral wall.

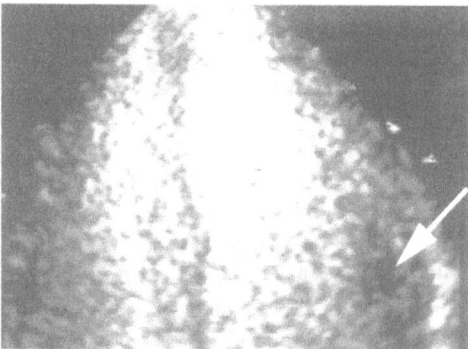

Figure 4. Apparent perfusion defect caused by attenuation from overlying contrast.

ity to incorporate all the segments within the ultrasound sector. Contrast in proximal segments may attenuate distal segments, as may contrast within the ventricular cavity (Figure 4). Off-axis views may be useful in overcoming the limitations posed by far-field attenuation, bubble destruction in the apex, and poor baseline visualization of the lateral and anterior walls. At present, therefore, as many views as possible should be obtained.

3. Contrast administration. Although all agents have been administered in bolus form, the free-flowing agents may also be administered as an infusion, in which case steady states are attained. The infusion rate may be titrated to minimize posterior attenuation. The other benefit of infusion is that, once administration is optimized, additional help from an assistant is not required.

Interpretation of myocardial contrast studies

1. Evaluation of perfusion defects. Assessment of myocardial perfusion from intravenous injections of contrast was feasible in only about one quarter of injections with first generation agents [20], using fundamental imaging. The use of harmonic imaging and second generation agents has increased the feasibility of myocardial contrast echocardiography, which may be evaluated qualitatively or quantitatively. Qualitative analysis is attractive because additional software and hardware would not be required in addition to standard echocardiographic imaging technology. However, this approach is limited by subjectivity, the need for adequate training, the ability to appreciate minor gradations of gray scale, and dependence on the technical quality of the image. Even when the echo image is optimized, the backscatter intensity from different walls may vary. If a wall is already bright on the pre-contrast image, an increment of brightness due to myocardial perfusion will be difficult to detect. Regional variations of echo contrast intensity may be unrelated to CAD, for example due to attenuation (Figure 4), or artifacts (Figure 3). Although a qualitative gray-scale approach has been found efficacious in expert hands, the technique has produced disappointing results in multicenter studies [21].

The use of post-processing may increase the feasibility of the visual analysis of myocardial contrast echocardiography. The first and simplest step is to acquire the data in digital format, which has the benefit of avoiding image degradation from video tape, as well as allowing interpretation of contrast activity in the context of the segmental activity on the resting image. The ability to compare segmental backscatter before and after contrast may reduce the impact of heterogeneous backscatter levels obtained from segment to segment. Digital acquisition also permits further steps in post-processing, such as averaging and subtraction of the baseline image [22]. The averaging of multiple cardiac cycles reduces the amount of noise in the image, and subtraction from baseline reduces the impact of gray scale levels in the resting image, so that only the effect of the contrast is seen in the subtracted image. The use of subtraction is only possible if no changes have been made in the power, gain and dynamic range settings between baseline and post contrast. Finally, because the eye is more able to discern colors than shades of gray, color coding of the resulting subtracted image may also facilitate visual analysis [23].

Although these steps may enhance the feasibility of visual analysis, this approach remains subjective. Myocardial perfusion defects may be quantified by analysis of videointensity or using radio-frequency data. Video intensity analyses may examine the maximum degree of reflectivity from a segment, the rate of appearance of contrast, or its speed of disappearance (Figure 1). Unfortunately, following intravenous injection, myocardial contrast agents do not act as good blood flow tracers. First, the contrast bolus is diluted before delivery to the myocardium; thus, the rate of appearance of tracer may reflect stroke volume as much as coronary flow [24]. Second, many microbubbles lack the traditional requirements of a blood flow tracer, such as inertness, stability, and passage as red blood cells [1], so that the transit time is itself influenced by the concentration of tracer. Third, time-intensity curves are also concentration dependent, and influenced by the thresholding and saturation points of different echocardiographic systems (Figure 1). Finally, the analogue-digital converter and the standard imaging display (dynamic range 30 dB) require focusing the larger dynamic range of the ultrasound system (approximately 70 dB) by logarithmic compression and nonlinear postprocessing. Consequently, the intensity of the displayed signal does not correlate with microbubble concentration. The recent development of acoustic densitometry minimizes this problem by use of linear acoustic data. However, the resulting time intensity curves reflect myocardial blood volume rather than regional flow because of the limitations discussed above.

The use of integrated backscatter measurements of unprocessed radio-frequency signals may permit identification of phase shifts of the returning ultrasound due to absorption of energy by microbubbles [25,26]. This approach is highly sensitive to the identification of small concentrations of contrast agents, and less for high concentrations [27]. However, the technique of examining phase shift is not feasible from video intensity because of distortion due to scan conversion and postprocessing. Unfortunately, due to the huge amounts of data that are obtained for radio-frequency analysis, and the extensive postprocessing requirements, the technique is unlikely to be useful in the clinical arena.

2. Quantitation of myocardial blood flow. Although the quantitation of myocardial perfusion is looked upon as an ultimate goal of contrast echocardiography, this has proved elusive. Initial studies examining the washout time and area under the contrast intensity-time curve showed poor correlation with coronary blood flow and flow reserve [28]. Reasons for this include the limitations of current injection techniques and analysis, and the mixture of both deposit and free-flowing characteristics of tracers [29]. However, Skyba has recorded correlation of background-subtracted peak intensity values with myocardial blood volume and blood flow when both are coupled, for example during inotropic stimulation [30]. As microbubbles demonstrate similar transit times and velocities to red blood cells [7], contrast echocardiography has the ability to identify both myocardial blood flow and myocardial blood volume.

A novel approach to measurements of myocardial blood flow with contrast agents is based upon the destruction and replenishment of microbubbles within the circulation [5]. Using this methodology, microbubbles are infused constantly. Exposure to ultrasound and one point in time may destroy most or all of the bubbles. As blood with new bubbles passes into the region of interest, the concentration of microbubbles increases. Intermittent imaging will document a commensurate increase of video-intensity, until the pulsing interval parallels the time needed to replenish the beam thickness with bubbles, at which time a plateau is attained (Figure 5). The rate of video-intensity increase reflects myocardial blood flow

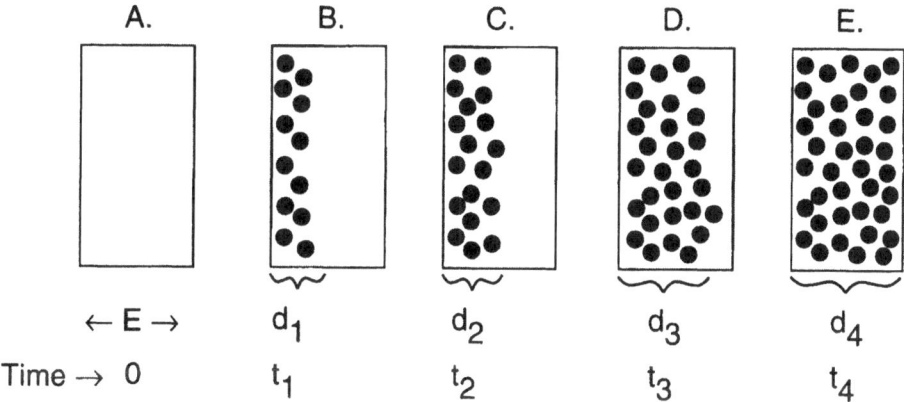

Figure 5. Destruction of microbubbles (t=0), followed by gradual filling of beam thickness after various intervals of time (d1-d4). The time required to refill the thickness of the beam is proportionate to coronary flow.

velocity. The procedure is performed by defining two triggers, one designed to destroy the bubbles, and the second to obtain images. The two will not be confused if imaging is performed in a uniform time during the cardiac cycle, for example in systole. Progressive increments of the pulsing interval are made until a plateau of contrast intensity is obtained.

Clinical applications of contrast echocardiography

Right heart contrast

As has been mentioned previously, the initial applications of contrast echocardiography were performed using microbubbles prepared by hand agitation. Although these large bubbles are filtered by the lungs, this technique facilitated evaluation of the right heart. In combination with either transthoracic or transesophageal echocardiography, right heart contrast studies may be used for identification of interatrial shunts or patent foramen ovale (especially small lesions not detected by color Doppler), atrial septal aneurysm, quantitation of pulmonary shunt in patients with liver disease, and enhancement of evaluation of tricuspid regurgitation. Aberrant caval drainage to the coronary sinus may also be identified. These continue to be clinically useful applications of contrast techniques.

LV opacification

Attenuation due to overlying chest wall or lung may cause variable image quality using transthoracic echocardiography. While it is unusual for a study to be completely uninterpretable because of inadequate images, failure to identify all segments of the myocardium is quite common [31-33], especially in the anterior and apical walls [34]. Studies specifically focused on this question have shown inadequate imaging in 30% of segments [35,36]. Newer echo machines reduce these problems of image quality, but nonetheless, incomplete visualization may be a significant problem, especially for stress echocardiography. This is not so much because the diagnosis of CAD or ischemia is missed, but rather because the localization, and particularly the detection of multivessel disease may be compromised. Additionally, failure to visualize segments precludes a quantitative approach to stress echocardiographic measurement, and increases inter-observer variability of qualitative interpretations [37].

First generation contrast agents, such as Albunex and Levovist have both been shown to improve the ventricular opacification during standard resting transthoracic echocardiography [31,38], especially in combination with color Doppler [39]. The studies showed improvement of endocardial definition in >80% of segments, as well as improvement of the confidence level of the investigators. It is likely that newer agents will produce more impressive changes. However, some expertise is needed; the contrast effect of these agents may be excessive and shadowing may reduce endocardial visualization (Figure 6).

Both of the first generation agents have also been combined with stress echocardiography [38,40], showing improvements of endocardial delineation especially in the lateral wall (Figure 7) and enhancement to video intensity levels in the ventricle. Other effects include improvement in the diagnostic certainty of the observers, and improvement in the accuracy of inexperienced observers [41]. Preliminary data have suggested an improvement of accuracy [42]. Similarly, the 2nd generation agents are likely to improve the feasibility of contrast stress echocardiography; excellent endocardial definition may permit development of quantitative wall motion analyses. However, the appropriate selection of patients for contrast stress echocardiography remains unclear. In the current health economy, the additional cost of the contrast agent is likely to double the procedural cost of performing a stress echocardiogram [43]. In the managed-care environment, reimbursement cannot be sought for this increment of cost. Moreover, some consideration needs to be given to the fact that the accuracy of stress echocardiography, which varies from 80-85% is quite satisfactory, and it is unlikely that contrast will improve this by >5-10%. From a cost standpoint, a 5% increase in specificity would be required to justify the cost of contrast (at >$100 per procedure), on the basis of saving a coronary angiogram costing approximately $2,000 [43].

While the combination of contrast with harmonic imaging may improve the distinction of the ventricular cavity and myocardium, it should be recognized that use of harmonic imaging alone may improve the quality of otherwise suboptimal studies. Other advances like tissue Doppler imaging may present the possibility of quantitation of stress echocardiography. It seems most likely that contrast stress echocardiography will become routine only if stress perfusion data can be combined with wall motion data (see below).

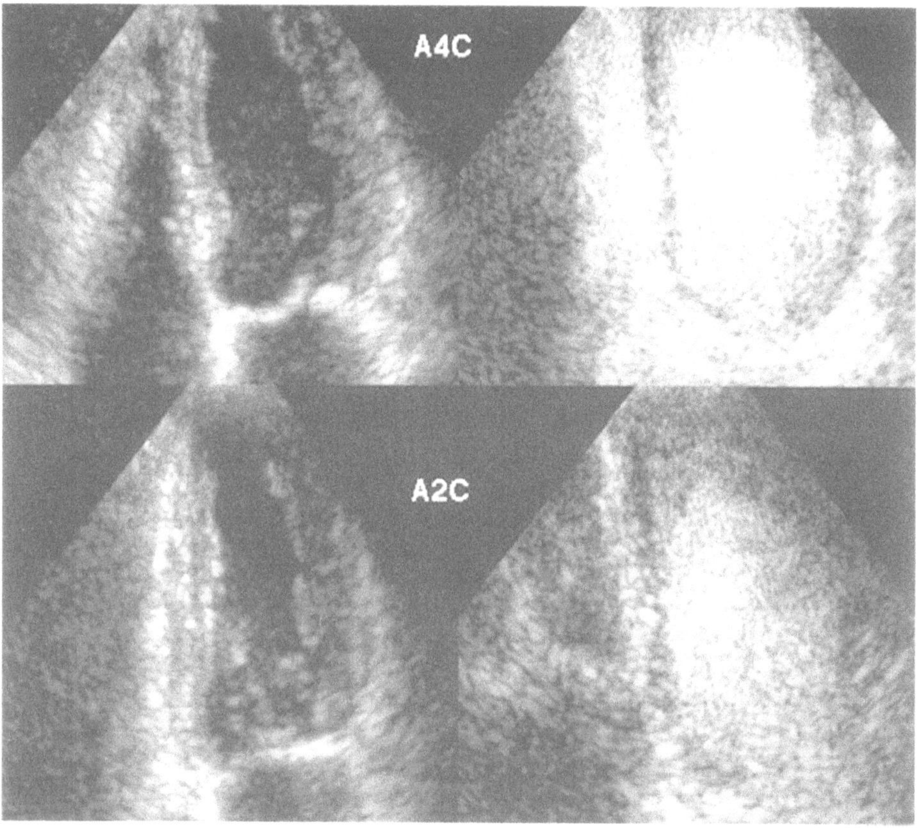

Figure 6. Contrast enhancement for LV opacification. Use of contrast may obscure delineation of the LV wall, especially early after injection when there may be shadowing. Reducing the gain settings may be useful.

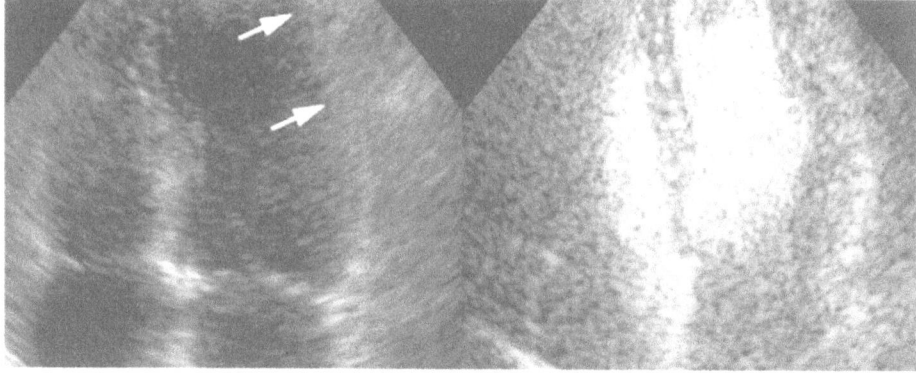

Figure 7. Enhancement of the lateral wall by echo-contrast enhancement of the LV cavity.

Doppler enhancement

The presence of microbubbles in stenotic and regurgitant jets may improve the signal to noise ratio of Doppler evaluation. Right heart contrast studies may be used to identify the presence of tricuspid regurgitation in situations where it is mild and not detectable by conventional techniques. Thus, estimation of pulmonary artery pressure may be obtained in circumstances when this cannot be identified without contrast enhancement [4]. Similarly, the assessment of mitral regurgitation using color flow mapping may be compromised by ultrasound attenuation between the chest wall and the left atrium, which is the deepest cardiac structure in the chest. The use of echo enhancement of the color jet may obviate the need for transesophageal imaging to assess jet severity and characteristics in patients with mitral regurgitation [44]. Finally, the evaluation of aortic stenosis is probably one of the most difficult lesions to assess in echocardiography, as accurate assessment is highly dependent upon alignment of the Doppler beam and the stenotic jet. The use of echo contrast may facilitate obtaining the maximal velocity.

Myocardial perfusion

Although the use of W to improve LV border delineation and enhance Doppler signals are both worthwhile objectives, the success of other technologies (e.g. tissue harmonic imaging) is likely to reduce the use of contrast agents for these purposes. This is not so of the evaluation of myocardial perfusion, which is looked upon as the ultimate goal for contrast echocardiography. However, the analysis of myocardial perfusion with echo contrast agents is complex, and although the lessons learned from nuclear perfusion imaging are pertinent, there are important differences between the techniques. The major clinical indications for myocardial contrast echocardiography are assessment of myocardial infarction, diagnosis of viable myocardium, and the detection of coronary disease using stress contrast perfusion imaging.

1. Myocardial infarction. In patients presenting with acute myocardial infarction, contrast echocardiography may be used to identify vessel patency, risk area, and infarct size. Contrast echocardiography is an attractive technique for use in acute myocardial infarction, due to its immediate availability, repeatability, safety, and portability to the coronary care unit and emergency room.

Patients presenting with chest pain are frequently admitted to the hospital because of uncertainty regarding the diagnosis of myocardial infarction. A number of strategies have been used to enhance the speed and accuracy of this diagnosis, including blood tests and even MIBI-SPECT [45]. The problem is that serum markers of myocardial infarction become positive after a delay of 4-6 hours, and SPECT imaging is expensive and rarely available in the emergency room. The use of contrast echocardiography may improve the identification of patients without perfusion defects, permitting either discharge with subsequent testing or immediate progression to other functional testing to identify if reversible ischemia had been the source of the initial presentation.

The detection of a perfusion defect presents important implications for therapy. In a patient with no previous history of myocardial infarction, in whom the diagnosis cannot be made on clinical and ECG grounds, the result may influence the selection of patients for thrombolytic therapy. Even in individuals in whom the diagnosis is clear, delineation of the risk area by contrast echocardiography may facilitate decision-making regarding use of thrombolytic therapy or primary PTCA, especially in situations where relative contraindications are present. Thus, determination of an extensive risk area would justify a lower threshold for aggressive therapy, while a small risk area could be used to justify a conservative approach. Moreover, defects may be followed sequentially over time [46]. Unfortunately, the detection of perfusion defects may be influenced by the presence of reactive hyperemia in adjacent non-infarcted tissue.

In patients who have undergone thrombolytic therapy, the critical issue relates to the detection of coronary patency following treatment. Unfortunately, with the exception of coronary angiography, techniques for demonstrating the success of lysis have been disappointing. Probably the most widely used are the resolution of chest pain and ST segment changes, but these rarely resolve completely. Contrast echocardiography may be of value in identifying restoration of coronary perfusion following lysis. Failure to achieve reperfusion may then prompt coronary angiography and rescue intervention.

Following acute coronary intervention, the return of epicardial coronary blood flow does not necessarily correlate with restoration of myocardial perfusion. A significant proportion of segments demonstrate the "no reflow" phenomenon [47], the causes of which are multifactorial, but include capillary plugging, and local edema. Contrast echo may identify the problem and permit selection of patients for additional medical therapy, or at least closer follow-up, as the risk of subsequent events is greater in this group [47].

2. Myocardial viability. Approximately 50% of segments showing wall motion abnormalities in association with coronary occlusion are not irreversibly damaged [48]. Early following infarction, much of this tissue shows regional dysfunction due to stunning [49]. Other regions may show dysfunction due to chronic ischemia, described as hibernation [50]. Contrast echocardiography may be valuable for the identification of viable tissue, based upon the preservation of the coronary microvasculature. Indeed, segments with flow-rates <0.15 mg/kg/min are associated with myocyte necrosis within 60 minutes.

Segments with severe malperfusion show no echo contrast enhancement, and are unlikely to recover during follow-up. However, the central infarct zone is usually surrounded by a functional border zone of viable myocardium, which may be identified by contrast echocardiography [51]. Segments showing echo enhancement are usually associated with residual viable tissue, and liable to recover after revascularization or with the passage of time [52]. However, in response to ischemic injury, the microvasculature is lost after the myocytes, and it is possible for the microvasculature to remain intact in the presence of necrotic muscle. In comparative studies with dobutamine echocardiography [53-57], contrast echocardiography has been shown to be a sensitive test for identifying viable tissue, but not highly specific. This pattern is similar to that associated with myocardial perfusion imaging [58]. The accuracy of contrast echocardiography after infarction may be increased by administering it in combination with dipyridamole [59] - this minimizes the effect of post-occlusion hyperemia.

3. Diagnosis of CAD with stress perfusion imaging. Myocardial perfusion imaging using nuclear techniques is the most sensitive non-invasive approach for the diagnosis of CAD. This should not be surprising, given that regional variations of myocardial perfusion constitute one of the earliest steps in the ischemic cascade. The problem with nuclear techniques is that they are expensive, technically demanding, and not available in all centers. The ability to perform rest and stress myocardial perfusion imaging with echocardiography would permit perfusion evaluations to be more widely performed, including in circumstances where SPECT cameras cannot easily be deployed, such as the coronary care unit and emergency room.

Studies comparing stress myocardial perfusion imaging with nuclear and echo contrast techniques should be divided into those performed in animals, and those performed in humans. The correlation is easier in animals, because the attenuation of ultrasound by the chest wall is usually less than in humans. Thus, using visual analysis, 12 of 16 animals with coronary stenoses were found to have echo contrast perfusion defects during hyperemia, correlating with the thallium area at risk [60]. Time-intensity curves of microbubble activity have been shown to correlate with coronary flow [61].

There are limited studies of stress contrast perfusion imaging in patients. Using coronary injection, Porter [62] described correlation of microbubble washout with flow reserve measurements obtained using a flow probe, in the setting of various degrees of coronary disease. In patients with single vessel disease involving the left anterior descending artery, the video intensity increased in the circumflex artery by about 50 percent, but decreased in the territory of the left anterior descending, giving a sensitivity and specificity of 91% for identification of coronary disease [63]. Also using coronary injection, Mesa showed good correlations between contrast activity after coronary injection with MIBI-SPECT [64].

Two previous studies have compared to intravenous contrast echocardiography and nuclear perfusion imaging in patients undergoing dipyridamole stress testing for the diverse of coronary disease [65,66]. In both studies, the presence, type (rest, stress or both) and location of perfusion defects were comparable. However, the echo data in both studies were postprocessed, with subtraction and color-coding, or video intensity measurements. As discussed above, the ability to perform myocardial contrast examinations of the examination of perfusion is unlikely to be realized using subjective evaluation alone.

4. Doppler assessment of coronary flow. Coronary flow may be measured echocardiographically in some coronary segments by transesophageal or transthoracic approaches. The most accessible by TEE is the proximal left anterior descending, which is aligned parallel to the Doppler beam from the transesophageal probe. The use of contrast has been shown to enhance the feasibility of flow measurements before and after vasodilator stress, thereby permitting the definition of coronary flow reserve [67]. New, high frequency transducers have permitted the assessment of coronary flow in the septal perforators and distal left anterior descending arteries using transthoracic echocardiography; these measurements are also more feasible after contrast enhancement [68]. These flow reserve measurements may improve the accuracy of stress echo results.

5. Intraoperative applications. Intraoperative echocardiography is most commonly applied to the evaluation of valvular lesions. Contrast echocardiography has permitted the application of echocardiography for the assessment of the coronary circulation in the operating room [69,70]. The most widely used applications focus on the evaluation of delivery of cardioplegia, detection of viable tissue in regions involved previously in myocardial infarction [71] and assessment of the adequacy of bypass grafting. In each situation, contrast solutions are injected into the aortic route, bypass, or coronary artery, and an evaluation is made of myocardial contrast effect. In patients with ventricular dysfunction following surgery, the technique may be valuable for distinction of stunning (where flow is preserved), and patients with ischemic injury.

Conclusions

Over the next few years, echo contrast enhancement is likely to become a routine component of the echocardiographic examination for some indications. As always, there is a trade-off of negative and positive considerations. The main negative aspect is cost, rather than risk, as the new contrast agents appear to be safe and effective. However, we must not lose sight of the place of ultrasound as a low cost diagnostic strategy, and avoid the addition of incremental variable costs. In addition to the technical challenges posed by contrast echocardiography, there exists an ongoing need to define the clinical indications where the technique adds most incremental value, and to focus its use in these areas.

References

1. Thomas JD. Contrast ultrasound for assessment of myocardial perfusion: promise and pitfalls. In: Van der Wall EE, Marwick TH, Reiber JHC, editors. Advances in imaging techniques in ischemic heart disease. Dordrecht: Kluwer; 1995. p. 101-11.
2. Villanueva FS, Glasheen WP, Sklenar J, Jayaweera AR, Kaul S. Successful and reproducible myocardial opacification during two-dimensional echocardiography from right heart injection of contrast. Circulation 1992;85:1557-64.
3. Gramiak R, Shah PM, Kramer DH. Ultrasound cardiography: contrast studies in anatomy and function. Radiology 1969;92:939-48.
4. Himelman RB, Stulbarg M, Kircher B *et al.* Noninvasive evaluation of pulmonary artery pressure during exercise by saline-enhanced Doppler echocardiography in chronic pulmonary disease. Circulation 1989;79:863-71.
5. Feinstein SB, Ten Cate FJ, Zwehl W *et al.* Two-dimensional contrast echocardiography. I. In vitro development and quantitative analysis of echo contrast agents. J Am Coll Cardiol 1984;3:14-20.
6. Sabia P, Afrookteh A, Touchstone DA, Keller MW, Esquivel L, Kaul S. Value of regional wall motion abnormality in the emergency room diagnosis of acute myocardial infarction. A prospective study using two-dimensional echocardiography. Circulation 1991;84(3 Suppl):I85-92.
7. Keller MW, Segal SS, Kaul S, Duling B. The behavior of sonicated albumin microbubbles within the microcirculation: a basis for their use during myocardial contrast echocardiography. Circ Res 1989;65:458-67.
8. Keller MW, Glasheen W, Smucker ML, Burwell LR, Watson DD, Kaul S. Myocardial contrast echocardiography in humans. II. Assessment of coronary blood flow reserve. J Am Coll Cardiol 1988;12:925-34.
9. Vuille C, Nidorf M, Morrissey RL, Newell JB, Weyman AE, Picard MH. Effect of static pressure on the disappearance rate of specific echocardiographic contrast agents. J Am Soc Echocardiogr 1994;7:347-54.
10. Padial LR, Chen MH, Vuille C, Guerrero JL, Weyman AE, Picard MH. Pulsatile pressure affects the disappearance of echocardiographic contrast agents. J Am Soc Echocardiogr 1995;8:285-92.
11. Kaul S. Myocardial contrast echocardiography. Curr Probl Cardiol 1997;22:555-635.
12. Keller MW, Glasheen W, Kaul S. Albunex: a safe and effective commercially produced agent for myocardial contrast echocardiography. J Am Soc Echocardiogr 1989;2:48-52.
13. Feinstein SB, Cheirif J, Ten Cate FJ *et al.* Safety and efficacy of a new transpulmonary ultrasound contrast agent: initial multicenter clinical results. J Am Coll Cardiol 1990;16:316-24.
14. Porter TR, Xie F. Visually discernible myocardial echocardiographic contrast after intravenous injection of sonicated dextrose albumin microbubbles containing high molecular weight, less soluble gases. J Am Coll Cardiol 1995;25:509-15.
15. Burns P. Potential advantages of harmonic imaging. Adv Echo-Contrast 1994;4:17-9.

16.   Tuchnitz A, Von Bibra H, Sutherland GR, Erhardt W, Henke J, Schomig A. Doppler energy: a new acquisition technique for the transthoracic detection of myocardial perfusion defects with the use of a venous contrast agent. J Am Soc Echocardiogr 1997;10:881-90.

17.   Vandenberg BF, Melton HE. Acoustic lability of albumin microspheres. J Am Soc Echocardiogr 1994;7:582-9.

18.   Porter TR, Xie F, Li S, D'Sa A, Rafter P. Increased ultrasound contrast and decreased microbubble destruction rates with triggered ultrasound imaging. J Am Soc Echocardiogr 1996;9:599-605.

19.   Ota T, Hillman ND, Craig D, Kisslo J, Smith PK. Contrast echocardiography: influence of ultrasonic machine settings, mixing conditions, and pressurization on pixel intensity and microsphere size of Albunex solutions in vitro. J Am Soc Echo 1997;10:31-40.

20.   Sanders WE Jr, Cheirif J, Desir R *et al.* Contrast opacification of left ventricular myocardium following intravenous administration of sonicated albumin microspheres. Am Heart J 1991;122:1660-5.

21.   Marwick TH, Nihoyannopoulos P, Pierard L, Vanoverschelde JL, Van der Wouw P, Lindvall K. How useful is contrast echo in patients after myocardial infarction? Comparison with wall motion and scintigraphy [abstract]. J Am Coll Cardiol. In press 1998.

22.   Halmann M, Beyar R, Rinkevich D *et al.* Digital subtraction myocardial contrast echocardiography: design and application of a new analysis program for myocardial perfusion imaging. J Am Soc Echocardiogr 1994;7:355-62.

23.   Davila-Roman VG, Barzilai B. Myocardial contrast echocardiography: enhancement of perfusion images by color coding. J Clin Ultrasound 1994;22:21-7.

24.   Firschke C, Lindner JR, Wei K, Goodman NC, Skyba DM, Kaul S. Myocardial perfusion imaging in the setting of coronary artery stenosis and acute myocardial infarction using venous injection of a second-generation echocardiographic contrast agent. Circulation 1997;96:959-67.

25.   Monaghan MJ, Metcalfe JM, Odunlami S, Waaler A, Jewitt DE. Digital radiofrequency echocardiography in the detection of myocardial contrast following intravenous administration of Albunex. Eur Heart J 1993;14:1200-9.

26.   Rovai D, Lombardi M, Taddei L *et al.* Flow quantitation by contrast echocardiography. Effects of intervening tissue and of the angle of incidence between flow and ultrasonic beam. Int J Card Imaging 1993;9:21-7.

27.   Meltzer RS, Ohad DG, Reisner S *et al.* Quantitative myocardial ultrasonic integrated backscatter measurements during contrast injections. J Am Soc Echocardiogr 1994;7:1-8.

28.   Ten Cate FJ, Silverman PR, Sassen LM, Verdouw PD. Can myocardial contrast echo determine coronary flow reserve? Cardiovasc Res 1992;26:32-9.

29.   Rovai D, Lombardi M, Distante A, L'Abbate A. Myocardial perfusion by contrast echocardiography. From off-line processing to radio frequency analysis. Circulation 1991;83(5 Suppl):III97-103.

30.   Skyba DM, Jayaweera AR, Goodman NC, Ismail S, Camarano G, Kaul S. Quantification of myocardial perfusion with myocardial contrast echocardiography during left atrial injection of contrast. Implications for venous injection. Circulation 1994;90:1513-21.

31.   Crouse LJ, Cheirif J, Hanly DE *et al.* Opacification and border delineation improvement in patients with suboptimal endocardial border definition in routine echocardiography: results of the Phase III Albunex Multicenter Trial. J Am Coll Cardiol 1993;22:1494-500.

32.   Freeman AP, Giles RW, Walsh WF, Fisher R, Murray IPC, Wilcken DEL. Regional left ventricular wall motion assessment: comparison of two-dimensional echocardiography and radionuclide angiography with contrast angiography in healed myocardial infarction. Am J Cardiol 1985;56:8-12.

33.   Visser CA, Kan G, David GK, Lie KI, Durrer D. Echocardiographic- cineangiographic correlation in detecting left ventricular aneurysm: a prospective study of 422 patients. Am J Cardiol 1982;50:337-41.

34.   Quinones MA, Waggoner AD, Reduto LA *et al.* A new, simplified and accurate method for determining ejection fraction with two-dimensional echocardiography. Circulation 1981;64:744-53.

35.   Bourdillon PD, Broderick TM, Sawada SG *et al.* Regional wall motion index for infarct and noninfarct regions after reperfusion in acute myocardial infarction: comparison with global wall motion index. J Am Soc Echocardiogr 1989;2:398-407.

36.   Panza JA, Laurienzo JM, Curiel RV, Quyyumi AA, Cannon RO 3rd. Transesophageal dobutamine stress echocardiography for evaluation of patients with coronary artery disease. J Am Coll Cardiol 1994;24:1260-7.

37.   Hoffmann R, Lethen H, Marwick T *et al.* Analysis of interinstitutional observer agreement in interpretation of dobutamine stress echocardiograms. J Am Coll Cardiol 1996;27:330-6.

38. Schroder K, Agrawal R, Voller H, Schlief R, Schroder R. Improvement of endocardial border delineation in suboptimal stress-echocardiograms using the new left heart contrast agent SH U 508 A. Int J Card Imaging 1994;10:45-51.

39. Agrawal G, Cape EG, Raichlen JS *et al.* Usefulness of combined color Doppler/contrast in providing complete delineation of left ventricular cavity. Am J Cardiol 1997;80:98-101.

40. Porter TR, Xie F, Kricsfeld A, Chiou A, Dabestani A. Improved endocardial border resolution during dobutamine stress echocardiography with intravenous sonicated dextrose albumin. J Am Coll Cardiol 1994;23:1440-3.

41. Armstrong WF, Marwick TH, Pellikka PA *et al.* Feasibility and clinical impact of intravenous Albunex injections during bicycle stress echocardiography. J Am Coll Cardiol. In press 1998.

42. Rubin DN, Haluska B, Morehead A, Marwick TH. Improving bicycle stress echo image quality with Albunex [abstract]. J Am Coll Cardiol 1997;29(Suppl A):260A.

43. Marwick TH. Combination of echo-enhancers with stress echocardiography: increasing feasibility or merely increasing cost? Adv Echo-Contrast 1996;4:74-81.

44. Von Bibra H, Becher H, Firschke C, Schlief R, Emslander HP, Schoming A. Enhancement of mitral regurgitation and normal left atrial color Doppler flow signals with peripheral venous injection of a saccharide-based contrast agent. J Am Coll Cardiol 1993;22:521-8.

45. Tatum JL, Jesse RL, Kontos MC *et al.* Comprehensive strategy for the evaluation and triage of the chest pain patient. Ann Emerg Med 1997;29:116-25.

46. Sakuma T, Hayashi Y, Shimohara A, Shindo T, Maeda K. Usefulness of myocardial contrast echocardiography for the assessment of serial changes in risk area in patients with acute myocardial infarction. Am J Cardiol 1996;78:1273-7.

47. Ito H, Maruyama A, Iwakura K *et al.* Clinical implications of the 'no reflow' phenomenon. A predictor of complications and left ventricular remodeling in reperfused anterior wall myocardial infarction. Circulation 1996;93:223-8.

48. Fudo T, Kambara H, Hashimoto T *et al.* F-18 deoxyglucose and stress N-13 ammonia positron emission tomography in anterior wall healed myocardial infarction. Am J Cardiol 1988;61:1191-7.

49. Kloner RA, Przyklenk K, Patel B. Altered myocardial states. The stunned and hibernating myocardium. Am J Med 1989;86:14-22.

50. Rahimtoola SH. The hibernating myocardium. Am Heart J 1989;117:211-21.

51. Nanto S, Masuyama T, Lim YJ, Hori M, Kodama K, Kamada T. Demonstration of functional border zone with myocardial contrast echocardiography in human hearts. Simultaneous analysis of myocardial perfusion and wall motion abnormalities. Circulation 1993;88:447-53.

52. Sabia PJ, Powers ER, Ragosta M, Sarembock IJ, Burwell LR, Kaul S. An association between collateral blood flow and myocardial viability in patients with recent myocardial infarction. N Engl J Med 1992;327:1825-31.

53. Meza MF, Kates MA, Barbee RW *et al.* Combination of dobutamine and myocardial contrast echocardiography to differentiate postischemic from infarcted myocardium. J Am Coll Cardiol 1997;29:974-84.

54. DeFilippi CR, Willett DL, Irani WN, Eichhorn EJ, Velasco CE, Grayburn PA. Comparison of myocardial contrast echocardiography and low-dose dobutamine stress echocardiography in predicting recovery of left ventricular function after coronary revascularization in chronic ischemic heart disease. Circulation 1995;92:2863-8.

55. Iliceto S, Galiuto L, Marchese A *et al.* Analysis of microvascular integrity, contractile reserve, and myocardial viability after acute myocardial infarction by dobutamine echocardiography and myocardial contrast echocardiography. Am J Cardiol 1996;77:441-5.

56. Bolognese L, Antoniucci D, Rovai D *et al.* Myocardial contrast echocardiography versus dobutamine echocardiography for predicting functional recovery after acute myocardial infarction treated with primary coronary angioplasty. J Am Coll Cardiol 1996;28:1677-83.

57. Agati L, Voci P, Autore C *et al.* Combined use of dobutamine echocardiography and myocardial contrast echocardiography in predicting regional dysfunction recovery after coronary revascularization in patients with recent myocardial infarction. Eur Heart J 1997;18:771-9.

58. Nagueh SF, Vaduganathan P, Ali N *et al.* Identification of hibernating myocardium: comparative accuracy of myocardial contrast echocardiography, rest-redistribution thallium-201 tomography and dobutamine echocardiography. J Am Coll Cardiol 1997;29:985-93.

59. Rovai D, Zanchi M, Lombardi M *et al.* Residual myocardial perfusion in reversibly damaged myocardium by dipyridamole contrast echocardiography. Eur Heart J 1996;17:296-301.

60.   Cheirif J, Desir RM, Bolli R *et al.* Relation of perfusion defects observed with myocardial contrast echocardiography to the severity of coronary stenosis: correlation with thallium-201 single-photon emission tomography. J Am Coll Cardiol 1992;19:1343-9.

61.   Mor-Avi V, Lang RM, Robinson KA *et al.* Contrast echocardiographic quantification of regional myocardial perfusion: validation with an isolated rabbit heart model. J Am Soc Echocardiogr 1996;9:156-65.

62.   Porter TR, D'Sa A, Turner C *et al.* Myocardial contrast echocardiography for the assessment of coronary blood flow reserve: validation in humans. J Am Coll Cardiol 1993;21:349-55.

63.   Agati L, Voci P, Bilotta F *et al.* Dipyridamole myocardial contrast echocardiography in patients with single-vessel coronary artery disease: perfusion, anatomic, and functional correlates. Am Heart J 1994;128:28-35.

64.   Meza MF, Mobarek S, Sonnemaker R *et al.* Myocardial contrast echocardiography in human beings: correlation of resting perfusion defects to sestamibi single photon emission computed tomography. Am Heart J 1996;132:528-35.

65.   Porter TR, Li S, Kricsfeld D, Armbruster RW. Detection of myocardial perfusion in multiple echocardiographic windows with one intravenous injection of microbubbles using transient response second harmonic imaging. J Am Coll Cardiol 1997;29:791-9.

66.   Kaul S, Senior R, Dittrich H, Raval U, Khattar R, Lahiri A. Detection of coronary artery disease with myocardial contrast echocardiography: comparison with 99mTc-sestamibi single-photon emission computed tomography. Circulation 1997;96:785-92.

67.   Caiati C, Aragona P, Iliceto S, Rizzon P. Improved Doppler detection of proximal left anterior descending coronary artery stenosis after intravenous injection of a lung-crossing contrast agent: a transesophageal Doppler echocardiographic study. J Am Coll Cardiol 1996;27:1413-21.

68.   Mulvagh SL, Foley DA, Aeschbacher BC, Klarich KK, Seward JB. Second harmonic imaging of an intravenously administered echocardiographic contrast agent: visualization of coronary arteries and measurement of coronary blood flow. J Am Coll Cardiol 1996;27:1519-25.

69.   Aronson S, Lee BK, Wiencek JG *et al.* Assessment of myocardial perfusion during CABG surgery with two-dimensional transesophageal contrast echocardiography. Anesthesiology 1991;75:433-40.

70.   Aronson S. Identifying stunned myocardium during cardiac surgery: the role of myocardial contrast echocardiography. J Card Surg 1993;8(2 Suppl):224-7.

71.   Hirata N, Shimazaki Y, Nakano S, Sakai K, Sakaki S, Matsuda H. Evaluation of regional myocardial perfusion in areas of old myocardial infarction after revascularization by means of intraoperative myocardial contrast echocardiography. J Thorac Cardiovasc Surg 1994;108:1119-24.

27.

State-of-the-Art.
Stress echocardiography
entering the next millennium

Otto Kamp, Gertjan Tj Sieswerda & Cees A. Visser

Summary

Stress echocardiography has entered the clinical domain and has improved the diagnostic capabilities of many echocardiographic laboratoria. Under certain conditions stress echocardiography has demonstrated to be safe and accurate. In experienced hands it has proven to be a valuable diagnostic tool in the management of patients with coronary artery disease. The availability of stress echocardiography permits assessment of myocardial ischemia and thus influences clinical management. Despite its relatively low costs, portability, absence of radiation, safety and its ability to determine the ischemic threshold, there are limitations for its widespread use, e.g. window limitation, subjective interpretation and learning curves being the most important amongst them.

Introduction

The clinical application of stress echocardiography has increased importantly since its introduction in the late 1970's [1] . Today, transthoracic stress echocardiography, especially with dobutamine, has gained increasing popularity for the evaluation of patients with known or suspected coronary artery disease because of a better sensitivity for single-vessel disease compared to dipyridamole [2]. Its use comprises assessment of myocardial ischemia in coronary artery disease to evaluate haemodynamic response in valvular or congenital heart disease. Furthermore, low-dose dobutamine echocardiography provides important clinical information in patients with left ventricular dysfunction, and is able to diagnose myocardial viability [3,4]. Therefore, common indications for stress echocardiography include: 1) evaluation of myocardial ischemia in patients with suspected or known coronary artery disease; 2) evaluation of myocardial viability in patients with left ventricular dysfunction; 3) risk assessment in patients after myocardial infarction or in patients undergoing noncardiac surgery; and 4) evaluation of ischemic mitral regurgitation or pulmonary hypertension in valvular or congenital heart disease.

The diagnostic hallmark and underlying mechanism of stress echocardiography is enclosed in the fact that ischemic myocardium shows new regional contractile dysfunction provoked by stress, even before electrocardiographic changes may occur and clearly prior to the onset of symptoms, and thus closely related with the onset of myocardial ischemia. In contrast, myocardial viability can be demonstrated, using low-dose dobutamine echocardio-

J.H.C. Reiber and E.E. van der Wall (eds.). What's New in Cardiovascular Imaging, 351–362.
©1998 Kluwer Academic Publishers.

graphy, by improvement of myocardial contractile dysfunction, being the basic concept for the diagnosis of either myocardial stunning or hibernation [3-5]. The mechanism for unmasking myocardial viability by low-dose dobutamine is that the inotropic effect of the drug is already nearly maximal at doses of 5 to 15 ug/kg/min [3-6]. Further differentation between myocardial stunning and hibernation can be made using high-dose dobutamine, in which a biphasic response (reduction of regional myocardial contractility compared with low-dose dobutamine) identifies myocardial hibernation, which only might improve after revascularization [5].

Experience from the Academic Hospital of the Free University, Amsterdam

Our experience with stress echocardiography started in 1986 with exercise echocardiography [7], and now includes 1032 stress echocardiographic procedures since the introduction of our database in 1989, using mainly dobutamine (82%), but also dynamic exercise (6%) and atrial pacing (12%). Most stress examinations were performed in the echocardiographic laboratory under strict ECG-monitoring using 6 or 12 leads ECG-recordings. Acquisition was performed by an ultrasound technician (79%) or a cardiologist (21%). If the technician performed the ultrasound examination, a fellow doctor supervised the stress procedure with back-up of a cardiologist. Furthermore, heart rate, blood pressure, symptoms and oxymetry (in selected patients only) were monitored during all incremental steps of dobutamine or non-dobutamine stress. In addition, emergency equipment was always present in the stress echocardiographic room. Dobutamine infusion was adjusted to body weight, and steps of 5 (first two doses) and 3 minutes duration were used with incremental doses of 5, 10, 20, 30 and 40 µg/kg/min. The infusion was stopped when severe chest pain or signs of myocardial ischemia (ECG or regional wall motion abnormality) was detected or, in absence of ischemia, at least 85% of age-predicted maximal heart rate had been achieved. Starting from 1992, atropine was added when the target heart rate was not reached. Analysis was done on-line and off-line, using a segmental left ventricular model (13 or 16 segments), and each segment was scored semiquantitatively as: 0= normal (normal motion excursion and wall thickening), 1= hypokinesia (moderate or severe reduction in motion excursion and wall thickening), 2= akinesia (absence of excursion and wall thickening), or 3 = dyskinesia (paradoxic outward motion in systole). Off-line analysis was done by reviewing the videotape as well as side-by-side display of selected images on a workstation. Final report was authorized by an experienced cardiologist and include site, extent, onset, duration and severity of wall motion abnormalities before, during and immediately after stress, as well as presence and severity of valvular or congenital disease. Our indications were similar to those reported from other institutions, although a higher proportion of patients were studied for ischemic mitral regurgitation due to research programs [8,9]. Indications for stress echocardiography are summarized in Figure 1. Our findings resulted in a change in clinical management in the majority of patients. Based on the results of the stress echocardiograms, the clinical decision to either avoid or to perform a diagnostic cardiac catheterization was made in the majority of the patients (86%). Interventions were guided by stress echocardiograms in 91 % of the patients. This included selective PTCA of the ischemia-related vessel or coronary artery bypass surgery. The overall rate of complications during stress echocardiography was low. Four serious complications (3.8 ‰) were reported (ventricular fibrillation in 1 patient, ventricular tachycardia in 3 patients) during the period and all were easily converted to sinus

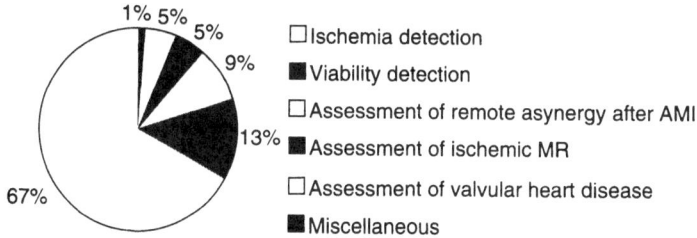

1% 5% 5%
9%
13%
67%

☐ Ischemia detection
■ Viability detection
☐ Assessment of remote asynergy after AMI
■ Assessment of ischemic MR
☐ Assessment of valvular heart disease
■ Miscellaneous

Figure 1. Indications for stress echocardiography in 1032 patients performed from 1989-1997 in the Academic Hospital Vrije Universiteit, Amsterdam. Significant proportion of the studies for ischemic mitral regurgitation, valvular heart disease and miscellaneous indications were performed in a research program.

rhythm. This is in accordance with earlier reports from the literature and underlines the conclusion that dobutamine stress echocardiography is safe [10].

Stress echocardiographic modalities

Diagnostic transthoracic window

Stress transthoracic echocardiography is performed using exercise, atrial pacing, vasodilators (e.g. dipyridamole), and inotropics (e.g. dobutamine). Nowadays, dobutamine is the most widely used pharmacologic agent for stress echocardiography. The popularity of dobutamine stress can be explained by its technically easier nature compared with exercise or pacing echocardiography showing similar levels of sensitivity (in the range of 80%) and specificity (in the range of 85%) in assessing myocardial ischemia in coronary artery disease. A further advantage of pharmacologic stress is, that it avoids submaximal stress testing in the large majority of patients. Compared with myocardial perfusion scintigraphy, accuracy of stress echocardiography is comparible (Table 1), apart from dipyridamole echocardiography which

Table 1: Diagnostic yield of pharmacologic stress echocardiography and myocardial perfusion scintigraphy for detection of coronary artery disease (myocardial ischemia)

	sensitivity		specificity	
	%	range %	%	range %
pooled echo data (21 studies, 2323 pat)	84	40-96	87	66-100
pooled nuclear data (56 studies, 6038 pat)	85	36-97	85	43-100

shows a significant lower sensitivity [2]. Dobutamine stress echocardiography has about similar specificity compared to nuclear imaging techniques (Table 1)[11-12]. In contrast, vasodilation nuclear perfusion imaging is superior to vasodilation echocardiography. Selection of the stress test should therefore be tailored to clinical circumstances.

In the setting of myocardial viability, nuclear imaging provides reliable information on regional perfusion, metabolism and cell membrane integrity, while echocardiography provides real-time visualization of myocardial thickening. However, using low-dose dobutamine echocardiography important functional information with regards to absence or presence of regional contractile reserve has become available.

Nondiagnostic transthoracic window

Because of limited image quality of transthoracic stress echocardiography in approximately 10-20% of patients, transesophageal stress echocardiography using atrial pacing or dobutamine is a valuable extention of diagnostic echocardiographic capabilities. Even when assessment of regional wall motion is feasible by the transthoracic window, measurement of myocardial thickening is not always possible due to incomplete endocardial visualization. In this regard, we evaluated the capability of simultaneous transesophageal echocardiography and atrial pacing. The technique has a high accuracy and diagnostic yield in assessing myocardial ischemia, multivessel coronary artery disease and ischemic mitral regurgitation [8,9]. Alternatively, dipyridamole and dobutamine are also used in transesophageal stress echocardiography [13,14] (Table 2). Potential indications for transesophageal stress echocardiography are:1) nondiagnostic transthoracic window; 2) ambiguous results from different tests; 3) accurate measurement of viability; 4) "unexplained" heart failure; 5) evaluation of dynamic mitral regurgitation; 6) measurement of coronary flow reserve; and 7) myocardial perfusion distribution with contrast agents.

Table 2: Sensitivity and specificity of transesophageal stress echocardiography for detection of coronary artery disease or viability

	sensitivity		specificity	
	%	range %	%	range %
coronary artery disease:				
pacing (3 studies,n=126)	91	83-91	96	93-100
dobutamine (2 studies, n=121)	89	82-89	100	93-100
dipyridamole (1 study, n=32)	92		100	
myocardial viability:				
dobutamine (1 study,n=42)	92		88	

Table 3: Indications for stress echocardiography for evaluation of myocardial ischemia

Nondiagnostic exercise-ECG, e.g. submaximal excersice or left bundle branch block

Females

Preoperative cardiac risk stratification

Risk stratification after myocardial infarction

Risk stratification in stable coronary artery disease

Current clinical indications

Evaluation of myocardial ischemia

Crucial to the evaluation of myocardial ischemia is the assessment of new or more severe wall motion abnormalities at peak exercise or at high-dose dobutamine. In severe coronary artery disease, reduction in wall motion can be detected early during the stress test, for example during low- or intermediate-dose dobutamine. At present, accepted indications in this catagory are summarized in Table 3. There are several reasons for a nondiagnostic or uninterpretable exercise electrocardiograms. Submaximal or inconclusive exercise is a clinical important indication for stress echocardiography and is responsible for the majority of indications as well as repolarization abnormalities on the resting ECG (e.g. digitalis effect, left ventricular hypertrophy or post myocardial infarction). Furthermore, the diagnostic value of stress echocardiography in patients with left bundle branch block has been clearly demonstrated [15]. Stress echocardiography in women is more accurate than exercise electrocardiography or exercise echocardiography with a high specificity, avoiding unnecessary coronary angiography in women [16]. Figure 2 illustrates the presence of myocardial ischemia in a patient with an inconclusive exercise ECG. However, in patients who are able to perform maximal exercise, with an interpretable resting ECG, routine exercise ECG remains the investigation of first choice. Nevertheless, in a meta-analysis using exercise ECG (ST depres-

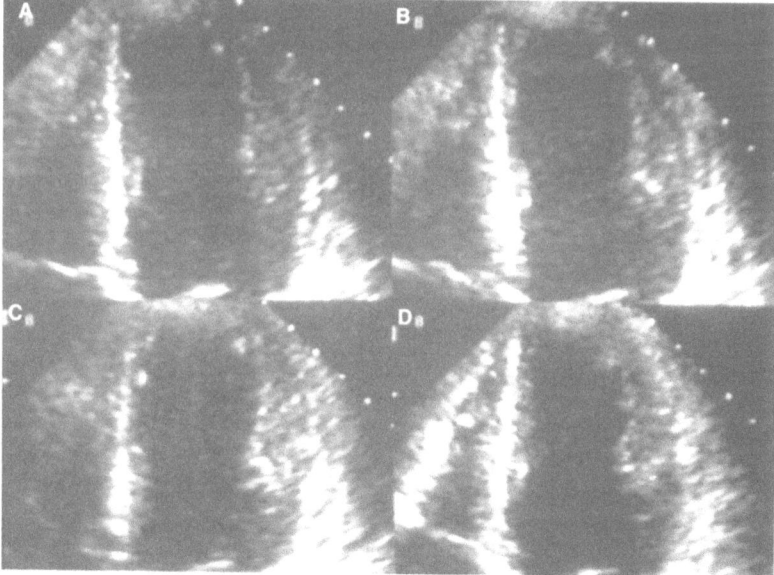

Figure 2. End-systolic stop frame images (apical four-chamber view) of dobutamine stress echocardiography obtained in a patient with a recent non-Q anterior myocardial infarction, significant residual LAD disease and inconclusive exercise ECG. A) at rest, hypokinesia of the distal inferoseptum is present. B) During low dose dobutamine augmented systolic myocardial thickening becomes apparent. C) At peak dose dobutamine however, this segment becomes akinetic, indicating a significant residual stenosis in the infarct related vessel. (D) During the recovery phase this ischemic response disappears.

sion) in the diagnosis of coronary artery disease, diagnostic yield was found to vary widely with a mean sensitivity of 68 ± 6% and a specificity of 77 ± 17%, reflecting significant variations in patient selection and exercise methodology [17].

Preoperative cardiac risk assessment

Pharmacologic stress imaging with echocardiography improves risk stratification for intermediate-risk patients having vascular or other major noncardiac surgery. Randomized, controlled trials have shown a survival benefit with perioperative use of beta-blockers in patients at risk for coronary artery disease. Therefore, evaluation of surgical patients undergoing vascular or other major surgery is recommended, because coronary artery disease represents an important risk. In this setting the accuracy of dobutamine echocardiography is comparable to dipyridamole-thallium scanning [18,19].

Evaluation of myocardial viability

Improvement of myocardial contractility or reversible myocardial dysfunction is the hallmark for myocardial viability. In a hypokinetic myocardial segment, a mixture of normal myocardium with scar or hibernating myocardium can both be present. However, only in hibernation the myocardial segments can be expected to improve after revascularization [20,21]. The presence of myocardial viability is dependent on infarct size, severity of infarct-related coronary artery stenosis and duration of infusion . Table 4 illustrates the pooled data

Table 4: Diagnostic yield of low-dose dobutamine echocardiography and FDG scintigraphy for detection of functional recovery (myocardial viability)

	sensitivity		*specificity*	
	%	*range %*	*%*	*range %*
pooled data LDDE[a] (16 studies,448 pat)	84	71-97	81	63-96
pooled data nuclear Tc-99m (10 studies,207 pat)	83	73-100	69	35-89
pooled data FDG-PET (12 studies,332 pat)	88	71-100	73	50-91

a. LDDE=low-dose dobutamine echocardiography, Tc-99m= technetium-99m sestamibi scintigraphy, FDG-PET=fluorine-18 fluorodeoxyglucose positron emission tomography

for the feasibility of low-dose dobutamine echocardiography and fluorine-18 fluorodeoxyglucose (FDG) scintigraphy for the detection of myocardial viability [22]. A case example from a patient after a recent myocardial infarction is shown in Figure 3.

Risk assessment after myocardial infarction

Evaluation of remote asynergy after myocardial infarction to predict multivessel disease is a classic indication to risk stratify patients after myocardial infarction [7]. However, in the thrombolytic era the detection of residual stenosis of the infarct-related artery became

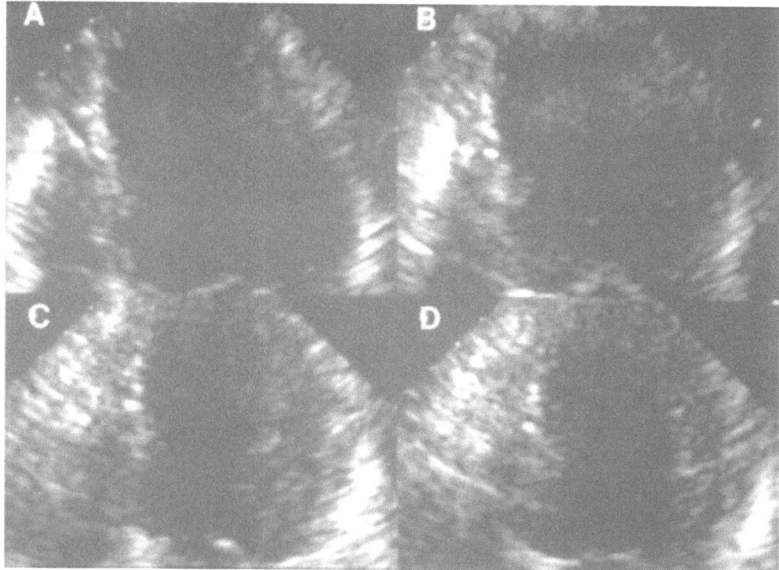

Figure 3. End-systolic stop frame images of illustrative echocardiograms obtained in a patient with recent inferior wall myocardial infarction. Apical four-chamber view is shown. (A) Akinesia of the basal lateral segment is present at rest. (B) Systolic myocardial thickening becomes apparent with low dose dobutamine (5 µg/kg/min). (C) At 10 µg/kg/min this systolic thickening becomes more pronounced, indicating myocardial viability (D). Same patient 10 weeks later. Note the functional recovery of the basal lateral segment.

increasingly important [23-25]. In addition to the assessment of new inducible myocardial ischemia (either detection of multivessel disease or a significant residual stenosis of the infarct-related artery), low-dose dobutamine echocardiogaphy can be used to assess myocardial viability and thus the presence of stunning or hibernation. This functional response to low-dose dobutamine is correlated with spontaneous recovery of regional function in the infarct area at follow-up [26].

Evaluation of valvular or congenital heart disease

Stress echocardiography provides an unique noninvasive means to evaluate cardiovascular function and hemodynamic response during increased cardiac workload. Thus, transvalvular and prosthetic valve gradient and right ventricular systolic pressure can be studied. Its clinical use in the evaluation of patients with mitral stenosis, dynamic mitral regurgitation or prosthetic valve dysfunction, aortic stenosis and impaired left ventricular function, and diseases associated with pulmonary hypertension or cor pulmonale have been reported [9,27]. To date, the importance of stress echocardiography in these patients and its effect on management need further to be defined.

Miscellaneous indications

Research is continuing in the field of heart failure, especially in patients with so called "unexplained" heart failure, that is clinical documentation of heart failure in normal or slightly impaired systolic left ventricular function, but also in patients with symptoms of dyspnea without any explanation on the resting echocardiogram. The number of studies in severe left ventricular systolic dysfunction and heart transplant recipients are also increasing [28]. Furthermore, new interventional techniques are evaluated using stress echocardiography, for example following transmyocardial laser revascularization.

Technical considerations

Hitherto, there is still a problem of considerable interobserver variability with stress echocardiography [29]. Improved image quality allowing better endocardial border definition, for example with contrast echocardiography, may diminish the subjective nature of interpretation and reduce interobserver variability . Analysis of wall motion is presently performed qualitatively, and requires experience and a significant learning curve, in order to reach high accuracy and high interobserver agreement [30]. Variability of image quality might lead to misinterpretation and thus patients with limited image quality should be excluded for stress echocardiography. This is about 10-20% of the unselected patients referred for stress echocardiography. The finding of regional asynergy is not only the result of significant coronary artery disease, but can be present with coronary spasm, cardiomyopathy, hypertrophy or coronary microvascular disease. Furthermore, abnormal septum activation may also cause false-positive results. The presence of tethering in regions adjacent to infarcted zones may lead to misinterpretation. An isolated wall motion abnormality in the basal inferior wall, close to the plane of the mitral valve, requires cautious interpretation. The definition of hypokinetic wall motion, ranging from mild to severe hypokinesia, might also cause variation between different observers and may sometimes be considered as normal and by others as pathologic. The use of a digital cineloop display in stress echocardiography is somewhat conflicting with studies supporting and others disproving its use. Selected images will simplify the analysis, however adjacent myocardial segments present on videotaped recordings are sometimes not captured in a cineloop display. Standardization in digital echocardiography is crucial to manage this problem.

The future of stress echocardiography

Developments already underway, for example contrast echocardiography, three-dimensional echocardiography, tissue Doppler and quantitative echocardiography, all will influence the future application of stress echocardiography. The administration of an ultrasound contrast agent results in clinically useful opacification of the left ventricle in the vast majority of low echogenic patients, especially when combined with new ultrasound equipment technology such as second harmonic imaging or transient response imaging. When applied to stress echocardiography, the use of contrast agents has been observed to improve confidence level in assessing left ventricular wall motion and thus interobserver variability (Figure 4) [31,32]. Better resolution of the endocardial borders promises the facilitation of quantitative evaluation of regional and global left ventricular function in combination with (semi) automatic contour detection systems (Figure 5). Although there seems to be a clear benefit in patients with limited echogenicity, routine use of contrast agents in stress echocardiography is still controversial, mainly due to pharmaco-economic considerations. Furthermore, newer and more stable intravenous contrast agents are expected to reach the market in the near future,

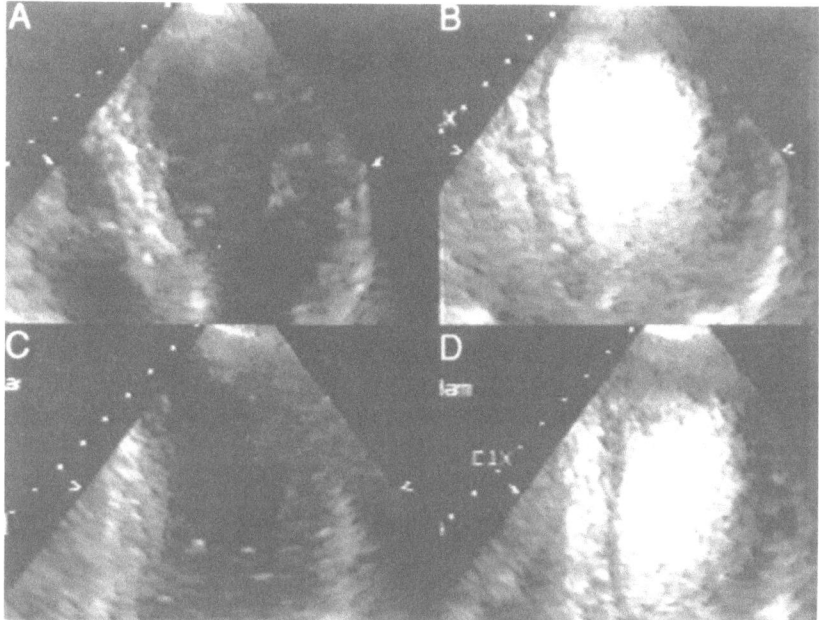

Figure 4. Contrast enhancement at peak stress in dobutamine echocardiography. (A) Non-enhanced four-chamber view, end-diastolic stop frame image. (B) Four-chamber view after administration of an intravenous echo contrast agent. (C) Non-enhanced two-chamber view, end-diastolic stop frame image. (D) Two-chamber view after intravenous contrast administration.

and are promising for myocardial perfusion assessment, the "holy grail" in contrast echocardiography. If combined with stress echocardiography the intriguing possibility of real-time dynamic assessment of both function and perfusion may become reality. It is also conceivable that stress echocardiography might take advantage of recent developments in three-dimensional echocardiography. The use of an intravenous contrast agent for myocardial contrast enhancement and three-dimensional information will make it a powerful stress modality.

Lastly, drug delivery and monitoring systems can be computer-controlled and are commercially available nowadays. Thus, the delivery of the stress agent can be adjusted to achieve a predefined heart rate rise and target.

Conclusions

The analysis of stress echocardiograms is still qualitative, and a more quantitative approach is mandatory to further enhance its clinical utility, e.g. with the help of automated contour techniques, in order to overcome the limitations of the inter- and intraobserver variability. Others reasons why stress echocardiography is not expanding as rapidly as has been expected are its time- and labor-consuming nature (presence of a physician or cardiologist is required) as well as the prerequisite to realize a good infrastructure. Contrast enhanced echocardiography using an intravenous agent with its ability to overcome suboptimal intra- and interobserver variability might lead to a more frequent use of stress echocardiography. To date, there is no proof that stress echocardiography is more cost-effective than nuclear perfusion

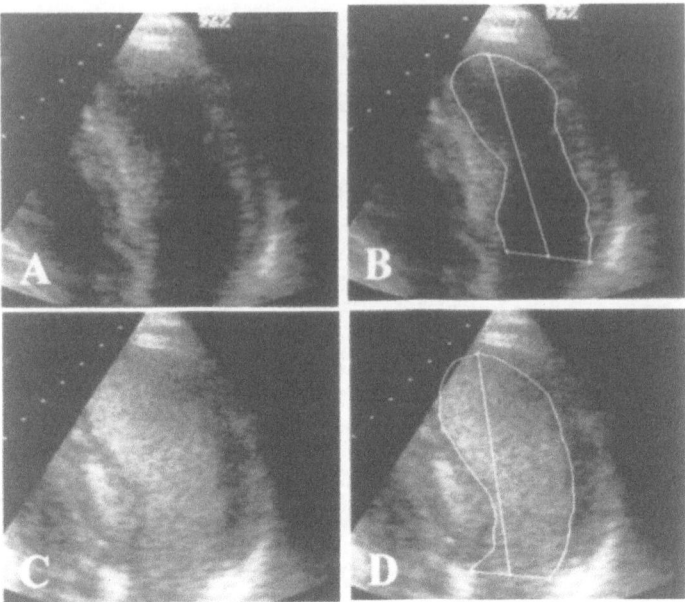

Figure 5. Case example of contrast enhancement of endocardial border visualization and automated border detection by ECHO-CMS (MEDIS medical imaging systems). End-diastolic stop frame images before (A) and after (C) intravenous contrast administration, and the automatically detected endocardial contours (B and D). (Images courtesy of J.G. Bosch, Leiden University Medical Center).

imaging techniques, despite the fact that costs for an ultrasound examination are significantly lower.

In conclusion, stress echocardiography increasingly influences our clinical management in patients, and in experienced echocardiographic laboratories the technique is as effective as nuclear perfusion imaging procedures.

Acknowledgements

We very much appreciated the great support from our ultrasound technicians, Irma Bekkering, Sylvia Bruinzeel and George Maas.

References

1. Wann LS, Faris JV, Childress RH, Dillon JC, Weyman AE, Feigenbaum H. Exercise cross-sectional echocardiography in ischemic heart disease. Circulation 1979;60:1300-8.
2. Previtali M, Lanzarini L, Ferrario M, Tortorici M, Mussini A, Montemartini C. Dobutamine versus dipyridamole echocardiography in coronary artery disease. Circulation 1991;83(5 Suppl):III27-31.
3. Cigarroa CG, deFilippi CR, Brickner ME, Alvarez LG, Wait MA, Grayburn PA. Dobutamine stress echocardiography identifies hibernating myocardium and predicts recovery of left ventricular function after coronary revascularization. Circulation 1993;88:430-6.
4. Afridi I, Kleiman NS, Rainzner AE, Zoghbi WA. Dobutamine echocardiography in myocardial hibernation. Optimal dose and accuracy in predicting recovery of ventricular function after coronary angioplasty. Circulation 1995;91:663-70.

5. Senior R, Lahiri A. Enhanced detection of myocardial ischemia by stress dobutamine echocardiography utilizing the "biphasic" response of wall thickening during low and high dose dobutamine infusion. J Am Coll Cardiol 1995; 26:26-32.
6. Rahimtoola SH. Hibernating myocardium has reduced blood flow at rest that increases with low-dose dobutamine. Circulation 1996;94:3055-61.
7. Jaarsma W, Visser CA, Kupper AJ, Res JC, Van Eenige MJ, Roos JP. Usefulness of two-dimensional exercise echocardiography shortly after myocardial infarction. Am J Cardiol 1986;57:86-90.
8. Kamp O, De Cock, CC, Kupper AJ, Roos JP, Visser CA. Simultaneous transesophageal two-dimensional echocardiography and atrial pacing for detecting coronary artery disease. Am J Cardiol 1992;69:1412-6.
9. Kamp O, De Cock CC, Van Eenige J, Visser CA. Influence of pacing-induced myocardial ischemia on left atrial regurgitant jet: a transesophageal echocardiographic study. J Am Coll Cardiol 1994;23:1584-91.
10. Picano E, Mathias W Jr, Pingitore A, Bigi R, Previtali M. Safety and tolerability of dobutamine-atropine stress echocardiography: a prospective, multicentre study. Echo Dobutamine International Cooperative Study Group. Lancet 1994;344:1190-2.
11. Detrano R, Janosi A, Lyons KP, Marcondes G, Abbassi N, Froehlicher VF, Factors affecting sensitivity and specificity of a diagnostic test: the exercise thallium scintigram. Am J Med 1988;84:699-710.
12. Marwick TH. Current status of stress echocardiography for the diagnosis of myocardial ischemia and viability. In: van der Wall EE, Marwick TH, Reiber JHC, editors. Advances in imaging techniques in ischemic heart disease. Dordrecht: Kluwer Academic Publishers; 1995. p. 83-99.
13. Agati L, Renzi M, Sciomer S et al. Transesophageal dipyridamole echocardiography for diagnosis of coronary artery disease. J Am Coll Cardiol 1992;19:765-70.
14. Panza JA, Laurienzo JM, Curiel RV, Quyyumi AA, Cannon RO 3rd. Tranesophageal dobutamine stress echocardiography for the evaluation of patients with coronary artery disease. J Am Coll Cardiol 1994;24:1260-7.
15. Mairesse GH, Marwick TH, Arnese M et al. Improved identification of coronary artery disease in patients with left bundle branch block by use of dobutamine stress echocardiography and comparison with myocardial perfusion tomography. Am J Cardiol 1995;76:321-5.
16. Secknus MA, Marwick TH. Influence of gender on physiologic response and accuracy of dobutamine echocardiography. Am J Cardiol 1997; 80:721-4.
17. Gianrossi R, Detrano R, Mulvihill D et al. Exercise-induced ST depression in the diagnosis of coronary artery disease. A meta-analysis. Circulation 1989;80:87-98
18. Poldermans D, Fioretti PM, Forster T et al. Dobutamine stress echocardiography for assessment of perioperative cardiac risk in patients undergoing major vascular surgery. Circulation 1993;87:1506-12.
19. Bach DS, Eagle KA. Dobutamine stress echocardiography. Stressing the indications for preoperative testing. Circulation 1997;95:8-10.
20. Vanoverschelde JL, Gerber BL, D'Hondt AM et al. Preoperative selection of patients with severely impaired left ventricular function for coronary revascularization. Role of low-dose dobutamine echocardiography and exercise-redistribution-reinjecting thallium SPECT. Circulation 1995:92(9 Suppl):II37-44.
21. Qureshi U, Nagueh SF, Afridi I et al. Dobutamine echocardiography and quantitative rest-redistribution 201Tl tomography in myocardial hibernation. Relation of contractile reserve to 201Tl uptake and comparative prediction of recovery of function. Circulation 1997; 95:626-35.
22. Bax JJ, Wijns W, Cornel JH, Visser FC, Boersma E, Fioretti PM. Accuracy of currently available techniques for prediction of functional recovery after revascularization in patients with left ventricular dysfunction due to chronic coronary artery disease: comparison of pooled data. J Am Coll Cardiol 1997;30:1451-60.
23. Smart SC, Sawada S, Ryan T et al. Low-dose dobutamine echocardiography detects reversible dysfunction after thrombolytic therapy of acute myocardial infarction. Circulation 1993;88:405-15.
24. Smart SC, Knickelbine T, Stoiber TR, Carlos M, Wynsen JC, Sagar KB. Safety and accuracy of dobutamine-atropine stress echocardiography for the detection of residual stenosis of the infarct-related artery and multivessel disease during the first week after acute myocardial infarction. Circulation 1997;95:1394-401.
25. Carlos ME, Smart SC, Wynsen JC, Sagar KB. Dobutamine stress echocardiography for risk stratification after myocardial infarction. Circulation 1997;95:1402-10.
26. Nijland F, Kamp O, Verhorst PMJ et al. Impact of myocardial viability on left ventricular dilatation following acute myocardial infarction [abstract]. J Am Coll Cardiol. In press 1998.
27. Schwammenthal E, Vered Z, Rabinowitz B, Kaplinsky E, Feinberg MS. Stress echocardiography beyond coronary artery disease. Eur Heart J 1997;18(Suppl D):1D30-7.

28.   Akosah KO, Olsovsky M, Kirchberg D, Salter D, Mohanty PK. Dobutamine stress echocardiography pre-
       dicts cardiac events in heart transplant patients. Circulation 1996;94(9 Suppl):II283-8.

29.   Hoffmann R, Lethen H, Marwick T *et al.* Analysis of interinstitutional observer agreement in interpretation
       of dobutamine stress echocardiograms. J Am Coll Cardiol 1996;27:330-6.

30.   Picano E, Lattanzi F, Orlandini A, Marini C, L'Abbate A. Stress echocardiography and the human factor:
       the importance of being expert. J Am Coll Cardiol 1991;17:666-9.

31.   Schroder K, Agrawal R, Voller H, Schlief R, Schroder R. Improvement of endocardial border delineation in
       suboptimal stress echocardiograms using the new left heart contrast agent SH U 508 A. Int J Card Imaging
       1994;10:45-51.

32.   Leischik R, Kuhlman C, Haude M, Ge J, Liu F, Erbel R. Improved reproducibility of quantitative analysis
       of left ventricular function during exercise echocardiography after intravenous injection of BY 936. J Am
       Soc Echocardiogr 1996;9:201-5.

28.

Overview of automated quantitation techniques in 2D echocardiography

Hans G. Bosch, Gerard van Burken, Francisca Nijland & Johan H.C. Reiber

Summary

Many methods for automated quantitation in two-dimensional echocardiography have been published, but few have gained practical importance. This chapter describes the problems and pitfalls of border detection in cardiac ultrasound, gives an overview of methods described in the literature and categorizes the applied techniques into a hierarchy of abstraction levels. Furthermore, a practical system for automated border detection (ECHO-CMS) and its evaluation will be discussed, and the chapter will be concluded with an overview of the general developments anticipated for the near future.

Introduction

Automated quantitation in two-dimensional (2D) echocardiography has been a field of continuous research since the advent of cardiac echo itself. Outlining the borders of the cardiac wall is essential for calculation of volumes, wall motion and thickness; automatic border detection (ABD), also known as contour detection or automatic delineation) would eliminate the tedious manual tracing, which is highly subject to inter- and intra-observer variability. Unfortunately, ABD in cardiac ultrasound (ABDU) is a difficult and underestimated task, partly due to the complexity and variability of the cardiac anatomy, partly due to limitations in image quality and problems specifically associated with ultrasound imaging. Many approaches for ABDU have been described in the literature, but few have made it into the real world. In this chapter we will discuss the problems in this unruly field, present a concise classification of developed methods, describe a practical system and sketch the anticipated developments in this field for the coming years.

Outline of the problems

Cardiac image analysis issues

Perception and interpretation of highly complex information like images is a very intricate task in general. Humans perform it extremely well; therefore they amply underestimate its

J.H.C. Reiber and E.E. van der Wall (eds.). What's New in Cardiovascular Imaging, 363–376.
©1998 Kluwer Academic Publishers.

complexity. Interpretation of medical images, especially of a complex, dynamic organ as the heart is still more difficult, as it requires expert knowledge of the three-dimensional anatomical structures in the heart, their dynamical behavior, pathology and anatomical variability between patients, and the intricacies of the imaging modality involved. This last point specifically is not to be underestimated for ultrasound.

Despite continuous efforts of numerous research groups, no 'silver bullet' technique for automatic quantitation in echocardiography has evolved yet. A number of useful and promising methods have been developed and have been used in clinical practice, but fully automated, unsupervised analysis of echocardiograms is still as distant a goal as automatic fluent speech recognition and computer reading of handwriting. Actually, the problems, the kind of (partial) successes and their limitations are very similar. These problems can be listed as follows:

1. The input is often incomplete, distorted, and open to multiple interpretations (this is especially appropriate for ultrasound, in comparison to other imaging modalities);
2. Quality of the input is variable, and may sink below the level where any recognition will fail or ambiguities cannot be resolved any more (in speech understanding, the point where humans would interrupt the speaker) or where we will have to guess or use our imagination to get to a reasonable result. One must also be prepared to revise interpretations as soon as new (context) information becomes available.
3. Different hierarchical levels of interpretation exist (for language: letters, syllables and words, sentences, signification; for cardiac images: pixel grey values, regions and edges, anatomical objects, total heart description, function and diagnosis). A fair amount of expert knowledge on each of these levels is necessary for consistent interpretations; in language, one has to know about alphabets, spelling, vocabulary, syntax and semantics, and ultimately about the subject of the text. Valid interpretations at any level should induce correction of mistakes or solving of ambiguities on other levels. In fact, this separation of the analysis problem in a hierarchy of abstraction levels serves well as a framework for automated image analysis systems in general and will be used in this chapter as a guideline for ordering ABDU methods.

Ultrasound specific problems

Ultrasound is an imaging modality with many problems and pitfalls of its own. Outsiders mostly find it hard to interpret, contrary to other tomographic modalities such as CT and MRI. Indeed, ultrasound suffers from several drawbacks, that also impede automated analysis:

1. There is no direct, simple physical relation between pixel intensity and any physical property of the tissue visualized, in contrast to the Lambert-Beer law for X-ray or the Hounsfield units for CT. In ultrasound, images are formed by sound reflection and scattering, resulting in a combination of interference patterns (ultrasound speckle patterns) and reflections at tissue transitions. Different tissues are often only distinguishable by subtle differences in texture (speckle patterns) or behavior of texture over time, rather than by different image intensity values.
2. Ultrasonic image information is very anisotropic and position-dependent, as reflection intensity, spatial resolution and S/N ratio are very dependent of both the depth and the angle of incidence of the ultrasound beam, as well as of the user-controlled Time Gain Compensation (depth gain) settings.

3. Image disturbances: artifacts caused by side lobes, reverberations, lateral and radial point spread functions, significant amounts of random noise. Many of these problems are associated with high gain settings, often necessary in obese or older patients. Speckle noise can be seen as an artifact as well; although it is an inherent part of ultrasound imaging, it often veils anatomical details.

4. Missing information: dropouts (for structures parallel to the ultrasound beam), shadowing (behind acoustically dense structures), scan sector limitations, limited echo windows. Still-frame images generally miss some information, that the human eye catches by viewing a sequence of images; it resolves ambiguities and interpolates the missing parts by exploiting the temporal behavior of structures and texture, which allows discrimination between noise, artifacts and anatomy.

5. Problems caused by the limited temporal resolution and the scanning process. The sequential scanning of lines combines information from different time moments into one image; for fast moving structures, this may lead to spatial distortion. When the scan frame rate is not equal to the video frame rate of 25 or 30 images per second, also sharp transitions between 'old' and 'new' scan line information may appear in still images. These effects are stronger for lower scan frame rates.

Furthermore, 2D ultrasound generally lacks any spatial reference information: no exact spatial localization of the cross section plane is known. In 3D techniques as MRI or CT, this information is often employed in model positioning for the detection. In cardiac ultrasound, the choice of the imaged cross section depends both on the skill and precision of the echo technician and the available echo window, which is limited by ribs (Transthoracic echo, TTE) or esophagus (Transesophageal echo, TEE). Apart from volume measurement errors, this may also result in detection problems if the ABDU method relies on assumptions of shape, distance between epicard and endocard, presence or absence of other structures like valves, papillary muscles, etc.

Overview of methods

We will not try to present a complete taxonomy of methods published: literally hundreds have been proposed. We will limit ourselves to an overview of the main classes of methods, while highlighting a few publications representing the major directions of research.

We are only addressing automated border detection techniques in 2D ultrasound here, either for single images or time sequences. We will not consider quantitation techniques for videodensitometry or methods dealing with Doppler or M-mode; optical flow or temporal correlation techniques generating motion vector fields rather than contours; nor methods that rely completely on manually drawn contours. For a broader overview that includes these fields, please refer to [1].

We will refrain from any comparisons on reported success scores, as there exist no standard test data sets for this purpose, nor standard test criteria. It is also very difficult to compare the type and extent of user interaction, reproducibility etc. Any success scores reported depend very much on the chosen inputs and their quality. As there exists no gold standard, contours are generally judged by an expert, or compared to contours manually drawn by one or more experts, or derived values like area or volume are compared to alternative measurements of these parameters. Most of these are hard to compare between studies. A rough measure for the value of a method could be the number of patients on which it has been tested;

methods that have been tested on less than 10 patients probably have no practical value (although their academic value may be high).

Abstraction level hierarchy

Methods can be divided based upon several criteria; we have chosen the hierarchical level (as described above) of the essential or most innovative part of the method. This division will be roughly equivalent to historical development. Older methods generally were limited to the lowest levels (edge and region finding), relying on user intervention or very simple models for all higher-level interpretation. More modern methods generally address higher levels.

The traditional image interpretation abstraction level hierarchy (Table 1) is sketched in some form in almost all papers on this subject [2,3].

Table 1: Abstraction level hierarchy

Level	General	Speech	Image	Cardiac	Associated operations
0	raw data	samples	pixels	pixels	image generation
1	features	amplitude, frequency	intensity, texture, gradients	intensity, texture, gradients	preprocessing, filtering, feature extraction
2	structures	phonemes	edges, regions	edge	linking, merging, matching, clustering
3	objects	words	world entities, borders, objects	cardiac structures (lumen, endocard, valve)	model relaxation, border finding, classification
4	object sets	sentences	scene	cardiac scene	scene modeling, inter-object relations
5	interpretation	significance	scene interpretation	interpretation and diagnosis	hi-level interpretation. Expert systems, rules

In general we can assume that all hierarchical levels are in some way present in all methods, but that methods have resolved part(s) of the problem by one of 3 ways:
1. implicitly or explicitly limiting themselves to a specific subset of the problem domain, for aspects like cross sections (e.g. only short-axis cross sections at the mid-papillary level),

anatomy (e.g. no congenital defects), image quality (no dropouts, selected images), or imaging equipment (e.g. only certain types of ultrasound machines, or specific requirements on the settings, scale, frequency, etc.)

2. implicitly or explicitly making certain simplifying assumptions on the solution (e.g. the short-axis contour is convex, the endocard is the strongest edge, the cardiac wall will not move more than x mm per frame)

3. relying on the user for preselections (e.g. center points, initial contours) and/or corrections.

To overcome the limitations and errors of their methods, every system relies to some extend on the intervention of the user (USER = Universal Solution for Error Recovery). While this is indeed the only practical way of getting a working system, this is far from ideal, especially when the user is required to correct for 'dumb' mistakes of the system.

However, in a situation where there is missing or distorted information, there is always room for multiple interpretations or 'truths', and in this the user definitely must have the final decision. Ideally, this is the only interaction the user should perform.

Rules for a well-behaved ABD method

With the above in mind, we can formulate a few criteria for a good and well-behaved ABD method.

First of all, the method should generate 'correct' contours. As this is highly subjective (in the light of multiple possible interpretations), a system should be able to adapt to the expert user's general ideas about correct contours.

Secondly, the contours should be reproducible; this seems obvious for an automatic system, but almost all systems require some type of user interaction (at least selection of the images to be analyzed) which will lead to some variability in results. This inter- and intra-observer difference should possibly be smaller than the considerable inter- and intra-observer variabilities associated with similar manual work.

From the viewpoint of user interaction, the following is of importance. A well-behaved method:

• should never generate physically or anatomically impossible solutions; unlikely solutions should be marked as such. It should supply alternative hypotheses (when relevant).

• should not override user-drawn contours etc., unless specifically asked to (apart from cleanup of minor imperfections).

• should allow for easy, intelligent control and correction (the intent of the correction should be applied throughout the whole image set).

Classification of techniques

For each level, the most basic technique is given first. This one is often applied by methods that focus on other levels.

Level 1. Preprocessing.
• Basic: filtering (smoothing, often heavy) for noise/speckle reduction [4]; Contrast stretching; Histogram equalization.
• Spatiotemporal smoothing [5].
• Morphological filters [6].

- Texture filters: Inverse Difference Moment [7]; Wavelet transforms [8]; Fourier- based filters [9].
- RF data processing: Integrated backscatter (AQ) [10].

Level 2. Edge/region detection.
- Basic: global or local thresholding [5,11] or simple edge detectors like difference- of-boxes [4,12,13].
- Advanced edge detectors: Marr-Hildreth [14,15]; Canny [16-18]; rank-based operator [19].
- Pattern or profile matching [20] (see paragraph ECHO-CMS below).
- Matched filters [21]; arc filters [22].
- Region detection: Region growing [9]; fuzzy clustering; resolution pyramids; neural nets; Markov Random Fields [23].

Level 3. Geometrical objects/models.
- Basic: implicit model: e.g. radial search + some candidate point selection, interpolation/linking, smoothing/shape filtering.
- classification of edge points by fuzzy reasoning [15].
- Dynamic programming, or minimum cost optimization [17,24-27].
- Simulated annealing [18]; Self-organizing maps (SOM, Kohonen) [19].
- Snakes/balloons/active contours/deformable contours etc. [13,16,17,28].
- Active shape models (ASM)[20].

Level 4. Anatomical structure and scene models.
- Basic: none, implicit, manually positioned or user-drawn.
- Single geometrical shape models; either 2D, 2D+T, 3D, 3D+T. e.g.:
  - Several model positioning/landmark finding techniques: row/column sums [12,15], arc filters [22], template matching; Hough transform [18]; Fuzzy Logic [8].
  - Shape parameters (2D+T) (see paragraph ECHO-CMS below).
  - 3D shape Neural Nets [29].
- Composite models (modeling several objects and their relation, e.g. the ventricles and the septum), either 2D, 2D+T, 3D, 3D+T. e.g.:
  - Point Distribution Models (2D) [20].
  - Fuzzy neural nets (2D) [30].

Level 5. Interpretation and higher-level knowledge.
- Basic: None, user correction of contours, etc.
- Adaptation of models to image under analysis and expert (see ECHO-CMS below).
- Use of patient group derived models: Neural nets [30], SOM [19], geometrical variations and eigenvectors (PDM) [20].
- Learning behavior over all cases analyzed.
- Rule-based analysis.
- Pathology awareness.
- Multiple hypothesis generation.

Of level 5, few true examples currently exist. The terms 'knowledge-based', 'intelligent' and 'model-driven' are widely misused, even for the most basic techniques at any level.

AQ and its limitations

The clinically most widespread system for ABDU is by far Hewlett-Packard's Acoustic Quantification® (AQ) method that is installed in several HP ultrasound machine models. It is not an ABDU system in the strict sense as described above, because it merely does a blood/border/tissue pixel classification (by thresholding) on the basis of the integrated backscatter energy of the RF ultrasound signal [10]. Therefore, it falls into the lower hierarchical levels. However, its use of the RF data, the on-line applicability and widespread availability make it a potentially valuable tool. It suffers from some serious drawbacks that we have described earlier [31], which may be summarized as follows:

- the AQ borders are very sensitive to gain (TGC, LGC) settings, and often difficult to control for the user.
- AQ uses a fixed, user-drawn ROI within which the blood pixels are counted; parts of the ventricle (the valve plane and/or septum) tend to move in and out of such a region through the cycle, resulting in considerable measurement errors because of missed parts of the ventricle or included parts of the atrium and the other ventricle.
- it is mostly impossible to eliminate tissue parts within the ventricle (like valve, papillary muscle, trabecular structures) or to exclude dropout regions from the ventricle, and noise and artifacts may cause serious problems, especially in difficult patients. Reported success scores in larger patient populations vary widely.

These problems are exemplary for a low-level method that does not use any knowledge about cardiac anatomy. Apart from these drawbacks, the use of RF data supplies superior basic information for blood-tissue classification and may well serve as a basis for higher-level developments, especially when the digital RF data becomes available for off-line postprocessing.

ECHO-CMS endocardial border detection

As an example of a practically applicable ABDU system, we will describe the ECHO-CMS® system that was developed in our laboratory and is being distributed by MEDIS medical imaging systems. ECHO-CMS is an off-line analysis system for automated border detection in echocardiographic image sequences. It consists of a high-end PC-based workstation with image acquisition hardware running Windows-NT and the ECHO-CMS analysis software. The system has been designed for practical use, with the main intent of quantifying endocardial wall motion and lumen volume over sequences of images (frame-to-frame). The system applies different semiautomatic contour detection strategies, that require various amounts of user interaction. Short-axis detection requires just the indication of a center point of the left ventricle, or the manual drawing of a first contour approximation. This type of detection was developed earlier and evaluated with good results: the automated contour areas showed to correlate very well with manually defined contours (Semiautomatic=1.01 * Manual + 5.58%; r=0.989, SEE=11.8) [24]. Furthermore, intra-observer variability of the automated method was significantly smaller than that of manual delineation.

In an evaluation of this technique as applied to epicardial 4-chamber views in an open-chest canine model, monoplane Simpson's rule volumes were calculated from the detected contours and compared with the true LV volumes measured with an intracavitary balloon.

ABD volume and EF correlated well with the true value (Volume: Y=0.88 * X + 3 cc, r=0.85, SEE=15 cc; EF: Y=1 * X - 2.3%, r=0.81, SEE=12%) [32].

User interaction for long axis views

A different border detection method requiring more user interaction is employed in the different long axis views (apical 4-chamber (4C), 2-chamber (2C) and parasternal long axis (LAX) views). Sets of 3 marker points defining the apex and mitral valve plane throughout the cycle are defined, possibly supplemented with one or more manual contours. The most practical approach requires the manual definition of endocardial contours for one end-diastolic (ED) and one end-systolic (ES) image.

After image digitization or import (containing one ore more complete beats), the phase must be defined, from ECG information and/or by indicating ED and ES images. One ED and ES contour must be manually drawn (Figure 1). Next, three landmark points characterizing the position of the LV (apex and mitral valve attachment points, which are the end points of the contour) are extracted from the contours and inter/extrapolated linearly over the cycle(s). The user is required to inspect these markers over the cycle(s) and may then redefine, if necessary, intermediate positions where the true position deviates from the estimated position. In general, this is rarely necessary in the systolic phase, in which motion behaves quite linearly; but it is generally necessary to do this in the diastolic phase, which is highly nonlinear. By dividing the diastolic phase in three subphases (rapid filling, diastasis and atrial filling) and by defining the markers at these phase transitions (start and end of dia-

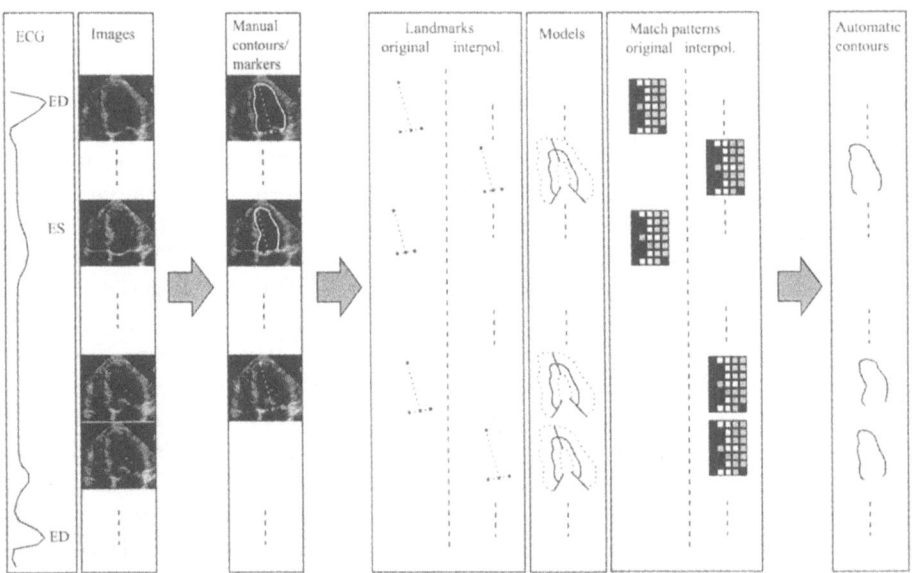

Figure 1. ECHO-CMS long-axis frame-to-frame border detection procedure. From left to right:
- ECG and original images;
- manual drawing of 2 contours and inspection of markers;
- generation of pose, shape and profile models;
- detected contours.

stasis, which can easily be identified in the images from mitral valve leaflet motion), the true valve plane and apex motion can be mimicked easily. This manual landmark positioning in three or more images is an obvious candidate for automation; in the past we have developed a method to do so, but evaluation showed it was slow and not reliable enough, so that it is not used in practice. This landmark tracking problem is now subject of new research using novel concepts.

Automated detection

After these manual stages, the automated contour detection is started. From the manually drawn ED and ES contours, models are extracted describing the geometrical shape of the ventricle over the cycle and the grey-value profiles in a neighborhood of the drawn contours. Phase and LV position are already known from the manual definitions described above. All models (phase, pose, geometry and edge profiles) are interpolated over the cycle and extrap-

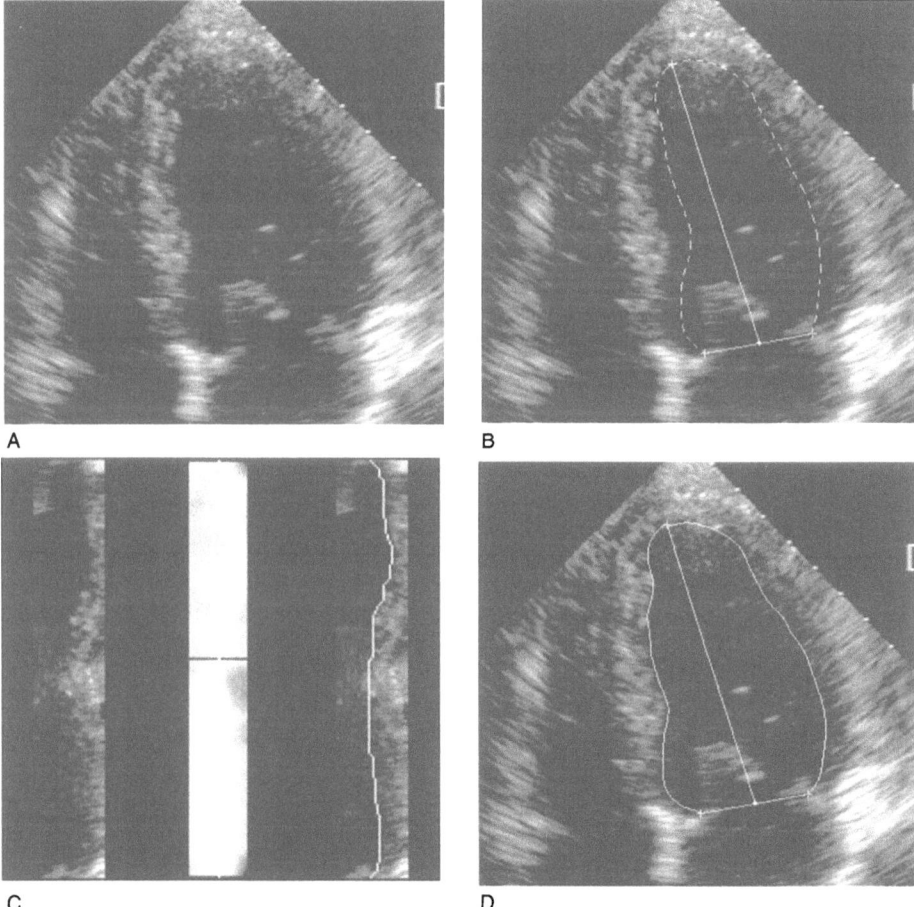

Figure 2. ECHO-CMS Minimum Cost border detection. A) Original image. B)Image with landmarks and shape model. C) Scan and cost value matrices and detected path. D) Image with detected contour.

olated over other cycles (Figure 1). The resulting geometry models are positioned over the images (Figures 2A, 2B), and in a neighborhood of the model, the image is resampled along straight lines perpendicular to the model. For each point of all scan lines (Figure 2C, left), a so-called cost value is calculated representing the likeliness of this point as a contour point: unlikely points will have high cost. The cost is calculated from a combination of edge detectors, match differences with the edge profile models, and local edge reliability measures. Through this rectangular array of cost values (Figure 2C, center), an optimal connective path is determined using a dynamic programming (Minimum Cost) approach. Cumulative costs for all connective paths are calculated, applying position-dependent penalties for deviation from a straight path. In this way, local stiffness of parts of the border are modeled. The path with overall lowest cost is selected as optimal (Figure 2C, right) and by inversion of the resampling process converted into a new contour (Figure 2D).

After detection of all contours, the user may apply any corrections by overdrawing part of a contour. Consequently, all models are updated with the extra user-defined information, which is interpolated and extrapolated over the sequence, followed by a redetection of all non-manual contours.

In short, this method uses full-cycle models for the 2D pose, shape and local stiffness properties of the wall, and for the intensity profiles of the edges. Case-specific and user-specific information is incorporated by collecting information from all user-defined contours.

Evaluation study

The long-axis border detection technique as described above was validated as part of a large clinical study on the impact of myocardial viability on left ventricular dilatation with low-dose dobutamine stress echocardiography (DSE) [33]. Goal of the study was to assess whether ventricular dilatation occurs less in patients with myocardial viability as shown by DSE. In 129 infarct patients from 2 different hospitals in Amsterdam, the Netherlands, 3 separate sets of apical 4-chamber (4C) and 2-chamber (2C) cross sections were recorded: at day 3±1 after acute myocardial infarction, in rest (DAY3); at the same day, with low-dose dobutamine applied (DOBU), and after 3 ± 1 months, in rest (3MTH). The sequences were recorded on VHS videotape. Single complete beats (ED to ED) for each of the 6 sequences were digitized from tape and analyzed. ED and ES contours were drawn manually by the expert user; point markers at next ED and start and end of diastasis were repositioned (and more if necessary to accurately track the marker motion), and the other contours were detected automatically. User corrections to the contours and markers were allowed and counted; redetection was applied after the correction. Contours were corrected until the user was content with all resulting contours. Approximate analysis time was about 20 minutes per sequence, including digitization, loop editing, review, manual drawing, marker correction, contour detection and corrections. Detection itself took approximately 20 seconds. This resulted in data on frame-to-frame biplane volume, local and regional wall motion over the complete heart cycle.

Evaluation results

Because of missing follow-up, not all 129 patients had 6 sequences; a total of 732 single-beat sequences were analyzed, with a total of 16,736 images and contours (Table 2). Apart from the 2 manually drawn contours, at the average less than 1 contour correction per sequence

Table 2: Evaluation results

Results (n=129 patients)	*#Frames / seq. (Average ± SD)*	*#Manual contours / seq.*	*#Manual points & contours / seq.*
4C, DAY3 (n=129)	23.0 ± 3.6	2.9 ± 0.8	6.8 ± 2.5
2C, DAY3 (n=129)	23.0 ± 3.7	2.8 ± 0.8	6.2 ± 2.1
4C, DOBU (n=129)	21.5 ± 3.9	3.1 ± 0.9	6.7 ± 2.4
2C, DOBU (n=128)	21.1 ± 3.8	3.0 ± 0.9	6.6 ± 2.3
4C, 3MTH (n=109)	24.5 ± 3.9	2.9 ± 0.9	6.9 ± 2.4
2C, 3MTH (n=108)	24.6 ± 3.9	2.8 ± 0.9	6.8 ± 2.4
All seq. (n=732)	22.9 ± 4.0	2.9 ± 0.9	6.7 ± 2.3
Corrected / above initial manual input		0.9 corrections above initial 2	1.7 above initial 5
Total # over all seq.	16,736	2,122 (12.7%)	4,865 (29,1%)
Total # corrected / above initial manual input		658 (3.9%)	1,185 (7.1%)

(0.9) was necessary (Table 2, column 3). The total number of frames per sequence requiring contour or marker interaction is listed in column 4 (on average 6.7/seq.). Initially, contours were drawn in 2 frames and markers positioned generally in 3 more, which leaves 1.7 frames/seq. for corrections and extra points. Although the time and effort for the marker manipulations is relatively low, these numbers suggest the processing time and user dependence of the method can be improved by automating this marker placement.

Contour detection was slightly better in the baseline sequences (DAY3 and 3MTH) than in the stress sequences (DOBU), and better for 2C than for 4C, but none of these differences were significant.

Overall, this proves that the ECHO-CMS system provides a practical and successful way of analyzing contours over the full cardiac cycle. In this study, no direct comparison with manually drawn contours was performed for practical reasons (the manual drawing of almost 17,000 contours), but there is no reason to assume that results would be inferior to those found in the earlier studies [24,32].

Future trends

Instrumentation developments

First of all, several ultrasound instrumentation developments will influence the feasibility of successful ABDU.

The current trend to apply digital signal processing in the ultrasound system front end (RF processing) will further contribute to image quality and thus to higher success rates in automated analysis.

Digital image storage will eliminate the image degradation inherent to VCR tape storage, allow inclusion of calibration and settings information that may help in accurate detection and will ultimately (when RF data is stored) allow digital postprocessing of RF data and use of this rich source of information for texture characterization, blood/tissue classification, and use of additional information like Tissue Doppler and Power Doppler for border detection and additional quantitative processing. With reference to Moore's Law, which states that computer storage capacity and speed doubles approximately every 18 months, we can expect general feasibility of RF data storage within 2 to 5 years.

3D and 4D echo, both from scanning/rotational probes and native 3D probes will certainly gain interest, and inherently 3D/4D border detection techniques will emerge, probably primarily evolving from similar developments in the MR and CT modalities. The great advantage for ultrasound ABD lies in the applicability of true 4D models, elimination of the cross section uncertainty and the possibility of resolving ambiguities and estimating 'missing' information from the extra dimension.

Concerning contrast echocardiography, we do not expect a direct impact on success of automatic contour detection; this is mainly due to the incomplete and irregular filling of the ventricle/tissue, the destruction of contrast bubbles because of the acoustic pressure, and the transient nature of the contrast. With technical contrast agent improvements, and the development of ABD techniques which are aware of the specific behavior of a certain contrast agent, this may provide new opportunities.

ABDU developments

Apart from these trends external to the field of ABDU, we can distinguish multiple interesting and promising developments, most of which lie at the higher hierarchical levels.

At the lower levels, not many spectacular developments may be expected; some improvements may result from the (still neglected) use of texture information, temporal correlation and the physical characteristics of the ultrasound image formation process.

At the higher levels, significant improvements are possible. The optimal detection of 3D and 4D complex geometrical structures is still an open problem with many directions of research (ASMs, 3D snakes, etc.). The modeling of 3D/4D complex anatomical scenes, complete with probability distributions and possibly available for normals, various types of pathology and congenital defects will be needed; this may emerge from extensions of CSG trees, adjacency graphs, PDMs, geometrical shape parameter stochastics, etc.

At the top level, the heuristics of interpretation and diagnosis, work is still in its infancy. Here we enter the dark realm of artificial intelligence. To evade the discussion on the ethical aspects of machines dealing with clinical decision making (instead of providing just measurements): we do not expect 'Deep Blue' to become a cardiologist.

Still, several aspects from this category will certainly come into view: the use of rule based expert systems and blackboards for high-level control of the system; systems employing combinations of many techniques and opportunistically choose an optimal detection strategy; systems generating multiple hypotheses with measures of confidence; the handling of pathological/congenital conditions as models or hypotheses in multiple hypothesis reasoning; model adaptation to patient in analysis and to expert; learning behavior by neural nets or rule-based systems.

Conclusions

Work on automated border detection for cardiac ultrasound is far from finished. Few clinically applicable systems exist, and automation is limited. Positive expectations exist for the future, both from outside and inside the field of ABDU; from the outside, on the basis of computer and ultrasound hardware improvements, integration of RF-based information into ABDU, advent of 4D echo; from the inside, by integration of several technologies at the higher hierarchical levels, especially better 3D/4D geometrical modeling, anatomical scene description and modeling of anatomical inter-patient variability and pathological conditions.

Acknowledgments

The work described has been supported by research grants (LGN92.1706 and LGN66.4349) from the Technology Foundation, The Netherlands.

References

1. Sher DB, Revankar S, Rosenthal S. Computer methods in quantitation of cardiac wall parameters from two dimensional echocardiograms: a survey. Int J Card Imaging 1992;8:11-26.
2. Cheng XS. Design and implementation of an image understanding system: DADS [dissertation]. Delft: Delft University of Technology; 1990.
3. Smets C. A knowledge-based system for the automatic interpretation of blood vessels on angiograms [dissertation]. Leuven; Catholic University Leuven; 1990.
4. Grube E, Mathers F, Backs B, Luderitz B. Automatische und halbautomatische Konturfindung des linken Ventrikels im zweidimensionalen Echokardiogramm. In-vitro Untersuchungen an formalinfixierten Schweineherzen. Z Kardiol 1985;74:15-22.
5. Ezekiel A, Garcia EV, Areeda JS, Corday SR. Automatic and intelligent left ventricular contour detection from two-dimensional echocardiograms. 1985:261-4.
6. Klingler JW Jr, Vaughan CL, Fraker TD Jr, Andrews LT. Segmentation of echocardiographic images using mathematical morphology. IEEE Trans Biomed Eng 1988;35:925-34.
7. Montilla G, Barrios V, Roux C, Mora F, Passariello G. Border detection in echocardiography images using texture analysis. Comput Cardiol 1992:643-6.
8. Setarehdan SK, Soraghan JJ. Automatic left ventricular feature extraction and visualisation from echocardiographic images. Comput Cardiol 1996:9-12.
9. Verlande M, Flachskampf FA, Schneider W, Ameling W, Hanrath P. 3D reconstruction of the beating left ventricle and mitral valve based on multiplanar TEE. Comput Cardiol 1991:285-8.
10. Perez JE, Waggoner AD, Barzilai B, Melton HE Jr, Miller JG, Sobel BE. On-line assessment of ventricular function by automatic boundary detection and ultrasonic backscatter imaging. J Am Coll Cardiol 1992;19:313-20.
11. Han CY, Lin KW, Wee WG, Mintz RM, Porembka DT. Knowledge-based image analysis for automated boundary extraction of transesophageal echocardiographic left-ventricular images. IEEE Trans Med Imaging 1991;10:602-10.
12. Monteiro AP, Marques de Sa JP, Abreu-Lima C. Automatic detection of echocardiographic LV-contours. A new image enhancement and sequential tracking method. Comput Cardiol 1988:453-6.
13. Hozumi T, Yoshida K, Yoshioka H et al. Echocardiographic estimation of left ventricular cavity area with a newly developed automated contour tracking method. J Am Soc Echocardiogr 1997;10:822-9.
14. Chu CH, Delp EJ, Buda AJ. Detecting left ventricular endocardial and epicardial boundaries by digital two-dimensional echocardiography. IEEE Trans Med Imaging 1988;7:81-90.

15. Feng J, Lin W-C, Chen CT. Epicardial boundary detection using fuzzy reasoning. IEEE Trans Med Imaging 1991;10:187-99.

16. Chalana V, Linker DT. A multiple active contour model for cardiac boundary detection on echocardiographic sequences. IEEE Trans Med Imaging 1996;15:290-8.

17. Dong L, Pelle G, Brun P, Unser M. Model-based boundary detection in echocardiography using dynamic-programming technique. Proc SPIE 1991:1445;178-87.

18. Friedland N, Adam D. Echocardiographic myocardial edge detection using an optimization protocol. Comput Cardiol 1989:379-82.

19. Belohlavek M, Manduca A, Behrenbeck T, Seward JB, Greenleaf JF. Image- analysis using modified self-organizing maps: automated delineation of the left-ventricular cavity in serial echocardiograms. Lecture Notes Comput Sci 1996;1131:247-52.

20. Cootes TF, Hill A, Taylor CJ, Haslam J. Use of active shape models for locating structures in medical images. Image Vision Comput 1994;12:355-65.

21. Detmer PR, Bashein G, Martin RW. Wall position and thickness estimation from sequences of echocardiographic images. IEEE Trans Med Imaging 1990;9:396-404.

22. Wilson DC, Geiser EA. Automatic center point determination in two-dimensional short-axis echocardiographic images. Pattern Recogn 1992;25:893-900.

23. Herlin IL, Nguyen C, Graffigne C. Stochastic segmentation of ultrasound images. In: Recognition A: Computer vision and applications. The Hague. IEEE Computer Society Press, 1992:289-92.

24. Bosch JG, Savalle LH, Van Burken G, Reiber JHC. Evaluation of a semiautomatic contour detection approach in sequences of short-axis two-dimensional echocardiographic images. J Am Soc Echocardiogr 1995;8:810-21.

25. Maes L, Delaere D, Suetens P, Aubert A, Van der Werf F. Automated contour detection of the left ventricle in short axis view and long axis view on 2D echocardiograms. Comput Cardiol 1990:603-6.

26. Gustavsson T, Molander S, Pascher R, Liang Q, Broman H, Caidahl K. A model- based procedure for fully automated boundary detection and 3D reconstruction from 2D echocardiograms. Comput Cardiol 1994:209-12.

27. Dias JMB, Leitao JMN. Wall position and thickness estimation from sequences of echocardiographic images. IEEE Trans Med Imaging 1996;15:25-38.

28. Cohen LD. Note on active contour models and balloons. CVGIP 1991;53:211-8.

29. Coppini G, Poli R, Valli G. Recovery of the 3-D shape of the left ventricle from echocardiographic images. IEEE Trans Med Imaging 1995;14:301-17.

30. Brotherton T, Pollard T, Simpson P, DeMaria A. Echocardiogram structure and tissue classification using hierarchical fuzzy neural networks. In: ICASSP 94 Proceedings. New York: IEEE; 1994. p. 573-6.

31. Bosch JG, Reiber JHC, Van Burken G, Savalle L, Maurincomme E, Helbing WA. Automated contour detection and acoustic quantification. Eur Heart J 1995;16(Suppl J):35-41.

32. Picard MH, Bosch HG, Morrissey RL, Reiber JHC. Automated echocardiographic ventricular volume quantitation: validation of a new border detection method [abstract]. Circulation 1994;90(4 Suppl):I608.

33. Nijland F, Kamp O, Verhorst PMJ, De Voogt WG, Bosch HG, Visser CA. Myocardial viability: impact on left ventricular dilatation after acute myocardial infarction. J Am Coll Cardiol. In press 1998.

29.   Doppler myocardial imaging

George R Sutherland

Summary

Imaging of the myocardium using Doppler techniques, based on either spectral or colour principles has been available for use in clinical cardiology for some six years. Despite early enthusiasm and some preliminary studies which indicated potential clinical applications for the technique, it has remained somewhat of a Cinderella among cardiac ultrasound techniques. It is, therefore, appropriate to review the reasons why there remains a clinical need for such a technique (given the profusion of competing new ultrasound modalities), how the technique has developed since its introduction and why there has not been greater interest in the technique leading to its widespread introduction into clinical practice, despite its many theoretical advantages over grey-scale imaging in a number of clinical situations.

Rationale for Doppler myocardial imaging - the quantification of regional myocardial motion to allow accurate and reproducible measurements of contraction at relaxation

The measurement of regional myocardial motion and indices of contractility has been the traditional role of M-mode echocardiography. However, the traditional M-mode technique has been limited in the number of myocardial segments it may be applied to as insonation must be at 90%. In addition, standard parasternal M-mode studies examine only circumferential contraction and do not take into account longitudinal shortening. The M-mode technique has been expanded to look at base-apex shortening by examining the motion of the fibrous atrio-ventricular valve plane throughout the cardiac cycle but this information is examining the global function of the underlying myocardial wall and cannot determine regional long-axis function. Thus, a new ultrasound modality which could determine regional myocardial long and short axis function during both systole and diastole for all myocardial segments could be an advantage during both resting and stress echo studies. Doppler myocardial imaging could form the basis of such a quantitative technique.

Doppler myocardial imaging - technical considerations

All current standard cardiac ultrasound techniques derive their information on myocardial function indirectly based either on parameters measured from the endo- and epicardial specular reflections or from blood pool Doppler indices. Doppler myocardial imaging is a technique in which Doppler signal processing is applied to the reflected ultrasound signals originating within the myocardium [1,2]. Information on myocardial function can be

J.H.C. Reiber and E.E. van der Wall (eds.). What's New in Cardiovascular Imaging, 377–390.
©1998 Kluwer Academic Publishers.

derived either from the use of either colour Doppler principles or by performing either spectral or power analysis of the pulsed Doppler signal derived from a sampler volume placed within the myocardium. In the colour Doppler approach, mean velocity estimation is based on the autocorrelation technique and quantifies regional intramural velocities by detecting consecutive phase shifts of the reflected echoes from myocardium. The use of Doppler techniques to interrogate myocardium motion is not a new concept. Pulsed Doppler recordings of myocardial motion using a single sample volume technique were first described by Isaaz et al. in 1989 [3]. Although deemed to be interesting, little clinical value was ascribed at that time to this approach. It was not until 1991 that McDicken et al. [4] first described the modifications required to standard Doppler signal processing which would allow visualisation of the motion of a tissue-equivalent phantom that the potential clinical value of colour Doppler recording of myocardial signals began to be appreciated.

In a conventional ultrasound machine, prior to blood pool Doppler signal processing the reflected ultrasound signals are passed through a high-pass (clutter) filter which rejects the high-intensity, low-frequency ultrasound signals arising from the myocardium. Thus to visualise only the myocardium, an ultrasound machine must be adapted. This is effected by changing the thresholding and filtering algorithms to reject the low amplitude echoes from the blood pool and to allow the high amplitude, low velocity information from the myocardium to pass to subsequent determination of the mean Doppler shift, and hence mean velocity, using standard colour Doppler autocorrelation methodology. The mean velocity information thus derived may be displayed in either a two-dimensional or M-mode format. From the mean velocity information, the machine can also be programmed to calculate and display in a 2-D format myocardial acceleration, regional phase information, amplitude of motion and regional synchronicity. In addition, a further myocardial Doppler parameter can be measured and displayed - the power (or energy) of the Doppler signal.

Doppler signal processing of myocardial ultrasound information has several theoretical advantages over standard grey scale imaging. Doppler processing has an intrinsically lower noise floor and higher signal to clutter ratio. Doppler processing allows the accurate measurement of differing mean myocardial velocities at a large number of neighbouring intramural sites. (This is inherently simpler, quicker and more reliable than the other alternative technique of tracking the speckle pattern within conventional B and M-mode images). In addition, as both spectral and colour Doppler techniques measure frequency shift rather than signal amplitude, any velocity image information thus obtained is less affected by tissue attenuation than grey-scale imaging. (Thus, it is frequently possible to obtain diagnostic image quality DMI images from patients who appear "poorly echogenic" on standard grey-scale imaging.) Where grey-scale imaging remains superior to colour Doppler imaging is in its inherent higher spatial resolution and (in current generation equipment) higher frame rates. Yet despite both current frame rate and resolution limitations, the colour Doppler technique already can provide clinical diagnostic information. Modern ultrasound data processing techniques allied to the digital signal pathway within the new generation of ultrasound machines allow colour Doppler images to be displayed with a frame rate of 50-80/ second. While image spatial resolution is inferior to grey-scale imaging, this approaches 1 x 1 mm at low colour Doppler frame rates and 2 x 2 mm at frame rates of 40-50/second.

Doppler myocardial imaging - in vitro studies on the accuracy of velocity estimation

A series of in vitro phantom studies have confirmed the accuracy of DMI velocity encoding over a range of velocities at which normal and abnormal myocardium would be expected to move [5]. Velocity estimation has been shown to be affected by target velocity, target material. system receive gain and the pulse train size but the inherent error is at worst ± 10% of the true mean velocity [5]. The spatial resolution of both the two-dimensional velocity and power maps is at best 1 m x 1 mm and at worst 3 x 3 mm with a slightly inferior axial resolution compared to standard grey-scale imaging but a similar lateral resolution [2]. This means that the DMI technique is a better real-time spatial discriminator than real-time MRI, Position Emission Tomography or current nuclear perfusion techniques.

Doppler power (energy) interrogation of the myocardium

The power (or signal strength) of reflected myocardial Doppler ultrasound information is related to the number of scatters within the tissue block insonnated. Thus measurement of regional Doppler power levels could provide information on tissue characterisation. The Doppler power signal is both velocity independent and angle independent as this measurement is independent of the phase-shift of the signal. Regional Doppler power can be displayed in two formats: as a two-dimensional image (currently with a dynamic range of 0-40 dB) or as the temporal variation in signal strength of the signal derived from a pulsed Doppler sample volume placed within the myocardium (but excluding the endocardial and pericardial specular reflectors). This latter measurement can be obtained by measuring the power of the new audio data (which is available on all ultrasound machines) using a specially developed on-line meter. The temporal variations in power levels can then be fed back into the machine via an auxiliary channel and displayed as a trace in real time simultaneously with the Doppler Myocardial velocity information. Raw audio data is relatively unprocessed ultrasound information obtained early in the signal processing path with the ultrasound machine - it has a wide dynamic range (typically 0-70 dB) and is linearly processed data. This should be the direct equivalent of integrated backscatter data derived from the myocardium. Using a similar Doppler power measurement technique, Schwartz et al. [6] have already demonstrated in a series of in vitro studies that single pulsed Doppler power measurement is the direct equivalent of integrated backscatter measurement in terms of changes in blood pool reflectivity produced by varying the concentrations of echo contrast agent.

DMI studies of normal myocardial function circumferential contractile function

To circumvent the temporal resolution problems inherent in the first generation of DMI systems in determining intramural velocities using the two-dimensional approach, DMI M-mode interrogation of intramural velocities was developed. This technique allows myocardial sampling at approximately 4 millisecond intervals with high spatial resolution but as with all M-mode techniques should only be carried out where insonnating the myocardium at 90°. Such M-mode velocity studies in normal patients have confirmed the presence of transmural systolic and diastolic velocity gradients across the left and right ventricular walls during the cardiac cycle [7,-10]. These velocity gradients are presumed to present circumferential contractile function only and are in accord with prior reports on intramural velocity gradients recorded by placement of a series of ultrasonic crystals within the myocardium during animal experiments. These latter studies have also recorded an early systolic transmural velocity gradient with higher velocities encoded in the sub-endocardial region and lowest velocities in the sub-epicardial region. A series of DMI M-mode velocity studies have confirmed the normal velocity distribution and timing peak velocity gradients within the left ventricular posterior wall and interventricular septum during the cardiac cycle. These studies have also identified predictable changes in intramural diastolic velocities which occur associated with ageing.

Longitudinal contractile function

DMI M-mode studies have also been used to interrogate long-axis shortening of the heart by aligning the M-mode beam along the apex-base of the interventricular septum or lateral left and right ventricular walls. These studies have demonstrated a base-apex longitudinal velocity gradient on both the septum and ventricular free walls with the highest long-axis shortening velocities recorded at the cardiac base and with almost zero velocities recorded at the apex. Thus the DMI technique has the potential to characterise long-axis function of the heart including regional abnormalities in long-axis contraction and relaxation. With respect to both circumferential and longitudinal contractile function, DMI velocities has also been shown to change in a predictable manner in response to both positive and negative inotropes in an animal model. In addition, single pulsed Doppler DMI velocity sample volume interrogation of the myocardium allows the determination of regional myocardial peak velocities and their temporal relationship to regional mechanical and electrical events in the heart.

Left ventricular diastolic and left atrial function

Current ultrasound parameters used to evaluate left ventricular diastolic function are indirect indices derived either from digitised M-mode traces of the endocardial surfaces of the left ventricle or from Doppler indices derived from blood flow through the left heart. DMI provides a direct measure of regional intramural velocities during left ventricular relaxation and hence may provide a better and more clinically relevant measure of diastolic function. Early studies have shown that DMI indices parallel transmitral Doppler blood flow measurements and normal changes in these latter indices associated with ageing [9]. Other studies have shown that measured DMI diastolic velocities of long axis lengthening to correlate with atrio-ventricular valve ring velocities during diastole [11,12]. In addition, DMI indices have been shown to correlate well with both left atrial wall function indices of left atrial appendage function [13,14]. To what extent these new indices provide more clinically relevant information remains to be determined but it is likely that such direct measurements may supplant current indirect measurements of left ventricular diastolic function.

DMI studies in cardiomyopathies and transplant patients

A series of comparative clinical studies in patients with dilated cardiomyopathies, hypertrophic cardiomyopathies, and patients with concentric left ventricular hypertrophy have determined a range of abnormalities in intramural velocities which could not be predicted from either standard grey-scale two-dimensional or M-mode studies. The results of these studies showed a significant decrease in mean velocity gradients during all systolic phases during atrial contraction in DCM patients [15]. In HCM patients, velocity gradients were significantly decreased or reversed in all systolic cardiac phases despite apparently normal M-mode fractional thickening indices [16]. These abnormalities are likely to be due to the abnormal myocardial architecture in HCM patients and may prove to be a new ultrasound marker specific for this condition. Similar studies in patients with infiltrative cardiomyopathies have demonstrated both Doppler velocity and reflectivity changes which seems to mirror the degree of myocardial involvement not always apparent on the grey-scale image. In transplant patients, similar changes in myocardial reflectivity have been shown to correlate well with biopsy-proven early moderate rejection but whether these changes are sufficiently sensitive indicators to be used in routine clinical practice remains to be proven. In addition, pulsed wave Doppler can be used to determine the contractile function of both donor and recipient atria.

DMI studies in ischaemic heart disease

That both colour and spectral DMI can determine a series of predictable changes in myocardial contractile function induced by ischaemia has been clearly documented [17,18] These have been determined both in animal models and in patients. The earliest ischaemia induced changes have been recorded using the DMI pulsed Doppler technique to identify regional velocity changes. In a dog model, significant early changes in regional diastolic velocities in the ischaemic zone were found after only 15 seconds of ischaemia, while diastolic velocities remained normal in the non-ischaemic territories. [19]. Later changes in systolic peak velocities were also observed which paralleled changes in the transmural velocity gradient obtained by two-dimensional DMI reduction in wall thickening on M-mode grey-scale imaging. Encouraging results have also been reported with regard to reversible ischaemic changes detected using the DMI single sample volume pulsed Doppler technique in conjunction with low-dose dobutamine infusions [20]. In areas where infarction has occurred, pulsed Doppler DMI studies of long-axis contractile function would appear to identify a specific and predictive bi-phasic pattern of low velocity myocardial systolic motion which is readily distinguished from the low velocity mono-phasic pattern induced by ischaemia and is present in viable myocardium. In addition, predictable changes in transmural velocities associated with a marked reduction in Doppler power signal strength have also been noted in patients with both acute ischaemia and infarction. These appear to parallel changes in integrated backscatter levels (see below).

Pulsed Doppler signal strength - a direct equivalent to integrated backscatter measurements? Normal and ischaemic studies

Measurement of variation in the power of the pulsed Doppler myocardial signal from normally contracting myocardium have shown this to demonstrate a cyclic variation in signal strength which parallels the temporal variation in standard integrated backscatter measurements. The largest variation in myocardial pulsed Doppler signal strength and highest signal intensities are recorded at the base of the heart with the lowest levels recorded at the apex. These findings again parallel integrated backscatter parameters. Clinical studies have also demonstrated that ischaemia blunts both the absolute peak signal levels and the cyclic variation of power of the myocardial pulsed Doppler signal. In infarct zones, there is no measurable cyclic variation in pulsed Doppler signal strength although the absolute level of the signal may vary depending on the relative amounts of oedema or fibrosis present in the infarct zone. Furthermore, the intensity of the pulsed Doppler myocardial signal can be increased by the presence of a myocardial contrast agent.

Doppler myocardial imaging vs. integrated backscatter data in the assessment of myocardial ischaemia

With increasing interest in the quantification of ultrasound images, the increasing availability of access to the raw ultrasound data and the increase in computing speed and power, attention is again paid to the acquisition and analysis of new and more complex ultrasound data sets which may add to our understanding of myocardial ischaemia and infarction. Both Doppler Myocardial Imaging (DMI) and the measurement of the Cyclic Variation in Integrated Backscatter (CVIB) have been invoked as new indices of myocardial contractile function. Animal and clinical studies have suggested that both can identify a range of normal and abnormal values for myocardial contractile function and both have the ability to identify specific changes in myocardial contractility associated with varying degrees of ischaemia. How do these two techniques compare and contrast and in which way, if at all, are they likely to add more information than standard grey-scale imaging to our quantification of myocardial function during ischaemic events?

Radiofrequency data is the raw, largely unprocessed ultrasound data which returns to the ultrasound machine from the transducer. This signal has a wide dynamic range and is non-logarithmically compressed. Two main forms of signal processing can be applied to this dataset; frequency domain analysis or time domain analysis. Analysis of the frequency information is a complex off-line procedure and is currently out with both the computing and manpower resources of most cardiac departments. A much simpler approach has been to average the signal strength of the returning radiofrequency data and to perform an analysis of regional variation in image signal strength in the time domain. This parameter is known as the cyclic variation in integrated backscatter and for the pre-determined region of interest is expressed in dB. It is a non-log compressed signal, typically with a dynamic range of 60-70 dB. It is based on signal processing via the grey-scale imaging signal path.

Doppler Myocardial Imaging data, in contrast, is obtained by processing the returning raw radiofrequency data from the transducer via the Doppler signal processing path. This may be done by using either spectral Doppler or more commonly, colour Doppler signal processing. The important information obtained by this technique is velocity information compared to the reflectivity information obtained by measuring integrated backscatter. However, Doppler power information which measures reflectivity can also be obtained.

The two techniques differ not only in their methods of processing the returning radiofrequency data set but also in the nature of the radiofrequency data set acquired. Grey-scale and Doppler insonation differ in both their method of insonating a target and in the average amount of acoustic energy delivered to the target thus creating differences in the returning radiofrequency signal. Furthermore, the two data sets differ in their noise floor with Doppler signal processing typically having a 15-35 dB lower noise floor than comparable grey-scale signal processing methodology.

Clinical studies

Despite using only information based on changes in the strength of the ultrasound signal returning from the myocardium, CVIB has been strongly suggested to be a good index of regional myocardial contractility. In normal patients, a base-apex gradient in peak IB levels has been found throughout the myocardium. A similar base-apex velocity gradient can be recorded in normals using Doppler Myocardial Imaging. Indeed, with the left ventricular posterior wall and septum, an endo-epicardial gradient in peak IB levels is present with the highest levels found sub-endocardially. This correlates well with the transmural velocity gradient found during M-mode DMI studies and could again tend to confirm that both IB and DMI measurements are examining similar aspects of contractile function.

With the onset of ischaemia, the CVIB is increasingly blunted with increasing degrees of ischaemia. With the onset of infarction, the CVIB is lost but differing studies have shown widely disparate changes in absolute backscatter levels. Our own experience would suggest that with irreversible ischaemic damage, absolute IB levels fall relatively quickly as muscle death occurs and only return to normal or increased levels some days or weeks later as tissue oedema settles and fibrosis occurs. It should be pointed out, however, that others have shown a marked increase in absolute IB levels during ischaemia despite a blunting of the CVIB.

DMI can show a similar pattern of changes during ischaemic injury. Spectral Pulsed Doppler DMI studies can demonstrate regional changes in diastolic function parameters prior to the onset of measurable changes in systolic function. Similar information can also be derived from colour Doppler information obtained from a high-frame rate acquisition system. The earliest change in systolic function which can be detached in diminution is the transmural colour M-mode gradient with a fall in sub-endocardial velocities. However, this technique is cumbersome to use and should be supplanted by colour Doppler mean velocity estimation of overall wall velocity. This again shows a progressive fall in peak mean systolic velocities with decreasing degree of ischaemia and is an index which can be used to quantify stress echocardiographic studies. With the next onset of acute infarction, in both animal model and in patients with acute infarction, the presence of tissue oedema decreases the reflectivity of the dead muscle and the returning DMI signal falls below the threshold of the DMI algorithm. Thus acute infarct zones may appear as "black holes" within the myocardial Doppler 2-D image. This again parallels the acute reduction in absolute IB levels during acute infarction.

In summary, the IB and DMI techniques appear to give similar information on both contractile function and tissue reflectivity. However, DMI has advantages in its robustness, ease of acquisition (being less dependent on chest wall attenuation, as the velocity information is based predominantly on phase-shift evaluation) and ease of post-processing. IB estimation currently provides more useful information on tissue reflectivity than DMI and thus should be looked on as a complementary rather than a competing technique.

DMI stress echocardiography - could this be feasible?

One initial hope was that with appropriate development, Doppler Myocardial Imaging would allow quantification of two-dimensional stress echo images by determining ischaemia indiced intramural velocity changes. The initial low frame rates present in the first generation of DMI two-dimensional imaging systems made such an approach unlikely to be clinically useful. Even with the development of a second generation of DMI instruments with frame rates equal to or greater than current standard 2-D grey-scale imaging, the problems associated with the Doppler angle of insonnation of the myocardium was thought initially to preclude off-line measurement of absolute mean systolic velocity changes during stress echo studies. However, initial DMI studies during low and high dose dobutamine stress echocardiography using the left parasternal window approach demonstrated a predictable dose dependent increase in mean systolic velocities in both the inferior and anterior left ventricular walls in normal patients while patients with coronary artery disease were shown to have impaired augmentation of systolic velocities [21].

With the recent development of a third generation high frame rate colour Doppler myocardial imaging system in which grey-scale and colour Doppler information can be acquired in parallel, stored and subsequently down-loaded to a personal computer for off-line analysis, quantifiable stress echocardiographic studies are now potentially possible. Indeed, initial clinical studies in normals and in patients with coronary artery disease undergoing either bicycle or Dobutamine stress studies have proved encouraging. DMI velocity data on long axis contraction velocities can be obtained from an apical transducer position using a combination of two and four chamber views and information on circumferential contraction velocities will be obtained by using parasternal long and short axis views. To a large extent, this approach circumvents the problem of angle of insonation, as for apical views, long axis contraction is aligned virtually parallel to the ultrasound beam, while circumferential contraction (= inward motion of the myocardium) velocities are at 90° and can essentially be discounted. The reverse is true of the parasternal views where circumferential contraction occurs parallel to the ultrasound beam and the direction of longitudinal contraction is almost at 90°.

In a series of normals studied, using bicycle ergometry as the stress agent, a consistent and predictable mean systolic velocity response could be obtained for each of the 16 segments of the standard model. In patients with coronary artery disease, abnormal responses in velocity increase proved to be highly predictive of the presence of significant coronary artery disease and correlated well with observed acquired abnormalities on the simultaneously acquired grey-scale images. This was equally true of both bicycle ergometry and dobutamine stress echo. It must be emphasised that these are preliminary results but they are highly encouraging. It remains to be seen if this technique will indeed provide quantifiable stress echocardiography but it appears likely. Additionally, the information provided by DMI on phase, amplitude of motion, a regional synchronicity has to be examined in terms of exercise-induced changes in wall motion to determine which, if any, of these parameters improves the sensitivity or specificity of the technique.

Doppler power (energy) evaluation of myocardial perfusion

Current opinion would suggest that the successful detection of regional myocardial perfusion by cardiac ultrasound requires the combination of an effective left heart contrast agent and an appropriate ultrasound detection technique. Grey-scale videodensitometric analysis is increasingly being shown to be inappropriate for myocardial contrast detection due to the inherent grey-scale processing and compression algorithms within the current generation of ultrasound machines. Radiofrequency data acquisition, second harmonic imaging and Doppler power (energy) data acquisition are all more appropriate imaging modalities because of their individual unique properties and linear processing algorithms. Doppler power has been shown to be effective in detecting the presence of a galactose-based left heart contrast agent within the myocardium in both a closed-chest animal model and in normal subjects [2]. Two-dimensional Doppler power imaging has also been shown to detect regional perfusion abnormalities, perfusion changes caused by concomitant dipyridamole infusion and myocardial reperfusion in an animal model [22]. Why should the Doppler power mode offer advantages over grey-scale imaging? Firstly, the mode of insonation is different. Doppler power is based on information derived from colour Doppler signal processing. To produce an image, the transducer is programmed to send out up to six impulses per line and then waits to receive the returning impulses for a longer period than for a corresponding grey-scale image. This has the effect of delivering more average acoustic power to the contrast agent and in a more intermittent manner than grey-scale imaging. As acoustic power is important in creating a non-linear response in contrast agent reflectivity, this may account in part for the greater sensitivity of Doppler power mode imaging. Another factor, which may be important, is the intrinsically lower noise floor of the colour Doppler system. It is thus possible that any signal enhancement brought about by the contrast agent may not be identified as it lies within the noise floor of grey-scale imaging but that the same level of signal enhancement would be detected by the Doppler system as it lies above the noise floor. What role any of the Doppler power modalities might play in a clinically effective ultrasound technique remains to be determined but currently it shows equal promise when compared to either radiofrequency data or second harmonic imaging and has a major advantage in its relative ease of implementation within an ultrasound system.

DMI evaluation of arrhythmias

As DMI can identify regional myocardial velocities and regional variations in myocardial acceleration, theoretically both normal and abnormal patterns of myocardial velocities and accelerations could be identified on a two-dimensional image as could the presence and precise location of foci of onset of abnormal ventricular contraction [23]. In addition, the higher temporal resolution of pulsed Doppler myocardial imaging could also be used to derive instantaneous regional myocardial contraction and relaxation velocities [24]. The normal right and left ventricular myocardial velocity and acceleration sequences during the cardiac cycle have been determined by DMI (2-D, pulsed and Doppler and M-mode)

modalities. This data has been compared with myocardial velocity and acceleration information from patients with abnormal ventricular depolarisation including patients with pacemakers and bundle branch block. In addition, patients with ventricular arrhythmias and
patients with functioning accessory bypass tracts have been studied. The combination of
DMI velocity and acceleration mapping using 2-D mode, M-mode and pulsed DMI techniques can identify specific normal and abnormal sequences of myocardial acceleration
which accurately reflected the mode and timing of electrical depolarisation. Abnormal early
regional changes in velocity or acceleration associated with either WPW bypass tracts, unifo-
cal VPBs, or sustained ventricular tachycardias have been accurately located as have the
immediate normalisation in depolarisation induced during the monitoring or radiofrequency ablation [24]. This information was only in part available from standard grey-scale
imaging. Thus DMI would appear to be an important new adjunct to the non-invasive
investigation of abnormal myocardial depolarisation including the real-time monitoring of
radiofrequency ablation.

Doppler myocardial imaging - 3-D reconstruction

3D echocardiography (3DE) is gaining increasing interest as a potentially superior technique
to standard 2D echocardiography in the assessment of both congenital and acquired heart
disease.

To date, 3DE has been applied in the clinical setting in the assessment of (1) left and
right ventricular function and volumes, (2) septal defects and (3) native and prosthetic atrio-
ventricular valves. Previous studies on 3D reconstruction have used either transoesophageal
or transthoracic standard grey-scale imaging (GSI) as their data source. A major limitation of
the transthoracic approach is the poor quality of the images acquired in a substantial proportion of patients. This is because the quality of a GSI image is mainly related to only one
parameter, i.e. the amplitude of the ultrasound signal returning from the interrogated myocardium which, in a substantial number of patients, is markedly attenuated by the chest
wall. The Doppler technique could be used as an alternative tissue-data acquisition technique to overcome problems with low signal to noise ratio. This is due to the fact that, in
contrast to GSI imaging, the quality of DMI images is dependent on two factors rather than
one: the amplitude of the returning signal (which is in turn, directly dependent on the attenuation) and the frequency shift of this signal which is relatively independent of the attenuation factor. Thus, it is this latter factor which gives rise to the potential of the Doppler
technique to provide more complete images of the myocardium than the standard GSI technique [25]. The first clinical case of 3D DMI reconstruction reported was a unique case of
an SLE mass causing acute mitral valve obstruction and mimicking mitral stenosis [26]. 3D
DMI information proved to be superior to that obtained from the 3D GSI. Thus, in this
case, standard 2D transoesophageal images proved unnecessary because the DMI images
obtained noninvasively from the precordial approach were of excellent quality, emphasising
the advantage of this technique. These images allowed both the correct quantification of
mass volume and determination of the morphology of the mass.

To validate 3 DMI technique and to assess the potential clinical application of DMI a
series of *in vitro* and *in vivo* studies were subsequently performed. To determine the accuracy
of 3D DMI imaging both a computer-generated virtual reality phantom and a dynamic tissue-mimicking phantom were used. The aims of these studies were to determine: (1) the

minimum size of an isolated crystal which could be determined and the minimum gap which could be seen in the 3-D image between 2 separate crystals and (2) the accuracy of 3D volume computation. The analysis of 3D images obtained from the virtual phantom showed that the 3D system could reconstruct structures of 0.3 mm size and identify a gap of 1 mm. 3D images of the tissue-mimicking phantom showed that a crystal of 1 mm could still be seen in both 3D GSI and DMI images. The minimum gap between 2 crystals which could be determined was 1.5 mm for GSI in the central part of the image and 2-3 mm in the peripheral part of the image. For DMI the values were 2 mm and 3 mm, respectively. Both 3D techniques underestimated the true volume of the phantom, but the systematic error was smaller for DMI than for GSI over the range of different sizes of true volume. This study has shown that although, the spatial resolution of the 3D images was virtually identical for both GSI and DMI, DMI is potentially more accurate acquisition technique in volume measurements. In vivo GSI and DMI 3D left ventricular volume measurements were performed in a group of sixteen patients and the results were correlated with those obtained from biplane cineventriculography [25-27]. In vivo, for grey-scale the end-diastolic volume mean difference was -12.6 ml and the limits of agreement were ±18 ml and for DMI the corresponding values were -4.2 and ±10.6 ml, respectively. The difference for end-systole was, for grey-scale -6.5 ± 10.6 ml and for the Doppler technique -1.5 ± 10 ml. The magnitude of the difference in volume measurement between 3D echocardiography and cineventriculography was significantly smaller using the Doppler technique for both end-diastole and end-systole.

To determine whether transthoracic 3D echocardiography could accurately define atrial septal defect (ASD) morphology 30 ASD patients were studied [28]. In each patient, two techniques were used to acquire 3D data: GSI and DMI. 3D images were constructed to simulate the surgeons view of the ASD. Measured parameters were: max. and min. vertical (V) and horizontal (H) ASD dimensions (D), distances to inferior- (IVC) and superior vena cava (SVC), coronary sinus (CS), tricuspid valve (TV). The max. ASD Ds were compared with Magnetic Resonance phase-contrast cine Imaging (MRI) and surgery [28]. This study has shown that 3DE accurately displays the varying morphology, size and spatial relationships of an ASD. As a DMI data-set it provides the optimum information on which to base patient management decisions.

Doppler imaging of skeletal muscle

Potential applications of DMI are not confined to cardiac imaging. Early validation work has demonstrated that DMI could be used to identify contracting skeletal muscle groups. Since then, a systematic examination of skeletal muscle contraction in healthy volunteers has been undertaken [29]. This study demonstrated the capability of DMI to identify tetanic skeletal muscle contraction, to differentiate between active contraction and passive muscle movement, and to characterise isotonic, isometric and reflex skeletal muscle contraction profiles. Thus, there may be considerable potential for further evaluation of DMI in neurological and musculoskeletal applications. In particular, DMI may have practical application in the design and validation of biomechanical assist systems such as latissimus dorsi cardiomyoplasty [30,31].

Perspectives

DMI developments are currently at a most exciting point. Pulsed Doppler evaluation of regional myocardial function at rest is entering clinical practice. The Colour Doppler technique is being further investigated in terms of new parameters to assess myocardial motion. From the colour mean velocity data, a whole series of new parameters of myocardial motion can be calculated. These include: regional acceleration, regional amplitude of motion at 90% to the insonnating beam, regional delay, regional phase, regional synchronicity. In addition, in-plane strain rates for any myocardial segments can be calculated and displayed, this information being derived from the colour Doppler data set. It remains uncertain, what new clinical information each of these parameters will contribute but this should be determined in the near future. Other new developments include the ability to acquire and display the Colour Doppler myocardial velocity data set in three dimensions using a free-hand 3-D acquisition technique. From this data set it is possible to visualise and measure the extent of in-plane velocity and strain rate abnormalities within the myocardium in three dimensions.

Conclusions

DMI is potentially a valuable addition to the clinical ultrasound investigative modalities providing new information not available from current standard echo techniques. However, at present, it remains a technique in development.

References

1.   Sutherland GR, Steward MJ, Grounstroem KWE *et al.* Colour Doppler myocardial imaging: a new technique for the assessment of myocardial function. J Am Soc Echocardiogr. 1994;7:441-58.
2.   Miyatake K, Yamagishi M, Tanaka N *et al.* A new method for the evaluation of left ventricular wall motion by color-coded tissue Doppler imaging: in vitro and in vivo studies. J Am Coll Cardiol 1995;25:717-24.
3.   Isaaz K, Thomson A, Ethevenot G, Cloez JL, Brembella B , Pernot C. Doppler echocardiographic measurement of low velocity motion of the left ventricular postrior wall. Am J Cardiol 1989;64:66-75.
4.   McDicken WN, Sutherland GR, Moran CM, Gordon L. Colour Doppler velocity imaging of the myocardium. Ultrasound Med Biol 1992;18:651-4.
5.   Fleming AD, McDicken WN, Sutherland GR *et al.* Assessment of colour Doppler tissue imaging using test phantoms. Ultrasound Med Biol 1994;20:937-51.
6.   Schwarz KQ, Bezante GP, Chen X. When can Doppler be used in place of integrated backscatter as a measure of scattered ultrasound intensity? Ultrasound Med Biol 1995;21:231-42.
7.   Fleming AD, Palka P, McDicken WN, Sutherland GR. Ultrasound Med Biol. In press 1996.
8.   Fleming AD, Xia X, McDicken WN, Sutherland GR, Fenn L. Myocardial velocity gradient by Doppler imaging. Br J Radiol 1994;67:679-88.
9.   Palka P, Lange A, Flemin AD, Sutherland GR, Fenn LN, McDicken WN. Doppler tissue imaging: myocardial wall motion velocities in normal subjects. J Am Soc Echocardiogr. 1995;8:659-68.
10.   Palka P, Lange A, Flemin AD *et al.* Age-related transmural peak mean velocities and peak velocity gradients by Doppler myocardial imaging in normal subjects. Eur Heart J 1996;17:940-50.
11.   Rodriguez L, Garcia M, Ares M, Leung D, Thomas JD, Griffin B. is mitral annulus motion during early diastole active of passive? Clinical evidence of elastic recoil [abstract]. J Am Coll Cardiol 1995;P57A.
12.   Rodriguez L, Garcia M, Nakatani S, Ares M, Griffin B, Thomas JD. Longitudinal axis diastolic dynamics in patients with left ventricular hypertrophy: a Doppler tissue imaging study [abstract]. J Am Soc Echocardiogr 1995;8:391.

13. Rodriguez L, Garcia M, Nakatani S *et al.* Quantitation of left atrial systolic function by doppler tissue imaging: clinical validation [abstract]. J Am Echocardiogr 1995;8:349.

14. Rodriguez L, Nakatani S, Leung D *et al.* Measurement of atrial appendage cycle length by transthoracic echocardiography using doppler tissue imaging [abstract]. J Am Soc Echocardiogr 1995;8:391.

15. Lange A, Palka P, Sutherland GR *et al.* Doppler tissue imaging assessment of systolic and diastolic transmural velocity gradients in dilated cardiomyopathy: a new diagnostic index [abstract]. Eur Heart J 1995;16(Suppl)298.

16. Palka P, Lange A, Sutherland GR *et al.* Doppler tissue imaging: assessment of systolic and diastolic transmural velocity gradients in hypertrophic cardiomyopathy. A new diagnostic index [abstract]. Eur Heart J 1995;16(Suppl):105.

17. Uematsu M, Miyatake K, Tanaka N *et al.* Myocardial velocity gradient as a new indicator of regions left ventricular contraction: detection by a two-dimensional tissue Doppler imaging technique. J Am Coll Cardiol 1995;26:217-23.

18. Stewart MJ, Sutherland GR, Moran CN, Fleming AD, Fenn LN, McDicken WN. Imaging of ischaemic and infarcted myocardium by Doppler tissue imaging [abstract]. Circulation 1993;88:I47.

19. Garcia-Fernandez MA, Azevedo J, Puerta M, Moreno E, Torrecilla E, San Roman D. quantitative analysis of segmental left ventricular wall dysfunction by pulsed doppler tissue imaging. A new insight into diastolic performance [abstract]. Eur Heart J 1995;16(Suppl):451.

20. von Bibra H, Tuchnitz A, Firschke C, Schühlen H, Schömig A. Doppler tissue imaging of left ventricular myocardium - initial results during pharmacologic stress [abstract]. J Am Coll Cardiol 1995;P57A.

21. Fontavet HL, Puleo JA, Davis MG, Lockely M. Quantitative dobutamine stress echo-cardiography utilising doppler tissue imaging. J Am Col Cardiol 1996;27(Suppl A):65A.

22. Sutherland GR, von Bibra H, Tuchnitz A, Henke J, Schönig A. transthoracic detection of regional myocardial perfusion abnormalities using a pervenous contrast agent - a comparative study of doppler energy and grey scale imaging. Br Heart J 1995;73(Suppl 3):57.

23. Yamagishi M, Tanaka N, Itoh S, Miyatake K, Yamayaki N, Hirama M. An enhanced method for detection of early contraction site of ventricles in Wolff-Parkinson-White syndrome using color coded tissue Doppler echocardiography [abstract]. J Am Soc Echocardiogr 1993;6:30.

24. Sutherland GR, Pons Llado GP, Carreras F *et al.* Doppler myocardial imaging in the evaluation of normal and abnormal ventricular depolarisation. Br Heart J 1995;73(Suppl 3):85.

25. Lange A, Palka P, Caso P *et al.* Doppler myocardial imaging versus b-mode grey scale imaging: a comparative in vitro and in vivo study into their relative efficacy in endocardial boundary detection. Ultrasound Med Biol. In press 1998.

26. Lange A. Wright RA, Al-Nafusi A, Sang C, Palka P, Sutherland GR. Doppler myocardial imaging: a new method of data acquisition for three-dimensional echocardiography. J Am Soc Echocardiogr. In press 1996.

27. Lange A, Bouki K, Fenn LN, Palka P, McDicken WN, Sutherland WN. A comparison study of grey scale versus Doppler tissue imaging left ventricular volume measurement using three dimensional reconstruction [abstract]. Eur Heart J 1995:16(Suppl):266.

28. Lange A, Palka P, Sutherland GR, Shaw TRD, Fox KAA, Godman MJ. Three- dimensional definition of dynamic atrial septal defect morphology by transthoracic echocardiography [abstract]. Eur Heart J 1996;17(Suppl):425.

29. Grubb NR, Fleming A, Fox KAA, Sutherland GR. Evaluation of Doppler tissue imaging for the assessment of skeletal muscle function in healthy volunteers. Radiology 1995;194:837-42.

30. Grubb NR, Sutherland GR, Campanella C. Optimisation of myostimulation in dynamic cardiomyoplasty. Eur J Cardio Thor Surg 1995;9:45-9.

31. Grubb NR, Fleming A, Sutherland GR, Campanella C, Fox KAA, Sinclair C. Assessment of latissimus dorsi muscle function after cardiomyoplasty using Doppler tissue imaging. Br Heart J 1994;71(Suppl):302-34.

30.

Carotid intima-media thickness measurement: predictor of future cardiovascular disease

Michiel L. Bots, Antonio Iglesias & Diederik E. Grobbee

Introduction

High-resolution B-mode ultrasonography enables us to accurately assess vessel wall characteristics of the carotid arteries in populations at large. This technique facilitates the evaluation of the lumen diameter, the intima-media thickness and the presence and extent of plaques of the carotid artery. In an increasing number of studies carotid intima-media thickness (CIMT) measurements are currently applied to study determinants of presence and progression of atherosclerosis in populations at large [1-8]. Furthermore, these studies allow for studying atherosclerosis as a risk factor for future cardiovascular disease.

In cross-sectional studies an increased CIMT has been associated with unfavourable levels of established cardiovascular risk factors, with prevalent cardiovascular and cerebrovascular disease and with atherosclerosis elsewhere in the arterial system. Based on these findings there is a growing belief that CIMT measurements can be regarded as an indicator of generalised atherosclerosis and may be used as an intermediate endpoint or proxy endpoint as a suitable alternative for cardiovascular morbidity and mortality [9]. This view is conditional on the observation that increased CIMT is related to future cardiovascular events.

Images, validation, reproducibility and distribution

A typical characteristic longitudinal ultrasound image of the distal part of the common carotid artery is shown in Figure 1. On this 2-dimensional ultrasound image, the anterior (near) and posterior (far) wall of the carotid artery are displayed as two bright white lines separated by a hypo-echogenic space. For the far wall the distance of the leading edge of the first bright line of the far wall (lumen-intima interface) and the leading edge of the second bright line (media-adventitia interface) indicates the intima-media thickness. For the near wall, the distance between the trailing edge of the first bright line (adventitia-media interface) to the trailing edge of the second bright line (intima-lumen interface) at the near wall provides the best estimate of the near wall intima-media thickness. The inner lumen diameter can be assessed as the distance between the intima-lumen interface at the near wall and

J.H.C. Reiber and E.E. van der Wall (eds.). What's New in Cardiovascular Imaging, 391–400.
©1998 Kluwer Academic Publishers.

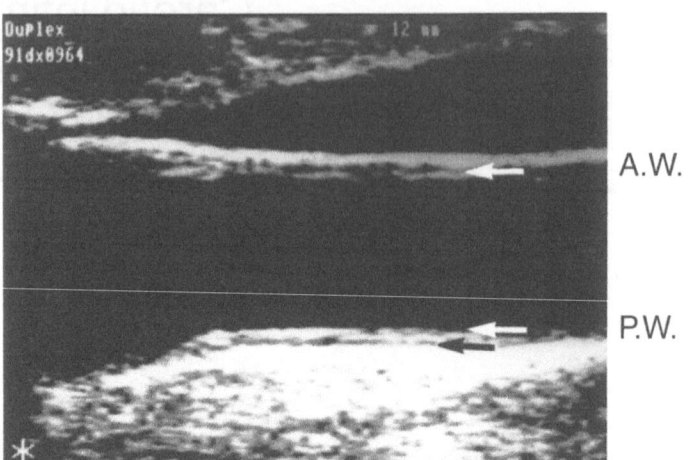

Figure 1. Characteristic longitudinal 2-D ultrasound image of the distal common carotid artery. AW = Anterior (near) wall of the carotid artery . PW = Posterior (far) wall of the carotid artery. Arrows from top to bottom indicate the leading edge of the intima-lumen interface at the near wall, the lumen-intima interfaces and the media-adventitia interface at the far wall, respectively.

the lumen-intima-interface at the far wall [10]. An image such as Figure 1 allows for measurement of common carotid (mean and maximum) intima-media thickness of the near wall and far wall and of the lumen diameter. The image is digitised, and displayed on a screen of a personal computer. The beginning of the carotid bifurcation (widening of the near and far wall) is the reference point from which the measurements start. With a cursor the interfaces of the near and far wall are marked over a length 10-mm to proximal. Dedicated computer software calculates the mean and maximum intima-media thickness and the mean and minimal lumen diameter over that segment. Recently a number of automated edge detection programmes have become available for measuring CIMT [11,12]. The first results look promising.

Validation studies, in which ultrasound measurements of intima-media thickness were compared with histology, showed that ultrasonic far wall intima-media thickness truly and accurately represents intima-media thickness [10,13,14]. In contrast, these studies have indicated that near wall intima-media thickness measurements may considerably underestimate the true intima-media thickness. Furthermore, the near wall measurement may be affected by the axial resolution and the gain settings of the ultrasound equipment. Based on these findings it has been argued that near wall measurements should not be used and that emphasis should be on far wall measurements.

In several studies the reproducibility of ultrasonographically assessed CIMT has been determined [14-17]. In general, the mean differences in repeated measurements between sonographers, between readers and between visits were small and a good correlation between paired measurements of CIMT was seen. The measurement variability was small in relation to the biological variability between subjects.

Currently, several noninvasive ultrasound protocols are being used to quantify the presence and extent of carotid atherosclerosis using CIMT measurements. In general, these approaches differ in four aspects, i.e., the length of the segment of the measurement (maximum or mean intima-media thickness); the artery (left or right); the site (common carotid artery, carotid bifurcation and internal carotid artery) and the location of the measurement (near and far wall). Similarly, the individual outcome variable, based on intima-media thickness measurements, differs across studies from a (weighted) average of all measurements at all sites and locations to site specific far wall measurements. At present it is not clear which approach is clearly superior for use in research into determinants of presence and progression of atherosclerosis and into atherosclerosis as a determinant of future disease.

Figure 2 presents the distribution of common CIMT measurements as observed among the first 1000 participants of the Rotterdam Study [4]. The mean far wall common CIMT was 0.77 mm (SD 0.19). Common CIMT was normally distributed with a small tail to the right. Similar distributions have been described for other studies and for intima-media thickness measurements in the carotid bifurcation and internal carotid artery [18]. Importantly, there appears to be no clear cut-off point to indicate at which common CIMT level a subject is diseased or not. All decisions to dichotomise subjects based on common CIMT measurements in groups of subjects with and without abnormalities are therefore arbitrary.

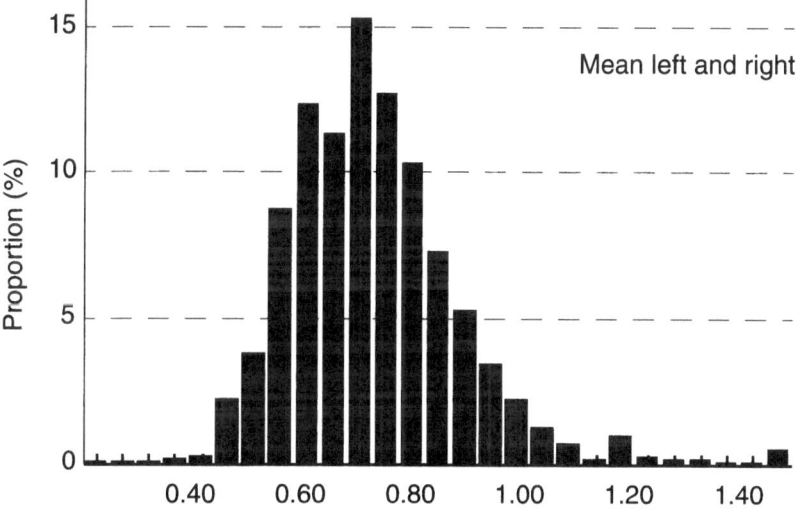

Figure 2. Distribution of common carotid intima-media thickness measurements in the first 1000 participants of the Rotterdam Study [4].

Cross-sectional findings

Several studies demonstrated that with increasing age common CIMT increases in both men and women. The estimates of change in common CIMT based on cross-sectionally obtained data were around 0.009 mm/yr for men and 0.009 mm/yr for women [1-8,19-21]. Common CIMT was increased in men compared to women for all ages, with a mean difference of around 5 to 10 %, which has been interpreted as differences in presence or extent of atherosclerosis. However, this difference is partly attributable to differences in end-diastolic lumen diameter and may therefore reflect differences in physiology rather than differences in atherosclerosis per se [22].

Subject with prevalent cardiovascular disease, such as myocardial infarction, angina pectoris, and stroke, have in general a 6 to 12% thicker common carotid intima-media compared to those without symptomatic cardiovascular disease [23-26]. A 15 to 20% increased CIMT has been observed in subjects with intermittent claudication compared to subjects without intermittent claudication [8]. Associations were similar for men and women. Strong and graded positive associations of common CIMT to left ventricular mass, measured by echocardiography, have been reported [27-29].

An increased common CIMT has been shown to be associated with presence of atherosclerosis elsewhere in the arterial system like plaques and stenosis in the internal carotid artery [5,19,26]. Presence of calcifications of the abdominal aorta was associated with a 18 % increase in common CIMT [30]. A gradual increase in common CIMT with decrease in ankle-arm index, as an indicator of atherosclerosis in the arteries of the lower extremities has been reported [8,31]. Subjects with peripheral arterial disease, defined as an ankle-arm index < 0.90 has a significantly 15% increased intima-media thickness compared to those without peripheral arterial disease (ankle-arm index Æ 0.90).

Elevated levels of established cardiovascular risk factors, such as LDL cholesterol, systolic blood pressure, body mass index, and a decrease in HDL cholesterol were associated with an increased intima-media thickness [1-3,6,7,9,20-22]. Additionally, subjects with presence of hypertension, smoking and diabetes mellitus have an 5 to 12 % increased CIMT compared to subjects without these conditions. At present limited information is present on the association between coagulation factors, such as fibrinogen, factor VII activity and factor VIII activity, and intima-media thickness.

Longitudinal findings

Intima-media thickness as predictor of future disease

Based on the findings in cross-sectional studies, there is a growing belief that CIMT measurements can be regarded as an indicator of generalised atherosclerosis and may be used as an intermediate endpoint or proxy endpoint as a suitable alternative for cardiovascular morbidity and mortality. This view is conditional on the observation that increased CIMT is related to future cardiovascular events.

At present we are aware of only three published reports that explored the possible association between CIMT and incident events. Salonen and co-workers, in a study carried out in a random sample (n = 1,257) of middle-aged Finnish men, reported that an increase of 0.1 mm in maximum far wall common CIMT was associated with 11% [95% CI 6,16] increase in risk of myocardial infarction [32]. This analysis was based on 36 coronary heart disease events that occurred after 1 to 3 years of follow-up.

Findings from the Atherosclerosis Risk In Communities (ARIC) study were recently reported based on 290 coronary heart disease events that occurred after a 4 to 7 years of follow up in 7289 women and 5552 men, aged 45-64 years [33]. In this study IMT was based on the mean far wall of the common carotid artery, the bifurcation and the internal carotid artery. The age adjusted risk of coronary heart disease increased gradually with increasing

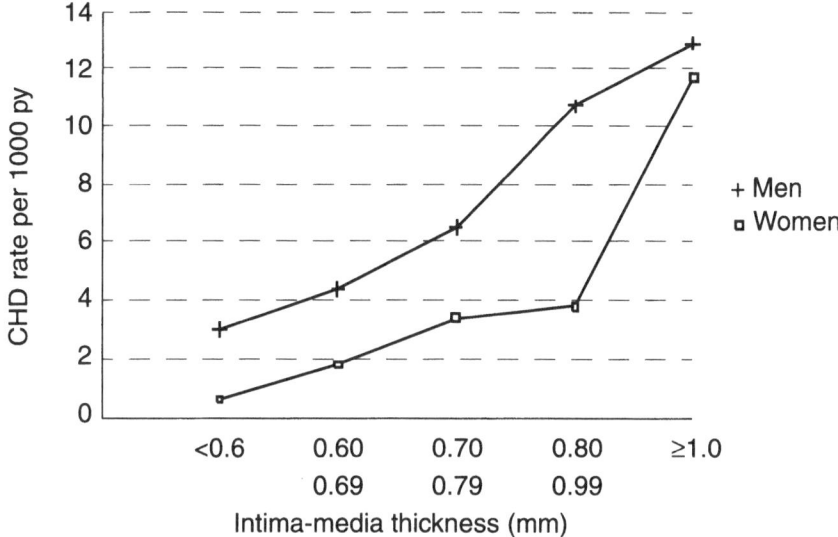

Figure 3. Risk of coronary heart disease by carotid intima-media thickness. Results from the ARIC study [33].

CIMT (Figure 3). Analyses with CIMT as a continuous variable indicated that the risk of CHD increased by 69% [95% CI 50%-90%] in middle-aged women and 36% [23%-51%] in middle-aged men per 0.19 mm increase in CIMT. Results for the common CIMT per 0.19 mm increase were 92% [95% CI 66%-122%] and 32% [95% CI 8%-23%], respectively. As expected, adjustment for several cardiovascular risk factors reduced the magnitude of the association.

In the Rotterdam Study a nested case-control design was used to evaluate whether common carotid IMT is related to future stroke and myocardial infarction among 7983 subjects aged 55 years and over participating in The Rotterdam Study [34]. The analysis was based on 98 myocardial infarctions and 95 strokes, and a sample of 1373 subjects who remained free from myocardial infarction and stroke during follow-up. The mean duration of follow-up was 2.7 years. CIMT was based on the average of the near and far wall of the left and right common carotid artery. The risk of stroke and of myocardial infarction gradually with increasing IMT (Figure 4). The odds ratio for stroke per standard deviation increase (0.163 mm) was 1.41 [95% CI 1.25-1.82]. For myocardial infarction, an odds ratio of 1.43 [95% CI 1.16-1.78] was found. When subjects with a previous myocardial infarction or stroke were excluded, odds ratios were 1.57 [95% CI 1.27-1.94] for stroke and 1.51 [95% CI 1.18-1.92] for myocardial infarction. Additional adjustment for several cardiovascular risk factors attenuated these associations: 1.34 [95% CI 1.08-1.67] and 1.25 [95% CI 0.98-1.58], respectively.

The important findings from these studies implicate that CIMT measures are strongly related to future coronary heart and cerebrovascular disease in middle-aged and elderly subjects. This predictive power remained even when established cardiovascular risk factors wee taken into account. These findings provide supportive evidence for the use of CIMT as an intermediate or proxy endpoint in observational and intervention studies.

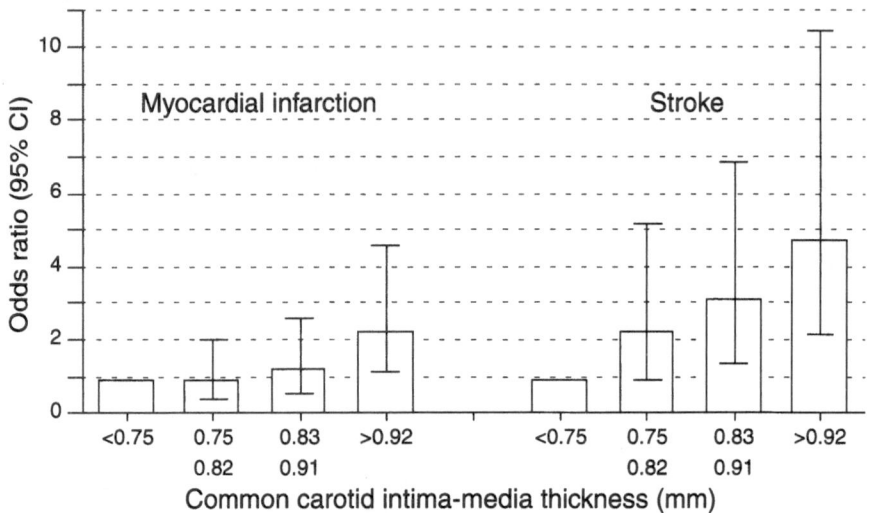

Figure 4. Association between common carotid intima-media thickness and risk of first stroke and myocardial infarction. Results from the Rotterdam Study [34].

Important current issues

Near wall versus far wall CIMT measurements

Several studies in which the ultrasound measurements were compared with histology have indicated that the ultrasonographic far wall intima-media thickness measurements reflect the true thickness [10,14,15]. The intima-media thickness measurement of the near wall of the carotid artery is at best an approximation of the true wall intima-media thickness. Moreover, the precision of the estimate of the near wall intima-media thickness depends on the axial resolution of the equipment used and on the gain setting. The near wall findings in the validation studies have lead to an intensive discussion on whether near wall intima-media measurements should be performed at all. At present there are two strong views [35]: 1) the near wall measurements should not be used, because they do not reflect the true thickness and therefore are invalid; 2) the near wall measurements are of value and should be used. The latter view recognises and respects the view that the near wall measurement not truly reflects its anatomical substrate, but there is evidence to argue in favor of the use of near wall CIMT measurements.

The reproducibility of the near wall CIMT measurements is similar as those reported for the far wall CIMT measurements [5]. In addition, recent cross-sectional results from the Rotterdam Study have indicated that the association between near wall intima-media thickness and prevalent cardiovascular disease is as strong and precise as compared to the association found for the far wall [36]. Combining information of the near wall and far wall common CIMT into one intima-media thickness estimate (average of four sites) provided the strongest association with cardiovascular disease in this study. Similar results were

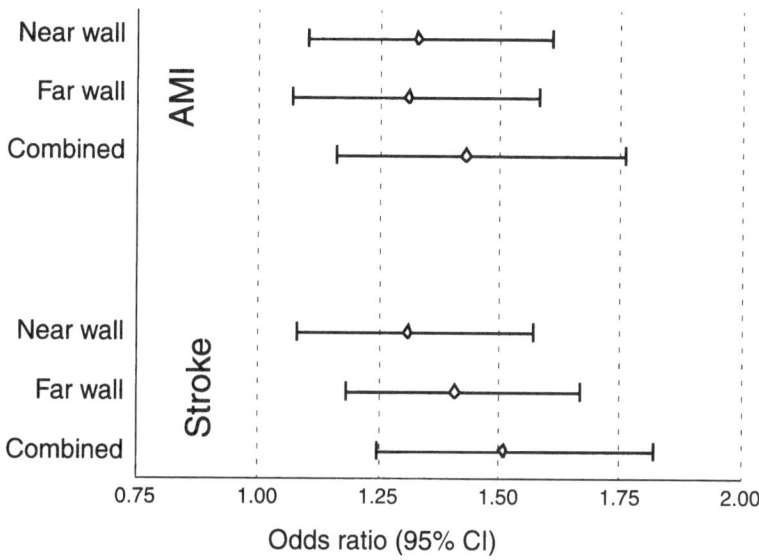

Figure 5. Association between near wall common carotid intima media thickness and far wall common carotid intima-media thickness and risk of myocardial infarction and stroke. Findings from the Rotterdam Study [34].

obtained for the association with lower extremity arterial disease. Longitudinal results from the Rotterdam study supported these cross-sectional findings: the association between near wall CIMT and stroke or myocardial infarction was as strong as that found for far wall CIMT [34] (Figure 5). The combined near and far wall intima-media thickness led to the strongest association. Findings in three randomised placebo controlled intervention studies among subjects receiving placebo treatment indicated that the progression rate of near wall common CIMT was similar to that for the far wall common CIMT [37]. Combining information of both near and far wall yielded estimates of progression rates with higher precision, i.e., smaller standard errors. The consequence is that the number of patients that is needed in an intervention study to demonstrate a treatment effect is smaller when CIMT is based on the average of near and far wall measurements compared with far wall measurements only. Thus, measurement of the near wall intima-media thickness yields valuable information, and should not be discarded easily.

However, one should realise that, in particular for the near wall measurement standardisation of gain settings and B-mode ultrasound technique across various sonographers is of utmost importance. In general, this is easier in single centre studies than in multicenter studies. Also, near wall measurements are more difficult to obtain compared to far wall measurements. For example, in the Rotterdam study near wall intima-media thickness measurements of at least one or both sides of the common carotid artery could not be obtained from the images in 8.9% of the subjects. For far wall measurements, data on either left, right or both sides were missing in 3.1% of the study population [36]. However, in analyses indicators of presence or absence of near wall measurements may add to the regression model, or a near wall estimate may be used based on the measurement of the side that is available, or a model may be used to impute missing values.

Should we use common CIMT measurements only?

A very frequent question that is put forward is whether one should limit the study to common CIMT measurements only or also should include measurements of the carotid bifurcation and internal carotid artery. The main approach to this question is to evaluate the balance between evidence showing differences in strength of associations of common CIMT and internal CIMT to cardiovascular disease and the practicalities involved, being time consumption, missing data, and reproducibility [2,20,23,33].

Several studies have indicated that combining the information from several sites of the carotid artery results in an estimate for carotid atherosclerosis with enhanced precision. Consequently, due to the increased precision of the measurement, the magnitude of the association under study should increase. The differences were however not statistically significant. Differences in quantifying presence and extent of carotid atherosclerosis across studies should be appreciated. At present, however, it cannot be answered satisfactorily, which approach provides the 'best' indicator of atherosclerosis for cross-sectional studies, for assessment of change over time, and for studies on determinants of progression of intima-media thickness.

Conclusion

An increased CIMT is associated with unfavourable levels of established cardiovascular risk factors, with prevalent cardiovascular disease and with atherosclerosis elsewhere in the arterial system. The available data indicate that the risk of coronary heart disease and stroke gradually increases with increasing CIMT. This predictive power of CIMT measurements remains after adjustment for cardiovascular risk factors. These findings support the view that CIMT measurements can be used as an endpoint as a suitable alternative for cardiovascular morbidity and mortality in observational and intervention studies. In particular in trials evaluating the efficacy of a treatment the use of CIMT measurements will result in a considerable smaller number of subjects needed than when using disease or death as an endpoint. Strict ultrasound protocols, training and monitoring of sonographer and reader performance are mandatory.

Whether CIMT measurements should be performed in all patients at high risk of future cardiovascular and cerebrovascular diseases in order to help in risk profiling of an individual patient needs to be studied.

References

1. Heiss G, Sharett AR, Barnes R, Chambless LE, Szklo M, Alzola C. Carotid atherosclerosis measured by B-mode ultrasound in populations: associations with cardiovascular risk factors in the ARIC study. Am J Epidemiol 1991;134:250-6.
2. O'Leary DH, Polak JF, Wolfson SK Jr *et al.* Use of sonography to evaluate carotid atherosclerosis in the elderly. The Cardiovascular Health Study. CHS Collaborative Research Group. Stroke 1991;22:1155-63.
3. Auperin A, Berr C, Bonithon-Kopp C *et al.* Ultrasonographic assessment of carotid wall characteristics and cognitive functions in a community sample of 59- to 71-year-olds. The EVA Study Group. Stroke 1996;27:1290-5.

4.   Bots ML, Hofman A, De Jong PT, Grobbee DE. Common carotid intima-media thickness as an indicator of atherosclerosis at other sites of the carotid artery. The Rotterdam Study. Ann Epidemiol 1996;6:147-53.

5.   Stensland-Bugge E, Bonaa KH, Joakimsen O. Reproducibility of ultrasonographically determined intima-media thickness is dependent on arterial wall thickness. The Tromso Study. Stroke 1997;28:1972-80.

6.   Mykkanen L, Zaccaro DJ, O'Leary DH, Howard G, Robbins DC, Haffner SM. Microalbuminuria and carotid artery intima-media thickness in nondiabetic and NIDDM subjects. The Insulin Resistance Atherosclerosis Study (IRAS). Stroke 1997;28:1710-6.

7.   Salonen R, Salonen JT. Carotid atherosclerosis in relation to systolic and diastolic blood pressure: Kuopio Ischaemic Heart Disease Risk Factor Study. Ann Med 1991;23:23-7.

8.   Allan PL, Mowbray PI, Lee AJ, Fowkes FG. Relationship between carotid intima-media thickness and symptomatic and asymptomatic peripheral arterial disease. The Edinburgh Artery Study. Stroke 1997;28:348-53.

9.   Grobbee DE, Bots ML. Carotid artery intima-media thickness as an indicator of generalized atherosclerosis. J Intern Med 1994;236:567-73.

10. Wendelhag I, Gustavsson T, Suurküla M, Berglund G, Wikstrand J. Ultrasound measurement of wall thickness in the carotid artery: fundamental principles, and description of a computerized analysing system. Clin Physiol 1991;11:565-77.

11. Wendelhag I, Liang Q, Gustavsson T, Wikstrand J. A new automated computerized analyzing system simplifies readings and reduces the variability in ultrasound measurement of intima-media thickness. Stroke 1997;28:2195-200.

12. Selzer RH, Hodis HN, Kwong-Fu H *et al.* Evaluation of computerized edge tracking for quantifying intima-media thickness of the common carotid artery from B-mode ultrasound images. Atherosclerosis 1994;111:1-11.

13. Li R, Cai J, Tegeler C, Sorlie P, Metcalf PA, Heiss G. Reproducibility of extracranial carotid atherosclerotic lesions assessed by B-mode ultrasound: the Atherosclerotic Risk in Communities Study. Ultrasound Med Biol 1996;22:791-9.

14. Wong M, Edelstein J, Wollman J, Bond MG. Ultrasonic-pathological comparison of the human arterial wall. Verification of intima-media thickness. Arterioscler Thromb 1993;13:482-6.

15. Gamble G, Beaumont B, Smith H *et al.* B-mode ultrasound images of the carotid artery wall: correlation of ultrasound with histological measurements. Atherosclerosis 1993;102:163-73.

16   Bots ML, Mulder PG, Hofman A, van Es GA, Grobbee DE. Reproducibility of carotid vessel wall thickness measurements. The Rotterdam Study. J Clin Epidemiol 1994;47:921-30.

17. Kanters SD, Algra A, van Leeuwen MS, Banga JD. Reproducibility of in vivo carotid intima-media thickness measurements: a review. Stroke 1997;28:665-71.

18. Howard G, Sharrett AR, Heiss G *et al.* Carotid artery intimal-medial thickness distribution in general populations as evaluated by B-mode ultrasound. ARIC Investigators. Stroke 1993;24:1297-304.

19. Howard G, Burke GL, Evans GW *et al.* Relations of intimal-medial thickness among sites within the carotid artery as evaluated by B-mode ultrasound. ARIC investigators. Atherosclerosis Risk in Communities. Stroke 1994;25:1581-7.

20. O'Leary DH, Polak JF, Kronmal RA *et al.* Thickening of the carotid wall. A marker for atherosclerosis in the elderly? Cardiovascular Health Study Collaborative Research Group. Stroke 1996;27:224-31.

21. Bots ML, Witteman JC, Hofman A, De Jong PT, Grobbee DE. Low diastolic blood pressure and atherosclerosis in elderly subjects. The Rotterdam study. Arch Intern Med 1996;156:843-8.

22. Bots ML, Hofman A, Grobbee DE. Increased common carotid intima-media thickness. Adaptive response or a reflection of atherosclerosis? Findings from the Rotterdam Study. Stroke 1997;28:2442-7.

23. Burke GL, Evans GW, Riley WA *et al.* Arterial wall thickness is associated with prevalent cardiovascular disease in middle-aged adults. The Atherosclerosis Risk in Communities (ARIC) Study. Stroke 1995;26:386-91.

24. Bots ML, Hofman A, Grobbee DE. Common carotid intima-media thickness and cardiovascular disease in the Rotterdam Study. A cross-sectional analysis. In: Koenig W, Hombach V, Bond MG, Kramsch DM, editors. Progression and regression of atherosclerosis. Vienna: Blackwell Scientific Publishers; 1995. p. 118-23.

25. Salonen R, Tervahauta M, Salonen JT, Pekkanen J, Nissinen A, Karvonen MJ. Ultrasonographic manifestations of common carotid atherosclerosis in elderly eastern Finnish men. Prevalence and associations with cardiovascular diseases and risk factors. Arterioscler Thromb 1994;14:1631-40.

26. Polak JF, O'Leary DH, Kronmal RA *et al.* Sonographic evaluation of the carotid artery atherosclerosis in the elderly: relationship of disease severity to stroke and transient ischemic attack. Radiology 1993;188:363-70.

27. Cuspidi C, Lonati L, Sampieri L *et al*. Left ventricular concentric remodelling and carotid structural changes in essential hypertension. J Hypertens 1996;14:1441-6.

28. Linhart A, Gariepy J, Giral P, Levenson J, Simon A. Carotid artery and left ventricular structural relationship in asymptomatic men at risk for cardiovascular disease. Atherosclerosis 1996;127:103-12.

29. Roman MJ, Saba PS, Pini R *et al*. Parallel cardiac and vascular adaptation in hypertension. Circulation 1992;86:1909-18.

30. Bots ML, Witteman JC, Grobbee DE. Carotid intima-media wall thickness in elderly women with and without atherosclerosis of the abdominal aorta. Atherosclerosis 1993;102:99-105.

31. Bots ML, Hofman A, Grobbee DE. Common carotid intima-media thickness and lower extremity arterial atherosclerosis. The Rotterdam Study. Arterioscler Thromb 1994;14:1885-91.

32. Salonen JT, Salonen R. Ultrasonographically assessed carotid morphology and the risk of coronary heart disease. Arterioscler Thromb 1991;11:1245-9.

33. Chambless LE, Heiss G, Folsom AR *et al*. Association of coronary heart disease incidence with carotid arterial wall thickness and major risk factors: the Atherosclerosis Risk in Communities (ARIC) Study, 1987-1993. Am J Epidemiol 1997;146:483-94.

34. Bots ML, Hoes AW, Koudstaal PJ, Hofman A, Grobbee DE. Common carotid intima-media thickness and risk of stroke and myocardial infarction: the Rotterdam Study. Circulation 1997;96:1432-7.

35. Wikstrand J, Wiklund O. Frontiers in cardiovascular science. Quantitative measurements of atherosclerotic manifestations in humans. Arterioscler Thromb 1992;12:114-9.

36. Bots ML, De Jong PT, Hofman A, Grobbee DE. Left, right, near or far wall common carotid intima-media thickness measurements: associations with cardiovascular disease and lower extremity arterial atherosclerosis. J Clin Epidemiol 1997;50:801-7.

37. Furberg CD, Byington RP, Craven TE. Lessons learned from clinical trials with ultrasound end points. J Intern Med 1994;236:575-80.

31.   What is the current role of electron beam computed tomography in coronary imaging?

John A. Rumberger, Axel Schmermund & Raimund Erbel

Summary

Electron beam computed tomography (EBCT) has emerged as a powerful means to examine and quantitate cardiovascular anatomy, function, and flow in patients presenting with a variety of diseases of the heart, coronary arteries, pericardium and great vessels. This brief discussion is focused on the developing use of EBCT to image the coronary arteries. There are currently two main areas of interest, i.e., the quantification of coronary calcium by EBCT and the use of peripheral contrast injections for coronary luminal opacification (intravenous EBCT coronary angiography). The amount of coronary calcium as determined by EBCT has been shown to be representative of coronary atherosclerotic plaque burden and thus offers a non-invasive approach to the delineation of coronary artery disease. In several thousands patients followed over one through 5 years, quantities of coronary calcium have been demonstrated to predict cardiovascular events and related mortality. Individuals with large amounts of coronary calcium have a high likelihood of at least one obstructive coronary lesion, require strict measures regarding modifiable risk factors, and may additionally be considered for further evaluations of potential myocardial ischemia. Intravenous EBCT coronary angiography has been performed by several independent groups of investigators and has yielded highly reproducible results. The proximal segments of the major coronary arteries are reliably visualized. High negative predictive values suggest that this technique may be of value for ruling out significant disease in patients undergoing clinical evaluation for obstructive versus non-obstructive coronary artery disease. As is true for any cardiac imaging modality, EBCT should be analyzed in the context of the patient's history and symptoms.

Introduction

In the past 50 years since the introduction of diagnostic coronary artery imaging into clinical practice there have been dramatic changes in the way we view the heart. Selective coronary arteriography and intravascular ultrasound are now commonplace and have provided diagnostic and prognostic information of significant benefit to the clinician. However, these techniques are invasive and carry a small but real potential for mortality and morbidity. Additionally, they are expensive, and require at least a brief admission to the hospital as well as the attendance of a team of physicians, nurses, and technologists. X-ray computed tomo-

J.H.C. Reiber and E.E. van der Wall (eds.). What's New in Cardiovascular Imaging, 401–410.
©*1998 Kluwer Academic Publishers.*

graphy (CT) of the chest was introduced in the early 1970's with imaging times as long as 30 minutes and image reconstruction times of comparable length. Today, imaging can be done using a scanning electron beam (EBCT) with rapid acquisition and reconstruction, to facilitate detailed studies of the heart and coronary arteries. Currently applications for EBCT are going beyond studies of cardiac chamber size, and myocardial function and perfusion, to a rapidly developing area of non-invasive coronary artery imaging. In the paragraphs to follow we briefly discuss the application of EBCT for direct imaging of the coronary artery mural and luminal surfaces.

Electron beam computed tomography

Electron beam computed tomography (EBCT) has emerged as a powerful means to examine and quantitate cardiovascular anatomy, function, and flow in patients presenting with a variety of diseases of the heart, coronary arteries, pericardium and great vessels. Details on the use of EBCT for quantification of left and right ventricular volumes and function [1-3], muscle mass [4,5], myocardial perfusion [6], diastolic function [7], and post-infarction remodeling [8,9] can be found elsewhere [10]. However, the purpose of this brief discussion is to focus on the developing use of EBCT to image the coronary arteries.

Coronary artery calcification

EBCT, unlike conventional and spiral body CT scanners, employs a stationary source/detector combination along with a rotating electron beam to produce serial, contiguous, thin section, 100 msec scans in synchrony with the heart cycle. Scanning of the entire heart can be completed in 1 or 2 short breatholds. Standardized methods for imaging, identification and quantification of coronary artery calcium using EBCT have been established [11]. Figure 1 shows representative EBCT tomograms at the base of the heart from two patients. Figure 1, upper panel, shows no calcification in the proximal and mid left anterior descending (Figure 1a) and in the proximal right coronary artery (Figure 1b) and is a negative scan. Figure 1, lower panel, demonstrates extensive "ossification" of mural arterial segments in the left anterior descending and left circumflex coronary arteries (Figures 1c,1d) and in the proximal right coronary artery (Figure 1e). The "calcium score" is a product of the area of calcification per coronary segment and a factor rated 1 through 4 dictated by the maximum calcium CT density within that segment [12]. A calcium score can be calculated for a given coronary segment, a specific coronary artery, or for the entire coronary system; however, most studies have reported data related to the summed or total "score" for the entire epicardial coronary system. The total calcium scores for the study shown on Figure 1, upper panel, was zero, and for Figure 1, lower panel, was >1000.

Coronary artery calcium is observed in variable degrees of atherosclerotic involvement, can denote an active process of plaque development, and is regulated in a manner similar to bone formation [11]. Its role in disease remains unclear, but may function to stabilize the plaque in response to the inflammatory cascade of developing coronary disease. Although quantification of segmental and total coronary calcium by EBCT affords only a measure of "calcified plaque", direct relationships have been established between coronary calcium as

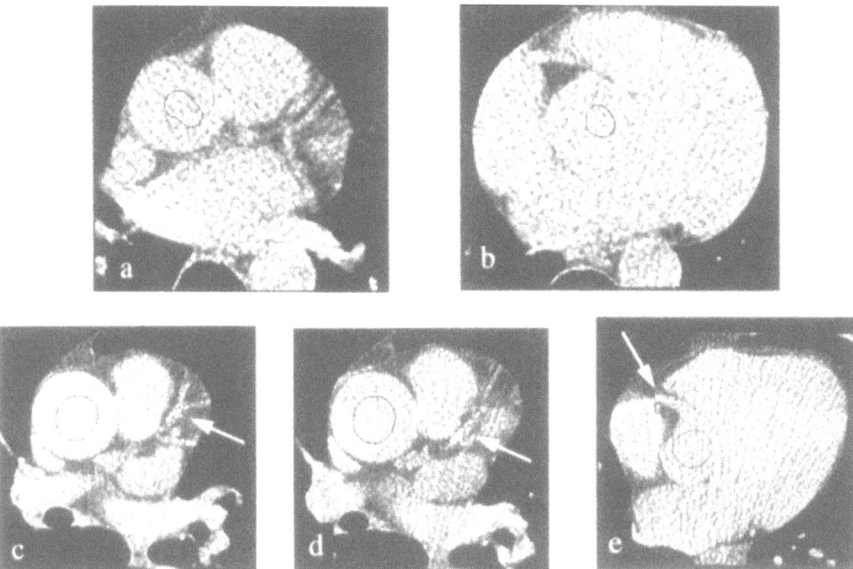

Figure 1. Representative electron-beam computed tomographic sections for quantification of coronary artery calcium. The upper panel shows sections from a patient with a total calcium score of 0. There are no dense lesions in the proximal and mid left anterior descending coronary artery (Figure 1a) or the proximal right coronary artery (Figure 1b). The lower panel shows sections from a patient with a total calcium score > 1000. The arrows point to extensive "ossification" of mural arterial segments in the left anterior descending and left circumflex coronary arteries (Figures 1c,1d) and in the proximal right coronary artery (Figure 1e).

measured by EBCT and histologic [13,14], ultrasonic [15], and angiographic [16-18] measures of coronary disease on a heart-by-heart, vessel-by-vessel, and segment-by-segment basis. Additionally, there is increasing evidence that the composite epicardial coronary artery "calcium score" has prognostic value in both symptomatic and asymptomatic patients [19-21].

There are two major areas where EBCT scanning for coronary calcification are likely to prove of significant clinical value [11,22]. A number of studies have confirmed that the vast majority of patients with fixed significant coronary stenoses [16-18] or those presenting with acute coronary syndromes due to significant stenoses [23] have identifiable calcium by EBCT. Subsequently the absence of calcification by EBCT (i.e. calcium score of zero) has been shown to have negative predictive values between 90% to 100% for a ≥50% fixed luminal coronary diameter stenosis. Clinical EBCT scanning can be done at a cost of less than one-half that of a stress echocardiogram, less than one third of a stress thallium examination, and at a fraction of the cost for diagnostic coronary arteriography [22]. A practical application of EBCT scanning could be realized in the patient with no prior coronary disease who presents to the emergency department with chest pain or a questionable ischemic syndrome, but a negative or non-diagnostic ECG and negative cardiac enzymes. Especially in a patient with a low to intermediate likelihood of significant fixed coronary disease, a negative EBCT could facilitate early dismissal from the emergency department or chest pain unit. This could also apply to ambulatory patients with "atypical" cardiac symptoms in whom the pretest likelihood for ischemic disease is considered by the clinician to be low (based upon age, gender, or absence of cardiovascular risk factors). Individuals with a zero calcium score could be reassured and further testing directed at non-cardiac sources of chest pain. Conversely, if the calcium score is consistent with moderate or severe atherosclerotic plaque development, then additional cardiac evaluation may be appropriate. But, issues specifically addressing whether the very high negative predictive value for EBCT offers economic and/or clinical advantages over other more conventional means to non-invasively diagnose fixed coronary disease have not been resolved.

Application of EBCT to define atherosclerotic plaque burden in asymptomatic individuals at risk for coronary disease, on the other hand, has received a fair amount of discussion [11,20-22,24] and is one of the areas of intense research. Arad and colleagues [20] followed 1173 initially asymptomatic patients (average age 53 ± 11 years) who had no known coronary disease for a mean of 19 months after a screening EBCT coronary calcium scan. Eighteen subjects had 26 cardiovascular events: 1 death, 7 non fatal myocardial infarctions, 8 coronary bypass grafting procedures, 9 coronary angioplasties, and 1 nonhemorrhagic stroke. The magnitude of the coronary calcium score at the time of the index EBCT scan was highly predictive of subsequently developing symptomatic cardiovascular disease during follow up. Odds ratios ranged from 20:1 for a calcium score of 100 to 35:1 for a calcium score of 160. These data along with the complimentary studies by Detrano [19] in symptomatic, middle aged adults, and Secci [21] in asymptomatic, elderly adults emphasize that the calcium score, as a surrogate to the total atherosclerotic plaque burden, can confer differential prognostic information.

Currently guidelines for use of EBCT as a screening test for coronary disease are under development but broad generalizations of these opinions can be offered. The absence of identifiable coronary calcium is consistent with no or at most minimal atherosclerotic plaque burden. Individuals in this group are likely to fall into a favorable prognostic group [11,22]. On the other hand, studies from our laboratory have shown that calcium scores exceeding 80-100 are highly consistent with at least non-obstructive coronary disease [22,25]. It is important to underscore that the presence of moderate, although non-obstructive coronary disease can engender an adverse long term prognosis. In a study of 521 patients undergoing initial diagnostic coronary angiography, Proudfit and colleagues [26] found the incidence of any cardiac events (death, arteriographic progression to obstruction, myocardial infarction) over the next 10 years was 2.1% in those with normal angiograms, increasing to 13.8% with a <30% stenosis, and was 33% in those with 30% to 50% maximal stenoses. Thus, the presence of moderate calcium scores in an otherwise asymptomatic individual suggests that further evaluations, including careful identification and aggressive treatment of modifiable risk factors, may be prudent. Individuals with significant coronary calcium (calcium score > 400-500) have a high likelihood of at least one obstructive coronary lesion [25], have advanced and substantial plaque disease, require strict measures regarding modifiable risk factors, and additionally should probably be considered for further evaluations directed to determining the potential for ischemia.

Intravenous coronary arteriography

X-ray CT, like MRI, acquires digital format data in parallel tomographic images thus lending itself to three-dimensional data analysis, data processing and display for quantification of cardiac and peri-cardiac anatomy. Moshage and colleagues [27] studied 27 patients with

EBCT who also underwent conventional coronary arteriography. Contiguous 3 mm thick EBCT scans were acquired during a single breath-hold, commencing at the root of the aorta with 2 mm table overlap during intravenous injections of non-ionic contrast medium (120-160 ml). In this preliminary study, 9 out of 11 (82%) of high grade stenoses and 5 out of 5 (100%) of occlusions in the proximal left anterior descending coronary artery as identified by selective arteriography were found on review of the EBCT scans by blinded observers. Five patients who underwent selective angioplasty after arteriography underwent repeat scanning with EBCT. In each case, the improvements in the arterial lumen dimensions were definable in the EBCT images. In addition, 3 of 5 (60%) of high grade stenoses were also visualized in the right coronary artery. However, recognition of stenoses of the left circumflex was more difficult, likely due to motion artifact or difficulty in segmentation of the left atrium and appendage from the vessels course in the atrio-ventricular groove. The same group from Erlangen, Germany, has expanded their initial studies of EBCT coronary angiography to greater than 100 patients undergoing selective coronary arteriography [28]. Although only 74% of all coronary segments were seen using EBCT, overall sensitivity and specificity were good (90% and 95%, respectively). In particular the left main and proximal and mid portions of the left anterior descending artery are generally quite well seen, but sections of the mid to distal right coronary artery and all but the most proximal sections of the left circumflex artery (compromised by overlying structures such as the coronary sinus and left atrial appendage) remain often problematic. Importantly, however, the negative predictive value for significant disease was quite high at 97%, suggesting that this may provide for an adequate screen for individuals in which a negative EBCT would obviate the need for invasive angiography.

Nakanishi and colleagues [29] from Japan have examined EBCT coronary angiograms using a multi-planar format in 37 patients. They were able to identify 89% of all coronary segments by EBCT, but reported both a lower sensitivity (74%) and specificity (91%) than the Erlangen group. Achenbach and Moshage [30] have recently expanded their studies to EBCT angiography of coronary bypass grafts. These vessels, which are often twice or more the size of native coronary arteries are quite well seen using EBCT angiography, and thus in vessels imaged, sensitivity and specificity for significant disease or graft occlusion was found to approach 100%.

Our laboratory has begun to examine this novel application of EBCT [31]. The availability of several commercial three-dimensional workstations specifically designed for studies using EBCT have greatly facilitated the analysis. Three dimensional data can be presented in a variety of formats which include the shaded surface display, the curved surface or multi-reformatted tomographic projection, and maximum intensity projections (which resemble conventional angiographic projections). Figure 2 shows an example of a three-dimensional EBCT shaded surface rendering of normal cardiac and coronary anatomy (Figure 2a) and the corresponding curved surface display views of the proximal and mid portions of the major coronary arteries (Figure 2b).

Figure 3 shows a three-dimensional EBCT rendering (left panel) as compared with selective coronary angiography (right panel) in a patient with a 60% stenosis of the left anterior descending coronary artery. In Figure 4, an EBCT shaded surface display of the major coronary arteries is shown (left panel) as compared with selective coronary angiography (right panel) in a patient with an intermediate severity tandem stenosis of the left anterior descending artery. Simultaneous opacification of both arteries and veins using intravenous contrast

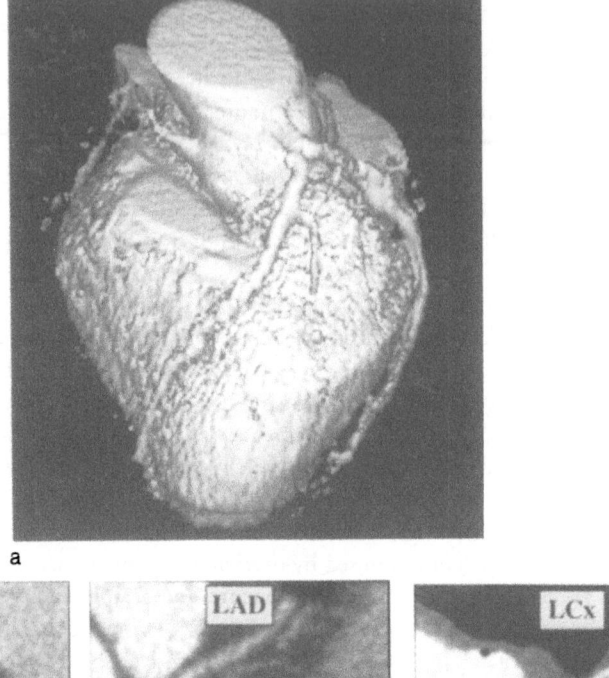

Figure 2. a) Three-dimensional electron-beam CT shaded surface rendering of normal cardiac and coronary anatomy. b) Corresponding curved surface display views of the proximal and mid portions of the major coronary arteries.

administration challenges interpretation, but although additional work is required to facilitate clinical entry of this application, the studies are easily feasible in the average, stable patient during a single breath hold, and the learning curve for interpretation is steep.

Conclusions

EBCT is a robust technology which can be used to image the heart regarding details of function, flow, and anatomy. In this Chapter, we have focused on its expanding applications to noninvasively image calcified plaque in the mural surfaces of the coronary arteries, as well as visualize (with the aid of iodinated contrast media) the luminal surface of the proximal coronary arteries and coronary bypass grafts. One of the major factors relating to EBCT is that

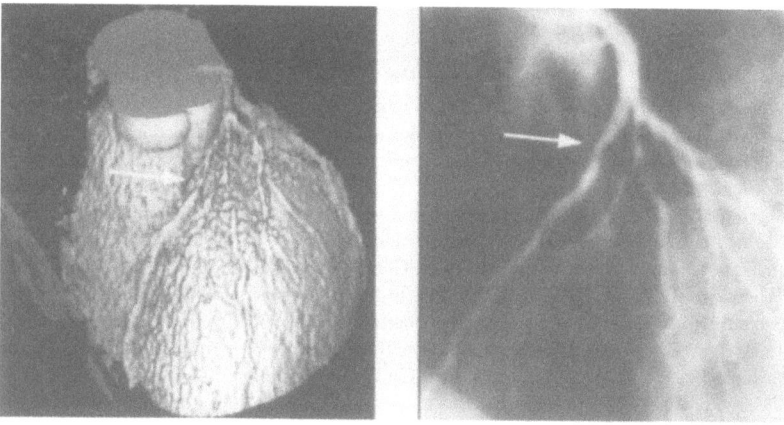

Figure 3. Three-dimensional electron-beam CT shaded surface rendering (left panel) as compared with selective coronary angiography (rigth panel) in a patient with a 60% stenosis of the left anterior descending coronary artery (arrows).

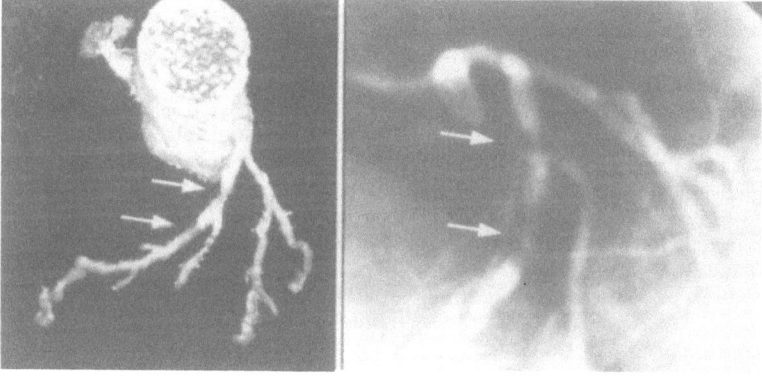

Figure 4. Electron-beam CT shaded surface display of the major coronary arteries (left panel) as compared with selective coronary angiography (right panel) in a patient with an intermediate severity tandem stenosis of the left anterior descending artery (arrows).

studies of coronary artery calcification and coronary arteriography have been reproducible and confirmatory in laboratories in which the technology is available. Commercially available workstations are now able to analyze data from both types of coronary artery scanning in minutes of completion of the examination. As the availability of EBCT expands, its utilization as a means to diagnose sub-clinical disease (coronary artery calcification) and/or as an adjunct to conventional coronary arteriography is likely to become a major influence in the care of patients with suspected or known coronary heart disease.

References

1. Reiter SJ, Rumberger JA, Feiring AJ, Stanford W, Marcus ML. Precision of measurements of right and left ventricular stroke volume by cine computed tomography. Circulation 1986;74:890-900.
2. Lanzer P, Garrett J, Lipton MJ et al. Quantitation of regional myocardial function by cine computed tomography: pharmacologic changes in wall thickness. J Am Coll Cardiol 1986;8:682-92.
3. Feiring AJ, Rumberger JA, Reiter SJ et al. Sectional and segmental variability of left ventricular function: experimental and clinical studies using ultrafast computed tomography. J Am Coll Cardiol 1988;12:415-25.
4. Feiring AJ, Rumberger JA, Reiter SJ et al. Determination of left ventricular mass in dogs with rapid-acquisition cardiac computed tomographic scanning. Circulation 1985;72:1355-64.
5. Hajduczok ZD, Weiss RM, Stanford W, Marcus ML. Determination of right ventricular mass in humans and dogs with ultrafast cardiac computed tomography. Circulation 1990;82:202-12.
6. Rumberger JA, Bell MR. Measurement of myocardial perfusion using electron- beam (ultrafast) computed tomography. In: Skorton DJ, editor. Marcus Cardiac imaging. (2nd Ed). Philadelphia: Saunders; 1996. p. 835-52.
7. Rumberger JA, Weiss RM, Feiring AJ et al. Patterns of regional diastolic function in the normal human left ventricle: an ultrafast computed tomographic study. J Am Coll Cardiol 1989;14:119-26.
8. Rumberger JA, Behrenbeck T, Breen JR, Reed JE, Gersh BJ. Nonparallel changes in global chamber volume and muscle mass during the first year after transmural myocardial infarction in humans. J Am Coll Cardiol 1993;21:673-82.
9. Sehgal M, Hirose K, Reed JE, Rumberger JA. Regional left ventricular wall thickness and systolic function during the first year after index wall myocardial infarction: serial effects of ventricular remodeling. Int J Cardiol 1996;53:45-54.
10. Rumberger JA, Sheedy PF, Breen JF. Use of ultrafast (cine) x-ray computed tomography in cardiac and cardiovascular imaging. In: Giuliani ER, Gersh BJ, Mc Goon MD, Hayes DL, Schaff HF. Mayo Clinic practice of cardiology. 3rd ed. St. Louis: Mosby-Year Book; 1996. p. 303-24.
11. Wexler L, Brundage B, Crouse J et al. Coronary artery calcification: pathophysiology, epidemiology, imaging methods, and clinical implications. A statement for health professionals from the American Heart Association. Writing Group. Circulation 1996;94:1175-92.
12. Agatston AS, Janowitz WR, Hildner FJ, Zusmer MR, Viamonte M Jr, Detrano R. Quantification of coronary artery calcium using ultrafast computed tomography. J Am Coll Cardiol 1990;15:827-32.
13. Mautner SL, Mautner GC, Froehlich J et al. Coronary artery disease: prediction with in vitro electron beam CT. Radiology 1994;192:625-30.
14. Rumberger JA, Simons DB, Fitzpatrick LA, Sheedy PF, Schwartz RS. Coronary artery calcium area by electron-beam computed tomography and coronary atherosclerotic plaque area. A histopathologic correlative study. Circulation 1995;92:2157-62.
15. Baumgart D, Schmermund A, Görge G et al. Comparison of electron beam computed tomography with intracoronary ultrasound and coronary angiography for detection of coronary atherosclerosis. J Am Coll Cardiol 1997;30:57-64.
16. Rumberger JA, Sheedy PF 3rd, Breen JR, Schwartz RS. Coronary calcium as determined by electron beam computed tomography, and coronary disease on arteriogram. Effect of patient's sex on diagnosis. Circulation 1995;91:1363-7.
17. Budhoff MJ, Georgiou D, Brody A et al. Ultrafast computed tomography as a diagnostic modality in the detection of coronary artery disease: a multicenter study. Circulation 1996;93:898-904.
18. Kajinami K, Seki H, Takekoshi N, Mabuchi H. Coronary calcification and coronary atherosclerosis: site by site comparative morphologic study of electron beam computed tomography and coronary angiography. J Am Coll Cardiol 1997;29:1549-56.
19. Detrano R, Hsiai T, Wang·S et al. Prognostic value of coronary calcification and angiographic stenoses in patients undergoing coronary angiography. J Am Coll Cardiol 1996;27:285-90.
20. Arad Y, Spadaro LA, Goodman K et al. Predictive value of electron beam computed tomography of the coronary arteries. 19-month follow-up of 1173 asymptomatic subjects. Circulation 1996;93:1951-3.
21. Secci A, Wong N, Tang W, Wang S, Doherty T, Detrano R. Electron beam computed tomographic coronary calcium as a predictor of coronary events: comparison of two protocols. Circulation 1997;96:1122-9.
22. Rumberger JA, Sheedy PF 2nd, Breen JF, Fitzpatrick LA, Schwartz RS. Electron beam computed tomography and coronary artery disease: scanning for coronary artery calcification. Mayo Clin Proc 1996;71:369-77.

23. Schmermund A, Baumgart D, Görge G *et al.* Coronary artery calcium in acute coronary syndromes: a comparative study of electron beam computed tomography, coronary angiography, and intracoronary ultrasound in survivors of acute myocardial infarction and unstable angina. Circulation 1997;96:1461-9.

24. Hoeg JM. Evaluating coronary heart disease risk. Tiles in the mosaic [published erratum appears in JAMA 1997;278:636]. JAMA 1997;277:1387-90.

25. Rumberger JA, Sheedy PF, Breen JF, Schwartz RS. Electron beam computed tomographic coronary calcium score cutpoints and severity of associated angiography lumen stenosis. J Am Coll Cardiol 1997;29:1542-8.

26. Proudfit WL, Bruschke VG, Sones FM Jr. Clinical course of patients with normal or slightly or moderately abnormal coronary arteriograms: 10-year follow-up of 521 patients. Circulation 1980;62:712-7.

27. Moshage WEL, Achenbach S, Seese B, Bachmann K, Kirchgeorg M. Coronary artery stenoses: three-dimensional imaging with electrocardiographically triggered, contrast agent-enhanced, electron-beam CT. Radiology 1995;196:707-14.

28. Achenbach S, Moshage W, Nossen J *et al.* Nichtinvasive Koronararterien- darstellung mittels Elektronenstrahltomographie - Vergleich zur Koronar-angiographie bei 100 Patienten [abstract]. Z Kardiol 1997;86:205.

29. Nakanishi T, Ito K, Imazu M, Yamakido M. Evaluation of coronary artery stenoses using electron-beam CT and multiplanar reformation. J Comput Assist Tomogr 1997;21:121-7.

30. Achenbach S, Moshage W, Ropers D, Nossen J, Bachmann K. Noninvasive, three- dimensional visualization of coronary artery bypass grafts by electron beam tomography. Am J Cardiol 1997;79:856-61.

31. Schmermund A, Rensing BJ, Sheedy PF 2nd, Bell MR, Rumberger JA. Intravenous electron-beam CT based angiography: segmental analysis of significant disease in the major coronary arteries [abstract]. Circulation 1997;96(Suppl1):I306.

32. Magnetic resonance and electron beam tomography coronary angiography

Pim J. de Feyter, Robert-Jan van Geuns, Peter van Ooijen, Fons Bongaerts,
Benno Rensing, Hein de Bruin, Pjotr Wielopolski & Matthijs Oudkerk

Summary

Recently, two non-invasive techniques Magnetic Resonance (MR) and Electron Beam Tomography (EBT) have been developed that are able to visualize the proximal and mid segments of the coronary arteries.

We studied 18 patients who underwent MR-EBT and diagnostic conventional coronary angiography. The proximal and mid segments of the coronary tree could be visualized with MR-CA in the majority of the patients and significant coronary stenoses were detected with a sensitivity and specificity of 69% and 92%, respectively.

Visualization of the proximal and mid segments of the coronary tree with EBT-CA is possible in the majority of the patients. The diagnostic accuracy to detect significant coronary stenoses is moderate with a sensitivity and specificity of 62% and 93%, respectively.

Conclusion: MR- and EBT-coronary angiography are diagnostic tools in progress, both with the potential to improve to a valuable clinical diagnostic technique.

Introduction

Imaging of the coronary arteries is the ultimate challenge for any noninvasive technique used to visualize arteries. The coronary arteries are small, 3 - 4 mm in diameter, tortuous, and run in a complex course so that they are difficult to catch in one plane, and extremely difficult to handle are the motion artifacts, caused by cardiac contraction and respiration. Ultrafast acquisition techniques, within 100 ms or preferably even less, obtained during diastole and

Table 1: Characteristics of MR- and EBT-coronary imaging

Signal	MR-CA	EBT-CA
Signal formation	Emission of radiofrequency	Transmission of X-rays
Signal intensity	Tissue T_1, T_2 relaxation	Attenuation of X-rays
	proton density	by tissue absorption
	blood flow characteristics	
Imaging	Any plane	Axial plane

J.H.C. Reiber and E.E. van der Wall (eds.). What's New in Cardiovascular Imaging, 411–418.
©*1998 Kluwer Academic Publishers.*

breathholding or using a respiratory gating technique are necessary to overcome these motion artifacts.

Technical innovations and the development of ultra-fast computers have made it possible to construct two basically different techniques that are able to visualize, noninvasively the coronary artery: magnetic resonance imaging (MRI) and electron beam tomography (EBT) (Table 1). Both imaging techniques have shown promising preliminary results, but still much improvement is necessary to make these techniques suitable for general clinical use. The strengths and limitations of both techniques will be discussed in the next paragraphs.

Magnetic resonance coronary angiography (MR-CA)

In conventional imaging, each radiofrequency (RF) excitation is accompanied by one-phase encoding and one frequency encoding thus acquiring one-line of raw data per excitation [1].

Per heart-beat one radiofrequency excitation is obtained at a fixed time window in diastole (100-150 ms) using R-wave ECG-triggering to reduce image distortion due to cardiac motion.

Hence, if we wish to acquire a full 256 x 256 pixel image from the same slice position through the heart this would require 256 heart beats. With a heart frequency of 72 beats per minute this would require approximately 3.6 minutes. However, uncontrolled patient motion and cardiac or respiratory motion occurring during this relative long period prevented reliable coronary imaging.

More rapid image acquisition is essential for application in coronary imaging. In the early nineties ultra-fast MR techniques became available which allowed more reliable visualization of the coronary arteries [2-6].

These rapid techniques, called turbo-Flash, differ from the conventional technique in that more than one RF-excitation and phase encoding is obtained per heart beat, so that an image is produced very rapidly. They make use of the gradient recalled echo (GRE) technique. Repetition times of RF excitations of 7-10 ms or even less can be achieved with modern high-performance MR-scanners. However, an image with a pixel matrix of 128 x 256 would require an acquisition time of around 1000 ms, so that even using these ultrafast techniques cardiac and respiratory motion still hamper image quality.

Other approaches are used to deal with these motion artefacts. To suppress cardiac motion data are collected in a relative cardiac motion free period of 100-150 ms during mid-diastole (using ECG triggering). Within this 100-150 ms motion free period one may be able to collect a set of up to 10 phase-encodings per heart beat. However, to acquire a clinical useful image one usually needs an image array of 128 x 128/256. Hence, more phase-encoding sets, from successive heart beats are needed. Using this technique of segmentation the phase encoding sets of several heart beats are used to produce one slice image. If for instance we would want to produce an image array of 128 x 128/256, and one acquires 8 phase encodings per segment one would require 16 successive heart beats. At a heart frequency of 60 beats/min, this would result in an imaging period of 16 s.

To reduce respiration artifacts one usually uses a breath-hold technique. In general, it appears to be well within the possibilities of patients to withhold their breath for a period of 20 seconds.

Reasonably reliable visualization of the coronary arteries and coronary stenoses has been achieved with this segmented, 2-dimensional Turboflash, one breathhold technique (Table 2) [2,6-8].

Table 2: Outcome of 2-D MR-coronary angiography

	Sensitivity (%)	*Specificity (%)*
Manning (1993)	90	92
Duerinckx (1994)	63	71
Post (1995)	33	89
Pennell (1995)	85	95

New approaches for MR-coronary artery imaging

Respiratory gating

Respiratory and cardiac motion continue to be the main enemies of MR-coronary imaging. Breathholding is not always reliable and may even be impossible in patients with chronic obstructive long disease or severe left ventricular dysfunction. An alternative approach is gating of the respiratory motion, which completely eliminates the need for breathholding maneuvers [9-13]. With this gating technique two navigator echo's intersect the diaphragm, and document the diaphragm position. This allows for data acquisition at a predetermined similar diaphragm position, which can be achieved during normal breathing. However, respiratory gating always require a finite "gate" which has a width varying between 1 to 5 mm, and thus accounts for minor inconsistency of positioning. Initial studies using this "gating technique" are promising, but improvements are necessary to generate consistent reliable coronary images.

Three-dimensional coronary imaging

Initially MR visualization was achieved by obtaining axial cross-sectional images (2-D MR-imaging), or by use of image acquisition obtained from double-oblique planes, which followed the course of the coronary arteries more accurately. However, due to the tortuous and complex course of the coronary arteries, they may easily run out of the imaging plane and thus may cause misinterpretation. Volume acquisition (3-D MR-imaging) should overcome this problem [4,5,9-15]. Three-dimensional MR-imaging sequences provide a higher signal-to-noise ratio, and generate more isotropic data sets, allowing accurate image reformatting in any plane. In contrast to 2-D MR-imaging, 3-D MR-imaging is less operator dependent and does not require ample knowledge and experience with selection of planes in which the coronary arteries run. However, problematic are the saturation effects in the large 3-D volume and the longer time needed to acquire these images. These 3-D volume acquisitions are obtained using respiratory gating techniques. Preliminary results with 3-D MR-coronary angiography are promising (Table 3) [9,14,15].

Table 3: Outcome of 3-D MR-coronary angiography

	Sensitivity (%)	Specificity (%)
Post (1996)	38	95
Woodard (1996)	80	n.a.
Müller (1996)	87	97
This study (1997)	69	92

Echoplanar imaging

Recently, after the introduction of high gradient performance systems and phased array coils [16,17], a new ultrafast imaging technique, echo-planar imaging (EPI) has been developed for clinical use [18,19]. This technique allows acquisition of an image with a matrix of 64 x 128 in less than 100 ms. EPI sequences can be obtained after one RF excitation (single shot). However, the signal to noise ratio is rather low. But this can be improved by using a multishot EPI scanning technique with data acquisitions from several consecutive heart beats (segmentation). This technique can be used to image the heart in a single breathhold, 3-dimensional segmented echoplanar imaging sequence [19]. However, EPI is prone to chemical shift artefacts, and is more sensitive to magnet inhomogeneity. The role of EPI in the use of coronary imaging is unsettled and more studies are needed.

Own experience

We have investigated the diagnostic capabilities of a variant of the above described techniques. We used a 3-D segmented Turbo-Flash sequence with retrospective navigator feedback. The field of view was 200 x 320 mm with acquisition of 3 slabs of 36 mm, and an overlap of 8 mm. The TR was 8 ms and TE: 2.7 ms. The inplane resolution was 1.4 x 1.4 mm with a contiguous slice thickness of 2 mm. The diastolic acquisition time window was approximately 150 ms. The acquisition per slab varied between 8 to 16 minutes.

We examined 18 symptomatic patients with a mean age of 56.1 years (range 28 to 82 years) all of whom were in sinus rhythm. All 18 patients underwent MR coronary angiography, EBT coronary angiography and conventional diagnostic coronary angiography. The data of conventional coronary angiography were considered as the golden standard, to which the noninvasive angiograms were compared. Three patients were excluded from further analysis because of technical problems, claustrophobia or inadequacy of breathholding. The coronary tree was divided in segments. The right coronary artery in 4 segments (proximal, mid, distal and descending posterior artery), the left main coronary artery, the left anterior descending coronary artery in 3 segments (proximal, mid and distal) and the circumflex coronary artery in 2 segments (proximal and distal). The number of segments which could be adequately visualized with MR-coronary angiography are shown in Figure 1. The figures to the left to the slash represent the percentage of segments adequately visualized. Clearly is shown that the distal segments of the RCA, LCX and LAD can only be visualized in a few

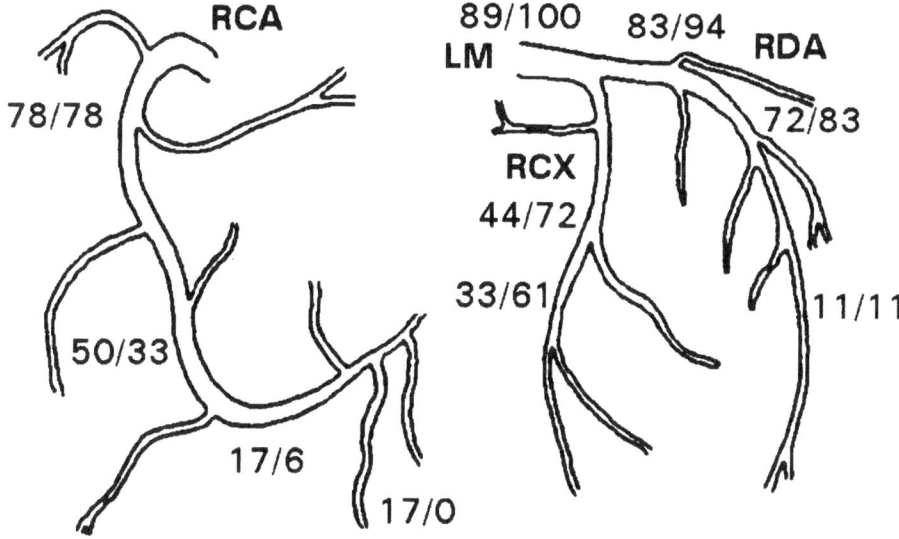

Figure 1. Number and location of coronary segments which can be adequately visualized by MR-CA (figures to the left of slash) and EBT-CA (figures to the right of slash).

patients. The left main and proximal and mid-segments of the LAD can most often be visualized. If we, more realistically, limit ourselves to the visualization of the proximal and mid coronary segments, and eliminate the distal segments from further analysis, we potentially have 126 coronary segments in 18 patients for analysis. Of these, 85 segments could be adequately visualized by MR-coronary angiography (Table 4). In the segments that were visualized we examined the diagnostic accuracy of the detection of a significant stenosis. A significant stenosis was considered as a more than 50% luminal diameter stenosis as determined by conventional coronary angiography. The sensitivity and specificity of MR-coronary angiography was 69% and 92%, respectively (Tables 3 and 4).

Table 4: Correlation CAG, MR-CA, and EBT-CA of visualized segments

	CAG					
	normal < 50%		*> 50%*			
	correctly	*overesti mated*	*correctly detected*	*not number*	*total number segments visualized*	*total segments*
MR-CA	65	6	9	5	85	126
EBT-CA	77	6	8	5	96	126

EBT-coronary imaging

Electron Beam Tomography (EBT), unlike conventional CAT-scanners, or spiral scanners, employs a stationary X-ray and detector system along with a rotating electron beam which produces X-rays [20]. This unique configuration is able to acquire axial tomograms at an extremely fast rate. EBT-coronary angiography is obtained in the high resolution mode which acquires axial slices in 100 ms per slice. The acquisitions are triggered to the electro-cardiogram and one slice per heart beat can be acquired during middiastole. The slice thickness is 1.5 mm and a maximum of 60 subsequent slices can be obtained.

The acquisitions are obtained during breathholding and depending on the heart frequency and duration of breathholding (in most instances approximately 20-30 s.) typically 30 to 40 slices can be acquired (depending on the heart frequency) thereby covering the heart from the aortic root to the apex over a distance ranging from 4.5 cm to 6 cm with a maximum of 9 cm (if 60 slices are acquired).

The complete human epicardial coronary trajectory running from the aortic root to the apex of this heart is 8 to 10 cm. The acquisitions are obtained after bolus injection of 180-200 ml of a contrast agent via the cubital vein at a flow rate of 4-6 ml s^{-1}.

EBT-coronary angiography is performed with a field of view of 15 to 22 cm, using a 512 x 512 matrix thus yielding in plane pixel dimensions of 0.3/0.45 x 0.3/0.45 mm.

Three-dimensional reconstruction from a stack of two-dimensional slice is performed.

The three-dimensional reconstruction of the heart and coronary arteries is rendered to a shaded surface display, maximum intensity projection or volume rendered display of the coronary arteries. So far, a few preliminary reports have shown that images of sufficient quality can be obtained in healthy volunteers and patients [21-23].

Also, these studies demonstrated that EBT-coronary angiography was able to identify significant coronary stenoses with a sensitivity varying from 79 to 90% and a specificity varying from 82 to 93%.

We have studied 18 patients with EBT-coronary angiography who also underwent MR-coronary angiography and diagnostic conventional coronary angiography(see section MR-angiography). An example is given in Figure 2. Visualization of the distal coronary segments is not possible. The proximal and mid coronary segments can be adequately visualized in the majority of the cases. The numbers to the right of the slash represent the percentage of adequately visualized coronary segments with EBT-coronary angiography (Figure 1). A total of 96 segments of 126 proximal and mid coronary segments could be adequately visualized (Table 4). The diagnostic accuracy of EBT-coronary angiography to detect a significant coronary stenosis (≥ 50% luminal diameter) was established. The sensitivity and specificity was 62% and 93%, respectively.

These preliminary results appear promising. Pitfalls of the technique are: motion artefacts due to cardiac contraction and respiration, incomplete coverage of the coronary arteries so that distal parts are not visualized, irregular heart rhythm causing triggering problems, contrast opacification problems due to inadequate timing of contrast transit time (time from vena cubiti to coronary artery) and finally overlap of close anatomic structures, in particular the obscuring of the circumflex artery by crossing or close proximity of the visualized coronary sinus venosus. Unique for EBT is that calcium may obscure underlying coronary anatomy and thus significant stenoses may pass undetected.

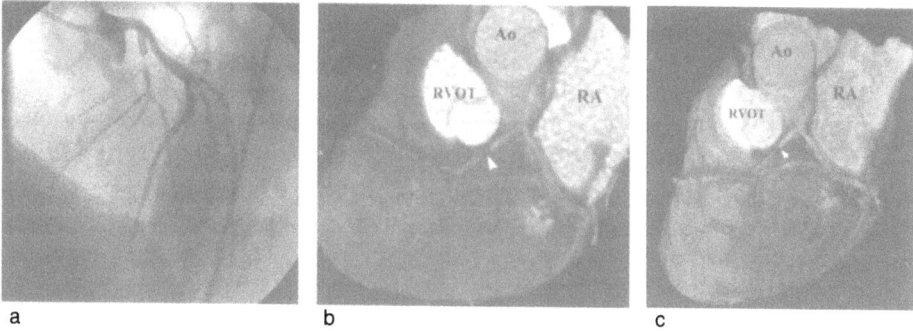

a   b   c

Figure 2a. Diagnostic conventional coronary angiography demonstrating a significant stenosis in proximal segment of the left anterior descending coronary artery (LAD). 2b) Electron beam tomography coronary angiogram of same patient with LAD stenosis (arrow). 2c) Magnetic resonance coronary angiogram of same patient with LAD stenosis (arrow). AO = aorta, RVDT = right ventricular outflow tract, RA = right atrium.

Comparison of MR- and EBT-coronary angiography

It appears that both techniques are able to visualize the proximal and mid coronary segments in the majority of the cases. EBT is slightly better than MR to adequately visualize coronary segments, but the diagnostic accuracy to detect a significant coronary stenosis is nearly similar. So far, both techniques, although promising, require significant improvements to more reliably visualize the coronary arteries.

Conclusion

MR-coronary angiography and EBT- coronary angiography are viable noninvasive coronary imaging techniques. Today both techniques should be considered as tools in progress. Technical improvements and developments of new sequence protocols are within reach, that should significantly increase the robustness and reliability of noninvasive coronary imaging.

References

1. Paulin S, Von Schulthess GK, Fossel E, Kraeyenbuehl HP. MR imaging of the aortic root and proximal coronary arteries. AJR Am J Roentgenol 1987;148:665-70.
2. Manning WJ, Li W, Edelman RR. A preliminary report comparing magnetic resonance coronary angiography with conventional angiography [published erratum appears in N Engl J Med 1993;330:152]. N Engl J Med 1993;328:828-32.
3. Pennell DJ, Keegan J, Firmin DN, Gatehouse PD, Underwood SR, Longmore DB. Magnetic resonance imaging of coronary arteries: technique and preliminary results. Br Heart J 1993;70:315-26
4. Paschal CB, Haacke EM, Adler LP. Three-dimensional MR imaging of the coronary arteries: preliminary clinical experience. J Magn Reson Imaging 1993;3:491-500.
5. Li D, Paschal CB, Haacke EM, Adler LP. Coronary arteries: three-dimensional MR imaging with fat saturation and magnetization transfer contrast. Radiology 1993;187:401-6.

6.   Duerinckx AJ, Urman M. Two-dimensional coronary MR angiography: analysis of initial clinical results. Radiology 1994;193:731-8.

7.   Pennel DJ, Bogren HG, Keegan J, Firmin DN, Underwood SR. Assessment of coronary artery stenosis by magnetic resonance imaging. Heart 1996;75:127-33.

8.   Post JC, van Rossum AC, Hofman MBM, Valk J, Visser CA. Protocol for two- dimensional magnetic resonance coronary angiography studied in three-dimensional magnetic resonance data sets. Am Heart J 1995;130:167-73.

9.   Post JC, van Rossum AC, Hofman MBM, Valk J, Visser CA. Three-dimensional respiratory-gated MR angiography of coronary arteries: comparison with conventional coronary angiography. AJR Am J Roentgenol 1996;166:1399-404.

10.   Müller MF, Fleisch M, Kroeker R, Chatterjee T, Meier B, Vock P. Proximal coronary artery stenosis: three-dimensional MRI with fat saturation and navigator echo. J Magn Reson Imaging 1997;7:644-51.

11.   Wang Y, Rossman PJ, Grimm RC, Riederer SJ, Ehman RL. Navigator-echo based real-time respiratory gating and triggering for reduction of respiratory effects in three-dimensional coronary MR angiography. Radiology 1996;198:55-60.

12.   Oshinski JN, Hofland L, Mukundan S Jr, Dixon WT, Parks WJ, Pettigrew RI. Two-dimensional coronary MR angiography without breath holding. Radiology 1996;201:737-41.

13.   Li D, Kaushikkar S, Haacke EM *et al.* Coronary arteries: three-dimensional MR imaging with retrospective respiratory gating. Radiology 1996;201:857-63.

14.   Woodard PK, Li D, Dhawale P *et al.* Identification of coronary artery stenoses with 3D MR retrospective respiratory gating [abstract]. AJR Am J Reontgenol 1996;166(3 Suppl):36.

15.   Mueller MF, Fleisch M, Kroeker R. Coronary arteries: three-dimensional MR- imaging with fat saturation and navigator echo [abstract]. Radiology 1996;201(P):274.

16.   Reeder SB, McVeigh ER. The effect of high performance gradients on fast gradient echo imaging. Magn Reson Med 1994;32:612-21.

17.   Constantinides CD, Westgate CR, O'Dell WG, Zerhouni EA, McVeigh ER. A phased array coil for human cardiac imaging. Magn Reson Med 1995;34:92-8.

18.   Edelman RR, Wielopolski P, Schmitt F. Echo-planar MR imaging. Radiology 1994;192:600-12.

19.   Wielopolski PA, Manning WJ, Edelman RR. Single breath-hold volumetric imaging of the heart using magnetization-prepared 3-dimensional segmented echo planar imaging. J Magn Reson Imaging 1995;5:403-9.

20.   McCollough CH, Morin RL. The technical design and performance of ultrafast computed tomography. Radiol Clin North Am 1994;32:521-36.

21.   Moshage WEL, Achenbach S, Seese B, Bachmann K, Kirchgeorg M. Coronary artery stenosis: three dimensional imaging with electrocardiographically triggered, contrast agent - enhanced, electron-beam CT. Radiology 1995;196:707-14.

22.   Achenbach S, Moshage W, Bachmann K. Coronary angiography by electron beam tomography. Herz 1996;21:106-17.

23.   Chernoff DM, Ritchie CJ, Higgins CB. Evaluation of electron beam CT coronary angiography in healthy subjects. AJR Am J Roentgenol 1997;169:39-9.

Color section

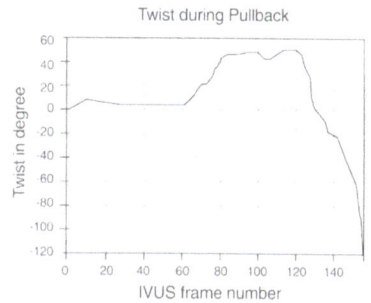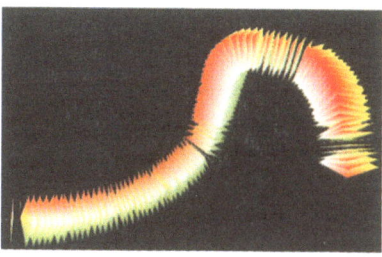

Figure 5.5. Catheter twisting during IVUS pullback. a) Analytically-determined catheter twist as scalar values along the pullback path. b) Visualization of the orientation of IVUS frames.

J.H.C. Reiber and E.E. van der Wall (eds.). What's New in Cardiovascular Imaging, 419–430.
©1998 Kluwer Academic Publishers.

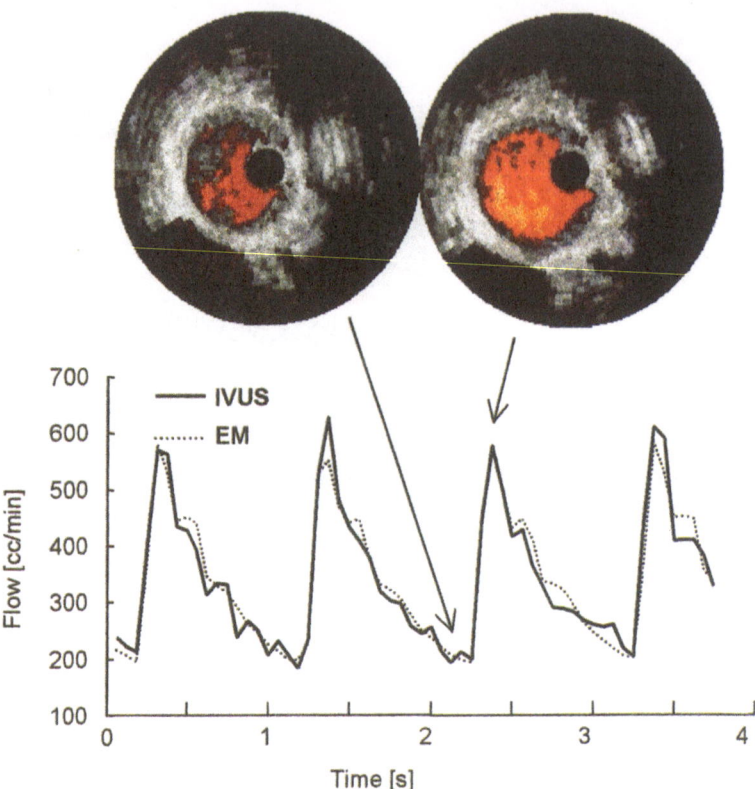

Figure 11.4. Upper panel: *In vivo* color flow mapping images obtained at low (left) and high (right) velocity settings. Lower panel: Flow curves of phasic EM-flow (dotted line) and IVUS-flow (solid line) showing an almost identical beat-to-beat change in blood flow volume.

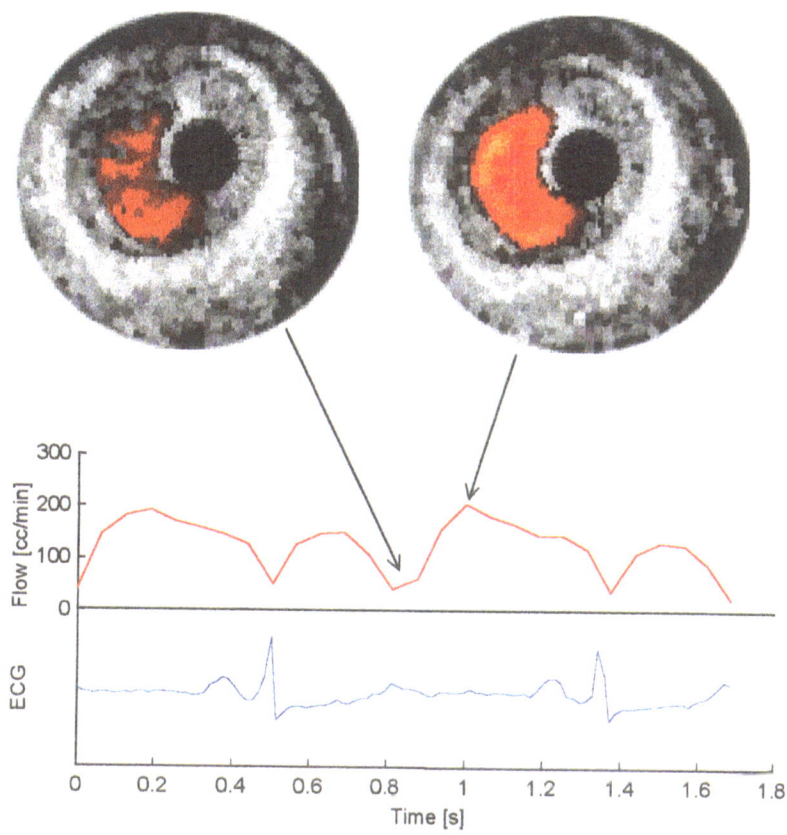

Figure 11.5. Upper panel: Coronary flow mappings obtained in patient for low (left) and high (right) flow rates during the cardiac cycle. Lower panel: IVUS-flow curve showing a typical 2-phasic diastolic flow pattern of a coronary artery in synchronization with the ECG signal.

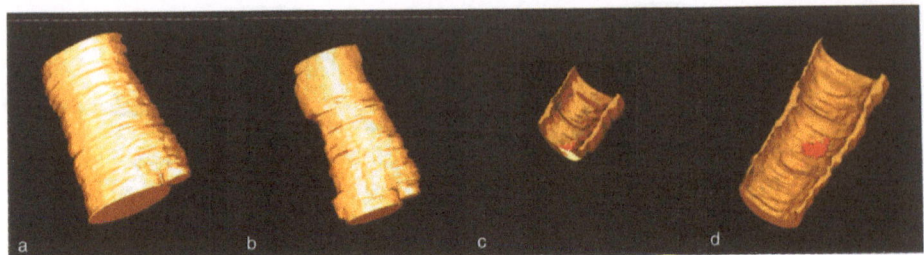

Figure 14.8. A 3-D reconstruction of a coronary vessel from a 14 mm pullback sequence. (a) Coronary wall reconstruction. (b) Lumen reconstruction. (c) Plaque composition within hard plaque. Hard plaque regions is dark and soft plaque regions are gray. (d) Plaque composition of the entire pullback sequence.

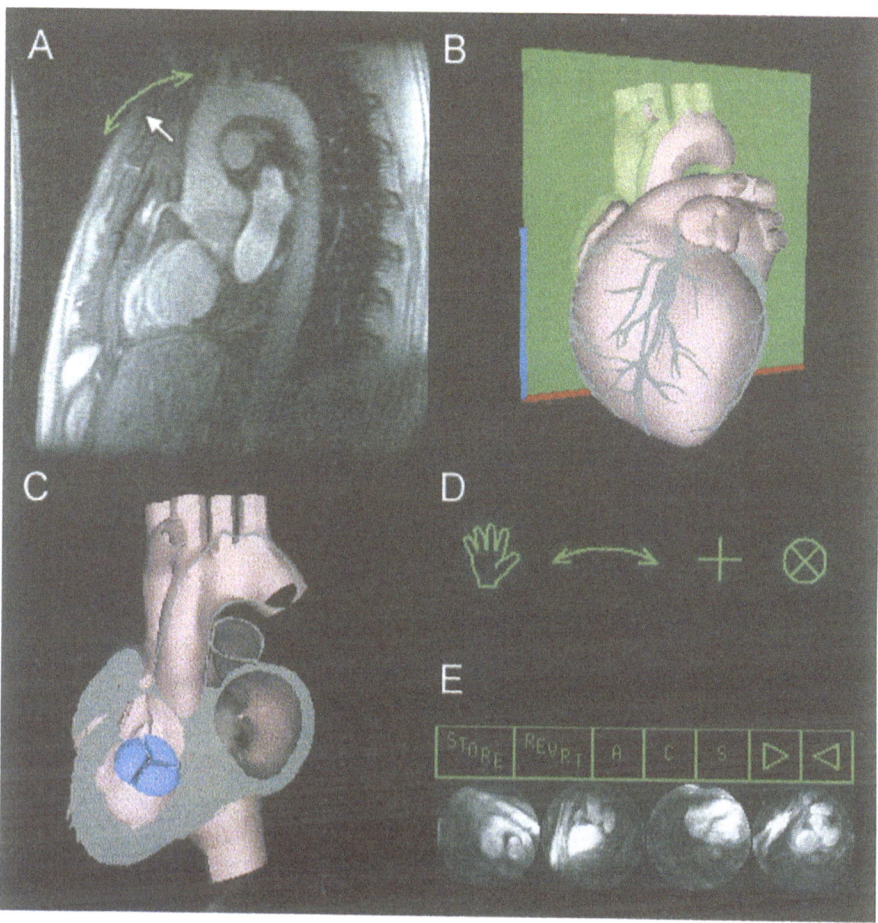

Figure 16.4. Graphical tools used for interactive cardiac MRI. Imaging window (A) shows current scan plane, whose position is continuously reflected in semitransparent embedded plane (B) or cut-away view (C) of colored 3D heart model. Colored icons (D) can be dragged across imaging window to rotate or offset scan plane, as shown in (A) for in-plane rotation. Scan-plane library (E) allows rapid storage and retrieval of scan locations.

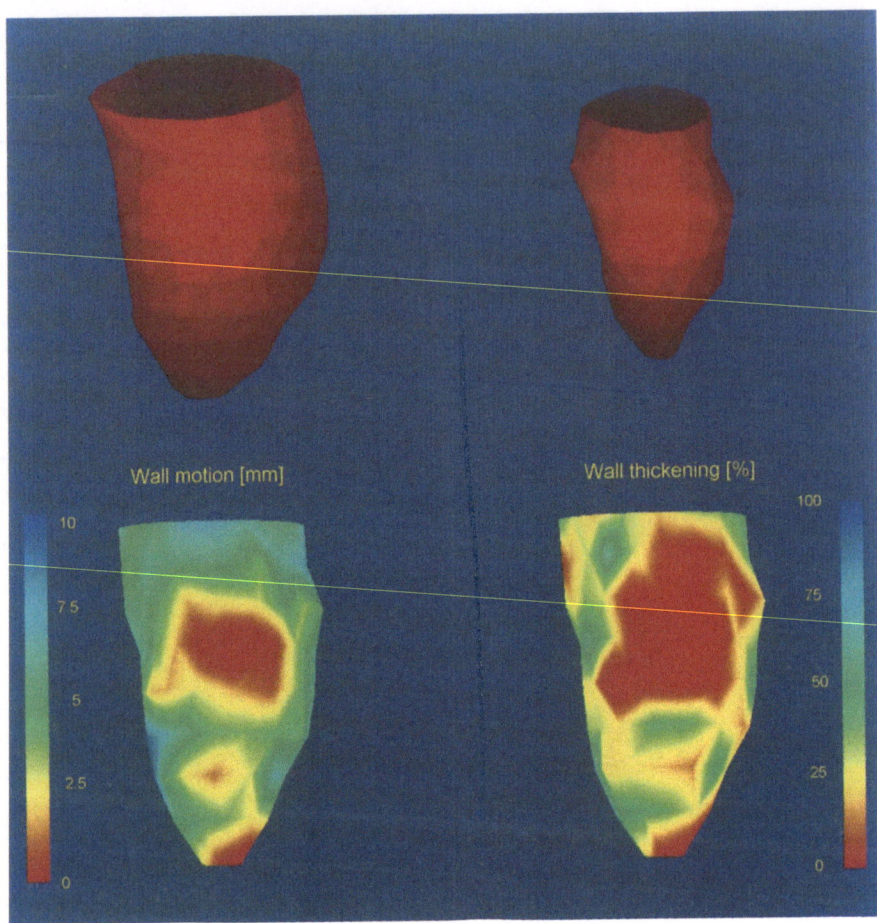

Figure 18.5. Surface rendered 3D-displays of the left ventricular endocardial surface of a normal volunteer in the ED (a) and ES (b) phases. The lower panel shows endocardial surfaces in the ES phase of an infarct patient. Functional information is projected on the surface by using a color coding scheme to display regional wall motion (c) and wall thickening (d).

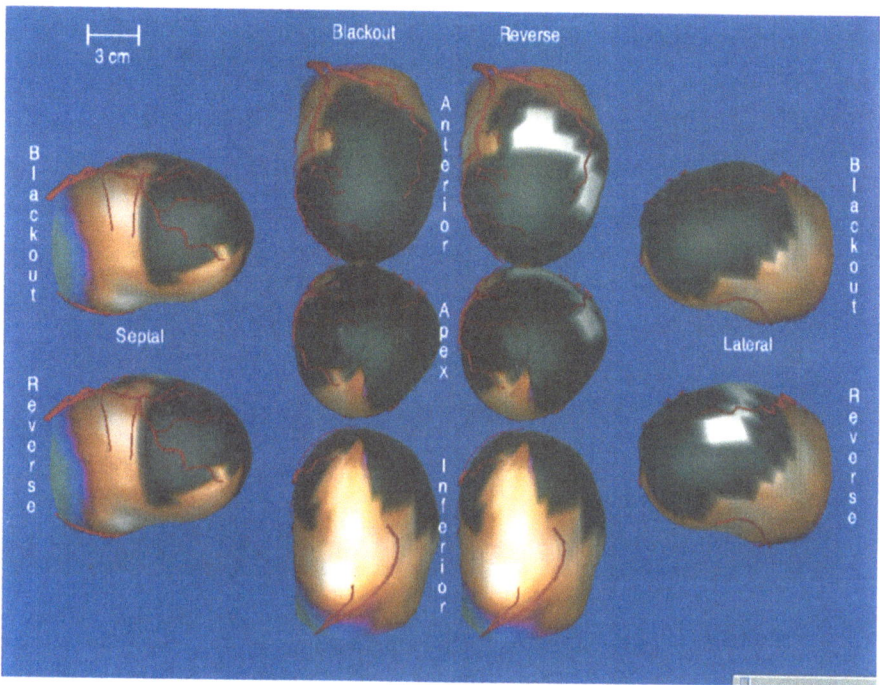

Figure 21.1. Three-dimensional display of the myocardial perfusion distribution. This is a 3-D display of a patient's myocardial perfusion distribution depicted from different orientations after the distribution has been compared to a dual isotope normal data base (Tc-99m sestamibi stress/ Tl-201 rest). The colors are indicative of the amount of tracer uptake which is related to myocardial perfusion with the lighter colors representing higher myocardial flow. The "Blackout" results highlights in black the regions of the stress study which were statistically abnormal. The "Reverse" results highlights in white the regions of the rest study that statistically improved at rest and were found at stress to be abnormal. Superimposed is a generic set of coronaries to be used as a road map to assign a region of the myocardium to a vascular territory. This patient exhibits extensive anterolateral and anteroseptal stress perfusion defects with partial reversibility at rest.

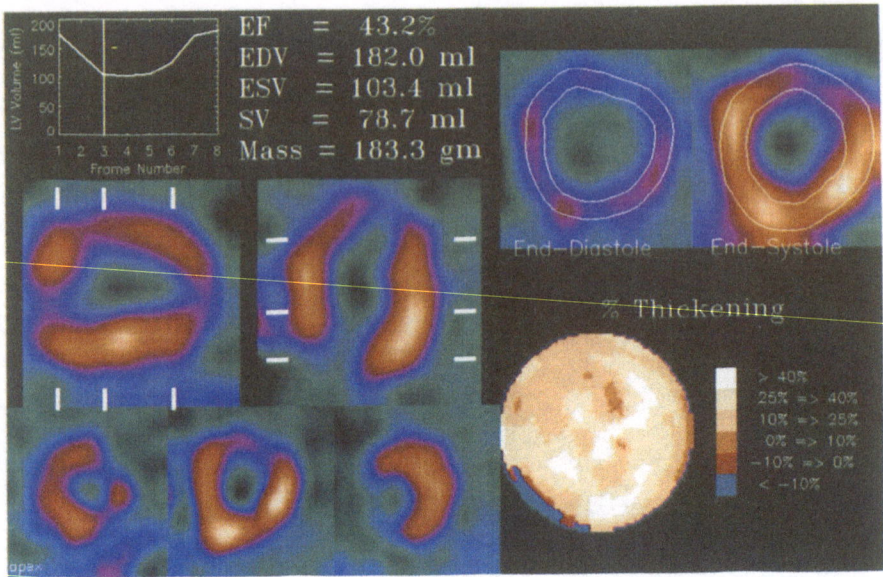

Figure 21.2. Display of myocardial function parameters for the patient shown in Figure 1. This comprehensive report includes the patient's LV volume-time curve, ejection fraction (EF), end-diastolic volume (EDV), end-systolic volume (ESV), stroke volume (SV) and total LV mass as calculated using the Emory CEqual-EGS approach. The report also includes in the lower right panel a polar map of myocardial thickening as measured using amplitude and phase analysis. The map is color coded to correspond to the % thickening color bar on its right. The lower left panel may be used for a cinematic display of the LV to visually assess wall motion and wall thickening.

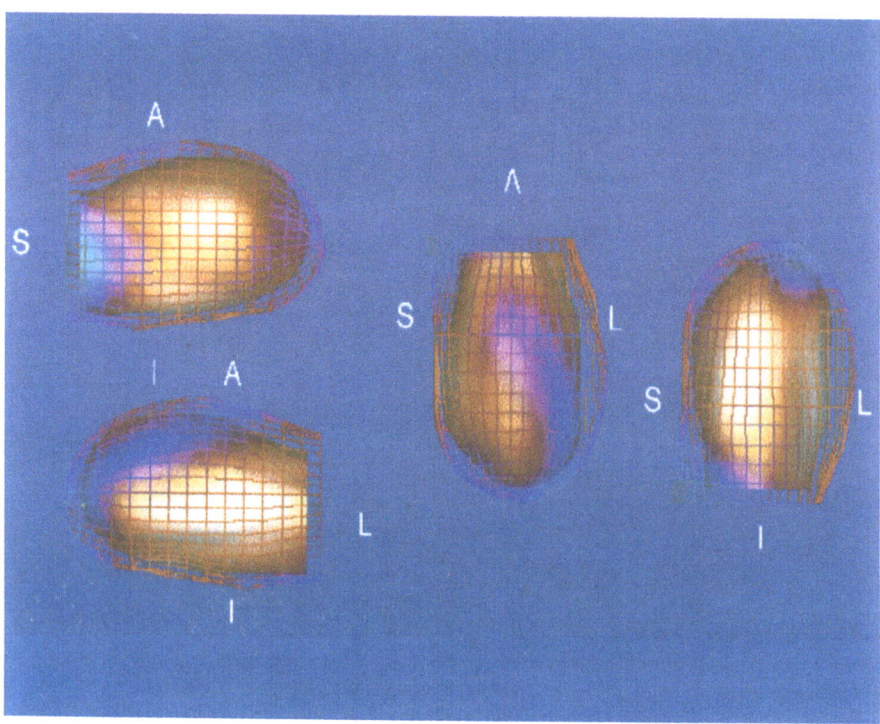

Figure 21.3. Three-dimensional display of myocardial function. This is a 3-D display of a patient's myocardial endocardial surface at end-diastole (mesh) and at end-systole (solid surface) depicted from different orientations. This display may be viewed in a dynamic fashion to visually assess wall motion as the excursion of the wall and wall thickening as the change in color. The color is a function of both myocardial perfusion and myocardial thickness. A myocardial segment that increases in color brightness indicates thickening and thus viable myocardium. This patient exhibits extensive anterolateral and anteroseptal resting wall motion and wall thickening abnormalities. (Abbreviations: A = anterior, S = septal, L = lateral and I = inferior).

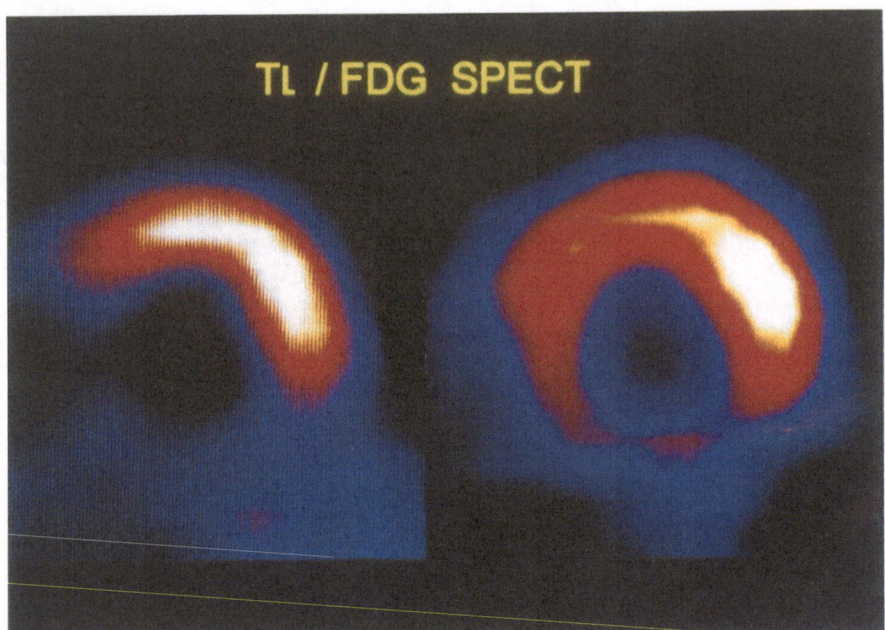

Figure 23.1. Corresponding short-axis slices of a patient with a perfusion defect on the early thallium-201 image (representing perfusion, left) in the infero-septal region and relatively increased FDG uptake (representing glucose utilization) in the septum. The area of FDG-perfusion mismatch represents viable myocardium (from reference 11, with permission) (For color figure, see color section).

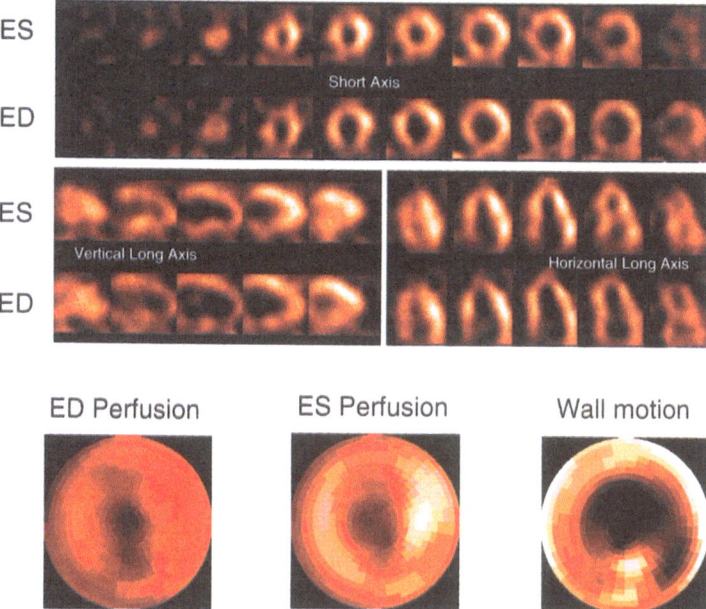

ED Perfusion   ES Perfusion   Wall motion

Figure 24.1. Gated myocardial perfusion SPECT. Corresponding end-systolic (ES) and end-diastolic (ED) slices are displayed as a report page. Additionally, software tools are applied to calculate polar maps of regional perfusion and wall motion (endocardial shortening), which may add to visual image analysis. As expected in this case of a patient with three vessel CAD; there is inhomogeneous perfusion as well as wall motion.

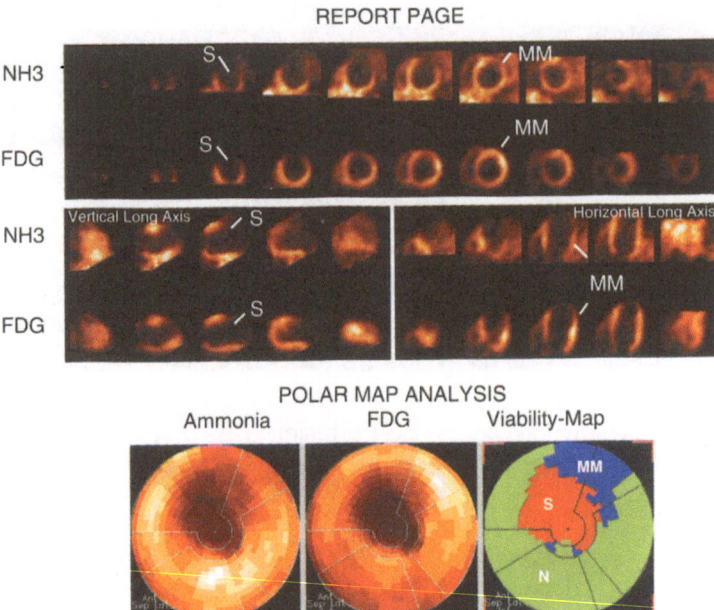

Figure 24.3. PET viability study of a patient with ischemic cardiomyopathy using (13N)- ammonia (NH3) as flow tracer, and (18F)-fluorodeoxyglucose (FDG) as metabolic tracer. Corresponding slices along the short and long axes of the ventricle are displayed on the top. In the basal area of the ante-rolateral wall , a markedly reduced flow (upper row) but preserved FDG uptake (lower row) was observed. This flow/metabolism mismatch (MM) indicates the presence of ischemically compromised but viable myocardium. In the apex and the distal anterior wall, a scar (S) with reduction of both flow and FDG uptake was observed. The polar-map analysis can be used to quantitate the size of abnor-malities. In this case, the mismatch area (MM) includes 15% of the left ventricle, while 31% are scar (S) and 54% are normal (N).

Index

Developments in Cardiovascular Medicine

28. B. Surawicz, C.P. Reddy and E.N. Prystowsky (eds.): *Tachycardias*. 1984
ISBN 0-89838-588-1
29. M.P. Spencer (ed.): *Cardiac Doppler Diagnosis*. Proceedings of a Symposium, held in Clearwater, Fla., U.S.A. (1983). 1983 ISBN 0-89838-591-1
30. H. Villarreal and M.P. Sambhi (eds.): *Topics in Pathophysiology of Hypertension*. 1984 ISBN 0-89838-595-4
31. F.H. Messerli (ed.): *Cardiovascular Disease in the Elderly*. 1984
Revised edition, 1988: see below under Volume 76
32. M.L. Simoons and J.H.C. Reiber (eds.): *Nuclear Imaging in Clinical Cardiology*. 1984 ISBN 0-89838-599-7
33. H.E.D.J. ter Keurs and J.J. Schipperheyn (eds.): *Cardiac Left Ventricular Hypertrophy*. 1983 ISBN 0-89838-612-8
34. N. Sperelakis (ed.): *Physiology and Pathology of the Heart*. 1984
Revised edition, 1988: see below under Volume 90
35. F.H. Messerli (ed.): *Kidney in Essential Hypertension*. Proceedings of a Course, held in New Orleans, La., U.S.A. (1983). 1984 ISBN 0-89838-616-0
36. M.P. Sambhi (ed.): *Fundamental Fault in Hypertension*. 1984 ISBN 0-89838-638-1
37. C. Marchesi (ed.): *Ambulatory Monitoring*. Cardiovascular System and Allied Applications. Proceedings of a Workshop, held in Pisa, Italy (1983). 1984
ISBN 0-89838-642-X
38. W. Kupper, R.N. MacAlpin and W. Bleifeld (eds.): *Coronary Tone in Ischemic Heart Disease*. 1984 ISBN 0-89838-646-2
39. N. Sperelakis and J.B. Caulfield (eds.): *Calcium Antagonists*. Mechanism of Action on Cardiac Muscle and Vascular Smooth Muscle. Proceedings of the 5th Annual Meeting of the American Section of the I.S.H.R., held in Hilton Head, S.C., U.S.A. (1983). 1984 ISBN 0-89838-655-1
40. Th. Godfraind, A.G. Herman and D. Wellens (eds.): *Calcium Entry Blockers in Cardiovascular and Cerebral Dysfunctions*. 1984 ISBN 0-89838-658-6
41. J. Morganroth and E.N. Moore (eds.): *Interventions in the Acute Phase of Myocardial Infarction*. Proceedings of the 4th Symposium on New Drugs and Devices, held in Philadelphia, Pa., U.S.A. (1983). 1984 ISBN 0-89838-659-4
42. F.L. Abel and W.H. Newman (eds.): *Functional Aspects of the Normal, Hypertrophied and Failing Heart*. Proceedings of the 5th Annual Meeting of the American Section of the I.S.H.R., held in Hilton Head, S.C., U.S.A. (1983). 1984
ISBN 0-89838-665-9
43. S. Sideman and R. Beyar (eds.): [3-D] *Simulation and Imaging of the Cardiac System*. State of the Heart. Proceedings of the International Henry Goldberg Workshop, held in Haifa, Israel (1984). 1985 ISBN 0-89838-687-X
44. E. van der Wall and K.I. Lie (eds.): *Recent Views on Hypertrophic Cardiomyopathy*. Proceedings of a Symposium, held in Groningen, The Netherlands (1984). 1985
ISBN 0-89838-694-2
45. R.E. Beamish, P.K. Singal and N.S. Dhalla (eds.), *Stress and Heart Disease*. Proceedings of a International Symposium, held in Winnipeg, Canada, 1984 (Vol. 1). 1985 ISBN 0-89838-709-4
46. R.E. Beamish, V. Panagia and N.S. Dhalla (eds.): *Pathogenesis of Stress-induced Heart Disease*. Proceedings of a International Symposium, held in Winnipeg, Canada, 1984 (Vol. 2). 1985 ISBN 0-89838-710-8
47. J. Morganroth and E.N. Moore (eds.): *Cardiac Arrhythmias*. New Therapeutic Drugs and Devices. Proceedings of the 5th Symposium on New Drugs and Devices, held in Philadelphia, Pa., U.S.A. (1984). 1985 ISBN 0-89838-716-7
48. P. Mathes (ed.): *Secondary Prevention in Coronary Artery Disease and Myocardial Infarction*. 1985 ISBN 0-89838-736-1
49. H.L. Stone and W.B. Weglicki (eds.): *Pathobiology of Cardiovascular Injury*. Proceedings of the 6th Annual Meeting of the American Section of the I.S.H.R., held in Oklahoma City, Okla., U.S.A. (1984). 1985 ISBN 0-89838-743-4

Developments in Cardiovascular Medicine

50. J. Meyer, R. Erbel and H.J. Rupprecht (eds.): *Improvement of Myocardial Perfusion.* Thrombolysis, Angioplasty, Bypass Surgery. Proceedings of a Symposium, held in Mainz, F.R.G. (1984). 1985   ISBN 0-89838-748-5

51. J.H.C. Reiber, P.W. Serruys and C.J. Slager (eds.): *Quantitative Coronary and Left Ventricular Cineangiography.* Methodology and Clinical Applications. 1986
                                ISBN 0-89838-760-4

52. R.H. Fagard and I.E. Bekaert (eds.): *Sports Cardiology.* Exercise in Health and Cardiovascular Disease. Proceedings from an International Conference, held in Knokke, Belgium (1985). 1986   ISBN 0-89838-782-5

53. J.H.C. Reiber and P.W. Serruys (eds.): *State of the Art in Quantitative Cornary Arteriography.* 1986   ISBN 0-89838-804-X

54. J. Roelandt (ed.): *Color Doppler Flow Imaging and Other Advances in Doppler Echocardiography.* 1986   ISBN 0-89838-806-6

55. E.E. van der Wall (ed.): *Noninvasive Imaging of Cardiac Metabolism.* Single Photon Scintigraphy, Positron Emission Tomography and Nuclear Magnetic Resonance. 1987
                                ISBN 0-89838-812-0

56. J. Liebman, R. Plonsey and Y. Rudy (eds.): *Pediatric and Fundamental Electrocardiography.* 1987   ISBN 0-89838-815-5

57. H.H. Hilger, V. Hombach and W.J. Rashkind (eds.), *Invasive Cardiovascular Therapy.* Proceedings of an International Symposium, held in Cologne, F.R.G. (1985). 1987   ISBN 0-89838-818-X

58. P.W. Serruys and G.T. Meester (eds.): *Coronary Angioplasty.* A Controlled Model for Ischemia. 1986   ISBN 0-89838-819-8

59. J.E. Tooke and L.H. Smaje (eds.): *Clinical Investigation of the Microcirculation.* Proceedings of an International Meeting, held in London, U.K. (1985). 1987
                                ISBN 0-89838-833-3

60. R.Th. van Dam and A. van Oosterom (eds.): *Electrocardiographic Body Surface Mapping.* Proceedings of the 3rd International Symposium on B.S.M., held in Nijmegen, The Netherlands (1985). 1986   ISBN 0-89838-834-1

61. M.P. Spencer (ed.): *Ultrasonic Diagnosis of Cerebrovascular Disease.* Doppler Techniques and Pulse Echo Imaging. 1987   ISBN 0-89838-836-8

62. M.J. Legato (ed.): *The Stressed Heart.* 1987   ISBN 0-89838-849-X

63. M.E. Safar (ed.): *Arterial and Venous Systems in Essential Hypertension.* With Assistance of G.M. London, A.Ch. Simon and Y.A. Weiss. 1987
                                ISBN 0-89838-857-0

64. J. Roelandt (ed.): *Digital Techniques in Echocardiography.* 1987
                                ISBN 0-89838-861-9

65. N.S. Dhalla, P.K. Singal and R.E. Beamish (eds.): *Pathology of Heart Disease.* Proceedings of the 8th Annual Meeting of the American Section of the I.S.H.R., held in Winnipeg, Canada, 1986 (Vol. 1). 1987   ISBN 0-89838-864-3

66. N.S. Dhalla, G.N. Pierce and R.E. Beamish (eds.): *Heart Function and Metabolism.* Proceedings of the 8th Annual Meeting of the American Section of the I.S.H.R., held in Winnipeg, Canada, 1986 (Vol. 2). 1987   ISBN 0-89838-865-1

67. N.S. Dhalla, I.R. Innes and R.E. Beamish (eds.): *Myocardial Ischemia.* Proceedings of a Satellite Symposium of the 30th International Physiological Congress, held in Winnipeg, Canada (1986). 1987   ISBN 0-89838-866-X

68. R.E. Beamish, V. Panagia and N.S. Dhalla (eds.): *Pharmacological Aspects of Heart Disease.* Proceedings of an International Symposium, held in Winnipeg, Canada (1986). 1987   ISBN 0-89838-867-8

69. H.E.D.J. ter Keurs and J.V. Tyberg (eds.): *Mechanics of the Circulation.* Proceedings of a Satellite Symposium of the 30th International Physiological Congress, held in Banff, Alberta, Canada (1986). 1987   ISBN 0-89838-870-8

70. S. Sideman and R. Beyar (eds.): *Activation, Metabolism and Perfusion of the Heart.* Simulation and Experimental Models. Proceedings of the 3rd Henry Goldberg Workshop, held in Piscataway, N.J., U.S.A. (1986). 1987   ISBN 0-89838-871-6

Developments in Cardiovascular Medicine

71. E. Aliot and R. Lazzara (eds.): *Ventricular Tachycardias.* From Mechanism to Therapy. 1987
    ISBN 0-89838-881-3
72. A. Schneeweiss and G. Schettler: *Cardiovascular Drug Therapoy in the Elderly.* 1988
    ISBN 0-89838-883-X
73. J.V. Chapman and A. Sgalambro (eds.): *Basic Concepts in Doppler Echocardiography.* Methods of Clinical Applications based on a Multi-modality Doppler Approach. 1987
    ISBN 0-89838-888-0
74. S. Chien, J. Dormandy, E. Ernst and A. Matrai (eds.): *Clinical Hemorheology.* Applications in Cardiovascular and Hematological Disease, Diabetes, Surgery and Gynecology. 1987
    ISBN 0-89838-807-4
75. J. Morganroth and E.N. Moore (eds.): *Congestive Heart Failure.* Proceedings of the 7th Annual Symposium on New Drugs and Devices, held in Philadelphia, Pa., U.S.A. (1986). 1987
    ISBN 0-89838-955-0
76. F.H. Messerli (ed.): *Cardiovascular Disease in the Elderly.* 2nd ed. 1988
    ISBN 0-89838-962-3
77. P.H. Heintzen and J.H. Bürsch (eds.): *Progress in Digital Angiocardiography.* 1988
    ISBN 0-89838-965-8
78. M.M. Scheinman (ed.): *Catheter Ablation of Cardiac Arrhythmias.* Basic Bioelectrical Effects and Clinical Indications. 1988
    ISBN 0-89838-967-4
79. J.A.E. Spaan, A.V.G. Bruschke and A.C. Gittenberger-De Groot (eds.): *Coronary Circulation.* From Basic Mechanisms to Clinical Implications. 1987
    ISBN 0-89838-978-X
80. C. Visser, G. Kan and R.S. Meltzer (eds.): *Echocardiography in Coronary Artery Disease.* 1988
    ISBN 0-89838-979-8
81. A. Bayés de Luna, A. Betriu and G. Permanyer (eds.): *Therapeutics in Cardiology.* 1988
    ISBN 0-89838-981-X
82. D.M. Mirvis (ed.): *Body Surface Electrocardiographic Mapping.* 1988
    ISBN 0-89838-983-6
83. M.A. Konstam and J.M. Isner (eds.): *The Right Ventricle.* 1988 ISBN 0-89838-987-9
84. C.T. Kappagoda and P.V. Greenwood (eds.): *Long-term Management of Patients after Myocardial Infarction.* 1988
    ISBN 0-89838-352-8
85. W.H. Gaasch and H.J. Levine (eds.): *Chronic Aortic Regurgitation.* 1988
    ISBN 0-89838-364-1
86. P.K. Singal (ed.): *Oxygen Radicals in the Pathophysiology of Heart Disease.* 1988
    ISBN 0-89838-375-7
87. J.H.C. Reiber and P.W. Serruys (eds.): *New Developments in Quantitative Coronary Arteriography.* 1988
    ISBN 0-89838-377-3
88. J. Morganroth and E.N. Moore (eds.): *Silent Myocardial Ischemia.* Proceedings of the 8th Annual Symposium on New Drugs and Devices (1987). 1988
    ISBN 0-89838-380-3
89. H.E.D.J. ter Keurs and M.I.M. Noble (eds.): *Starling's Law of the Heart Revisted.* 1988
    ISBN 0-89838-382-X
90. N. Sperelakis (ed.): *Physiology and Pathophysiology of the Heart.* Rev. ed. 1988
    3rd, revised edition, 1994: see below under Volume 151
91. J.W. de Jong (ed.): *Myocardial Energy Metabolism.* 1988 ISBN 0-89838-394-3
92. V. Hombach, H.H. Hilger and H.L. Kennedy (eds.): *Electrocardiography and Cardiac Drug Therapy.* Proceedings of an International Symposium, held in Cologne, F.R.G. (1987). 1988
    ISBN 0-89838-395-1
93. H. Iwata, J.B. Lombardini and T. Segawa (eds.): *Taurine and the Heart.* 1988
    ISBN 0-89838-396-X
94. M.R. Rosen and Y. Palti (eds.): *Lethal Arrhythmias Resulting from Myocardial Ischemia and Infarction.* Proceedings of the 2nd Rappaport Symposium, held in Haifa, Israel (1988). 1988
    ISBN 0-89838-401-X
95. M. Iwase and I. Sotobata: *Clinical Echocardiography.* With a Foreword by M.P. Spencer. 1989
    ISBN 0-7923-0004-1

Developments in Cardiovascular Medicine

96. I. Cikes (ed.): *Echocardiography in Cardiac Interventions.* 1989
ISBN 0-7923-0088-2
97. E. Rapaport (ed.): *Early Interventions in Acute Myocardial Infarction.* 1989
ISBN 0-7923-0175-7
98. M.E. Safar and F. Fouad-Tarazi (eds.): *The Heart in Hypertension.* A Tribute to Robert C. Tarazi (1925-1986). 1989 ISBN 0-7923-0197-8
99. S. Meerbaum and R. Meltzer (eds.): *Myocardial Contrast Two-dimensional Echocardiography.* 1989 ISBN 0-7923-0205-2
100. J. Morganroth and E.N. Moore (eds.): *Risk/Benefit Analysis for the Use and Approval of Thrombolytic, Antiarrhythmic, and Hypolipidemic Agents.* Proceedings of the 9th Annual Symposium on New Drugs and Devices (1988). 1989 ISBN 0-7923-0294-X
101. P.W. Serruys, R. Simon and K.J. Beatt (eds.): *PTCA - An Investigational Tool and a Non-operative Treatment of Acute Ischemia.* 1990 ISBN 0-7923-0346-6
102. I.S. Anand, P.I. Wahi and N.S. Dhalla (eds.): *Pathophysiology and Pharmacology of Heart Disease.* 1989 ISBN 0-7923-0367-9
103. G.S. Abela (ed.): *Lasers in Cardiovascular Medicine and Surgery.* Fundamentals and Technique. 1990 ISBN 0-7923-0440-3
104. H.M. Piper (ed.): *Pathophysiology of Severe Ischemic Myocardial Injury.* 1990
ISBN 0-7923-0459-4
105. S.M. Teague (ed.): *Stress Doppler Echocardiography.* 1990 ISBN 0-7923-0499-3
106. P.R. Saxena, D.I. Wallis, W. Wouters and P. Bevan (eds.): *Cardiovascular Pharmacology of 5-Hydroxytryptamine.* Prospective Therapeutic Applications. 1990
ISBN 0-7923-0502-7
107. A.P. Shepherd and P.A. Öberg (eds.): *Laser-Doppler Blood Flowmetry.* 1990
ISBN 0-7923-0508-6
108. J. Soler-Soler, G. Permanyer-Miralda and J. Sagristà-Sauleda (eds.): *Pericardial Disease.* New Insights and Old Dilemmas. 1990 ISBN 0-7923-0510-8
109. J.P.M. Hamer: *Practical Echocardiography in the Adult.* With Doppler and Color-Doppler Flow Imaging. 1990 ISBN 0-7923-0670-8
110. A. Bayés de Luna, P. Brugada, J. Cosin Aguilar and F. Navarro Lopez (eds.): *Sudden Cardiac Death.* 1991 ISBN 0-7923-0716-X
111. E. Andries and R. Stroobandt (eds.): *Hemodynamics in Daily Practice.* 1991
ISBN 0-7923-0725-9
112. J. Morganroth and E.N. Moore (eds.): *Use and Approval of Antihypertensive Agents and Surrogate Endpoints for the Approval of Drugs affecting Antiarrhythmic Heart Failure and Hypolipidemia.* Proceedings of the 10th Annual Symposium on New Drugs and Devices (1989). 1990 ISBN 0-7923-0756-9
113. S. Iliceto, P. Rizzon and J.R.T.C. Roelandt (eds.): *Ultrasound in Coronary Artery Disease.* Present Role and Future Perspectives. 1990 ISBN 0-7923-0784-4
114. J.V. Chapman and G.R. Sutherland (eds.): *The Noninvasive Evaluation of Hemodynamics in Congenital Heart Disease.* Doppler Ultrasound Applications in the Adult and Pediatric Patient with Congenital Heart Disease. 1990
ISBN 0-7923-0836-0
115. G.T. Meester and F. Pinciroli (eds.): *Databases for Cardiology.* 1991
ISBN 0-7923-0886-7
116. B. Korecky and N.S. Dhalla (eds.): *Subcellular Basis of Contractile Failure.* 1990
ISBN 0-7923-0890-5
117. J.H.C. Reiber and P.W. Serruys (eds.): *Quantitative Coronary Arteriography.* 1991
ISBN 0-7923-0913-8
118. E. van der Wall and A. de Roos (eds.): *Magnetic Resonance Imaging in Coronary Artery Disease.* 1991 ISBN 0-7923-0940-5
119. V. Hombach, M. Kochs and A.J. Camm (eds.): *Interventional Techniques in Cardiovascular Medicine.* 1991 ISBN 0-7923-0956-1
120. R. Vos: *Drugs Looking for Diseases.* Innovative Drug Research and the Development of the Beta Blockers and the Calcium Antagonists. 1991 ISBN 0-7923-0968-5

Developments in Cardiovascular Medicine

121. S. Sideman, R. Beyar and A.G. Kleber (eds.): *Cardiac Electrophysiology, Circulation, and Transport.* Proceedings of the 7th Henry Goldberg Workshop (Berne, Switzerland, 1990). 1991 ISBN 0-7923-1145-0
122. D.M. Bers: *Excitation-Contraction Coupling and Cardiac Contractile Force.* 1991 ISBN 0-7923-1186-8
123. A.-M. Salmasi and A.N. Nicolaides (eds.): *Occult Atherosclerotic Disease.* Diagnosis, Assessment and Management. 1991 ISBN 0-7923-1188-4
124. J.A.E. Spaan: *Coronary Blood Flow.* Mechanics, Distribution, and Control. 1991 ISBN 0-7923-1210-4
125. R.W. Stout (ed.): *Diabetes and Atherosclerosis.* 1991 ISBN 0-7923-1310-0
126. A.G. Herman (ed.): *Antithrombotics.* Pathophysiological Rationale for Pharmacological Interventions. 1991 ISBN 0-7923-1413-1
127. N.H.J. Pijls: *Maximal Myocardial Perfusion as a Measure of the Functional Significance of Coronary Arteriogram.* From a Pathoanatomic to a Pathophysiologic Interpretation of the Coronary Arteriogram. 1991 ISBN 0-7923-1430-1
128. J.H.C. Reiber and E.E. v.d. Wall (eds.): *Cardiovascular Nuclear Medicine and MRI.* Quantitation and Clinical Applications. 1992 ISBN 0-7923-1467-0
129. E. Andries, P. Brugada and R. Stroobrandt (eds.): *How to Face 'the Faces' of Cardiac Pacing.* 1992 ISBN 0-7923-1528-6
130. M. Nagano, S. Mochizuki and N.S. Dhalla (eds.): *Cardiovascular Disease in Diabetes.* 1992 ISBN 0-7923-1554-5
131. P.W. Serruys, B.H. Strauss and S.B. King III (eds.): *Restenosis after Intervention with New Mechanical Devices.* 1992 ISBN 0-7923-1555-3
132. P.J. Walter (ed.): *Quality of Life after Open Heart Surgery.* 1992 ISBN 0-7923-1580-4
133. E.E. van der Wall, H. Sochor, A. Righetti and M.G. Niemeyer (eds.): *What's new in Cardiac Imaging?* SPECT, PET and MRI. 1992 ISBN 0-7923-1615-0
134. P. Hanrath, R. Uebis and W. Krebs (eds.): *Cardiovascular Imaging by Ultrasound.* 1992 ISBN 0 7923-1755-6
135. F.H. Messerli (ed.): *Cardiovascular Disease in the Elderly.* 3rd ed. 1992 ISBN 0-7923-1859-5
136. J. Hess and G.R. Sutherland (eds.): *Congenital Heart Disease in Adolescents and Adults.* 1992 ISBN 0-7923-1862-5
137. J.H.C. Reiber and P.W. Serruys (eds.): *Advances in Quantitative Coronary Arteriography.* 1993 ISBN 0-7923-1863-3
138. A.-M. Salmasi and A.S. Iskandrian (eds.): *Cardiac Output and Regional Flow in Health and Disease.* 1993 ISBN 0-7923-1911-7
139. J.H. Kingma, N.M. van Hemel and K.I. Lie (eds.): *Atrial Fibrillation, a Treatable Disease?* 1992 ISBN 0-7923-2008-5
140. B. Ostadel and N.S. Dhalla (eds.): *Heart Function in Health and Disease.* Proceedings of the Cardiovascular Program (Prague, Czechoslovakia, 1991). 1992 ISBN 0-7923-2052-2
141. D. Noble and Y.E. Earm (eds.): *Ionic Channels and Effect of Taurine on the Heart.* Proceedings of an International Symposium (Seoul, Korea , 1992). 1993 ISBN 0-7923-2199-5
142. H.M. Piper and C.J. Preusse (eds.): *Ischemia-reperfusion in Cardiac Surgery.* 1993 ISBN 0-7923-2241-X
143. J. Roelandt, E.J. Gussenhoven and N. Bom (eds.): *Intravascular Ultrasound.* 1993 ISBN 0-7923-2301-7
144. M.E. Safar and M.F. O'Rourke (eds.): *The Arterial System in Hypertension.* 1993 ISBN 0-7923-2343-2
145. P.W. Serruys, D.P. Foley and P.J. de Feyter (eds.): *Quantitative Coronary Angiography in Clinical Practice.* With a Foreword by Spencer B. King III. 1994 ISBN 0-7923-2368-8

Developments in Cardiovascular Medicine

146. J. Candell-Riera and D. Ortega-Alcalde (eds.): *Nuclear Cardiology in Everyday Practice*. 1994   ISBN 0-7923-2374-2
147. P. Cummins (ed.): *Growth Factors and the Cardiovascular System*. 1993
                                                                ISBN 0-7923-2401-3
148. K. Przyklenk, R.A. Kloner and D.M. Yellon (eds.): *Ischemic Preconditioning: The Concept of Endogenous Cardioprotection*. 1993   ISBN 0-7923-2410-2
149. T.H. Marwick: *Stress Echocardiography*. Its Role in the Diagnosis and Evaluation of Coronary Artery Disease. 1994   ISBN 0-7923-2579-6
150. W.H. van Gilst and K.I. Lie (eds.): *Neurohumoral Regulation of Coronary Flow*. Role of the Endothelium. 1993   ISBN 0-7923-2588-5
151. N. Sperelakis (ed.): *Physiology and Pathophysiology of the Heart*. 3rd rev. ed. 1994
                                                                ISBN 0-7923-2612-1
152. J.C. Kaski (ed.): *Angina Pectoris with Normal Coronary Arteries: Syndrome X*. 1994
                                                                ISBN 0-7923-2651-2
153. D.R. Gross: *Animal Models in Cardiovascular Research*. 2nd rev. ed. 1994
                                                                ISBN 0-7923-2712-8
154. A.S. Iskandrian and E.E. van der Wall (eds.): *Myocardial Viability*. Detection and Clinical Relevance. 1994   ISBN 0-7923-2813-2
155. J.H.C. Reiber and P.W. Serruys (eds.): *Progress in Quantitative Coronary Arteriography*. 1994   ISBN 0-7923-2814-0
156. U. Goldbourt, U. de Faire and K. Berg (eds.): *Genetic Factors in Coronary Heart Disease*. 1994   ISBN 0-7923-2752-7
157. G. Leonetti and C. Cuspidi (eds.): *Hypertension in the Elderly*. 1994
                                                                ISBN 0-7923-2852-3
158. D. Ardissino, S. Savonitto and L.H. Opie (eds.): *Drug Evaluation in Angina Pectoris*. 1994   ISBN 0-7923-2897-3
159. G. Bkaily (ed.): *Membrane Physiopathology*. 1994   ISBN 0-7923-3062-5
160. R.C. Becker (ed.): *The Modern Era of Coronary Thrombolysis*. 1994
                                                                ISBN 0-7923-3063-3
161. P.J. Walter (ed.): *Coronary Bypass Surgery in the Elderly*. Ethical, Economical and Quality of Life Aspects. With a foreword by N.K. Wenger. 1995 ISBN 0-7923-3188-5
162. J.W. de Jong and R. Ferrari (eds.), *The Carnitine System*. A New Therapeutical Approach to Cardiovascular Diseases. 1995   ISBN 0-7923-3318-7
163. C.A. Neill and E.B. Clark: *The Developing Heart: A 'History' of Pediatric Cardiology*. 1995   ISBN 0-7923-3375-6
164. N. Sperelakis: *Electrogenesis of Biopotentials in the Cardiovascular System*. 1995
                                                                ISBN 0-7923-3398-5
165. M. Schwaiger (ed.): *Cardiac Positron Emission Tomography*. 1995
                                                                ISBN 0-7923-3417-5
166. E.E. van der Wall, P.K. Blanksma, M.G. Niemeyer and A.M.J. Paans (eds.): *Cardiac Positron Emission Tomography*. Viability, Perfusion, Receptors and Cardiomyopathy. 1995   ISBN 0-7923-3472-8
167. P.K. Singal, I.M.C. Dixon, R.E. Beamish and N.S. Dhalla (eds.): *Mechanism of Heart Failure*. 1995   ISBN 0-7923-3490-6
168. N.S. Dhalla, P.K. Singal, N. Takeda and R.E. Beamish (eds.): *Pathophysiology of Heart Failure*. 1995   ISBN 0-7923-3571-6
169. N.S. Dhalla, G.N. Pierce, V. Panagia and R.E. Beamish (eds.): *Heart Hypertrophy and Failure*. 1995   ISBN 0-7923-3572-4
170. S.N. Willich and J.E. Muller (eds.): *Triggering of Acute Coronary Syndromes*. Implications for Prevention. 1995   ISBN 0-7923-3605-4
171. E.E. van der Wall, T.H. Marwick and J.H.C. Reiber (eds.): *Advances in Imaging Techniques in Ischemic Heart Disease*. 1995   ISBN 0-7923-3620-8
172. B. Swynghedauw: *Molecular Cardiology for the Cardiologist*. 1995
                                                                ISBN 0-7923-3622-4

Developments in Cardiovascular Medicine

Developments in Cardiovascular Medicine

Previous volumes are still available

KLUWER ACADEMIC PUBLISHERS – DORDRECHT / BOSTON / LONDON